Operating Theatre Technique

*To
My Wife
Anne
and Son
Nigel*

Operating Theatre Technique

A Textbook for Nurses, Technicians,
Operating Department Assistants, Medical Students,
House Surgeons and others associated
with the Operating Theatre

RAYMOND J. BRIGDEN, S.R.N.

Nursing Officer,
Department of Health and Social Security,
London
Formerly Senior Nursing Officer,
Northwick Park Hospital, Harrow, Middlesex

Third edition

CHURCHILL LIVINGSTONE
EDINBURGH AND LONDON 1974

CHURCHILL LIVINGSTONE
Medical Division of Longman Group Limited

Distributed in the United States of America by
Longman Inc., New York, and by associated companies,
branches and representatives throughout the world.

First edition 1962
Second edition 1969
Third edition 1974

ISBN 0 443 01058 7

Library of Congress Catalog Card Number 73-85891

Printed in Great Britain

Preface to Third Edition

It is now twelve years since the first edition of *Operating Theatre Technique* was published. With continuing new developments and changes in surgical techniques the objectives remain unchanged: to provide a comprehensive textbook to which nurses, technicians, operating department assistants and medical staff can refer to supplement their practical experience.

The extensive revision is again mainly in the first ten chapters, those which deal with theatre technique. Some additional surgical procedures have been included, but not the more sophisticated such as transplant operations. The chapter on Plaster of Paris has been brought up to date.

In Chapter 1 an opportunity has been taken to include an outline of operating department management procedures and the role of the operating department assistant. This is based on the recommendations of the Lewin Report. Chapter 2 now includes a section on electromedical equipment, the definition of 'earth free' equipment, and relevant safety procedures.

Ligature and suture materials are now graded in metric sizes with the BP sizes in parenthesis. Throughout the new edition, whenever possible, metric measurements are given prominence. Where exact sizes are essential, i.e. drills, screws, etc., these are given. In other cases, e.g. instruments, readers will find that metric sizes are rounded up or down. In most instances this is because the relevant instrument has not yet been manufactured in a metric size: for example, an 8 inch forcep is described as 20 cm.

The preset tray method of preparing instruments is still favoured in the chapter on Sterilisation. Methods of sterilisation described include sub-atmospheric steam/formaldehyde and ethylene oxide under pressure. The use of chemicals for disinfection of instruments is deplored.

Perhaps the greatest change is in the format of the book, which is quite different from the previous editions. My thanks are due to the publishers, Churchill Livingstone, who I am certain readers will agree have improved the format in keeping with modern presentation. The larger type area has permitted a reduction in the number of pages whilst at the same time still allowing an increase in content. Many of the illustrations have been replaced and where appropriate are presented as a series in proximity to the relevant text.

Once again I must express my grateful thanks to all those who have helped in some way during the preparation of the new edition. Many individuals have co-operated in providing material for inclusion and this applies particularly to the manufacturers whose instruments are depicted throughout the book.

Space does not permit inclusion by name of everyone who has helped in this work, but nevertheless grateful thanks are due to all. Of special mention must be colleagues and staff at Northwick Park Hospital, Harrow, who provided facilities for preparing many of the illustrations in the first ten chapters.

This revision would not have come to fruition if it were not for the patience and encouragement of my wife at all times. As usual, the staff of Churchill Livingstone steered me carefully through the intricate, laborious process of revision, and I appreciate their helpful attention at all times.

It must be clearly understood that the contents of this book and the opinions expressed do not necessarily reflect the policy of the Department of Health.

LONDON, 1974   RAYMOND J. BRIGDEN

Preface to the First Edition

For some time now the author has felt there is a need for a comprehensive textbook on Theatre Technique to which nurses, technicians and medical students can refer and supplement their practical experience.

This book is written primarily for personnel who intend to specialise in theatre duties, but is hoped that house surgeons and others who may be associated with this work may derive some benefit also.

Theatre technique is now a very complex subject, and it would be impossible to include all the operations and procedures associated with the various specialities without producing a rather unwieldy volume. The author appreciates that techniques vary considerably and wishes to impress upon the reader that this book must be regarded as a basis for practical experience and study in individual units. It is hoped that advantage will be taken of the various references which have been listed if a more detailed study of a particular subject is required.

The chapters on Electricity and Static Electricity have been included because it is felt that these subjects are of increasing importance to theatre staff. A better understanding of electrical apparatus and lighting will ensure a sensible approach to the use of such equipment in a modern operating theatre.

Emphasis has been placed upon a packet system of sterilisation and the use of heat rather than chemicals whenever possible. Although nylon has been described as a wrapping material, it is accepted that many units are using paper or linen for this purpose. This is, of course, a matter of individual preference.

The chapter on Ligature and Suture Materials has been made comprehensive in order that it may be used for reference. The sizes and technical data quoted are in accordance with BP standards.

'Assisting the Surgeon and Draping the Operation Area' is intended to help the reader to understand how this is done, combined, of course, with practical instruction from the surgeon, theatre superintendent or charge nurse. Again, methods of draping the operation area must be adapted to individual needs, but those described, if carried out correctly, will ensure the drapes remain in position during the course of operation.

The instruments described for various operations are those in common use and are arranged in sets. Substitution of instruments may be necessary according to a surgeon's individual preferences, but those shown should be adequate for the particular procedure. The outline of procedure for each operation is not intended to replace the many excellent textbooks on operative procedure, but it is hoped will act as a general guide and handy source of reference. The reader is referred to the appropriate surgery textbook if further details are required.

The Appendix of Instruments is an extraction of those in common use from the multitude illustrated in the surgical instrument catalogues. An opportunity has been taken to list technical data of orthopaedic implants as this information is not easily available from other sources at present.

COVENTRY, 1962   RAYMOND J. BRIGDEN

Contents

1
The Theatre or Operating Department

When describing the theatre or operating department for the purpose of a textbook it is usual to list those features which are considered to be ideal. Hundreds of new operating departments have been built during the last decade but nevertheless many hospitals have still to utilise facilities which are not ideal, despite extensive upgrading schemes. But even new departments cannot be expected to fulfil all theoretical requirements, as new ideas are constantly being developed, and by the time they are incorporated into building, fresh ones take their place on the drawing board. Definitions of the terms operating department, suite and theatre are as follows:

1. *Operating Department.* This is a unit consisting of one or more operating suites together with the ancillary accommodation including such common-use rooms as changing and rest rooms, reception, transfer and recovery areas and circulation space.

2. *Operating Suite.* This comprises the operating theatre or room together with its immediate ancillary areas such as anaesthetic room; sterile lay-up or preparation room; disposal room; a scrub-up and gowning area; and an exit room or area which may be part of the circulating space of the operating department.

3. *Operating Theatre.* This is the room in which surgical operations and certain diagnostic procedures are carried out.

OPERATING DEPARTMENT PERSONNEL

All personnel must aim to reach the highest possible standard, taking into consideration the equipment available, the limits of the operating department facilities and the surgical specialties. Strict asepsis would perhaps not be achieved during tonsillectomy operations as compared with a bone graft, but the same amount of care must be taken during the preparation of each. Speed and accuracy, with absolute efficiency are the goals to which all must aim. The ability of professional nurses to work in an operating team and create a happy professional atmosphere helps toward the attainment and maintenance of the high standard so desired.

The pattern of staffing will depend to some extent on local preferences and circumstances. Due consideration must be given not only to the overall shortage of nurses and particularly trained theatre nurses but also to the difficulties of recruiting suitable ancillary staff, often in competition with industry for their services. For many years the operating department was regarded almost exclusively as the domain of nurses; ancillary staff were usually restricted mainly to orderlies, porters and domestics. It is, perhaps, ironical that changes in composition of the theatre team are due both to an increased complexity in the technical aspects of surgery and an increasing shortage of nursing staff. Without entering too deeply into the controversy in some quarters of nurses versus technicians (or operating department assistants), a sensible approach is to acknowledge that each has an important role in the modern theatre team.

Whether or not the nurse will continue to co-ordinate the services of the operating department will depend upon sufficient numbers wishing to pursue a career in operating department management. The nurse's role, however, must be clearly defined and some interchangeability of present duties should enable better deployment of trained nurses in the operating department where it is considered their skills are essential. Trained operating department technicians or assistants can play an increasingly full part as members of the team including responsibility for acting as the 'scrub or instrument assistant' and assisting the anaesthetist. (Already highly trained technicians provide special services such as the operation of cardiological equipment including cardio-pulmonary by-pass procedures. These technicians are generally members of departments normally outside the jurisdiction of the operating department manager but providing a service to the theatre team when required. The term 'manager' refers to the person in charge of/accountable for the operating department services. It could apply equally to a nursing officer, superintendent, supervisor or sister).

In order to ensure a continuing high standard of care for patients undergoing surgery it is essential to set up well-planned induction and training programmes for all grades of operating department staff. Student and pupil nurses should, as part of their training, have adequate experience in the operating department and be taught pre- and post-anaesthetic care of patients and acquire some understanding of surgical procedures. The General Nursing Council 1969 syllabus indicates that student nurses may either spend two weeks in operating departments as observers only or eight weeks with participation in operating department work. In Scotland this is different in that student nurses must have four weeks experience and eight statutory lectures in theatre technique.

When student nurses are in the department for only two weeks, hospitals should regard them as supernumerary to the establishment and even when they are there for longer it is important to maintain a practical ratio between trained and untrained staff. Although the General Nursing Council for Scotland does not stipulate the period of time pupil nurses should gain experience in the operating department, the GNC for England and Wales suggest that pupil nurses should receive eight weeks practical experience either in the operating department or in the accident/emergency or in the out-patient departments.

An understanding of work carried out in the operating department is important if nurses are to be encouraged to undertake a 'theatre' career when their training is completed.

Ancillary staff

In all operating departments, irrespective of age or size, a critical appraisal should be made of the duties undertaken by skilled staff. Whenever possible, duties not requiring their skills should be delegated to clerical and ancillary staff (Lewin Report, 1970). Some clerical assistance for the operating department manager is essential and where there are four or more operating theatres it may be necessary to employ a full-time receptionist in addition to a clerk/typist (see Appendix, p. 558 for duties).

The development of Central Sterile Supply Departments (CSSD), Hospital Sterilising and Disinfection Units (HSDU) and Theatre Sterile Supply Units (TSSU) adjacent to the operating departments enable theatre staff to be relieved of the task of cleaning and re-processing instruments. Where such facilities exist these duties should be performed by ancillary staff, after appropriate in-service training, their work being supervised by skilled staff. These units may or may not be under the jurisdiction of the operating department manager but obviously the closest co-operation must be established.

Whilst preparation of the operating theatre between cases and operating sessions will be the responsibility of the team of nurses, technicians/assistants and other immediate ancillary staff, major cleaning including walls, ceilings and 24-hour cleaning in the operating department should be carried out under arrangements made with the domestic manager or supervisor. Domestic staff should be employed to care for staff changing rooms, rest rooms and offices and where necessary for serving refreshments to staff. 'Care' in this context includes duties such as disposal of used items, replenishment of supplies including linen and general tidiness. These are not duties for which skilled operating department staff should be employed.

Tasks undertaken by operating department porters vary considerably from hospital to hospital. In some cases their duties may be restricted to the transfer of patients between wards and theatres, in others their work extends to duties which may normally be carried out by technicians/assistants. Specification of their role is of course a matter for local arrangement, but where there is a strict demarcation between the 'outside' and 'clean' zones a practical solution is to employ 'outside' duty porters from the general portering pool and retain portering or orderly services exclusive to the 'clean' zone.

Operating department manager

The person in charge of an operating department influences to a great extent the degree of co-operation between members of the team (Douglas, 1962; Yeager, 1965). This person essentially should be a good leader with a generally placid nature and qualifications of kindness, tolerance and a sense of responsibility. The capability of planning ahead with good judgment, and the ability to take orders and accept constructive criticism are very important. There should always be a willingness to adapt to developments in surgery and operating theatre technique. Loyalty to the patient, surgeon, co-worker and hospital is vital and obvious. In short, a good 'manager' but essentially a leader of a nursing and technical team.

The visible signs of good leadership can be summed up in seven observable qualities (McKenzie, 1971).

1. A leader should be able and willing to assist his team and individual members of the team to carry out their roles, and in so doing think out clearly what are the roles and functions of all members of the team and then facilitate their carrying out of these functions.

2. He is capable of thinking out and bringing about *desirable* changes, for not all changes result in progress.

3. Since changes may be resisted, the leader will know the most acceptable and effective method of introducing them.

4. He will be seen and known to assist the team and members of the team to overcome difficulties and hardships.

5. The leader will observe and develop initiative and potentialities of members of his team.

6. He will preserve and transmit those appropriate features of the team pattern which are desirable.

7. Finally, the leader will encourage and help the members of his team to express, whether in words or actions, their hopes, desires, apprehensions and wishes.

The manager of an operating department will ensure delegation of tasks which staff are adequately trained to perform. He or she will ensure also that a suitable working environment is established in the operating department so as to secure the safety and welfare of staff and in addition review local rules from time to time to avoid the imposition of unnecessary restrictions upon staff.

An essential quality for an operating department manager, indeed any nurse or technician/assistant working in the operating theatre, is the ability to assimilate practical, mechanical and electronic information related to the correct use and simple maintenance of surgical instruments and equipment. It is probably for this reason that men are particularly attracted towards a career in operating theatre work.

MANAGEMENT

A multiplicity of textbooks devoted to management techniques exist. Many of these are equally as applicable to the operating department as to hospital management in general. A list of suitable books are included in the bibliography on page 31 and readers may seek specialised information from these. However, the organisation and management of operating departments does include aspects which are not readily available from these sources and it is useful to mention some at this stage.

It should be unnecessary to stress that operating departments cannot be organised in isolation from the work of the hospital as a whole. An obvious example is that the provision of surgical facilities must relate to surgical bed turn-over, admission and theatre requirements from diagnostic and other departments of the hospital (Lewin Report, 1970). The organisation of the department must relate to the overall policy decisions of the hospital and for this reason there must be close liasion between the operating department manager and administrative, medical and nursing colleagues responsible for other areas of the hospital. The establishment of a good management structure along the lines of the Salmon and Cogwheel Reports (Salmon, 1966; Cogwheel, 1967), should contribute towards this liaison. A link with administrators is probably best established by a member of the hospital's administrative staff having a special interest in the operating department. The formation of an 'Operating Department Committee' will help to preserve liaison with surgeons, anaesthetists and others who are directly concerned with day-to-day matters.

Operating department committee

Although the operating department manager has overall accountability for the service provided, there is a need for a broadly based operating department committee to advise on the overall organisational requirements of the users. Where the hospital is large it will require its own committee but in the case of smaller hospitals it may be more practical to arrange for one committee to serve a number of hospitals in a group.

The function of this committee will vary according to local circumstances. Essentially the committee is advisory to the operating department manager but it may have an executive function also. Examples of executive function include ensuring the most effective use of facilities and staff; to keep under review the incidence of infection; recommending the purchase of new instruments and equipment within financial restraints and a general monitoring of the standards of care and skill in the department. In their advisory role the committee could, for example, make proposals for changes in the organisation of the department which may effect other departments in the hospital or group; advise on staffing patterns and training programmes.

The chairman of this committee should be a surgeon or other suitable person nominated by the Medical Executive Committee. A small committee is more efficient and therefore it is suggested that the remaining members would normally be restricted to the operating department manager, a representative of the anaesthetic staff, a representative of the surgical staff, a member of the junior surgical staff and a senior member of the administrative staff. Other members can be co-opted as required, for example representatives of the general nursing service, CSSD manager, microbiologist, pharmacist, radiologist, domestic supervisor and hospital engineer. It is important that these specialists are invited to attend when matters of particular concern are being discussed and similarly they should also have access to the committee to bring up any matters affecting their own specialty. The committee should meet regularly, at least once a quarter. Minutes should be kept and circulated to interested parties.

Pattern of work

The pattern of work in an operating department should be arranged so as to achieve the most effective utilisation of accommodation, operating time and manpower consistent with the best interests of patients and staff.

Preparation of operation lists by medical staff in collaboration with the operating department manager and ward sisters should ensure that typed copies are available for distribution to all departments concerned not later than the afternoon previous to the operations taking place. The schedule drawn up should be realistic and one which can reasonably be expected to be completed by the surgeons within a defined period. The Lewin Committee (1970) considered that the average length of an elective operating session should be three and a half to four hours, with the afternoon session starting at a time which allows it to finish ideally before 17.00 hours.

Abbreviations should never be used on an operation list which should be typed and include the following information:

1. Surname and first name(s) of patient
2. Age
3. Sex
4. Registered hospital or unit number
5. Nature, site and side of operation
6. Ward or unit
7. Date and time of operation
8. Name of surgeon
9. Name of anaesthetist
10. Special requirements.

Self adhesive labels incorporating identity information, and suitable for attachment to request and other forms, are being used increasingly in hospitals. In the preparation of operation lists these are eminently suitable for indicating the information listed under items 1 to 4. They are an additional safeguard in avoiding errors of transcription.

Last minute changes in operating lists cause concern and possible risk or error. A distinct policy should be laid down by the Operating Department Committee for the procedure to be adopted for any changes to the operation list, in order that all relevant operating department, ward and other personnel are informed. Procedures for checking the identity of patients undergoing surgery are described in Chapter 10.

Records

It is of vital importance that adequate records of operations performed and personnel involved are maintained. The records should be entered and *numbered serially* either in a bound book or filed in a specially designed loose leaf folder. The latter procedure is of particular use where there are a number of theatres in an operating department and a separate page can be used for each. The information should include the following:

1. Surname and first name(s) of the patient
2. Age and sex
3. Registered hospital or unit number
4. Operation serial number
5. Nature of the operation
6. Ward
7. Special remarks (e.g. drug therapy, drainage tubes)

8. Names of surgeon, anaesthetist and assistants
9. A record of staff present during an operation, which can be of value in monitoring sources of cross infection
10. Type of anaesthetic
11. Signatures of two persons checking swabs and instruments.

It is valuable also to keep some record of theatre utilisation and although the day-to-day responsibility for the maintenance of records of this kind rests with the operating depart-department manager, the system employed should be kept under periodic review by the Operating Department Committee. Operation records and swab checking procedures are discussed further in Chapter 5.

DESIGN

Nowadays the need is recognised to group together operating department facilities in a hospital, for this provides the maximum economic use of equipment and skilled personnel. Many planners advocate the centralisation of all intensive care facilities, with operating theatres and labour suites immediately adjacent to the intensive therapy unit and near to the accident/emergency and X-ray departments. Planning restraints may preclude this in entirety but the relationship between these departments, surgical wards, CSSD and laboratory facilities are important.

The operating department should be constructed so that it is separate from and independent of general traffic and air movement in the rest of the hospital (Medical Research Council, 1962; DHSS, 1968). In the past the department was often placed on the top floor of a tall building but in order to reduce solar heat-gain, a position at a lower level is now favoured. Noise transmission from ventilation plants sited on the roof is also reduced as they are no longer immediately above the operating department.

Clean and dirty streams of traffic in an operating department should as far as practicable be segregated. Although adequately bagged soiled equipment can be routed via a clean corridor without risk of bacteriological contamination, the provision of a separate disposal corridor has distinct advantages. Such a corridor provides direct access to the point of disposal and reduces traffic congestion in the clean circulation areas.

There should be a transfer or changeover section at the entrance to an operating department providing the first stage entry/exit to the sterile zone. This 'protective' zone includes also the recovery area, plaster room and changing rooms for staff and other personnel. The recovery area can be sited just outside the protective zone, possibly incorporated in the intensive therapy unit, although with such a design there are problems of access for the anaesthetist working in the clean zone and some barrier gowning procedure must be devised for him to enter and leave these zones.

Rooms of the department should be so arranged that there is a continued progression from the entrance through zones that increasingly approach sterility to finally the operating theatre and sterile preparation room. The 'clean' zone consists of scrub room and gowning, anaesthetic room, exit lobby, clean movement and rest areas and sterile store. The operating theatre and lay-up or sterile preparation room form the 'sterile' zone. The least clean area of the whole department is the disposal or sluice room and disposal corridor; this is termed the 'disposal' zone.

The clean zone must include adequate storage rooms for equipment or general supplies in addition to sterile packets; an X-ray darkroom may be provided. Various offices, conference rooms and teaching accommodation are usually sited in the vicinity of changing rooms outside the protective zone although there may be a need for a floor office in the clean zone of a large department.

If possible the processing and sterilisation of drape and instrument packets should be

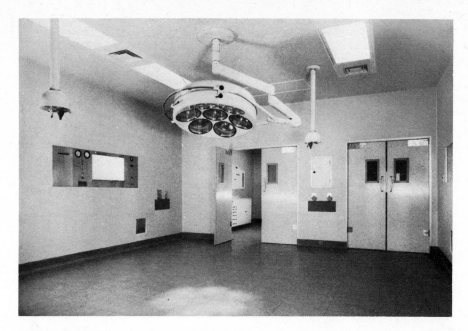

Figure 1   Single theatre suite, type 3. On the left, the surgeon's equipment panel with ventilation controls; in the background anaesthetic and recovery rooms, note the 'through' drug cupboard just above the socket outlets; and the ceiling pendants for oxygen, nitrous oxide, vacuum and compressed air. (Newcastle Regional Hospital Board.)

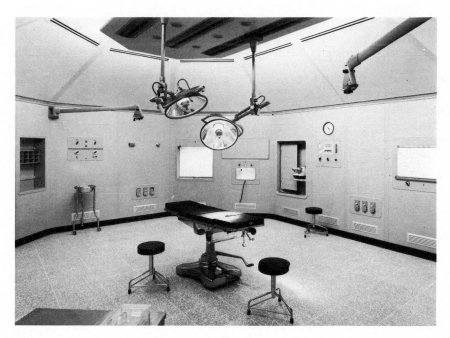

Figure 2   A Venesta modular operating theatre showing wall mounted equipment which allows clear space for the surgical team. (Venesta Hospital Systems.)

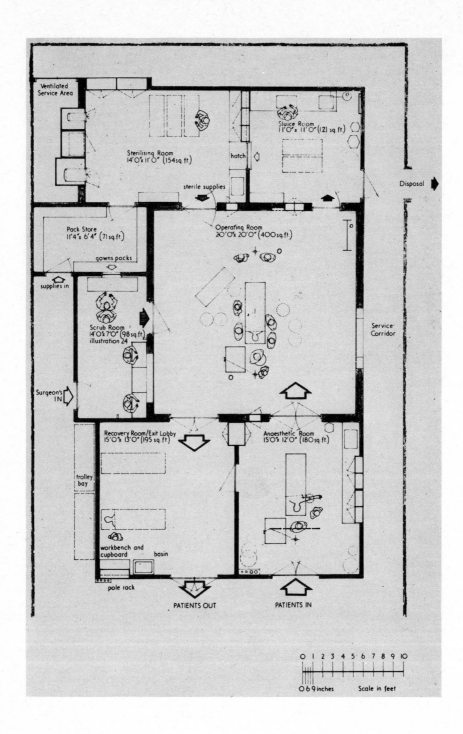

Figure 3   Sketch plan of single theatre suite, type 3. (Newcastle Regional Hospital Board.)

centralised in a Theatre Sterile Supply Unit built either adjacent to the operating department or forming part of the main hospital Central Sterile Supply Department. (Buxton Hopkin, 1962; DHSS, 1968).

Personnel working within the department should be able to move from one clean area to another without having to pass through unprotected or traffic areas. Ventilation should be on the principle that the direction of air-flow is from the clean to the less clean areas (Medical Research Council, 1962). Heating and ventilation should also allow comfortable climatic conditions for the patient, surgeons, anaesthetists and other personnel. There should be no movement of air between one theatre suite and another.

The construction must be such that a high standard of cleanliness may be obtained (Houghton and Hudd, 1967). All surfaces should be washable and all joins between walls, ceilings and floors curved to minimise the collection of dust.

Types of operating departments

The general layout is frequently dependent on the total hospital plan. Sometimes the operating department may have been built after the hospital was established, and in this case may probably have been fitted into an existing space. One assumes that active steps have been taken to upgrade these facilities and it is taken for granted that such improvements include the elementary features of an adequate ventilation system. Operating departments constructed in new buildings or extensions to buildings should be of a more satisfactory and compact layout. Readers will find, however, that operating departments may generally be classed in five main categories:

1. The now rather outdated single theatre with combined sterilising and utility accommodation. There are the usual ancillary rooms such as anaesthetic accommodation and exit lobby.

2. Similar to the above but arranged as a twin theatre suite with shared ancillary accommodation.

3. The single theatre suite containing operating theatre; scrub-up and gowning area; anaesthetic room; sterile preparation room; exit lobby and disposal area. Ancillary accommodation within and outside the clean areas includes storage space, rest rooms, probably an X-ray darkroom, changing rooms, offices, conference and teaching rooms (Figs. 2, 3).

4. The two theatre suite with facilities similar to number 3 but with duplicated ancillary accommodation immediate to each operating theatre; sharing other accommodation such as changing rooms and offices etc.

5. Multiple theatre departments of three or more operating suites with ancillary accommodation similar to numbers 3 and 4.

Construction

The operating theatre itself should have walls of an impervious semi-matt surface (Jolly, 1950). The finish can be laminated plastic sheet, vinyl sheet or an epoxy resin type of paint. If the latter is used then the plaster should be a high impact type incorporating fibre glass. Tiles are not ideal due to the crevices formed between each. The most important point is that the surface be easily washable and withstand the repeated application of disinfectants in general use.

A semi-matt wall surface reflects less light than a highly gloss-finish and is less tiring to the eyes of surgeons and staff. With this in mind the colour is important also, pale blue, grey or green being the most generally suitable colours.

The floor should be impervious also, either of terrazzo, rubber or vinyl. The same considerations should apply regarding the colour, and the floor must be of an anti-static composition, or tiling which is well earthed to minimise the danger of an explosion due to

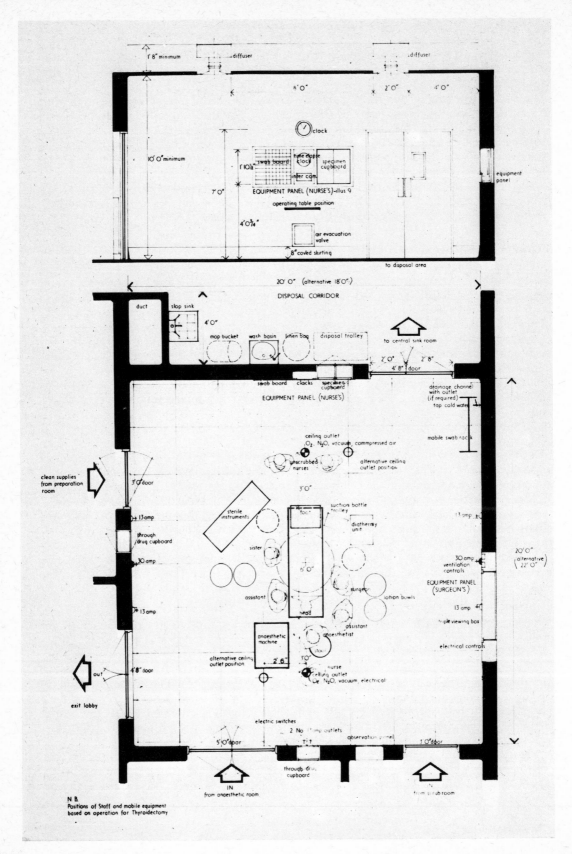

Figure 4   Layout and fittings of a single theatre. (Newcastle Regional Hospital Board.)

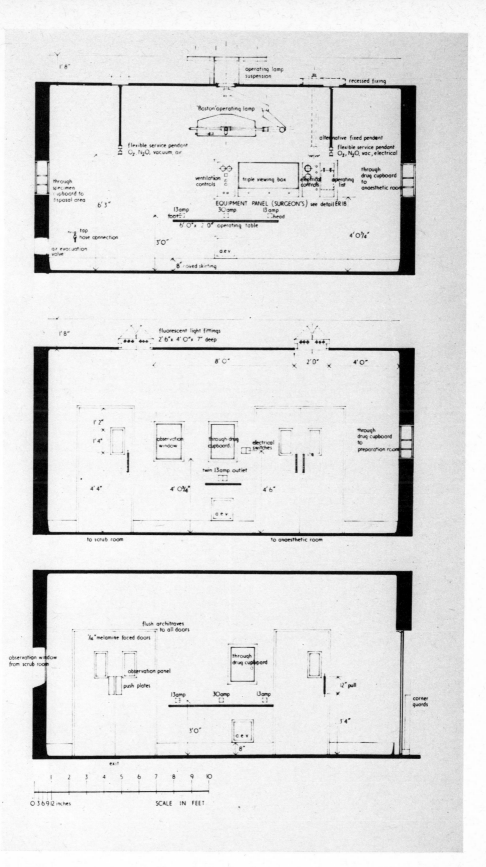

Figure 4—continued.

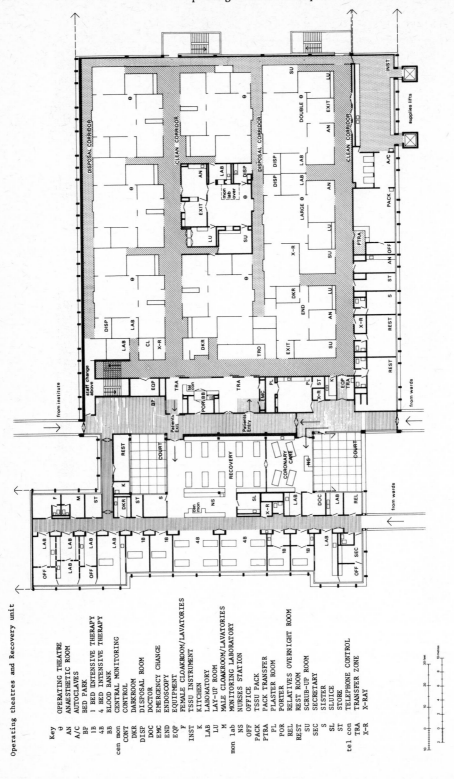

Operating theatres and Recovery unit

Key	
ᶿ	OPERATING THEATRE
AN	ANAESTHETIC ROOM
A/C	AUTOCLAVES
BP	BED PARK
1B	1 BED INTENSIVE THERAPY
4B	4 BED INTENSIVE THERAPY
BB	BLOOD BANK
cen mon	CENTRAL MONITORING
CONT	CONTROL
DKR	DARKROOM
DISP	DISPOSAL ROOM
DOC	DOCTOR
EMC	EMERGENCY CHANGE
END	ENDOSCOPY
EQP	EQUIPMENT
F	FEMALE CLOAKROOM/LAVATORIES
INST	TSSU INSTRUMENT
K	KITCHEN
LAB	LABORATORY
LU	LAY-UP ROOM
M	MALE CLOAKROOM/LAVATORIES
mon lab	MONITORING LABORATORY
NS	NURSES STATION
OFF	OFFICE
PACK	TSSU PACK
PTRA	PACK TRANSFER
PL	PLASTER ROOM
POR	PORTER
REL	RELATIVES OVERNIGHT ROOM
REST	REST ROOM
SU	SCRUB-UP ROOM
SEC	SECRETARY
S	SISTER
SL	SLUICE
ST	STORE
tel con	TELEPHONE CONTROL
TRA	TRANSFER ZONE
X-R	X-RAY

Figure 5   Sketch plan of Northwick Park Theatres. (Llewelyn-Davis, Weeks, Forestier-Walker and Bar.)

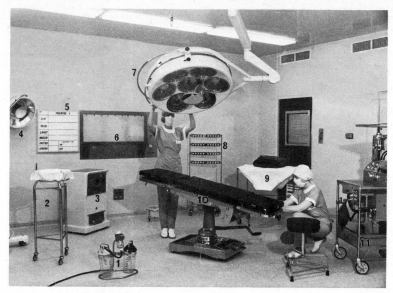

Figure 6   Picture of interior of theatres depicted in Figure 5.
  1. Pipeline suction apparatus.
  2. Stand with unopened packet containing sterile hand lotion bowl.
  3. Diathermy machine.
  4. Mobile supplementary operating light fitting.
  5. Swab count board.
  6. X-ray viewing screen.
  7. Main shadowless operating light fitting.
  8. Swab or sponge checking rack.
  9. Trolley with packet containing sterile instruments and drapes, outer layers only have been opened.
  10. Operation table.
  11. Anaesthetic machine.

electrical static sparks. The dangers of static electricity are dealt with more fully in Chapter 3.

Well established in Europe is the prefabricated modular operating theatre. This is constructed from factory-made prefabricated sections consisting of a framework of interlocking metal members and panels of a specially developed plastic core material faced with synthetic plastic finishes. The unit which is basically hexagonal can be erected relatively quickly either within existing buildings or a simple standard shell.

The unit is designed to take the maximum advantage of the space available. Several variations in layout can be achieved ranging from the single operating theatre to a complete unit of ancillary rooms also. The method provides a speedy means of improving facilities in an existing, outdated operating suite.

Lighting

At one time it was considered important to have windows large enough to admit good diffused daylight into the operating theatre. However, as all operations are performed with the aid of artificial light this is no longer important; indeed too much daylight is rather distracting.

If windows are fitted they should be small to reduce the amount of solar gain or loss and facilitate the control of heating and ventilation, and provision must be made to black-

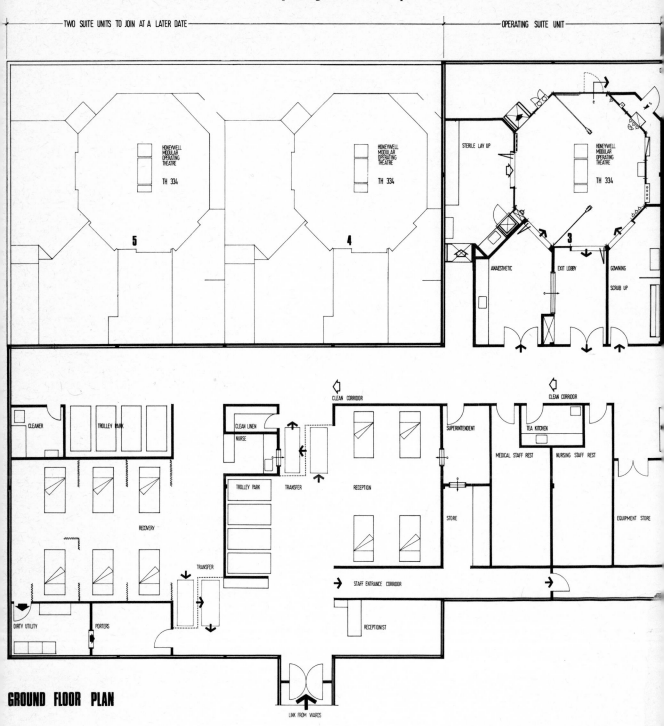

TWO SUITE UNITS TO JOIN AT A LATER DATE

OPERATING SUITE UNIT

HONEYWELL MODULAR OPERATING THEATRE

TH 334

5

HONEYWELL MODULAR OPERATING THEATRE

TH 334

4

STERILE LAY UP

HONEYWELL MODULAR OPERATING THEATRE

TH 334

3

ANAESTHETIC

EXIT LOBBY

GOWNING

SCRUB UP

CLEANER

TROLLEY PARK

CLEAN LINEN

NURSE

TROLLEY PARK

TRANSFER

RECOVERY

TRANSFER

DIRTY UTILITY

PORTERS

CLEAN CORRIDOR

RECEPTION

SUPERINTENDENT

CLEAN CORRIDOR

TEA KITCHEN

MEDICAL STAFF REST

NURSING STAFF REST

STORE

EQUIPMENT STORE

STAFF ENTRANCE CORRIDOR

RECEPTIONIST

LINK FROM WARDS

GROUND FLOOR PLAN

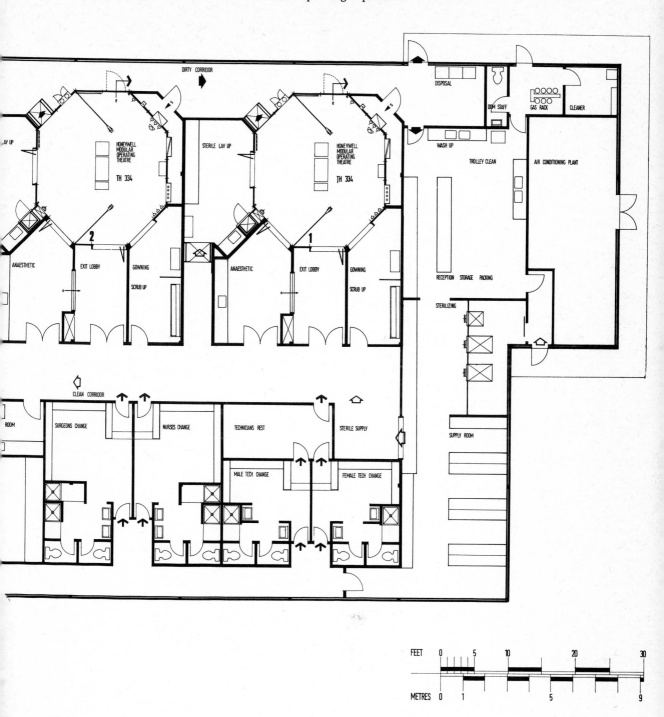

Figure 7   Sketch plan of an operating department, type 5, with multiple theatre suites and having provision for additional suites to be added at a later date. (St. Mary's Hospital, Portsmouth). (Venesta Hospital Systems.)

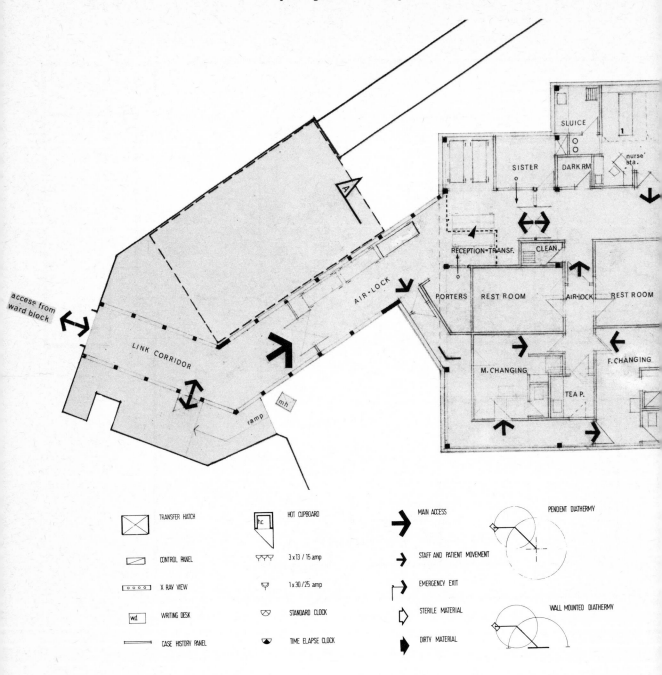

Figure 8   Sketch plan of an operating department, type 4, with twin theatre suites. (Prince of Wales General Hospital, Tottenham, London.) (Venesta Hospital Systems.)

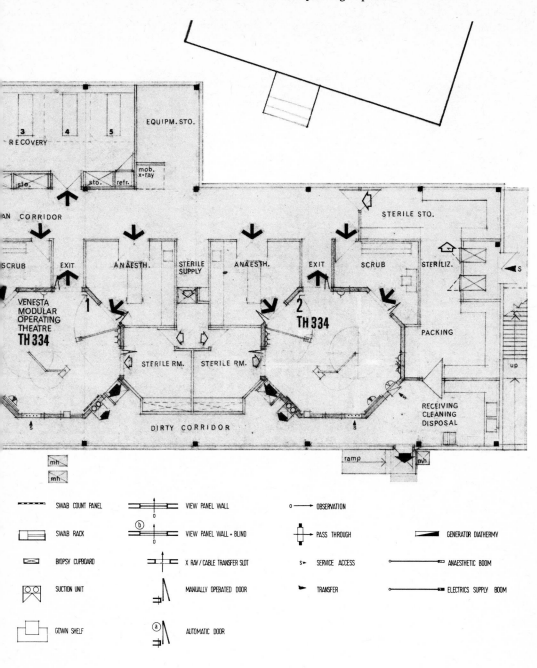

	SWAB COUNT PANEL		VIEW PANEL WALL	o—	OBSERVATION
	SWAB RACK		VIEW PANEL WALL + BLIND		PASS THROUGH		GENERATOR DIATHERMY
	BIOPSY CUPBOARD		X RAY / CABLE TRANSFER SLOT	s▸	SERVICE ACCESS		ANAESTHETIC BOOM
	SUCTION UNIT		MANUALLY OPERATED DOOR	▸	TRANSFER		ELECTRICS SUPPLY BOOM
	GOWN SHELF		AUTOMATIC DOOR				

out the operating areas if endoscopic operations are to be performed. This is best achieved by dust enclosed blinds, preferably between windows, or alternatively by a power-operated roller blind fitted exteriorly.

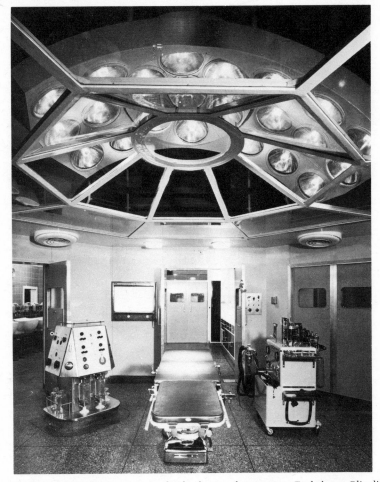

Figure 9   One of four theatres in a multiple theatre department. Each has a Blin lighting system consisting of multiple spotlights which is described in Chapter 2. A viewing gallery for students and visitors is provided also. (St James Hospital, Balham, London.)

An efficient system of artificial lighting which incorporates adequate emergency measures is absolutely essential. If the mains or fuses fail there must be sufficient light to complete the operation, and in emergency commence others. The emergency system must be fully automatic.

Ventilation

An efficient ventilation system should be provided in the operating department to achieve three functions: (1) to supply heated or cooled, humidified, contamination-free air to the operating theatre and adjacent clean areas; (2) to introduce air into these rooms so that it removes the contaminants liberated therein; and (3) prevent the entry of air from adjacent contaminated areas.

The minimum bacteriological requirements are:

1. The air delivered should not contain detectable *Clostridium sp.* or coagulase-positive *Staphylococcus aureus*. Aerobic cultures on non-selective medium should indicate not more than 35 bacteria-carrying particles in 1 m^3 (1 per ft^3) of ventilating air.

2. During surgical operations the concentration of bacterially-contaminated airborne particles in the operating theatre averaged over any 5-minute period should not exceed 180 per m^3 (5 per ft^3), although it is recognised that for some special types of surgical operations, e.g., orthopaedic and transplantation procedures, higher standards of air cleanliness may be justified (Medical Research Council, DHSS, Regional Engineers' Association, 1972).

A certain division of opinion exists in respect to the best method by which this can be achieved. An improvement in the reduction of surgical sepsis over the last decade is probably due to some extent to the installation of plenum ventilation (Bourdillon and Colebrook, 1946; Blowers and Crew, 1960; *Lancet*, 1956, 1958, 1968). More recently the development of high and medium velocity laminar or linear flow ventilation and the high-input/high-exhaust enclosure has emerged (Charnley, 1964, 1970).

Plenum turbulant air flow system. A medium velocity system of this type is the method most commonly employed at present. If it is maintained and balanced correctly the system is reasonably efficient (coupled with good theatre discipline and correct protective clothing for personnel). Air at roof level is drawn by means of a fan through a series of filters, is humidified, cooled or warmed and forced into the operating theatre through high-level diffusers fitted into the walls or ceiling.

Filters must be changed regularly. Some installations incorporate a system of continuous-feed filters which move on automatically as they become clogged. Micro-organisms such as *Pseudomonas sp.* often multiply on cooling coils, eliminator plates and in water reservoirs of humidifying apparatus and may contaminate the air. The addition of bacteriocides to water reservoirs does not necessarily discourage the growth of bacteria and should therefore never be used. Humidification should preferably be by steam injection, although if this is not possible fresh soft water from spinning discs may be used. Easy access for routine cleaning of these components by maintenance staff is essential.

The air pressure in the operating theatre should be slightly greater than that outside the suite (Medical Research Council, 1962). The greatest pressure of air is always in the sterile preparation room followed by the operating theatre in which the pressure is only slightly less. The volume of air supplied to the theatre should maintain a pressure in the order of $+25\mathrm{Nm}^{-2}$ to ensure that contaminated air does not enter from other areas. It is relatively easy to maintain an outward flow of air through the gaps around a closed door. The difficulty arises when one or more doors are open, for it is not generally appreciated that providing temperature differences between rooms are within 1°C, an air flow of about 10 m^3 per minute for each 1 m^2 (30 ft^3 per minute for each ft^2) of open doorway is needed to maintain an acceptable outward air flow. In practical terms a double door demands about 35 m^3 (1200 ft^3) of air per minute and to allow for various other air leaks, the air volume to an average theatre should be between 45 and 60 m^3 (1,500 and 2,000 ft^3) per minute, providing 20 to 30 changes of air per hour at a velocity of between 3 m and 12 m (10 ft and 40 ft) per minute. *If several doors to a theatre remain open during operations this may seriously interfere with the outward-flow air pattern.* Approximately 10 per cent of the air volume will be provided by air flowing from the sterile preparation room (pressure $+35\ \mathrm{Nm}^{-2}$) the operating theatre being its only outlet.

Extraction of air from the operating theatre is not mechanically aided. Air flows through the small gaps around closed doors and also spills via balanced flaps or valves set in the walls or lower part of doors. These flaps are hinged and weighted so that air is allowed to pass in one direction only—any tendency for a back-flow of air from the less sterile areas will cause them to close. When a theatre door is opened these flaps close and direct all outflowing air through the open doorway, thereby maintaining a degree of pressurisation.

The next highest pressure of air should be in the scrub-up (6 m^3 or 200 ft^3 per minute), anaesthetic (12 m^3 or 400 ft^3 per minute) and the clean circulation areas. Approximately 50 per cent of the air volume for the anaesthetic room flows from the operating theatre and 80 per cent of the supply in the scrub-up and clean circulation zone derives from the most sterile part of the suite. Extraction is again via gaps around doors and by balanced flaps from room to room. The pressure is in the region of $+5$ to $+15$Nm^{-2}.

Only a small positive pressure of air ($+2\cdot5$Nm^{-2}) is needed in the protective zone, i.e. transfer section at the entrance to the operating department, recovery area and changing rooms. Virtually all the air is supplied by progressive flow from the sterile parts of the suite. Extraction here is again by balanced flaps except if there is a primary air-lock between the transfer and main hospital corridors. In this instance extraction can be by fan and should be in the order of 8 m^3 (260 ft^3) per minute. There is no mechanical input into the air-lock.

The lowest pressure in an operating department should be in the disposal area, disposal corridor and plaster room (-5 Nm^{-2}). Input is received only from the more sterile areas such as the operating theatre and extraction is by fan at approximately 15 m^3 (500 ft^3) per minute.

It was thought at one time that extraction of air at floor level helped to dissipate anaesthetic gases thereby avoiding an accumulation of inflammable gases which could ignite under favourable circumstances. However, the zone of risk associated with flammable anaesthetics is now recognised as being an area extending for 25 cm around any part of the anaesthetic circuit or the gas paths of an anaesthetic apparatus; flammable gas mixtures escaping from anaesthetic breathing circuits rapidly dilute to a non-flammable level within a few centimetres of the point of escape (DHSS, 1971). A typical flow pattern for a theatre ventilation system is illustrated in Figures 10 and 11.

Care must be taken to check regularly the efficiency of the operating department ventilation. In addition to bacteriological sampling either by slit samplers or exposure of culture plates, the pressure differentials from room to room can be checked visually by tracing air-flows. This is performed by using a smoke test.

One method is to use glacial acetic acid and cyclohexylamine, holding the bottles close together with the tops removed. As the fumes rise from the bottles they mix and produce a smoke, enabling air currents to be traced. Alternatively an applicator, covered lightly at one end with cotton wool is dipped first into one bottle and then the other to create a flow of smoke. Any solution splashed on the skin should be washed off immediately.

Air currents should be checked at tops and bottoms of doors—both open and closed. If there is any backflow or air currents seem to flow from the less clean to the clean areas, this may indicate either a mechanical fault or that the filters are blocked and insufficient air is being forced into the suite.

An alternative to glacial acetic acid and cyclohexylamine is smoke generating tubes. In the United Kingdom these can be obtained from the Mine Safety Appliance Co. Ltd., Glasgow, E.3.

Laminar/linear flow ventilation systems. These originate from developments in the construction of 'clean rooms' for the assembly of electronic components in the aerospace industry. Advances in surgery have resulted in longer operations on patients who formerly may have been regarded as unsuitable for surgery. In orthopaedic or transplant procedures, for example, reconstructive operations may take several hours and stringent precautions must be taken to avoid bacterial contamination, particularly if the patient is receiving immunosuppressive drugs. Hence the need for ultra clean environments in

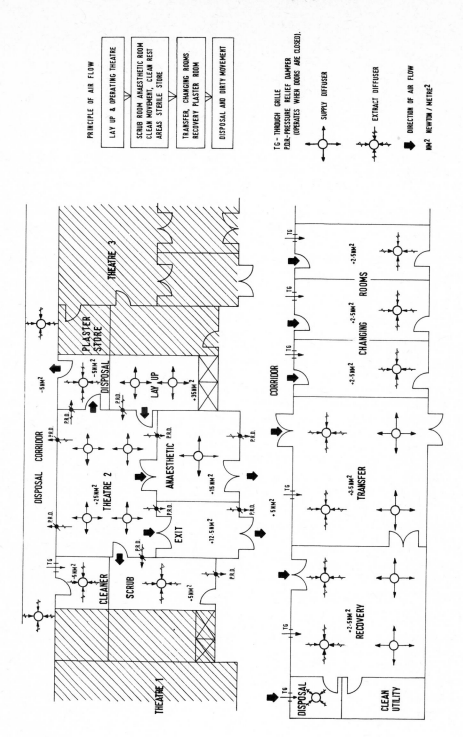

Figure 10   Typical airflow pattern for a theatre suite.

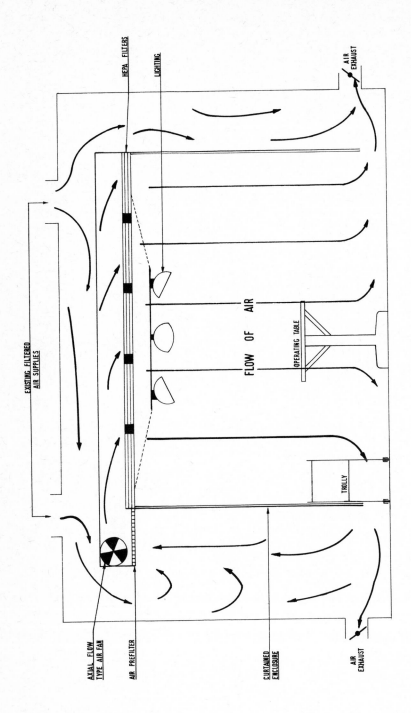

Figure 11   Method of upgrading existing operating theatre utilising vertical laminar/linear air flow.

operating theatres (Voda and Withers, 1966; Whitcomb and Clapper, 1966; U.S. Department of Health, Education and Welfare, 1967; Scott, 1970; Scott *et al.*, 1971).

The term laminar flow is rather a misnomer for the correct definition refers usually to a horizontal, parallel linear pattern of air flow with characteristics of low velocity, low humidity, low temperature and low turbulence. These aerodynamic conditions are not fulfilled in an operating theatre and as most conditions are not fulfilled in an operating theatre and as most installations provide a vertical flow arrangement it is more appropriate to use the term linear flow as a preferable alternative.

The fundamental difference between plenum turbulent ventilation and laminar/linear flow can be summarised as follows. In the former, a downward displacement or turbulent flow is created. Limitation on the liberation of contamination from within the room (e.g. shedding of bacteria laden skin particles) due to rising convection and eddy currents of air, is largely controlled by wearing special clothing such as Ventile/Scotchguard fabric suits and restriction of the number and movement of personnel. Pressurisation of the theatre prevents entry of air from outside and thereby reduces the incidence of contamination from this source. Between 20 and 30 changes of air per hour at a velocity of between 3 m and 12 m (10 ft and 40 ft) per minute are provided by this system which is relatively efficient if maintained adequately.

Laminar/linear flow utilises highly filtered air directed towards the operation area through a filter bank consisting of an entire wall or ceiling. The volume of air moves at a velocity in the region of 30 m (98 ft) per minute at approximately 10 changes per hour, making only a single transit over a given area. When a solid object is encountered, the air flows round the object interrupting the laminar/linear flow only momentarily. Surgery is carried out in a uniform flow of clean air and contaminants are flushed away as they are released.

The system incorporates High Efficiency Particulate Air (HEPA) Filters developed to a specification of the U.S. Atomic Energy Commission and which are 99·999 per cent efficient at the 0·3 μ and larger particle size which is more than adequate to stop bacteria-carrying particles. Air returned to the periphery of the room, plus a suitable amount of added air depending on the number of people present, is led back to the fans via a battery of disposable prefilters. The final HEPA filters ensure that recirculation presents no bacteriological hazard. Slight pressurisation of the operating theatre is maintained, as in the plenum turbulent system, to prevent ingestion of air from contaminated areas outside.

A disadvantage of some laminar/linear flow systems may be the noise created by the fans and the constant downward or horizontal flow of air may prove trying to the operating team, but unpleasant odours are quickly removed and the risk of contamination is reduced to minimal. Sampling has shown that virtually no bacteria are allowed to collect in the sterile area, whereas settling counts in a control operating theatre with conventional ventilation have ranged from four to 19 colonies per culture plate after only one hour's exposure. Before the system becomes generally accepted, further research is necessary, for example, in the design of overhead operating lights which cause minimal turbulence to air flows passing round them.

High input/high exhaust enclosure. This was first developed by Mr John Charnley in 1962; since that time further improvements have resulted in the Charnley-Howorth sterile enclosure which is considered by some to be a better alternative than laminar/linear flow.

The enclosure is installed in an existing operating theatre and provides a highly filtered, turbulent air flow at a velocity of 12 m (40 ft) per minute with up to 300 air changes per hour. It is fabricated from a metal frame with three transparent sides and a fourth through which three quarters of the operating table and patient is made to enter;

the fourth side is closed by sterilised curtains. The enclosure may be floor mounted and permanent with hinged access for emergency equipment, or ceiling suspended with completely removable walls of lightweight plastic panels. Fans draw air from the operating theatre into the plenum chamber at the top of the enclosure. With suitable silencing devices this air is then discharged into the enclosure through HEPA filters and then through non-return valves and specially designed fabric sleeves which prevent entrainment of surrounding air. The flow of air passes out of the enclosure via gaps under the walls and is recirculated after passing through the filter system (Fig. 12).

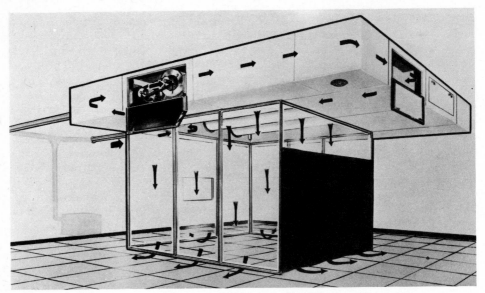

Figure 12   Air flow pattern of the Charnley-Howorth sterile enclosure.

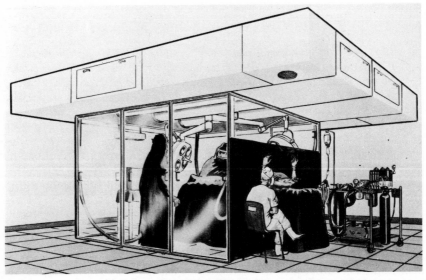

Figure 13   The Charnley-Howorth sterile enclosure in use.

The sterile enclosure is used in conjunction with the Charnley Body Exhaust System which is specifically designed to remove the body convection currents and exhaled breath of the operating team which is a major source of infection in operating theatres. A surgical gown of Ventile/Scotchguard fabric (see Chapter 5) prevents the transmission of bacteria-carrying skin particles which are continually being shed by the operating team. Air from under the gown is constantly extracted via the exhaust mask at $1\cdot5$ m^3 (5 ft^3) per minute taking away skin scales and exhalations in addition to cooling the wearer thereby preventing perspiration, and reducing fatigue by continuous ventilation. A communication system integral with the mask is available, enabling the team to talk to each other more easily, also to lecture to spectators outside the enclosure (Fig. 14).

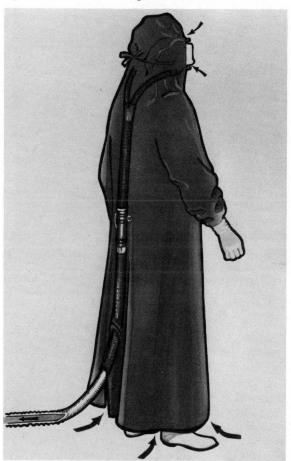

Figure 14   Charnley Body Exhaust System to reduce transmission of bacteria carrying skin particles.

The largest size of enclosure available is 10 feet square by just over 7 feet high. The objective is to isolate the surgical team and patient from circulating personnel and spectators. The anaesthetist can remain outside the enclosure as illustrated in Figure 13. Instruments needed for the operation can be carefully programmed beforehand and the separate trays presented in the order they are needed. The trays are sterilised in separate packets and, when required, the contents are introduced through an open service hatch at the foot end of the enclosure without the contents coming into contact with the air which is shared by the circulating personnel, anaesthetist and spectators. Alternatively, a conventional instrument trolley technique can be employed.

The main disadvantage levelled at the body exhaust system is that the special suits exercise considerable restraint on the numbers and mobility of the surgical team. Certain adaptation to the suits is necessary but against this must be weighed the statistics of infection produced by Charnley (Fig. 15). Some authorities consider however that further bacteriological evaluation of the separate roles of the enclosure, special clothing and surgical technique are necessary before this system is accepted for general use.

System	Year	Air Changes/hr	Colonies/Plate/hr	Number of Operations	Total Number of Operations	Infection %	Total Infection %
Open theatre exhaust ventilation	1959 −61		80–90	190	190	8·9	8·9
First prototype enclosure. Electrostatic precipitation	1962	10	25	108	108	3·7	3·7
Second prototype enclosure. Howorth-donated system	1963 1964 1965	80	1·8	1,079	1,079	2·2	2·2
First Howorth permanent enclosure	1966			410		1·7	
	1967	300	0 (limit of accuracy)	673	1,929	1·9	1·5
	1968			846		0·9	
	1969	300	0 (limit of accuracy)	1,039	2,152	0·6	0·5*
	1970			1,113		0·5	

*In both 1969 and 1970 the infections were caused independently of the enclosure. But the final infection rate cannot be decided until 3 years have elapsed since the operation.

The effects of the body exhaust system are not fully apparent because the system has been in constant use only since the second half of 1970. But no infections have so far been encountered from the 500 operations performed while wearing the equipment.

IMPORTANT NOTE: Pre-operational 'umbrella' injections of antibiotics are **not** used at Wrightington. The figures above, therefore, reflect directly the effectiveness of the Charnley-Howorth Enclosure System.

Figure 15   Comparative figures compiled by Pathological Department, Wrightington Hospital, 1971.

Humidity

As the air passes through the spinning water discs or steam humidifier in the ventilation plant its humidity is increased (Yates, 1967). The altered air must not be too dry and must have a humidity of between 50 and 60 per cent for optimum comfort and to lessen the tendency for static electricity formation.

Humidity is controlled by an electronic sensor switch situated in the operating theatre.

An instrument called an hygrometer is available to measure this humidity level.

Heating

Combined with background heating, a ventilation system is a very satisfactory way of rapidly adjusting the temperature in the operating theatre.

Before entering through ceiling diffusers the air is passed over steam pipes within the duct. The amount of steam flowing through these pipes is controlled by an automatic mechanical valve which is operated by an electrical thermostat in the theatre. By adjusting this thermostat a reasonably constant temperature is obtainable, and in extreme variations of hot or cold weather rapid alteration of temperature is possible. The temperature of an operating theatre should be maintained at between 18·5° C (65°F) and 22° C (72° F) generally, *except* during hypothermia anaesthesia when it may be necessary to keep it below this level.

Background heating is best obtained by pipes or panels within the wall or ceiling. The heating provided by this source should be limited, for experience has proved that heating entirely by panels can be very oppressive particularly in the theatre. Another disadvantage is that it takes some time for pipes to heat up or cool down and therefore makes it impossible to vary temperatures rapidly.

Open radiators or pipes for heating the operating theatre are totally inacceptable; they are dust and bacteria traps.

Equipment and furniture

An operating theatre should contain only the minimum of equipment necessary for operating. Scrubbing and gowning-up should take place in a separate adjacent room. If due to old design these actions take place in the theatre they should be as far away from the operating areas as possible. Splashing is the most likely source of contamination whilst scrubbing up under these circumstances, and a careful watch on the water-tap pressure is advisable.

With pre-set tray packet systems for instruments, trolleys can be prepared in the operating theatre itself just before the operation starts. However, during a list or series of operations, and when a good deal of activity occurs (for example, positioning of the patient for a complicated operation), the sterile packets should be opened in the sterile preparation or lay-up room.

All theatre furniture must be of hygenic finish. Stainless steel or aluminium are ideal materials for trolleys, lotion bowl stands, etc., although nylon-covered mild steel is quite suitable where expense is of primary consideration.

Small supplementary supplies e.g. sterile packets, strapping, lotions, etc., should be kept either in a recessed cupboard or on easily washable plastic laminate shelves in a corner of the room.

A wall desk 45·5 cm by 61 cm (18 inches by 24 inches) fitted under the X-ray viewing boxes will be found useful for writing up notes and swab registers, etc.

Adjoining the operating theatre are the anaesthetic, scrub-up, disposal and sterile preparation rooms. These must have adequate, wide connecting doors and be of the same hygienic finish as the operating room itself.

Anaesthetic room

The anaesthetic room is described in more detail in Chapter 10. Quietness is essential and it should be reasonably soundproof to minimise transference of general preparation sounds from the operating theatre. This important department must have adequate equipment which is maintained to a high standard and always ready for immediate use.

The post-anaesthetic recovery room must be sited for convenient access of the anaesthetists. It can be in the operating department or associated with the Intensive Therapy Unit if this is nearby. The services provided by this unit vary according to local requirements. It may be used for short-term recovery of patients after operation, indeed until they have recovered consciousness only. Alternatively it may be staffed to provide a 24-hour service and intensive care after operation.

The scrub-up area

This should be sufficiently large to allow gowning and gloving in addition to scrubbing up. The wash basins can be either the conventional type a trough or an adjustable angled plate-glass sheet which channels water into a waterpipe.

The most important basic requirement is a wash basin of sufficient depth and height to minimise splashing the scrub clothes of those using it. Taps should be of the elbow- or foot-operated type, mixing hot and cold water into a single faucet and preferably controlled by a thermostatic mixing valve.

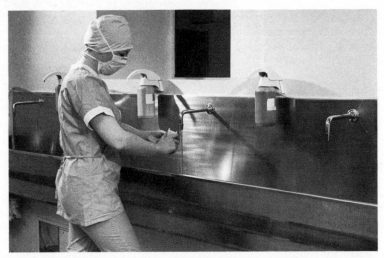

Figure 16   Three position 'scrubbing up' trough with foot operated tap and 'Nunk' liquid dispenser. (Northwick Park Hospital.)

There should be a clock or other timing device fitted in a convenient position near to the wash basins. Individual clean nail brushes are supplied from a suitable dispenser which can be refilled with brushes afterwards and then autoclaved for terminal disinfection.

Scrub-up solution, e.g. PHisoHex, Betadine, etc., is supplied from dispensers, foot or elbow operated either individually or piped from a central source.

The gowning section must be located as far away from the wash basins as possible. Gown packets can be opened either on a suitable trolley or a cantilever shelf fitted to the wall and having a 15 cm (6 inch) space at the rear to facilitate opening out the wrappings.

Adjustable shelves are suitable for storing packets of sterile gloves and gowns providing these are of a reasonable quantity. The basic stock should be kept in cupboards or preferably in the central sterile store.

Disposal room

This may also be called the sluice or sink room. Although basically its role is to handle the soiled instruments and dressings, etc., after operation, the extent depends on whether a Theatre Sterile Supply Unit (TSSU), CSSD or HSDU is available.

If a TSSU provides a full service, used trays of instruments may be simply over-wrapped with the trolley drapes and returned to the centre for processing (Harvey, 1958; Bowie et al., 1963). In this case the disposal room will be utilised only for disposing of soiled linen and dressings. The room will require a suitable wash basin and slop hopper. It will probably be utilised also for cleaning equipment and storing cleaning apparatus for the operating room.

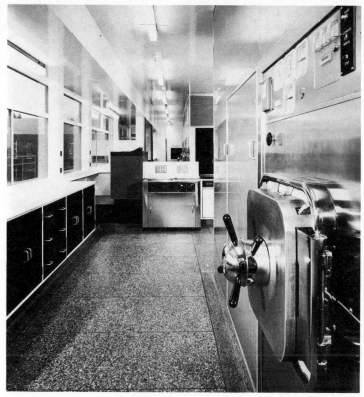

Figure 17 The disposal room of a four theatre department. In the foreground is a double-ended autoclave connecting with the sterile preparation room serving two of the theatres. This arrangement is repeated in the far background. In the centre are the ultrasonic cleaners and to the left of these, the supervisor's desk. (St James Hospital, Balham, London.)

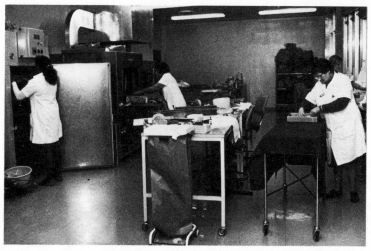

Figure 18 Theatre Sterile Supply Unit. Note washing machine and instrument drying cabinet on left; pre-set instrument trays being prepared on right.

Where processing of instruments is done at operating theatre level the disposal room may be equipped with suitable work surfaces, cupboards for supplies, and ultrasonic cleaner and dryer.

It should be possible to dispose of soiled items without taking them through clean areas such as the sterile preparation or sterilising room (Fig. 13).

Sterile preparation room

This room serves only for the storage of sterilised instruments or drape packets, supply of lotions and other items which may be required immediately in the operating theatre, and preparation of sterile trolleys.

Other ancillary rooms

The surgeons', nurses', and technicians' changing rooms should be equipped with lockers or clothes racks for outside clothes. They should have showers and toilet facilities. As mentioned previously, planning of the department should arrange that personnel and visitors can change into protective clothing before actually entering the operating section.

A separate office should be provided for the operating department manager or supervisor, and in large departments, an office for the anaesthetic service also. These offices are best positioned near to the entrance of the department as they are often used for interviewing representatives and others.

Adequate storage facilities, particularly for bulky equipment, are essential. A central sterile store should keep the main bulk of sterile supplies for the various operating suites.

The department may include an X-ray darkroom, small laboratory, blood storage facilities, and rest rooms for the surgeons and staff to avoid the necessity of personnel entering the changing rooms except at the beginning and end of operating sessions.

STERILISATION

Sterilising facilities may be provided either limited, or sufficient for the sterilisation of all instruments and equipment needed. Where a pre-set tray system is used and supplied

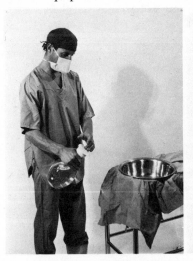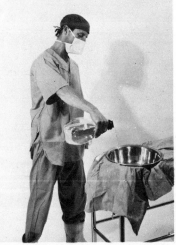

Figure 19   Sterile saline in Macbic flasks, checking the integrity of the vacuum by tapping the sealed cap. If the seal is unbroken and a vacuum present, there will be a characteristic water-hammer sound.

Figure 20   Dispensing sterile saline dropped into a hand lotion bowl.

sterile from the TSSU, CSSD or HSDU any autoclaves provided need only be adequate for the dropped instrument.

Regretably some operating suites are *still* disinfecting their instruments by boiling; there is no place for this in a modern department. The time has now come to deplore such techniques for even in remote areas where finance is limited, instruments can be sterilised by steam, utilising a portable autoclave or pressure-type cooker.

Sterile saline or water

The most suitable methods of supplying this for use as hand lotion are sealed flasks prepared by the pharmacy or a continuous running water press (Bowie, 1956; Medical Research Council, 1959; Gordon, 1963; Tallett, 1963; Wells and Lynch, 1963; Howie and Kelsey, 1963; Medical Research Council, 1968). The multi-supply tank or water boiler cannot be guaranteed to produce a safe, sterile solution. Even if the process of sterilisation is adequate, it is virtually impossible to avoid recontamination when drawing off the solution. In addition the water sterilised in the tank at the best is chemically softened and certainly *not* non-pyrogenic.

This is described in greater detail in Chapter 6.

Further reading on management useful in the operating department
BAKER, R. J. S. (1967) The Art of Delegation. *Journal of Royal Institution of Public Administration.*
BROWN, W. (1960) *Exploration in Management.* London: Heinemann.
DRUCKER, P. F. (1961) *The Practice of Management.* London: Heinemann.
GOWERS, E. (1970) *The Complete Plain Words.* London: Penguin.
JUDSON, A. S. (1966) *A Manager's Guide to Making Changes.* New York: Wiley.
REVANS, R. W. (1964) *Standards for Morale.* Oxford University Press.
SCHURR, M. (1968) *Leadership and the Nurse.* London: English University Press.
STEWART, R. (1963) *The Reality of Management.* London: Heinemann.
STEWART, R. (1967) *Managers and their Jobs.* London: Heinemann.

REFERENCES

BLOWERS, R. and CREW, B. (1960) *Journal of Hygiene,* **58**, 427.
BOURDILLON, R. B. and COLEBROOK, L. (1946) *Lancet,* **i**, 561, 601.
BOWIE, J. H. (1956) *Lancet,* **ii**, 45.
BOWIE, J. H., CAMPBELL, I. D., GILLINGHAM, F. J. and GORDON, A. R. (1963) *British Medical Journal,* **ii**, 1322.
BUXTON HOPKIN, D. A. (1962) *Lancet,* **ii**, 245.
CHARNLEY, J. (1964) *British Journal of Surgery,* **51**, 195.
CHARNLEY, J. (1970) *Lancet,* **i**, 1053.
COGWHEEL (1967) *Report of the Joint Working Party on the Organisation of Medical Work in Hospitals.* London: HMSO.
DEPARTMENT OF HEALTH AND SOCIAL SECURITY (1968) Article on Operating Departments. *Hospital Management,* September.
DEPARTMENT OF HEALTH AND SOCIAL SECURITY (1971) *Hospital Technical Memorandum No. 1.* London: HMSO.
DOUGLAS, D. M. (1962) *Lancet,* **ii**, 245.
GORDON, A. R. (1963) *Nursing Times,* March 1, 353.
HARVEY, J. (1958) In *Medical Electrical Equipment,* p. 61. Edited by R. E. Molloy. London: Newnes.
HOUGHTON, M. AND HUDD, J. (1967) *Aids to Theatre Technique,* 4th edn., chap. 1. London: Baillière, Tindall and Cassell.
HOWIE, J. W. AND KELSEY, J. C. (1963) *British Medical Journal,* **i**, 187.
JOLLY, J. D. (1950) *Operating Room Procedure for Nurses,* 3rd edn, pp. 13, 14. London: Faber.
Lancet (1956) Leading article. Ventilation of operating theatres. **ii**, 1197.
Lancet (1958) Annotation. Air contamination and layout of theatre suites. **i**, 203.
LEWIN (1970) *Report of a Joint Subcommittee of the Standing Medical and Nursing Advisory Committees on the Organisation and Staffing of Operating Departments.* London: HMSO.

McKenzie, N. (1971) *The Professional Ethic and the Hospital Service*, p. 5.

Medical Research Council (1959) Working Party. *Lancet*, i, 425.

Medical Research Council (1962) Operating Theatre Hygiene Subcommittee. *Lancet*, ii, 945.

Medical Research Council (1968) Aseptic Methods in the operating suite. *Lancet*, i, 763.

Medical Research Council, DHSS, Regional Engineers' Association (1972) Joint Working Party: *Operating Theatre Requirements*.

Salmon (1966) *Report of the Committee on Senior Nursing Staff Structure*. London: HMSO.

Scott, C. C. (1970) *Lancet*, i, 989.

Scott, C. C., Sanderson, J. T. and Guthrie, T. D. (1971) *Lancet*, i, 1288.

Tallett, E. R. (1963) *Lancet*, i, 489.

U.S. Department of Health and Education and Welfare (1967) May, Circular.

Voda, A. M. and Withers, J. E. (1966) *American Journal of Nursing*, 66, 2454.

Wells, C. and Lynch, P. F. (1963) *Lancet*, i, 57.

Whitcomb, J. G. and Clapper, W. E. (1966) *American Journal of Surgery*, 112, 681–685.

Yates, J. (1967) *Hospital World*, 6, 4, 5.

Yeager, M. E. (1965) *Operating Room Manual*, 2nd edn, p.3. London: Putnam.

2
Operating Theatre Lighting and Electromedical Equipment

The complexity of electromedical equipment used in the operating theatre has increased greatly during the past few years. Unless great care is taken in the maintenance and operating of this sophisticated equipment, potentially hazardous electrical situations can be created for patients and staff. Biomedical engineers and manufacturers have achieved a good deal in minimising these hazards, for example by developing 'earth-free' equipment where the patient is isolated electrically from earth or ground. Nevertheless, there must be an understanding by all working in the operating theatre of the principles involved and simple safety precautions to be observed.

The amount of electricity used in an operating department is often quite considerable, especially in a large unit, and provision is made for heavy loads.

The mains voltage supplied in the United Kingdom is between 220 and 240 V, 50 Hz, A.C. Emergency lighting is provided either from batteries at a low voltage, (12–24 volts) or by a supplementary generator which provides electricity at the standard mains voltage. In this case it is likely that the generator will supply a proportion of the electrical needs for the operating department through the existing mains wiring system. It is important to ascertain the maximum loading from such a system. Upon mains failure, there is usually a delay of up to 20 seconds before the generator comes into action. An automatic change-over switch is generally installed to ensure a temporary uninterrupted supply from batteries to the main operating light until the generator takes over (DHSS, 1974). Where special low voltage lamps are fitted exclusively for the emergency battery system great care must be taken to avoid interchanging with lamps used on the normal electricity supply.

In 1969 the Department of Health issued a recommendation that switches and socket outlets installed on the walls of operating theatres and anaesthetic rooms should *not* be of a sparkless type, regardless of the fixing height. Apparently, a review of explosion incidents had shown that the danger is confined to anaesthetic breathing circuits and the area immediately surrounding expiratory or other leakage outlets from anaesthetic equipment. Tests carried out under typical working conditions showed that flammable gas concentrations exist only in an area extending for 25 cm from the points where leakage occurs and gases quickly dilute to a non-flammable level beyond this. Thus, ignition risks associated with wall switches and socket outlets is negligible under normal working conditions. This does not apply to portable electromedical equipment which is liable to be used close to anaesthetic equipment and switches on such equipment should continue to be of a gastight sparkless type.

A gastight sparkless switch consists essentially of a short glass tube containing a small quantity of mercury. When the switch is operated, the tube tilts, causing the mercury to flow between two electrodes connected to the tube (Fig. 21). Any sparks which do occur when the current begins to flow or is interrupted are contained within the glass tube and do not come into contact with the atmosphere. All of this mechanism is concealed behind a plate or metal case of the apparatus and is operated by an insulated knob or toggle switch.

The framework of electrical apparatus, including portable light fittings and electro-medical equipment, must be earthed directly through the earth pin of the plug mechanism. Electric flex to such apparatus contains three insulated wires—brown, blue and green/yellow. The brown wire is connected to the live terminal and the blue wire to the neutral terminal. The green/yellow wire is always connected to the longer (earth) pin at the plug top at one end and to the metal frame of the apparatus at the other. (Previously the colour coding was red—live, black—neutral and green—earth). If a fault to earth occurs, the electric current has a safe passage to earth and not through an unfortunate person who may inadvertently touch the apparatus.

A nurse should not disconnect or reconnect any wiring, as this is the responsibility of the electrician, and if any electrical connection or wire is obviously loose the apparatus must not be used until thoroughly checked by the electrician.

Electric plugs

Sparkless electric sockets contain a mechanism to prevent the accidental withdrawal of the plug when the current is switched on.

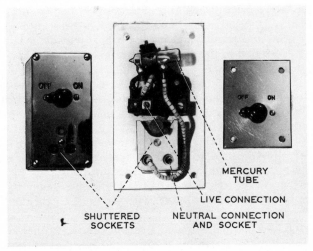

Figure 21   A spark-free electric plug socket and wall switch.

This mechanism usually consists of a specially mutilated earth pin which forms part of the interlocking device, or a device to prevent unauthorised electrical equipment being used in the anaesthetising area. Present experience points to the advantages of standardisation of mains socket outlets throughout the hospital, which is considered more important as this will allow any mains operated equipment to be used on the supply in emergency.

Where special plug sockets have been installed great care must be taken to avoid using an apparatus *which does not possess the correct type of locking-plug top*. If a plug top is used without the special locking slot or hole, undue force will result in damage to the internal mechanism of the socket. At one time special X-ray sockets were installed. Nowadays, utilising 30A ring circuits, a 13A *unfused* plug top connected to X-ray apparatus will only take high power from the circuit during a fraction of a second's exposure.

No moisture must be allowed to collect on the plug-top pins. If this should occur the moisture must be dried off thoroughly before the plug is inserted. Apparatus should be disconnected from the socket by grasping the plug top and not the flex. The use of adaptors for interchanging plug tops of different sizes is not a good practice, flexes can become frayed and connections loose.

THEATRE LIGHTING

When describing lighting equipment it is better to use the terminology usual with lighting engineers.

1. *Lamp.* This refers to the filament lamp, which is generally known as the bulb.

2. *The Light fitting.* This refers to the complete shadowless light fitting suspended from the ceiling, and includes the reflectors and the suspension gear. It also refers to mobile equipment, and is then described as a mobile light fitting or 'spot light'.

3. *The light field.* This is the area, usually circular illuminated by the light fitting.

The general lighting of the theatre may be provided by fluorescent tubes or filament lamps. These must be arranged to produce an even illumination with no glare, and are recessed in the ceiling, or alternatively in a dust-proof cornice surrounding the theatre at ceiling level.

The most important consideration, however, is the provision of a shadowless illumination of the actual operation area. This light fitting (or fittings) should be connected to a special switch incorporating an electrical relay which connects the emergency supply automatically upon mains or filament failure (Stevens, 1951; Smith, 1958).

Shadowless lighting is produced by directing the light on to the operation area (light field) from several angles to minimise shadows from the operator and his assistants.

Types of shadowless light fittings

Amongst the shadowless light fittings in common use are the single-reflector types, including the original scialytic with multiple mirrors, the metal reflector type and the

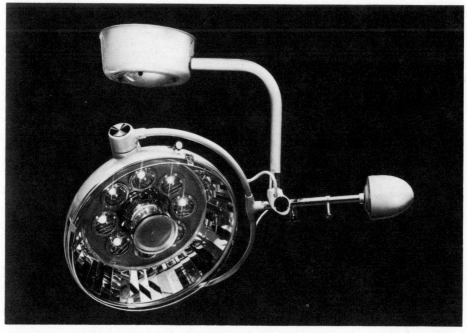

Figure 22   Scialytic operating light fitting with combined multi-reflector system. (Technical Lights & Equipment Ltd.)

multi-reflector type either contained in a single light fitting or set into a curved wall or in a domed ceiling at one end of the theatre.

The Scialytic Light Fitting. This consists of an optical lens, similar to a lighthouse lantern, surrounding a single lamp of 100 to 150 watts. Rays from the lens are projected on to a circle of mirrors which are set at 45 degrees to an imaginary perpendicular line running through the centre of the lens and which surround the inner circumference of the light fitting. These rays are then focused as a circular light field on the operation area.

Focusing of the light field is accomplished by sliding the lampholder up or down inside the lens. Release of a thumb screw at the top of the light housing will enable the metal tube (attached to the lampholder) to slide in or out of the supporting mount until the correct focus is achieved. This thumb screw must be retightened after focus adjustment. Alternatively adjustment of focus is controlled by a cam which is connected to a single external knob.

To focus, the operation table is raised to the height most generally used and the lamp position adjusted until the smallest possible spot of light illuminates the table. This should ensure that the light area will remain in focus as a spot when the table is raised or lowered between 15 and 23 cm (6 and 9 in) from this point to suit the individual surgeon.

The efficiency of this shadowless light, as with all light fittings, will depend to a large extent upon regular cleaning of the lens and mirrors. This may be the responsibility of the electrician, but if performed by the theatre staff care must be taken to ensure that the light is switched off before cleaning is commenced. *Do not* use any harsh cleanser which may scratch the highly polished surfaces. Soap and water or a window cleanser are quite suitable, followed by polishing with a soft lint-free cloth.

Another factor affecting the efficiency is dimming of the lamp due to over-heating. As the light fitting is designed to be dust proof, ventilation is often poor. This will affect the life of the lamp, which sometimes needs changing before it actually burns out.

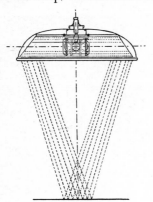

Figure 23   Sketch of the optical system in a scialytic light fitting.

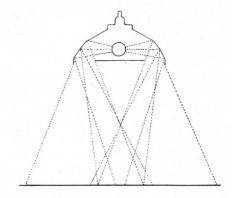

Figure 24   Sketch of optical system in metal reflector operating light fitting.

Shadowless light fittings may be fixed rigidly to the ceiling, but most are mounted on a swivel, counterbalanced arm or wires, which allow adjustment of position in relation to the operation area. It is possible also to mount the light on rails fixed to the theatre ceiling which allow movement across the theatre.

The Metal Reflector Light Fitting. This is basically the same as the scialytic lamp in respect of performance, but instead of mirrors the reflector consists of a concave, highly polished surface, either plain or made up of a number of facets. The lamp is situated at the central focal point and is adjustable in a similar manner to the scialytic type.

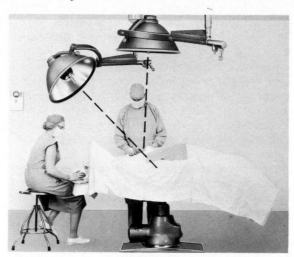

Figure 25   The AMSCO shadowless twin light fitting, metal reflector type. One lamp gives a broad general beam and the other a more concentrated narrow beam. Each can be adjusted to requirements. (American Steriliser Co.)

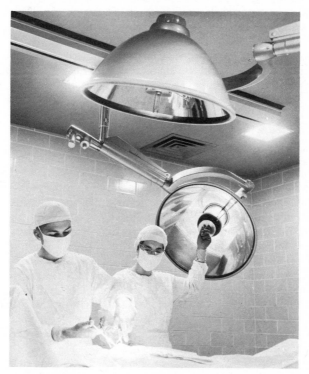

Figure 26   The AMSCO light fitting showing the use of a sterilisable handle, for easy adjustment by the operation team. (American Steriliser Co.)

A clear lamp should not be used in this type of light because it will give a small circle of highly concentrated light in the operating area. This light field may be only 5 or 7 cm (2 to 3 inches) in diameter, and is generally too small and certainly very tiring to the surgeon. Another important factor is that the depth of focus is very small and any adjustment in the operation table height will throw the light out of focus and produce poor illumination.

A pearl or opal lamp is more satisfactory for these reasons.

The larger the source of light *in the fitting*, the larger the diameter of the light field, and considerable adjustment of operation table height is possible before loss of focus occurs, thereby increasing the depth of focus. However, if this larger light source produces too much heat in the light field, the lamp may be surrounded with a heat-absorbing filter made from Chance glass. This filter absorbs most of the heat rays with only fractional reduction of the intensity of the light.

It must be remembered that the same considerations regarding the cleaning of reflectors apply as with other types of light fittings.

The Multi-Reflector Light Fitting. This has six to nine separate lights in the light fitting instead of one lamp and special reflectors. These 'spot' lights are focused simultaneously on the operation area by manipulating a single knob fitted to the light housing.

The lamps used in these 'spot' lights are smaller than those used in the light fittings just described. In one type of light fitting, the Hannulux (Fig. 27), they are of a lower wattage (40 W) and a lower voltage (24 V), and it is claimed produce a source of light which when used in conjunction with heat-absorbing filters is the best approximation to the colour of daylight possible with artificial lighting.

Although each 'spot' light is of relatively lower intensity compared to the lamp in the single-reflector fittings, the cumulative effect of the six or nine lights is very efficient, with the great advantage that should one lamp fuse the intensity of the light as a whole is only fractionally reduced.

The light field produced by the Hannulux Boston light fitting can be adjusted by a knob to between 16·5 cm (6·5 inches) and 34·9 cm (13·75 inches) in diameter. The maximum intensity of light at 16·5 cm (6·5 inches) is approximately 8,500 foot candles (90,000 lux) and at 34·9 cm (13·75 inches) diameter approximately 4,200 foot candles (45,000 lux).

Provision can be made in this lamp for a television camera or alternatively an automatic camera which, combined with a built-in electronic flash mechanism, enables photographs to be taken during operation.

Another development in this field is the Castle/Daystar light fitting which, it is claimed, produces a light of 6,000° K equivalent almost to perfect daylight colour (Fig. 29). The lamphead, measuring 101·6 cm (40 inches) in diameter, incorporates six pod 30·5 cm (12 inch) reflectors using incandescent quartz halogen lamps. The light is in focus at any distance from 76·2 cm to 152·4 cm (30 to 60 inches) from the cover glass; the prime focus being 106·7 cm (42 inches) from the glass providing a light field of about 40·6 cm (16 inches) in diameter. The maximum intensity at the centre of the light field at this distance is 5,000 foot candles (53,500 lux) and 1,200 foot candles (12,848 lux) at the edges; a dimming device is provided to reduce this intensity by up to half.

The heat rise from the fitting is 3°F (1·67°C) for each 1,000 foot candles of intensity, or 15°F (8·35°C) for 5,000 foot candles of intensity. This is achieved by the following:

A dichroic coating on the reflectors creates a 'cold mirror' that separates heat from light transmitting 80 per cent of the infra-red energy up through the reflectors, whilst reflecting colour corrected light energy downward;

Colour correcting cylinders cover each of the six lamps;

The skeletal configuration of the pod design takes advantage of upward air currents created by the infrared rays being transmitted through the reflectors.

In the event of a mains electricity failure a 24 V emergency system composed of six 24 V quartz halogen lamps comes into operation. Illumination is focused over the entire area of the operation table, with shadow reduced light in the centre of the light field which will penetrate cavities.

Multi-Reflector Wall Lights. With these a shadowless effect is produced by mounting a number of 'spot' lights in the wall and ceiling surrounding the operation table. These lights (up to 40 in number) are permanently focused on one spot in the centre of the theatre

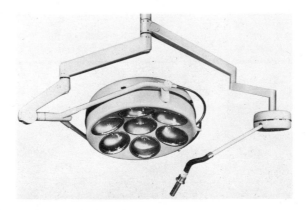

Figure 27 · A multi-reflector light fitting, the Hannulux Boston model with separate fibre-light satellite which gives a perfectly cool beam ideally suited to neurosurgery. (Sierex Ltd.)

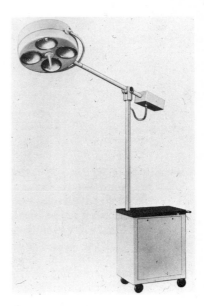

Figure 28   Mobile multi-reflector Hannulux spotlight.
(Sierex Ltd.)

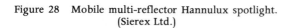

and may be independently switched in sets of six or eight according to the angle from which the light is required (Fig. 9 page 18, and Fig. 30 page 41).

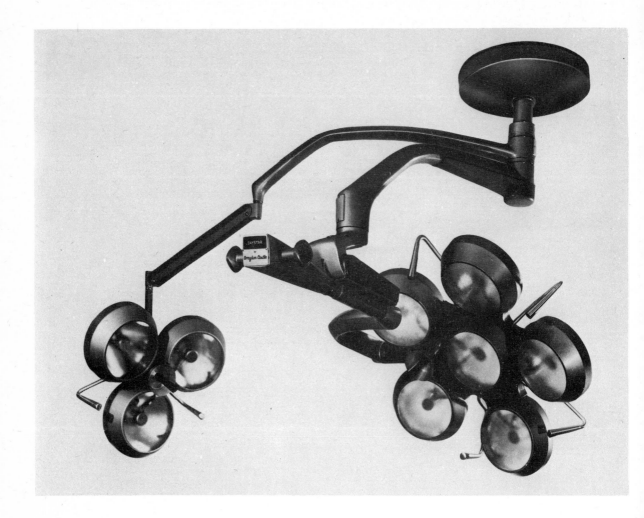

Figure 29   Daystar shadowless light fitting.

Changing operating light lamps

A spare lamp for the main light fitting and any mobile lights ('spot' lights) must always be easily available and placed in an accessible position. It is desirable for all members of the staff to become familiar with the method of changing a lamp in emergency.

The light must **always be switched off at the wall switch** before attempting to change a lamp.

Generally speaking, the lamp may be reached either by a raised panel in the region of the electric flex entrance on the top of the light fitting or through a removable panel in the glass or plastic cover on the front of the fitting.

In the former case the panel may be removed by unscrewing one or two remaining thumb screws and turning the panel in a clockwise or anti-clockwise direction to free it from any retaining pins. The cover may then be detached together with the lampholder and fused lamp, or will provide access for removal of the lamp from the lampholder.

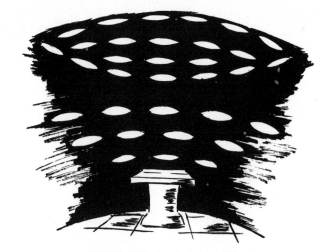

MULTIPLE SPOT LIGHTS SET IN THE
THEATRE WALL AND CEILING

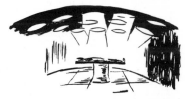

LAPAROTOMY ILLUMINATION

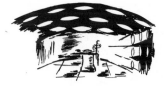

LITHOTOMY ILLUMINATION

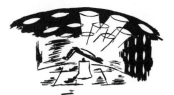

TRENDELENBURG ILLUMINATION

Figure 30

Access to the lamp through the glass or plastic cover at the front of the light fitting requires the release of three or four thumb screws, which allows the removal of the small central panel. There are no large modern operating light fittings requiring the removal of the complete front panel to reach the lamp. If the complete panel is ever removed for cleaning or other purposes the light fitting must be secured beforehand, as this will alter the counterbalancing and cause the whole assembly to spring upward towards the ceiling.

Where low-voltage or special lamps are used care must be taken to ensure that the correct lamp is fitted into the lampholder. A lamp should screw or plug into the holder easily and with no force. It should be remembered that certain lamps may be designed to burn efficiently in a particular position. A lamp which is suitable for burning in the portable 'spot' light fitting used mainly in a nearly horizontal position may burn out very quickly if used in the overhead vertical light, and vice versa. The cause of short life in a lamp may well be due to this reason as well as overheating which has been described.

Emergency lighting

The emergency lighting in the main overhead light fitting has already been discussed on page 33. These lamps come into operation automatically upon mains or fuse failure when the light is in use.

Emergency lighting should be tested regularly to ensure absolute reliability. During an emergency the supply must be switched off as soon as practicable and the use of unnecessary lights in the ancillary rooms carefully avoided. This will help to reduce the generator load, or 'drain' on batteries which are usually designed to give three or four hours' illumination on 'full loading'.

Sometimes portable emergency light fittings are provided in the theatre. The apparatus may contain only a battery, which must be recharged regularly by the electrician. With more modern apparatus a special trickle charger is incorporated within the unit and connected to a convenient plug socket when not in use. This mechanism keeps the batteries continually charged and the light ready for immediate use.

Low-voltage apparatus

There is a large amount of apparatus in the theatre which uses a low-voltage current. To mention just a few, these include laryngoscopes, bronchoscopes, cystoscopes, head lamps and illuminated retractors (Smith, 1958). To some extent low voltage illumination is being replaced by fibre optics (page 353).

It would be very true to say that no other type of apparatus can cause so many headaches for the theatre staff as the low-voltage equipment. It often seems to go out of action just when needed, and unless a careful step by step check of the circuit is made, much time can be wasted. The efficiency of such apparatus depends to a great extent on regular checking of batteries, lamps and electrical contacts together with knowledge of simple circuit testing to trace faults.

A low-voltage circuit may be likened to a circle of electric current flowing from the positive terminal of a battery, along an insulated wire, through the lamp filament and along another insulated wire thus completing the connection to the negative terminal of the battery. Apparatus such as torches, cystoscopes, bronchoscopes, etc., often use the outer metal case as the electrical return path to the battery instead of a second wire.

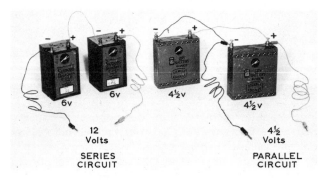

Figure 31   The principle of series and parallel battery circuits.

Generally a low-voltage circuit for theatre use may range from $1\frac{1}{2}$ V for apparatus such as bronchoscopes to 10 V for a surgeon's headlamp. The electric current may be supplied from batteries or a transformer which reduces the mains voltage to the required level. A transformer may be a separate item of equipment or may be incorporated in apparatus such as the diathermy machine.

In the case of batteries, two or more may be joined together either to give an increased voltage (series circuit) or prolong the period of supply (parallel circuit).

It is quite possible that when batteries or a transformer are working at full-power output the voltage given may be higher than that required for a particular lamp in an apparatus, and using a higher than necessary voltage may burn the lamp out immediately or reduce its life. It is usual in this case to introduce a rheostat into the circuit, which enables the voltage to be varied at will. The batteries or transformer may then be used for a variety of apparatus operating on different voltages.

A rheostat is an electrical resistance operated by turning a knob which when set at the required voltage reduces the slightly higher current to the required level. The rheostat should always be set at zero before switching on and connecting the apparatus.

Parallel lamp circuits

If any item of apparatus has more than one lamp it is usual to connect the lamps so that should one burn out the others will still illuminate. This is especially necessary in the case of an illuminated abdominal retractor which may have three or more lamps.

The basic method of connection can be illustrated with the example of a retractor with three lamps. Each of the lamps can be connected to the batteries by three separate sets of insulated wires. However, the most universal way is for each of the two wires leading from the battery or transformer terminals to be split into three, giving three positive and three negative wires. One positive and one negative wire is then connected to each of the lamps thereby allowing simultaneous illumination.

Care of apparatus

In order that a low-voltage circuit may operate satisfactorily all connections must be kept clean, dry and free from corrosion. After sterilisation, heat processed apparatus must be well dried before storing away. Good contact of the connections must be maintained and loose soldered contacts repaired immediately they are detected. Lamps must be securely screwed in position and the current source should, if possible, remain fairly constant. With batteries this means a careful watch for battery exhaustion.

Batteries left too long in a metal case tend to sweat, especially in humid atmospheres, causing corrosion and the discharge of power. All batteries not in actual use should be stored under dry conditions.

When a rheostat is connected in the power circuit it is preferable to switch on the full current slowly by commencing at nil volts and raising the current to the required level. This warms up the lamp filament before it receives the full current and increases its life considerably – a very important point as specialised lamps are often expensive and have a comparatively short life.

Checking a suspected faulty low-voltage circuit

This is a simple process if taken stage by stage, especially if a test lamp and battery are available. The test set consists essentially of a 1·5 V battery to which are connected two insulated wires, having rigid metal points at each of the two free ends, and a small low-voltage lampholder and lamp to which are also connected similar insulated wires. (A diagram of the circuit and illustration are shown on page 553.)

The battery is used for testing circuits and lamps, the lamp for testing faulty batteries. It is a simple matter for a carpenter to arrange these two items together in a box or on a movable board.

Irrespective of the type of apparatus tested (after connecting the apparatus correctly and switching on, as in the case of a laryngoscope, etc., it is found to be out of order) it is usually possible to check the faults as follows:

1. In the case of a transformer especially ensure that it is connected to the wall socket and is switched on correctly.

2. Check that the lamp is firmly screwed into position.

3. Check that all electrical connections appear to be in good contact and are not obviously broken. Where the apparatus has batteries in the handle, ensure that the inside of the case is free from any corrosion. Should there be corrosion, slight scraping of the contacts or tightening of loosened screws will usually suffice.

4. In the absence of a test battery try one or more new lamps in the lampholder or carrier. Small lamps can sometimes vary in size and length of the screw part. Should this be so, the centre contact at the base of the lamp may not reach the contact in the lampholder and it will appear that the lamp is out of order. These lamps should not be discarded as faulty until they have been tried with the test battery or in another lampholder or carrier.

Sometimes the centre contact of the lamp is made of a compressed coil of wire. Should the lamp not function in the apparatus but appear satisfactory on test with the testing unit, it may be advantageous to lengthen the contact by pulling out this coil of wire a fraction of an inch. When re-inserting the lamp be careful that the amount of lengthening is minimal, for if too much this contact may be pushed out of centre during screwing into position. This will then cause the wire to short-circuit across the inside of the lampholder, allowing the current to flow straight back to the battery or transformer and the lamp will still not light or may flicker.

5. If the lamp appears in order, check the batteries by connecting them with another apparatus known to be in working order, or use the test lamp, connecting it directly to the batteries. If the test lamp will not illuminate it is most probable that the batteries are exhausted.

6. Should the lamp still not function it is possible that the wires leading from the batteries or transformer to the lampholder or carrier may be broken somewhere within the insulation. These wires may be checked by connecting to other light carriers or lamps which are known to be in working order, or by using the test apparatus. The test is made by connecting the suspected faulty wires between the test battery and the two wires joined to the test lampholder.

ELECTROMEDICAL EQUIPMENT

The importance of earthing the metal framework of electrical apparatus has already been emphasised (page 34). This protects staff from electrocution should a fault occur and they inadvertently touch exposed metal parts of the apparatus. Unfortunately, earthing does not always give absolute protection to the patient, for if he is connected to 'earthed' electromedical apparatus it is possible under certain fault conditions for an electric shock to occur. This is particularly so in the presence of intracardiac catheters and pacemakers – a current of only a few millionths of an ampere could cause ventricular fibrillation and death. *Leakage is the term used in connection with electric current inherent in the system that is usually from the primary winding of the mains transformer in the apparatus.*

One risk is when the earth connection to the apparatus is accidentally broken; the leakage current may find its way to earth (ground) through other equipment connected to the patient or through some earthed object which the patient may be touching. Another path to earth could be through an attending nurse or doctor, who, standing on the floor, touches the patient and allows the leakage current to flow through both patient and nurse or doctor.

Another risk associated with the previous one is when the patient is connected to two or more pieces of 'earthed' apparatus, *i.e. utilising separate electrical sockets*. Each instrument will possess a protective device such as a fuse or circuit breaker in the electrical supply system. If a fault occurs whereby the live cable comes into contact with some part of the earth system, either the metal framework of the instrument or elsewhere in the building, the patient could momentarily be at risk. This is because the fuse or circuit breaker does not interrupt the supply quickly enough to prevent electric currents flowing momentarily along the earth system and through the patient. An inter-earth current is said to occur, that is, the voltage existing momentarily between two or more separate electrical sockets, via the earth wires, at the time of the fault (Fig. 32).

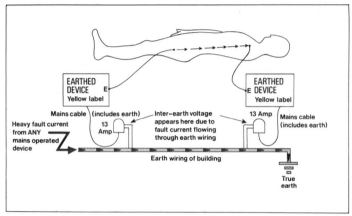

Figure 32   Current through patient. Due to inter-earth resistance, momentary fault current and use of several earthed devices. (Figures 32–37 reproduced with permission from Electrical Equipment Booklet – Patient Safety MO97–72 Northwick Park Hospital & Clinical Research Centre.)

Earth free patient circuits

Although the above mentioned risks are unlikely to occur they can be overcome by using equipment having 'earth free' patient circuits. The electrical design of the inside of 'earth free' equipment allows connections to the patient to be separated from earth. Consequently, the patient is on a 'floating' electrical circuit and *not* connected directly to the earth (Figs. 33 and 34). As a further explanation we can say that the inside of each apparatus is split into two halves – one half going to the patient and the other half obtaining electrical power and being connected to the hospital electrical supply. The equipment is so designed that an electrical failure would not be injurious to the patient. Completely 'earth free' equipment is therefore safe for connection to the patient, both internally and externally. The patient and all attachments to equipment, are 'separated' from earth (Fig. 35).

It is possible that both 'earth free' and 'earthed' equipment may have to be used on a patient at the same time. Although such a combination is not as safe as exclusively 'earth free' equipment, certain precautions will minimise danger of electric shock (Fig. 36).

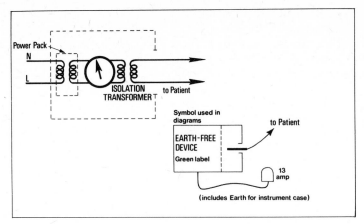

Figure 33   Basic earth-free equipment.

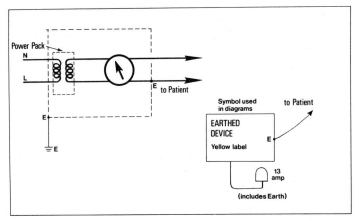

Figure 34   Basic earthed equipment.

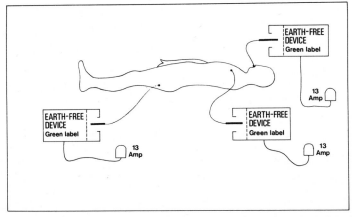

Figure 35   All earth-free devices. Patient completely protected against current flow through body.

Earthed patient circuits

If more than one piece of 'earthed' apparatus is connected to the same patient, e.g. 'earthed' diathermy machine and 'earthed' e.c.g. machine, it is possible for an inter-earth current to occur. To avoid this, external earth terminals should be fitted to each apparatus and when in use linked together with an approved safety earth wire which must be kept as short as possible (Fig. 37), this connects the patient to a common earth.

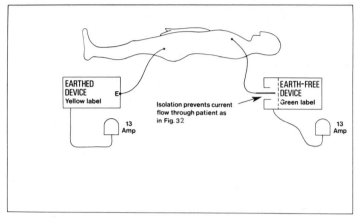

Figure 36   Single earthed instrument with other earth-free devices. (Generally satisfactory intermediate standard but shock from live object is possible because of one direct earth.)

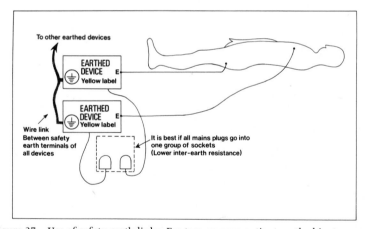

Figure 37   Use of safety earth links. For two or more patient earthed instruments.

It is worth noting that when the expression 'earth free' is applied to a diathermy machine it is relative; in a fault condition there is no danger of electrocution by external contact, but there is insufficient protection when intravascular catheters are in place. A safety earth should be connected if other 'earthed' equipment is in use. In the practical situation, therefore, diathermy machines should *not* really be regarded as 'earth free'.

Safety precautions

Guidance and care are necessary to minimise the risk of injury to patients and staff when using electromedical equipment. Much of the preceding information follows the work of a Safety Committee formed at Northwick Park Hospital and Clinical Research Centre, Harrow, England. This multidisciplinary group consists of doctors, biomedical and hospital engineers and nurses who meet to discuss developments in electromedical equipment and all aspects of electrical safety. The group formulated a safety guidance document (Northwick Park Hospital and Clinical Research Centre, 1972) and it is useful to reproduce the main points below:

Take care and think!

1. Do not place wet cloths, bottles of fluid or cups etc., on electrical equipment. Liquid seeping into the equipment could not only cause damage but also dangerous short circuits.

2. Never touch exposed pacemaker terminals, intracardiac catheters, or guide wires with one hand while making instrument adjustments or contacting electrically operated devices with the other hand. Wear rubber gloves when touching catheter connected metal fittings (except possibly in emergency).

3. Remove dried out saline solutions or jellies and always reapply the recommended amount of conducting material before placing electrodes on a patient.

4. Ensure that your hands are dry before touching the patient or electrical equipment; moisture allows more current to flow.

5. Disconnect from the patient any electrical equipment which is faulty.

6. Do not touch the patient and any kind of electrical equipment at the same time. You will provide the electrical link between the two, and there could be a fault.

7. Follow the manufacturer's instructions at all times.

8. If both 'earth free' and 'earthed' equipment is in use, then some means of identification is necessary. A useful system is to apply green labels with appropriate wording and use green plugs for 'earth free' and yellow labels and plugs for 'earthed' equipment. (This is the system used at Northwick Park Hospital.) Connect the *safety earth wire* provided between the *safety earth terminals* of all 'yellow label' equipment, when two or more of this type of apparatus are in use. This should be done before connection to the patient.

9. Ensure that electrical equipment is securely mounted so that it cannot be dislodged by the patient. Unexpected movement could cause breakage of wires, physical injury to the patient or even electrocution if the equipment is damaged.

10. Check all connections to the patient and equipment:

Look for:

        loose plugs
        kinks in wires
        worn or frayed wires
        electric cables touching hot surfaces.

Do not use mains extension cables and if in doubt call immediate attention to a suspected fault.

11. Take especial care with 'high power' apparatus, e.g. defibrillators, e.c.t. and diathermy machines. If misused, these can cause serious shock or burns to both patient and staff. *Never test* a defibrillator by power discharge when a synchroniser lead is connected to the patient – use an e.c.g. simulator for test purposes.

12. Use surgical diathermy 'indifferent electrodes' exactly as instructed by the manufacturers. The dry type of plate must make effective contact over a large flat surface of skin; separate small areas of contact could result in high-frequency electrical burns. Metallic rings worn by patients in operating theatres must be covered with water-proof, non-absorbent insulating material.

Monitoring equipment

Observation and recording a cardiac and respiratory function is called monitoring. A

wide range of equipment and systems are available to monitor data such as electrocardiograph wave form, arterial pressures, venous pressures and heart rate, to mention
just a few. It is beyond the scope of this book to describe these in detail and the reader
who seeks this information will find a number of recommended books listed on page 65.
However, the theatre nurse may be concerned in the use of some portable equipment; the
safety precautions already enumerated in previous paragraphs are equally as applicable
in the operating theatre as in the intensive care situation.

It is common now to manufacture modular equipment which allows maximum
flexibility in deciding the range of measurements to be undertaken. Various items of
equipment are designed so that they can be interconnected and plug-in units allow the
simple replacement of defective parts. The type of apparatus which the theatre nurse is
most likely to meet are the cardiac monitor (electrocardiograph), peripheral pulsometer,
cardiac pacemaker, and defibrillator.

The cardiac monitor or electrocardiograph. This is an apparatus which records the
electrical currents which are associated inseparably with cardiac impulses. As an electric
current is conducted readily through the body (for tissue fluids contain electrolytes,
mainly chlorides of sodium and potassium in fairly high concentrations), the electrical
currents generated by the heart are carried to the peripheral parts of the body. These can
be conducted to the cardiac monitor or electrocardiograph via wires or leads connected to
electrodes placed in contact with the skin; thus an electrical circuit is completed. The
electrical currents are led from certain paired parts of the body surface, and any pair of
electrodes (or rather parts of the body to which they are attached), with their connecting
wires are referred to as a 'lead'. Up to 12 pairs of leads may be used in diagnostic electrocardiography, but for monitoring purposes there are generally not more than 3 or 5
pairs.

Fundamentally the cardiac monitor or cardioscope consists of an electronic amplifier
which amplifies the electrical currents of the heart and displays them, either as a trace on
an oscilloscope or a continuous band of paper in a writing device. Figure 38 shows a

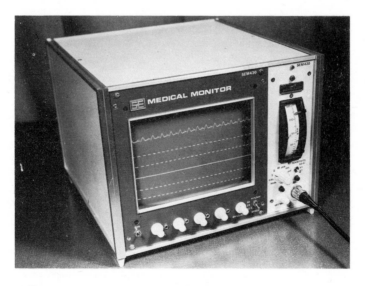

Figure 38   4-Channel cardiac monitor, only one ECG channel in use.
(S. E. Laboratories [Engineering] Ltd.)

modular system consisting of a four channel oscilloscope, e.c.g. amplifier and heart rate meter; only one channel is in use. Addition of further amplifiers enables the remaining three channels to be utilised and Figure 39 illustrates such an arrangement. This provides e.c.g., arterial pressure, peripheral pulse and temperature, each of which can be presented as a meter reading or wave form display on the oscilloscope. The four signals can be received from one patient, or the monitor may be used as the basis of a central

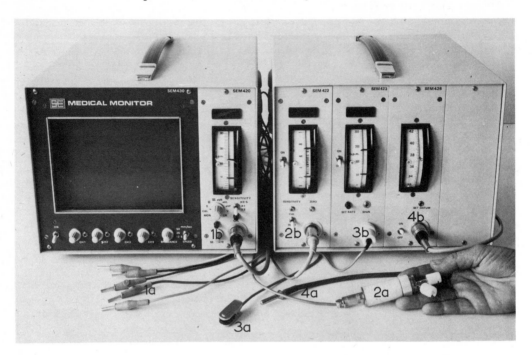

Figure 39   4-Channel cardiac monitor – all channels connected for use – oscilloscope display and meter readings available. (S. E. Laboratories [Engineering] Ltd.)

1a. ECG leads for connection to skin electrodes.
1b. Amplifier and rate meter (ECG).
2a. Pressure transducer (arterial pressures).
2b. Amplifier for pressure display.
3a. Ear lobe plethysmograph (pulse rate).
3b. Amplifier and rate meter (pulse rate).
4a. Thermometer probe (temperature).
4b. Amplifier and meter (temperature).

monitoring system whereby e.c.g. signals from four different patients are displayed on the four channels of the oscilloscope; a separate e.c.g. amplifier would be required for each channel. For a permanent record of traces, a writing device can be connected to any of the channels.

The basic characteristics of a cardiac monitor are:

1. Power supply; either from the electrical mains or batteries which may be rechargeable or replaceable.

2. Patient monitor cable dividing into three or five different coloured leads with terminals for connecting to the patient electrodes.

3. The oscilloscope screen (which may be green or covered with an orange filter) on which the e.c.g. trace or traces are displayed and may have an overlay grid scale.

4. A selector switch allowing the use of a number of channels (usually up to six) to select the most suitable trace.

5. Control knobs for height of trace (gain), brightness, focus, position and speed of trace (usually 12·5 mm, 25 mm and 50 mm per second).

6. Adjustable high/low alarm system which emits visual or audible signals if the heart rate exceeds above or below a pre-set range, e.g. 50 to 110 beats per minute.

7. A recording device or pen writer which records the e.c.g. trace on a continuous band of paper, either at predetermined intervals, e.g. every 15 minutes, when the alarm system actuates or when a button is pressed. This device may be part of the monitor or added as an accessory when required.

The monitor requires some adjustment to achieve optimum viewing conditions. The theatre nurse should first seek a demonstration of the various controls and then adjust them one at a time until the action of each is fully understood. The brightness and focus control in particular may require adjustment; if the trace is surrounded by a ring as it travels across the screen it is too bright, the minimum amount of brightness acceptable should always be selected to avoid burning the screen of the oscilloscope. According to how long each configuration of the wave or complex is required on the screen, so the speed of the trace traverse is adjusted. Generally four to six configurations should be present on the screen as the trace travels across.

The channel should be selected so that the trace appears as a thin line rather than a fuzzy one which may obscure smaller waves. If necessary, the size of the waves may be increased by adjusting the gain control. So long as the waves are clearly identifiable, it is not generally important whether they are upright or inverted on the screen (Figs. 40 and 41). Monitor observation is described further in chapter 10.

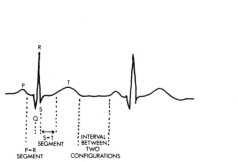

Figure 40   Normal ECG.

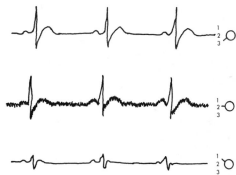

Figure 41   Selecting the most suitable channel.

Limb electrodes. These may be oblong brass plates 4 cm by 2 cm, slightly curved, plated with nickel or chrome. A screw socket is incorporated on the top side to which the lead is attached. The electrode is held in place by a band of rubber passing round the limb; one electrode is placed on each limb usually above the wrist or ankle. The leg electrode is positioned on the lateral aspect of the limb to avoid scratching the opposite leg with the screw (Fig. 42). Self-adhesive electrodes for limbs are available also.

Chest electrodes. These consist of small circular metal discs about 1 cm in diameter, mounted on a polythene disc and secured to the chest wall with non-irritant adhesive or adhesive tape such as Micropore (3Ms) or Dermacel (Johnson & Johnson). Usually three or four electrodes are used and positioned over the heart; the exact position of these is not critical and to some extent will be determined by the presence of surgical incisions and the best type of trace produced on the oscilloscope. Suitable sites are on or at either side of the sternum, below the nipples or below the clavicles (Figs 43 and 44).

Care must be taken in the correct application of electrodes to the skin.

1. It is no use applying chest electrodes over hairy areas, this will prevent a good electrical contact; shave if necessary.

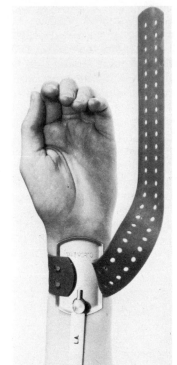

Figure 42   Limb electrode.

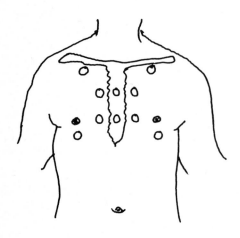

Figure 43   Sites for chest electrodes.

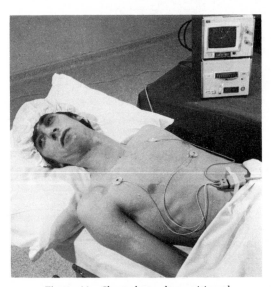

Figure 44   Chest electrodes positioned.

2. The skin must be cleaned thoroughly with ether meths or other solvent to remove traces of perspiration and grease.

3. Be certain that the surface of each electrode is perfectly clean and free from green corrosion; dirty electrodes should be cleaned with ether meths or methylated spirits.

4. A small quantity of a proprietory non-irritant jelly such as Cambridge (blue tube) should be applied to the contact surface of the electrode. With chest electrodes it is particularly important not to smother the electrode with jelly otherwise it may ooze on to the adhesive or fixing tape and prevent a good electrical contact and secure attachment to the chest. (Note: The electrically conductive pastes with a high salt content used for routine diagnostic electrocardiography are not suitable for long periods of monitoring. These pastes tend to produce skin reactions and excoriation over extended periods.)

5. After attachment to the limbs or chest the electrodes connected to the leads and thence to the monitor. It is important to ensure that the leads of the monitor cable are secured to the limb, or chest with a suitable non-irritant tape, to avoid pulling the electrodes.

6. In the ward or intensive care situation, the electrodes are checked daily for correct position, security, cleanliness and irritation. If these are all satisfactory, and provided that the trace displayed on the screen is acceptable, the electrodes will be left undisturbed, although generally it will be found necessary to renew them after a period of five to seven days. An interference or absence of a trace may not be due to a faulty electrode. Assuming that the patient's condition is otherwise satisfactory, interference artifacts may occur with movement of the patient and it is better to check all connections and leads thoroughly before removing a suspect electrode. An interference artifact appears on the trace as irregularly interrupting spikes of varying height.

Peripheral pulsometers. These consist essentially of a photoelectric plethysmograph (which is a device for measuring peripheral blood flow in the earlobe or fingertip) a receiver and an amplifier (Fig. 39). The plethysmograph is clamped to the ear lobe or held in contact with the tip of the finger by means of a Velcro strap. Signals are conveyed by a lead to the receiver/amplifier which may be mains or battery operated. The pulse rate per minute is displayed on a scale or meter and may be monitored also by a bleep from a built-in loudspeaker or buzzer.

Very careful positioning of the electrode is important, the plethysmograph is delicate and sensitive to movement artifacts. Care must be taken to secure the leads and avoid strain on the connections.

Cardiac pacing

The pacemaker is an apparatus which produces a series of electrical shock impulses to stimulate the heart ventricles to contract. Cardiac pacing is generally used for complete heart block although less commonly in the emergency situation it may be used for cardiac asystole applying the shock across the chest wall to cause contraction of the ventricles. In this situation, during surgery if the chest is open the electrodes may also be applied directly to the heart. External pacing requires an apparatus capable of producing in excess of 20 V as compared to up to 9 V with internal pacemaking.

The apparatus is powered by replaceable mercury batteries or a rechargeable nickel cadium battery. It has a series of controls allowing adjustment of:

1. Pulse rate per minute, generally 30–160 although models are available with a range of 80–120 per minute.

2. Voltage 0–9 V.

3. Pulse width i.e. duration, 1–2 milliseconds.

4. Selection of continuous or on demand impulses; continuous pacing impulses to

stimulate the ventricles are supplied at a fixed or constant rate; the demand setting only supplies pacing impulses as they are needed, for example, if the heart beat is too slow. If the time interval between two QRS configurations is too long then the apparatus supplies a pacing impulse to cause ventricular contraction thereby increasing the heart rate. When the heart rate is faster than the selected rate on the pacemaker then no pacing impulses are produced.

5. Battery level indicator.

6. Terminals for the active and indifferent electrode leads.

7. A pulse output indicator in the form of a neon lamp and/or buzzer.

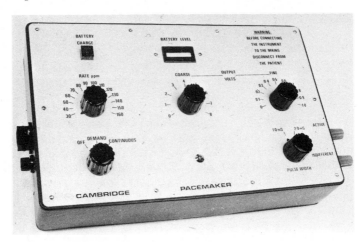

Figure 45   MP16 Demand/Continuous Pacemaker.
(Cambridge Scientific Instruments Ltd.)

An insulated wire or endocardial catheter electrode is passed under local anaesthesia into a suitable vein in the arm or neck and from there, under X-ray control, through the right atrium to the right ventricle where the tip is wedged against the wall of the cavity. This forms the active electrode; the indifferent electrode consists of a wire loop buried subcutaneously near the skin incision. The two wires can then be connected to the terminals of the pacemaker apparatus.

With the epicardial technique, the electrodes are sewn onto the epicardial or outer surface of the heart exposed at thoracotomy. The wires are brought out through the chest wall for connection to the pacemaker.

Alternatively, the wires can be passed subcutaneously to the axilla and connected to a small battery-powered pacemaker buried beneath the skin. When the batteries become exhausted the patient requires a further operation under general anaesthesia to replace the complete pacemaker; this however, does not need to be done very often. Developments have taken place in the production of nuclear powered pacemakers for implantation, which provide power almost indefinitely.

The impulses of a heart being paced if viewed on a cardiac monitor show that each QRS-T configuration, instead of being preceded by a P wave is now preceded by a pacing impulse (Fig. 46). The pacing impulse may appear as a narrow, bright vertical line immediately before each QRS-T configuration which is often wide and large but constant in shape. Points to note are whether the pacing impulse is present or absent; that the QRS-T shape is constant and immediately preceded by the pacing impulse; that the heart rate is correct and regular; whether any extra pacing impulses or QRS-T configurations are present.

Finally, it is important that theatre staff familiarise themselves with the type of pace-maker in use, particularly whether the power supply is from batteries or rechargeable cells, the method of adjusting controls and the method of attaching electrode leads, especially in the emergency situation.

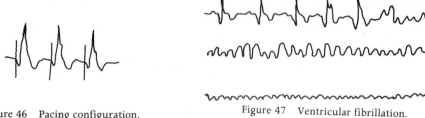

Figure 46   Pacing configuration.

Figure 47   Ventricular fibrillation.

Defibrillator

This apparatus enables a single electric shock to be applied to the heart to correct ventricular or atrial fibrillation. The apparatus may be mains or battery operated with a facility to discharge the shock through the chest wall or via electrodes placed directly in contact with the walls of the heart.

When switched on, the difibrillator charges a condenser to a maximum energy of 400 J. The level of discharge can be pre-set in steps between 15 and 400 J and this is released in a pulse duration of about 2·5 milliseconds. In the case of atrial fibrillation the defibrillator is coupled with an electrocardigraph connected to the patient. The defibrillation discharge is delivered in synchronisation, normally 40 milliseconds delay after the peak of the R wave of the patient's e.c.g.

Although different makes of defibrillators vary slightly in the method of operation,

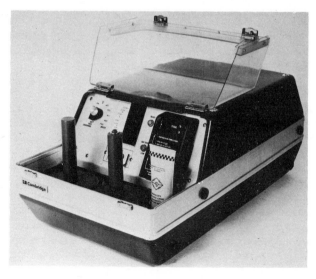

Figure 48   Cambridge Defibrillator – Synchronized with external electrodes.
(Cambridge Scientific Instruments Ltd.)

basically the same technique is used. The following is a description of the method of using a Cambridge defibrillator; although instructions are printed on the control panel.

External defibrillation. The apparatus is equipped with electrodes which can quickly be withdrawn from the front for use. The controls associated with synchronised cardioversion (atrial fibrillation) are mounted behind the black lid on the front panel to avoid any possible confusion during emergency use of the equipment for ventricular fibrillation.

1. *Keep black lid shut.* Closing this lid automatically switches the machine from synchronised to emergency.

2. Apply electrode jelly liberally to electrode surfaces but avoid smearing on hands or from the electrode surface up on to the handle.

3. *Set output to 400 J for adult and 50–200 J for a child.*

4. *Apply electrodes firmly to patient,* one at the upper sternum and one over the heart apex; jelly must not be allowed to spread to make contact between the two electrodes.

5. *Instruct those present to stand well clear* of patient, bed and any connecting leads, etc.

6. *When stored energy meter reads required output, press prime button.*

7. *Press fire button on handle within 10 seconds,* this will discharge the shock to the patient and the apparatus will recharge immediately. If the defibrillator is not used within the 10 seconds period, the prime button must be pressed again in order to prepare the apparatus for use, this is a safety cut-out to avoid accidental discharge. After use switch off apparatus which effects a safe discharge of any stored energy.

Synchronised cardioversion. Open the black lid on the front panel of the apparatus and set switch to synchronise position.

1. *Connect the synchronisation lead from the e.c.g. monitor* to the three-pin socket which is normally covered by the black lid.

2. *Connect the e.c.g. to the patient in the normal way* and adjust gain so that the R waves not less than 1 cm high are displayed on the screen. Upward or downward waves are equally acceptable.

3. *Set output to required energy.*

4. The loudspeaker in the defibrillator will now bleep in synchronisation with each R wave.

5. Apply electrode jelly liberally to electrode surfaces as previously described.

6. *When stored energy meter reads required output*, press prime button.

7. *Instruct those present to stand well clear* of patient, bed and any connecting leads.

8. *Apply electrodes firmly to patient as previously described.*

9. *Press fire button* within 10 seconds of prime button and keep pressed until discharge occurs i.e. on the next synchronised bleep. After discharge the defibrillator will immediately recharge, but will not fire again until the prime button has been pressed.

After use, switch off apparatus, which effects a safe discharge of any stored energy. Clean the electrodes and return them to their storage space. If synchronisation defibrillation has been used, remove e.c.g. synchroniser lead and close black lid. Connect defibrillator to charger unit.

Again, a final point of importance; although difibrillation apparatus is designed for safe operation it is important that regular checks are made to ensure that it is in working order. Special testing devices are available to check the level of discharge between the two electrodes, under no circumstances should a test consist of placing the two electrodes in direct contact and arcing between them. A defibrillator is *not* a piece of apparatus to be stored away in some obscure cupboard and forgotten, because every second may count when it is needed during cardiac resuscitation. Its whereabouts must be known to *all* who work in theatre, and *all* must familiarise themselves with the correct method of operation of the particular apparatus in use.

Surgical diathermy

Surgical diathermy is a high frequency electric current. When this current is passed through the patient's body between two electrodes, the effect is to produce a concentration of current at the electrode being used by the surgeon. As the surgeon applies his 'live' electrode to the tissues, the current passes through the adjacent tissue cells and owing to their electrical resistance, heat is generated at this point. The effect is localised because the current from the 'live' electrode spreads out in the patient's body and travels to the 'indifferent' electrode which is a large electrode placed in contact with the patient's body. A high density of current occurs only immediately beneath the live electrode because further away (except under fault conditions) the current density is too small to have any heating effect.

When a higher frequency electro-section or cutting current is selected and used with a needle electrode, an arc is struck between the point of this electrode and the underlying tissues. The arc is very hot (in excess of 1000° C) and causes tissue cells to disintegrate instantly in front of the electrode which may be moved with a cutting effect.

Blood vessels which are cut may continue to bleed and it is necessary to apply the diathermy current specifically to the vessel to effect coagulation. The vessel is gripped with artery forceps and an electro-coagulation current is applied via the artery forceps until sufficient heat is generated to cause coagulation of the blood and arrest further bleeding.

Electricity direct from the mains could achieve coagulation of blood, but the current needed to do this at 50 Hz per second (the mains frequency) would cause intense activation of muscle, thereby preventing the surgeon from working. Also, such a current is likely to cause ventricular fibrillation (page 44) and probable death of the patient. A diathermy current operates at high frequencies and although about 200 mA (milliamperes) may be used, the current can pass through the tissues without activating muscles.

Diathermy machines generate currents within the range of 400 kHz (400,000) to 3 MHz (3,000,000). In one type of machine, the energy for diathermy is created by an electrical discharge across a spark gap. The spark is produced in bursts of 50 to 100 per second, each burst oscillating at about 4 kHz per second although the energy can vary over a very wide band of frequency. (Fig. 49A.)

The valve generator machine usually produces bursts of energy 50 times per second, each burst oscillating at between 1·6 and 3 MHz per second (Fig. 49 B and C). Usually the lower frequencies are suitable for coagulation and the higher frequencies more suitable for cutting of tissue. This is not entirely correct however, for such factors as the composition of the oscillating wave affect its working characteristics and are beyond the scope of this book.

These two systems may cause severe interference with certain electromedical recording apparatus. This is caused by the fact that both machines release their energy in pulses at 50 or 100 times per second which is broadcast through electric wiring and through the air. This frequency lies within the frequency reception band for such apparatus as e.c.g. and e.e.g. This means that even with efficient radio supression, e.g. mains electrical filters, the pulse repetition of the diathermy energy will be detected, amplified by the electromedical recording apparatus and obliterate any physiological data. A type of machine is now available which releases its energy either continuously, or at a frequency of 20,000 to 60,000 bursts per second (each of 1·75 MHz) which is outside the necessary frequency band for physiological instruments (Fig. 49D). This enables the use of electrical filters and screened cables to supress any possible interference (Fig. 50).

The essential working parts of a diathermy machine are two electrodes connected by heavy insulated wire to the terminals on the machine, the rheostat adjustment for current strength and the spark-free footswitch, which may have separate sections to control coagulation and cutting currents. Alternatively the coagulation and cutting currents may be selected by turning a switch on the diathermy machine itself. There is usually a switch fitted to the machine to control the mains supply.

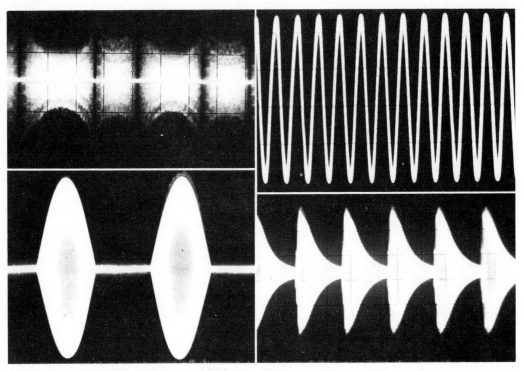

Figure 49   Oscilloscope traces of diathermy output.
A. Spark generated diathermy, 50/100 bursts per second at about 4 KiloHertz.
B. & C. Valve generated diathermy, 50/100 bursts per second at between 1·6 and 3 Mega-Hertz.
D. Valve generated diathermy, modulated at 20,000 to 60,000 bursts per second at 1·75 MegaHertz. (A. K. Dobbie.)

The live electrode which is used in the operating areas, is sterilised before connecting to the live terminal on the machine. There is a variety of different shaped electrodes ranging from a slender needle to a disc or ball-type point. These are connected to an insulated handle which is then coupled to the wire. Changing of these electrodes is made simple by the provision of a socket on the operating end of the wire.

The purpose of the indifferent electrode is to provide a surface of sufficient area to avoid any physiological effects at the site of application. This is because the indifferent electrode is in contact with hundreds or even thousands more cells than the live electrode which results in a correspondingly lower density of current in each cell. If the electrode is applied correctly, negligible heat is generated in this area.

The indifferent electrode at one time consisted of a lead plate wrapped in layers of lint soaked previously in a 15 to 20 per cent solution of salt. These electrodes are messy and inconvenient to apply to the skin. It has been known for diathermy burns to occur if the lint cover is either insufficiently damped at the outset, or becomes dried out during the course of an operation. Another disadvantage is that the strong solution of salt can cause a reaction to sensitive skin.

Nowadays, the commonest types of electrodes are flexible metal plates. The thin flexible metal plate electrode can either be placed under the patient's body or carefully bandaged round the thigh to ensure even contact with the skin. It is unnecessary to use electrode jelly, though if a hairy site is chosen for application, shaving beforehand is advisable – the hair acts as an electrical resistance. If the patient's skin is dry, moistening with water or saline can be done with advantage before applying the plate. Care must be taken to renew a plate electrode which becomes buckled otherwise areas of irregular contact with the skin which result could allow points of high current density and risk of burns. The electrode is connected to the diathermy machine indifferent or earth terminal by a heavy insulated wire.

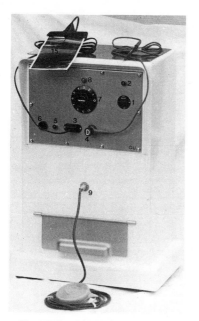
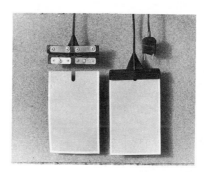

Figure 50   Diathermy machine. (Genito-Urinary Manufacturing Ltd.) Inset shows disposable indifferent electrode and connecting cable.

Key to Figures 50 and 51.
1. Mains switch.
2. 'Mains on' indicator lamp.
3. Monitored indifferent electrode socket.
4. Diathermy active terminal.
5. Monitor indicator lamp.
6. Audible warning device.
7. Power output control.
8. Power output indicator lamp.
9. Footswitch plug and socket.
10. Monitor circuit.
11. Valve.
12. Oscillator coil.
13. D.C. power supplies.
14. Footswitch relay.
15. Flexible indifferent plate electrode.

Another satisfactory type of electrode consists of aluminium foil half a thousandth of an inch thick backed with paper. A sheet of foil about 45.5 cm^2 (18 inches) square is placed under the patient's body and connected to the insulated wire with stainless steel clips. It has the advantages that it is cheap, can be autoclaved and is transparent to X-rays. The foil electrode is particularly suitable for use with infants.

It is important that electrodes are connected correctly to the terminals on the diathermy machine. The connections being reversed will almost certainly result in diathermy burns to the patient; modern diathermy machines incorporate non-interchangeable connections to avoid this danger.

It is vital that the indifferent electrode remains in electrical continuity with the patient and diathermy machine. If there is a defect and a break in this continuity, the patient is exposed to grave risk of diathermy burns. Failure of the return path to the earth terminal of the diathermy machine causes the patient's body to rise to a high voltage when diathermy is used. If any part of the patient then makes contact with earthed metal or a large mass of metal, e.g. the operation table, then a burn is likely to occur at the point of contact. This is why it requires great caution if hypodermic needles are used as e.c.g. electrodes – the current density occurring at the needles with diathermy can be very high even with 'earth free' e.c.g. apparatus which does not 'float' at diathermy frequencies; it is much safer to use the correct electrodes.

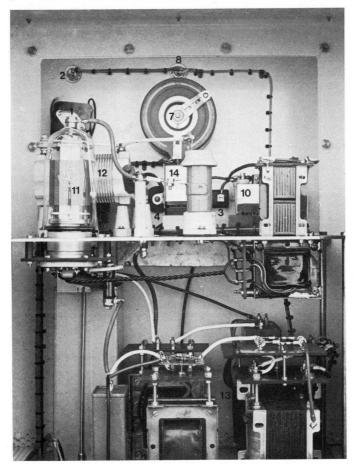

Figure 51   Components (rear view) of diathermy machine illustrated in Figure 50.

To detect a possible break in continuity of the indifferent electrode connection, a monitoring system is usually incorporated in the diathermy machine. The wire connection from the indifferent electrode consists of two separate insulated wires. A low voltage electrical current is passed out to the plate electrode via one wire and back by the other thereby ensuring an earth return path for the diathermy current from the patient. Failure of one wire normally activates an audible alarm and may cut off the generation of a diathermy current.

As a precaution the patient should be protected by a **thick** layer of insulating material such as rubber sheeting if there is a danger of his coming into contact with metal parts of the table. Thin layers of rubber are of no use as it is possible for a diathermy current to flow through them.

DIATHERMY MACHINE NOT WORKING

If a diathermy machine will not work when connected the following should be checked:

1. *After switching off at the wall socket,* check the wire leading from the plug top to ensure that there are no loose wires.

2. Ensure that the ON/OFF switch on the machine is correctly positioned; check with another socket.

If the machine will still not work consult an electrician. However, if an audible hum is made by the machine as it is switched on, but the current does not flow between the electrodes, the diathermy circuit should be checked:

1. *After switching off at the wall socket,* check that the electrode wires are connected correctly and securely to the machine.

2. Check that the insulated wires are still firmly soldered to both of the terminal connections in addition to the electrode handle and the plate connection. If a plate monitoring device is fitted, a broken indifferent electrode wire will be detected under 2. above.

3. Check that the metal connections are not corroded.

4. Check that the indifferent electrode is in good contact with the patient's skin.

Any further checks on the machine circuit are beyond the scope of theatre staff, and the electrician should be consulted.

The strength of current required depends upon the purpose for which diathermy is being used and on the type of machine. As a general rule maximum output is not usually needed, and for most cases one-third to a half of the maximum will often be sufficient. This current setting must of course be checked by the 'scrub nurse' assisting at the operation.

Surgical cautery

An electric cautery consists of a platinum wire loop or point which is raised to red heat by means of an electric current. This heated cautery point is then applied to the tissue area to cause coagulation.

The current may be produced by a low-voltage battery or transformer, although the transformer is preferable, as the output is more constant than that of a battery. The transformer has a rheostat knob which may be adjusted to alter the voltage applied to the platinum point. The cautery must not be used any hotter than at red heat, as too high a current will cause rapid burning out of the cautery point.

The cautery points, of which there is a varied selection, are mounted in a heat-resisting handle to which are connected two wires. These wires are then connected to the trans-former *which must be switched off at the wall socket.* Sometimes a transformer has two sets of low-voltage output terminals, one set being marked *Lights,* the other set being marked *Cautery.* The cautery must not be connected to the lights terminals as this may overload the transformer and cause it to burn out. After connecting the wires the transformer may then be switched on.

CAUTERY APPARATUS NOT WORKING

If the cautery will not work check the circuit in the following order, *after switching off at the wall socket:*

1. Inspect the cautery points to see if they are broken, the most usual points of breakage being where the platinum wire joins the thicker mount.

2. Check through all of the electrical connections – cautery point to handle, handle to wire, wire to transformer terminals – to see if they are clean and not corroded. Corrosion may cause poor electrical contact and failure of the current to flow to the cautery point. Cleaning of the points on these low-voltage connections with a small piece of emery cloth is often all that is necessary.

3. Check that the cautery ON/OFF switch is correctly positioned.

4. See that the cable leading from the transformer to the plug socket has not been pulled away from its connections. This may be done by manipulating the cable a little to see if any wires are loose at the points of connection to the transformer and plug top.

5. Re-connect the transformer and switch on. If it still does not operate, the plug socket may be tested by connecting another item of apparatus, such as a portable light fitting which is known to be in working order.

Should this reveal that the socket is operating correctly, it is advisable to have the apparatus checked by an electrician.

Electric suction units

These are a vital part of the theatre equipment for aspirating fluid, e.g., from the abdominal cavity or nasopharynx, etc.

The suction may be obtained with a portable machine or a larger central pump unit, connected by a pipe line system to wards and operating suites (Burns, 1958). With the pipe system coupling sockets are placed conveniently in the operating theatre, anaesthetic and recovery rooms, etc., for connection to a portable suction bottle unit in which aspirated fluids are collected (Fig. 52) (DHSS, 1972).

Portable suction machines are mainly of two types: (1) the high vacuum rotary compressor pump, and (2) the reciprocating pump. The first type is most suitable for use in theatre and recovery room as it has the advantage of producing a good vacuum at a high rate of free air displacement, that is, rapid suction of large quantities of fluid. The second type is more suitable for ward use, for although the vacuum produced is reasonably high the displacement of free air is much less, and the speed of suction is correspondingly reduced.

Any portable suction machines used in the operating theatre must have a spark-free switching mechanism and a flame-proof motor. All the well-known makes of rotary compressor or reciprocating pumps fulfil these requirements, and as the former are the most suitable for use in operating theatres they will be dealt with in more detail.

Although the various machines differ somewhat in design, they are basically similar in the method of fluid collection. The pump creates a vacuum in the glass suction bottle, into which the aspirated fluid is collected. This jar, which should be of 1·5 litre capacity for use in theatre, is provided with some method of quick release from its sealing cap. In some cases this will be a quick-release removable cap, and in others a method of securing the jar against a fixed metal cap which has a rubber washer or liner.

Incorporated in this cap are internal connections to the pump unit, and one or two external connections for suction tubing. Where two external connections are fitted, it is usual to have a selective tap to enable two suction tubes to be connected to the machine at once, e.g., one for the anaesthetist and one for the operation area. The tap is then positioned correctly for the suction tube in use at that particular time. Ideally, of course, it is preferable to have two suction machines for this purpose as both the surgeon and anaesthetist may require suction simultaneously.

In addition to the external suction tube connections a negative pressure gauge is fitted to the unit indicating the degree of vacuum, controllable by an adjacent screw valve. The degree of vacuum obtainable with the rotary compressor vacuum pump is about 66 cm (26 inches) of mercury, which is ideal for the rapid aspiration of large quantities of fluid. However, as in the case of suction required for neurosurgical and other delicate operations, this must be considerably less, about 13 cm (5 inches) of mercury, hence the value of the adjustable screw valve.

To avoid the danger of foreign matter entering the pump unit should the bottle become overfilled an automatic cut-out is fitted at some point between the bottle and the pump. This generally consists of a float which rises as the bottle contents approach overflow and seals off the connection to the pump. A spare suction bottle is usually provided and some

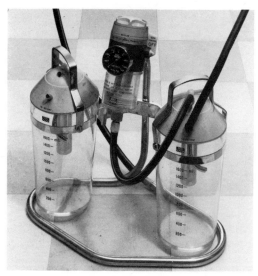

Figure 52   Pipeline suction apparatus. (British Oxygen Company Ltd.)

Safety features
Several safeguards are included in the design of the suction controller and the receiver jar in order to prevent over-filling and contamination of the pipeline:
1. A tangential inlet tube in the receiver jar minimises frothing in the aspirated liquid.
2. A float valve in the receiver jar prevents transfer of liquid to the controller unit.
3. If the receiver jar is inadvertently re-assembled without the float valve, a secondary valve in the controller unit protects the mechanism and the pipeline from contamination.
4. A disposable filter of non-absorbent cotton wool is incorporated in the control unit.

Ease of sterilisation
All components which can become contaminated are easily sterilised. After sterilisation, re-assembly is simple and straightforward.
Before sterilising, the equipment should be dismantled and all component parts cleaned thoroughly. The receiver jars, float valves and associated tubing are best sterilised by soaking in a suitable antibacterial solution (e.g. Cidex).
The control unit should be sterilised with hydrogen peroxide using an ultrasonic nebuliser, or by using ethylene oxide.

Performance
High Suction Controller Evacuates 1·5 litre receiver jar to 400mmHg vacuum in under 4 seconds. Variable control from 50 to 500mmHg vacuum.
Low suction controller Evacuates 1·5 litre receiver jar to 140mmHg vacuum in under 2 seconds. Variable control from 0 to 140mmHg vacuum. Safety valve setting at 180mmHg.

machines incorporate a quick change-over device between the two bottles (Fig. 53). The exhaust outlet from the pump should be fitted with a filter to prevent dissipation of contaminated air into the atmosphere. Modern rotary compressor pumps have an exhaust system which safeguards the machine to a certain extent in this respect, but nevertheless unnecessary strain should be avoided whenever possible.

The machine is mounted on strong antistatic castors and is connected with durable electric cable to a plug top.

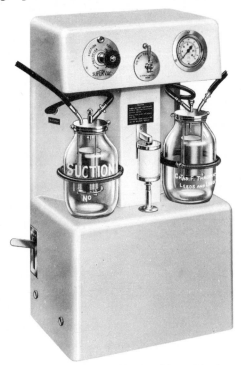

Figure 53   High vacuum rotary pump suction machine with change-over device between bottles. (Chas. F. Thackray Ltd.)

POINTS TO OBSERVE WHEN USING SUCTION UNITS

1. The suction tubing must be of adequate bore to avoid blockage and collapse. The size will depend upon the tubing connections fitted to the machine and the suction nozzles used, but generally an antistatic tubing of 0·75 cm ($\frac{5}{16}$ inch) bore and 0·3 cm ($\frac{1}{8}$ inch) wall will suffice.

2. The tubing must be in good condition, without punctures and with a clean lumen.

3. The degree of suction required is regulated initially by compressing the tubing (after switching on the machine) whilst setting the adjustable valve at the necessary position, e.g., to maintain a suction of 25 cm (10 inches) of mercury.

4. If the aspirated fluid 'froths up', the froth may be reduced by turning the suction tube connection tap so that the other unused connection is opened to the atmosphere, or alternatively opening fully the suction control valve. If this is not done, the froth may overflow and operate the cut-out mechanism prematurely.

5. The suction bottle must be emptied when the fluid reaches a pre-determined mark. If, by accident, it is overfilled thereby operating the cut-out, the machine is switched off, vacuum broken by opening the suction control valve and the bottle emptied before replacing and recommencing suction. If the cut-out is fitted in a separate chamber adjacent to the suction bottle, it may be necessary to empty this chamber before recommencing suction again.

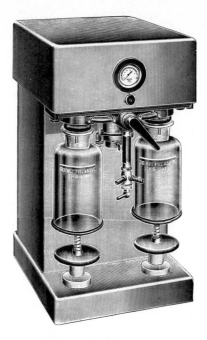

Figure 54 Another type of high vacuum rotary pump suction machine fitted with a twin bottle-holder which allows either bottle to be filled by changing the position of a lever. In addition the complete bottle unit including the overflow valve can be easily removed and dismantled for cleaning. (Genito-Urinary Manufacturing Ltd.)

6. Do *not* cause excessive strain to a suction pump by maintaining a constant high vacuum which occurs, for example, when the tubing is accidentally compressed or when the suction nozzle becomes occluded by contact with a towel.

7. After use, the bottle, cap, float and float chamber must be washed with an anti-bacterial agent (Chapter 6) and thoroughly dried. Movable taps, etc., must be lightly oiled at frequent intervals.

8. A final caution – do not leave a residual vacuum in the suction bottle after switching off. Possible cause: kinks in a coil of suction tubing wound round pegs fitted to the machine so that it is ready for emergency use. This may cause a back aspiration of oil from the vacuum pump with 'drying out' of the mechanism and consequent loss of efficiency. It is possible to lose half a pint, or more, of oil in this way.

REFERENCES

ARNOLD, V. F. (1958) In *Medical Electrical Equipment*, p. 177. Edited by R. E. Molloy. London: Newnes.
BURNS, J. T. (1958) In *Medical Electrical Equipment*, p. 229. Edited by R. E. Molloy. London: Newnes.
DEPARTMENT OF HEALTH AND SOCIAL SECURITY (1974) *Hospital Technical Memorandum No. 11*. London: HMSO.
DEPARTMENT OF HEALTH AND SOCIAL SECURITY (1972) *Hospital Technical Memorandum No. 22*. London: HMSO.
DOBBIE, A. K. (1969) *Biomedical Engineering*, 4, No. 5 p.p. 206–216.
Northwick Park Hospital and Clinical Research Centre. (1972) Electrical Equipment Booklet. *Patient Safety* (M097–72). London: Holborn Press.
SAVAGE, B. (1954) *Preliminary Electricity for the Physiotherapist*. London: Faber.
SMITH, A. C. (1958) In *Medical Electrical Equipment*, p. 156. Edited by R. E. Molloy. London: Newnes.
SMITH, E. A. (1958) *In Medical Electrical Equipment*, p. 30. Edited by R. E. Molloy. London: Newnes.
STEVENS, W. R. (1951) *The Principles of Lighting*. London: Constable.

3
Static Electricity

From the previous chapter the reader will realise the importance of using spark-free electrical apparatus in the immediate vicinity of anaesthetic apparatus. Even if a great deal of attention is paid to the safety of electrical apparatus and the elimination of naked flames from the operating suite, explosion risks are not entirely obviated, for there remains the danger of a spark caused by static electricity.

The extent of the risk of electrostatic sparks causing anaesthetic explosions was set out in a report from the Department of Health (1956). The report described an investigation of 36 anaesthetic explosions occuring during a seven year period, 1947 to 1954. Of these 36 accidents, 22 were almost certainly due to an electrostatic spark. The report recommended that antistatic precautions should be taken in all areas where anaesthetic apparatus employing a closed or partially closed breathing circuit is used with flammable anaesthetics. In the light of further experimental evidence, these recommendations have now been updated (DHSS, 1971a, b).

What is static electricity, how does it occur and why should it be of so much concern when electrostatic explosions are relatively infrequent? (Well over three million anaesthetics are administered each year without an explosion mishap.) It is very true that the majority of operating department staff complete their careers without being witness to a single anaesthetic explosion. However, this is no excuse for overlooking simple precautions which will result in these small risks being almost entirely eliminated.

The generation of static electricity

The formation of this condition is a very simple matter and occurs whenever two dissimilar materials are separated. It is not necessary to cause friction, although this will increase the amount of static electricity produced. The surface of one material or object becomes positively charged and the other negatively charged, but to what degree depends not only on the briskness of separation of the surfaces (friction) but also on the ability of the material to absorb moisture readily from the atmosphere and in this way become antistatic for all practical purposes.

These charges of electricity can continue to build up an electric potential or pressure on the surface of the object and will remain there until earthed or the object comes into contact with another object of a different potential. When this occurs the discharge of static between the two can cause a spark. It is as if the object stores up the static charge like a condenser and when earthed discharges the static as a spark which may be capable of igniting a flammable anaesthetic mixture.

Very high voltages can be created under favourable conditions, especially in a dry atmosphere, e.g., a person walking on a dry floor wearing ordinary rubber-soled shoes is capable of acquiring or being charged with a potential of 30,000 volts; the act of 'whipping off' a blanket lying on a rubber sorbo pad covering a trolley can produce a similar charge.

These dangers may be very real and steps which should be taken to minimise the formation of dangerous charges of static electricity are:

1. The elimination of materials which predispose towards the formation of static.

2. Allowing the charges to leak away to earth as they are generated and before high potentials are built up.

1. STATIC FORMING MATERIALS

Some materials are more inclined to form static electricity than others. High on this list are most plastics and woollen blankets, which are a grave potential source of sparks.

The following list indicates the materials which may be found in the vicinity of an operating theatre. The order of the list shows that each becomes positively electrified when rubbed with any of the materials following, but negatively when rubbed with any of the materials preceding. The list also indicates that the further apart the materials are on the list the greater the charge produced upon rubbing together.

(a) Nylon   (e) Cotton and linen
(b) Flannel and wool (f) Dry skin
(c) Viscose reyon   (g) Wood
(d) Glass   (h) Rubber
           (i) Various plastics.

Of the materials listed, cotton, linen and viscose rayon are certainly ideal for theatre clothing and towels, blanket covers, etc., unless they have been specially treated to render them water repellent. They have to be quite dry to generate a charge under normal atmospheric conditions, as they readily absorb moisture. It is this property which makes them excellent for theatre use. The only blankets which should be brought into the operating theatre are those of the cotton cellular type, which do not predispose towards the formation of static electricity and are easily sterilised.

2. THE DISSIPATION OF STATIC CHARGES

If all objects and persons were conductive to electricity and all floors conductive, static electricity would be dissipated as rapidly as it formed; unfortunately this is not so.

All ordinary rubber articles are very highly insulating and many items of theatre equipment are made from rubber, including sorbo trolley mattresses and wheels, macintoshes and tubing, etc. The use of ordinary rubber in the manufacture of these articles will prevent the leakage away to earth of any electrostatic charges which may form on the object. These charges will build up potential and leak away slowly unless they are earthed suddenly and dissipated as a spark.

In the past an attempt to overcome this problem consisted of trailing brass chains fitted to the metal work of the trolley, etc., and earthed brass strips set into the theatre floor, dividing it into sections. Theoretically the chains maintained the earth contact with the brass strips and all was well. In practice the chains quickly became coated with verdigris or grease from the floor and the result was non-conductivity and a false sense of security.

The answer to this problem has been the discovery that, if during the manufacture of rubber, carbon black is finely dispersed through it the resultant rubber is electrically conductive to a degree, dependent on the quantities of carbon present.

This antistatic rubber has sufficient insulation to ordinary mains electricity, but does allow electrostatic charges to dissipate rapidly as they are formed. Unfortunately antistatic rubber is necessarily black, and in order to distinguish this rubber from other types all antistatic rubber components have a distinctive yellow mark.

The risk of an electrostatic ignition is now considered to be confined to an area extending for 25 cm around the anaesthetic gas circuit or gas paths. Flammable gas mixtures escaping from anaesthetic breathing circuits rapidly dilute to a non-flammable level within a few centimetres of the point of escape. All equipment used in this danger zone must be antistatic and all metal parts must be electrically continuous with the floor, e.g. by fitting antistatic castors or feet. All rubber must be antistatic and have effective contact with metal connections used in the breathing circuit of the patient.

Although plastics are regarded as highly electrostatic, it is not practicable to eliminate them entirely from anaesthetic apparatus. The degree of electrostatic risk depends upon the size of the component and whether, due to its position, an electrostatic charge may be formed by the component being rubbed or brushed against. Rotameters, for example, although consisting of some clear plastic parts, do not constitute a great risk due to their location. Plastic soda lime canisters, on the other hand, may be located where they can be brushed against with clothing very easily. In order to minimise a charge building-up on the surface of the canister it is prudent to incorporate an electrically conductive mesh, either buried in the plastic or in contact with the inner or outer surface. This mesh must be made electrically continuous with other antistatic components which are in discharge contact with the floor.

Antistatic polish applied to plastic has a limited effect. The polish is liable to get rubbed off and requires reapplication following cleaning or sterilisation.

As endotracheal tubes are moist in use they need not be made from an antistatic material. There is very little electrostatic risk associated with plastic transfusion tubing although the metal supports associated should have a satisfactory antistatic contact with the floor.

Diathermy quivers are intended to insulate a live electrode from possible shorting through towels or with metal/antistatic equipment. They should be made from either ordinary rubber or plastic; the electrostatic risk with these items is negligible.

The efficiency of antistatic rubber is calculated by measuring the electrical resistance in ohms. This ohmic resistance is in effect the degree of insulation to electricity, the higher the ohms figure, the more insulative is the rubber.

A normal high insulation rubber will have a high electrical resistance probably in the region of 150 million ohms (150 MΩ), whereas antistatic rubber in service should have a resistance not exceeding 100 MΩ (DHSS 1971). This ohmic resistance is determined by measuring the amount of electricity which the rubber will pass under test.

Two insulated wire conductors, connected to a 500 V D.C. tester generator (Megger) are placed separately on two moistened areas of approximately 6·25 cm^2 (1 in^2), but 5 cm (2 in) apart, on the surfaces of the rubber being tested. By turning the handle on the tester a voltage of 500 V is generated and the amount of electricity passing between these conductors through the rubber will move a pointer on the tester scale, indicating the resistance in ohms.

There are many ways of testing various rubber objects and these are listed in the Department of Health circular (DHSS, 1971a) on static electricity.

The more common tests include the following:

(a) Rubber boots and shoes; the resistance is measured between the inside of the sole or heel and the under sole.

(b) Rubber tubing, etc.; the resistance is measured between spacings of every 1·5 m (5 ft) if the tubing exceeds this length.

(c) Furniture feet; the resistance is measured between the surface at the bottom of the cavity, and that normally in contact with the floor.

(d) Castors are tested by placing on a wet metal plate, and measuring the resistance between the plate and the metal framework of the trolley or hub of the wheel. When testing a castor fitted to a trolley, etc., the other castors should be insulated from the floor during the test.

(*e*) Sorbo pads or mattresses are tested by measuring the resistance between the top and underside, the electrodes being opposite.

(*f*) On thin sheeting the test areas should be on the same surface with approximately 50 mm (2 in) dry spacing between. (Measurements made through the thickness of thin sheeting are unreliable as they may be affected by small areas of conductivity.)

The recommended resistance limits for new equipment are as follows:

Anaesthetic tubing connecting machine to patient, per 1·5 m (5 ft) length: 25,000 Ω minimum, 1 MΩ maximum.

Mattresses or pads: 5,000 Ω minimum, 1 MΩ maximum.

Rubber boots and shoes: 75,000 Ω minimum, 10 MΩ maximum.

Castor tyres and other antistatic items: no lower limit but 10,000 Ω maximum.

The electrical resistance of some antistatic rubber items may increase with use. The maximum permitted electrical resistance of equipment in service is 100 MΩ and equipment exceeding this level should be replaced as having lost its antistatic properties.

All rubber operating theatre equipment, including tubing, sheeting, anaesthetic accessories, operation table mattresses, etc., should be made from an anti-static material and it is important to note that if the surfaces of these are damped, the electrical conductivity will be greater.

Antistatic Floors. If the surface of antistatic rubber is kept clean, the static charges will leak away to earth as they are formed, but the floor must also be antistatic. The efficient dissipation of static does depend a great deal on the provision of a suitable antistatic floor which has a resistance of not more than 2 MΩ or less than 50,000 Ω measured between two separate electrodes placed 60 cm (2 ft) apart.

The most satisfactory materials for theatre floors from the antistatic aspect are *in situ* terrazzo or terrazzo tiles (DHSS, 1971a) laid upon a metal mesh. A direct-to-earth connection for antistatic floors has been found unnecessary. If the floor is laid correctly and has satisfactory antistatic properties, it is capable of equalising any electrostatic charges which are likely to develop on persons or objects which are in electrical contact with the floor.

Wood, linoleum or composition floors are not satisfactory in the theatre suite but antistatic PVC containing granules of carbon may be used. Damp mopping of the floor regularly during an operation list will increase the electrical conductivity considerably. Even if the surface dries rapidly, some moisture will be retained by the floor to a degree dependent on its composition, e.g. a tiled floor will be more absorbent than a PVC one.

3. HUMIDITY

A highly humid atmosphere is a deterrent to the formation of static electricity, but should not be regarded as a guarantee against it. Humidity is much less effective as an antistatic measure with moist plastics or synthetic fibres which have an inherent tendency to be moisture repellent.

The relative humidity in an operating theatre should be between 50 and 55 per cent, or compatible with comfort.

Steam 'wafting' into the theatre from a steriliser will not maintain a constant and equal humidity throughout the room.

The humidity should be maintained with special apparatus incorporated within the air-conditioning plant in the form of a humidifier, which has already been described in Chapter 1. This system can be automatic, being coupled directly to a hygrometer or may be controlled manually in conjunction with direct reading 'gold beater' hygrometers situated in the theatre and anaesthetic room. These hygrometers which indicate the relative humidity as a direct reading on a scale should be checked periodically against a wet/dry bulb thermometer.

Conclusion

The simple precautions necessary to minimise the dangers of a static electricity explosion do not inconvenience the work of an operating suite.

All rubber components should be of antistatic rubber, tested regularly and renewed when the electrical resistance exceeds 100 MΩ.

Non antistatic rubber or plastic components such as tubes, airways, etc., should be moistened inside and out before use.

No one should enter the theatre unless wearing antistatic shoes or boots and their clothes covered with a cotton or linen gown. This will reduce the amount of personal static electricity produced by walking.

All theatre clothing, etc., should be made of a relatively antistatic material, such as cotton or linen.

Woollen blankets must never be used, cotton cellular blankets are very suitable from an antistatic as well as a bacteriological aspect. Hot blankets are more likely to generate a static charge than cold or warm ones; in no case must a blanket be 'whipped off' a trolley.

REFERENCES

DEPARTMENT OF HEALTH (1956) *Report of a Working Party on Anaesthetic Explosions.* London: HMSO.
DEPARTMENT OF HEALTH (1971a) Hospital Technical Memorandum no. 1. *Antistatic Precautions: Rubber, Plastics and Fabric.* London: HMSO.
DEPARTMENT OF HEALTH (1971b) Hospital Technical Memorandum no. 2. *Flooring in Anaesthetic Areas.* London: HMSO.

4
The Operation Table and Positions Used for Surgery

The modern operation table is an apparatus capable of adjustment to give a variety of positions for surgery. Some tables are designed for specific types of operations, but most are made as an all-purpose apparatus suitable for general and some specialised procedures.

It is essential that all members of the theatre staff familiarise themselves with the operation table and its accessories which must be easily available and ready for immediate use. The whole apparatus must be maintained in good working order and checked before each operation list.

The general operation tables illustrated in Figs. 55, 56 and 57 are all-purpose tables which can be adapted for specialised procedures by the addition of suitable accessories. All have an oil pump fitted into the base for raising and lowering the table top, Trendelenburg and lateral tilting mechanisms, adjustable head and foot ends, back or kidney elevator, and a full range of accessories. The table top of each is covered with a sectional sponge rubber mattress which is removable for cleaning. This mattress is covered with anti-static rubber as described in the previous chapter.

Figure 55 illustrates an operation table which has a 'break back' in the centre section to produce trunk flexion of the table for thoracic surgery, and conversion to a neurosurgical

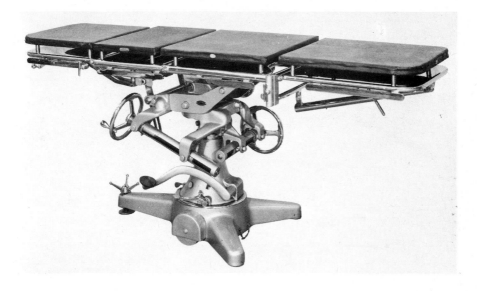

Figure 55   General operation table. (Chas. F. Thackray Ltd.)

chair. This table movement obviates the use of a back or kidney elevator, although it is incorporated in the table top for use if desired. The foot-brake mechanism is operated by one capstan wheel at the head of the table and provides good immobilisation even on moist floors.

Figure 56 illustrates an electro-hydraulic five-section operation table with telescoping

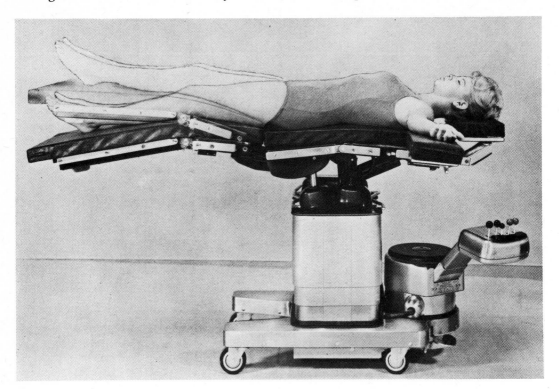

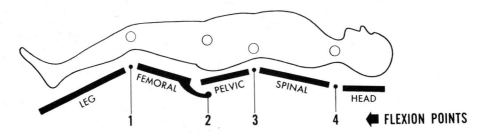

5-Section Table

Figure 56   Electrohydraulic five-section operation table. (Drayton Castle Ltd.)

spinal and femoral sections. The advantages claimed for this table are that each articulating section is in 'contour-correspondence' with the five anatomical regions. The table top has a head section, telescoping spinal section accommodating different lengths from the cervical spine to the lumbar arch, a pelvic section with a cut-out under the patient's perineum, a telescoping femoral section to ensure good popliteal flexion and a leg section.

This adjustment allows precise positioning for patients short or tall; always with head on headrest, lumbar arch over table break, perineum over perineal cut-out and popliteal space over the knee break. The head section is movable from side to side through a 180° arc. Hydraulic control of height, Trendelenberg/reverse Trendelenberg, lateral tilt and flexion of the spinal and femoral sections are through a control head incorporating five

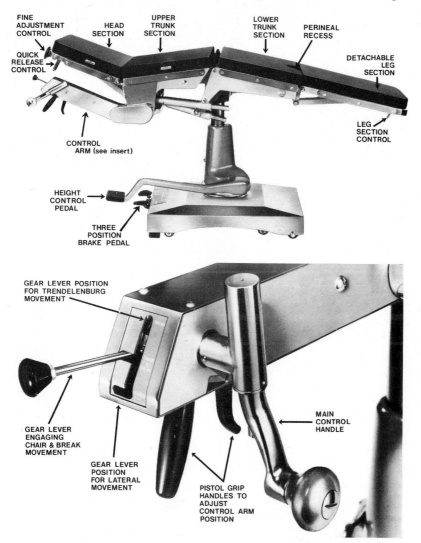

Figure 57   General operation table. Matburn 'break back' type. (Matburn Surgical Equipment Ltd.)

levers which automatically return to a neutral position. The operation table is connected to an electric socket outlet with flexible cable and there is provision for emergency manual hydraulic control.

Figure 57 illustrates a heavy-base table similar to Figure 55, but the Trendelenburg tilt, lateral tilt and 'break back' or chair mechanisms are operated by one control knob and gear lever at the head end of the table. The back or kidney elevator is also controlled from the head end by a hand control. The accessories illustrated show lithotomy stirrups and shoulder rests. This operation table is illustrated as a neurosurgical chair in Figure 70.

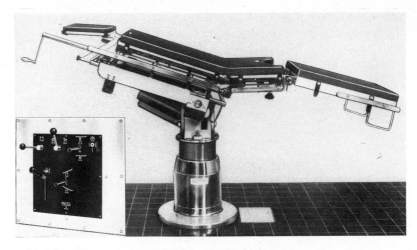

Figure 58   The Kifa hydraulically driven operation table. The fixed base is connected with the wall mounted control panel via underfloor tubes. Adjustment of various positions is accomplished by moving the appropriate lever. Insert shows control panel fitted onto wall. (Sierex Ltd.)

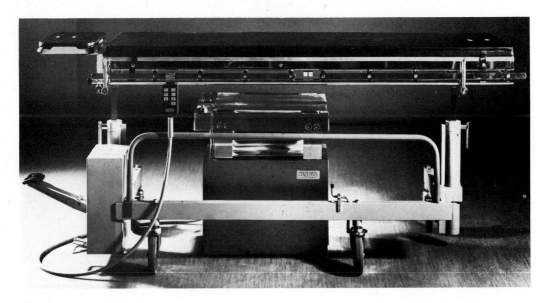

Figure 59   The Kifa H3 operation table base is the latest version of the Kifa table. Everything is contained in the rectangular base – there is no remote pump unit or control panel built in the wall. The Kifa operation table top is interchangeable between the fixed base and a transfer trolley. This trolley is used to transport the patient between the changeover area and the operating theatre. It avoids unnecessary lifting for the patient is placed on the table top on entering the operating suite and remains on it until leaving. By using a further transfer trolley in the changeover area the patient can be taken back to the ward still on the table top. The divided type of table top can also be used in this way. (Sierex Ltd.)

POSITIONS USED FOR SURGERY

Careful and correct positioning of the patient is very important, not only to provide good access for surgery but to prevent harm to the patient due to pressure, especially on nerves and bony prominences. These positions which are described can only be learned by repeated practical demonstrations, but the illustrations show essential points to be noted for various operations. The drapes have been omitted in order that these points are easily discernible (Jolly, 1950; Houghton and Hudd, 1967; Pearce, 1967).

Supine or dorsal recumbent position

This and most of the following positions are demonstrated on a combined general and orthopaedic operation table which incorporates the majority of the features described already, plus accessories for orthopaedic procedures.

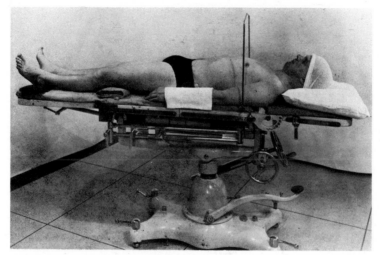

Figure 60   Supine or dorsal recumbent position. Plaistow 'all purpose' operation table. (M.S.A. Ltd.)

The position is used for many operations, including those on the eye, ear, face, chest, abdomen, legs or feet, and with modifications is suitable for operations on the breast and arms or hands, which may be placed across the chest or extended on an arm table.

Operations on the flexed knee are performed by lowering the foot end of the table with the division between the centre and foot sections situated at the point of knee flexion. Alternatively the foot end of the table can be removed completely.

An anaesthetic screen can be used for this and other positions when it is desirable, for local anaesthetics, or to isolate the anaesthetist from the operative field (Chapter 9, Fig. 216).

IMPORTANT POINTS

1. The arms should be at the sides and secured by L-shaped arm retainers which are slipped under the mattress. This applies unless of course otherwise indicated by surgery or for transfusion. Alternatively the arms may be secured across the chest by pinning the operation gown around them.

2. Pressure points to watch and protect with folded towels or soft pillows are: the heels and the forearms where the arm retainer is in contact with the skin. A soft pillow

behind the knees (which should be slightly flexed) will prevent hyperextension of the knee joints which may have painful consequences postoperatively.

Trendelenburg position

This position, a modification of supine, is used for intrapelvic operations, the object being to allow the intestines to displace away from the pelvic cavity by gravity towards the upper abdomen. They may then be packed off readily to leave easier access to the pelvic organs.

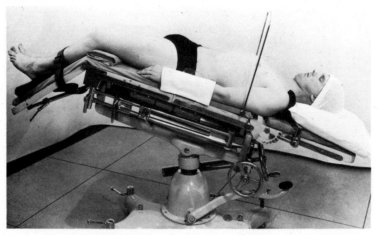

Figure 61   Trendelenburg position.

IMPORTANT POINTS

1. The arms are at the sides and secured in the usual manner.

2. The flexion of the knees must be directly over the junction of the foot and central sections of the table.

3. Pressure points to watch and protect are: the heels, leg strap (folded towel between the strap and legs has been omitted from the illustration in order to show the heel pad), behind the knees and the shoulders.

The well-padded shoulder rests must be positioned to the point of the shoulders. On no account must they be placed at the root of the neck, because this would cause pressure upon the brachial plexus and result in paralysis. These rests must prevent the patient from slipping and becoming suspended by flexed knees, which would cause pressure on the lateral popliteal nerve.

Alternatively, well-padded pelvic supports or a Langton Hewer corrugated ribbed mattress (in direct contact with the patient's exposed skin) may be used to retain the patient in position. These avoid the danger of pressure on the brachial plexus.

Gall-bladder and liver position

This is another modified supine position which is used for operations on the gall-bladder or liver. The patient is positioned over the back elevator which is raised to produce extension, and thereby push the gall-bladder towards the anterior abdominal wall. One arm is shown extended on an arm table for transfusion. Alternatively the patient can be positioned over the hinged section of a 'break back' table which when flexed produces a similar effect.

IMPORTANT POINTS

1. Both arms may be secured in the usual manner, or one extended on an arm table as illustrated, but the abduction must not exceed 90 degrees to the body otherwise the brachial plexus may be stretched.

2. Pressure points to watch and protect are: the heels, behind the knees and at the point where the arm is extended from the table.

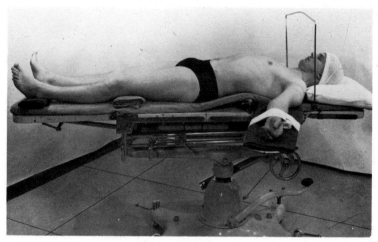

Figure 62   Gall-bladder or liver position.

Lateral position of extension

This is used for operations on the kidney and chest, but may be modified slightly for operations on the hip. For the former operations the patient is positioned over the kidney elevator which is raised to extend this region. Alternatively if an operation which incorporates a 'break back' is used extension is achieved by positioning the patient over the division in the centre section before adjusting the angle of the table top.

For hip operations in the lateral position the patient lies on his side in a similar manner to that illustrated, but with no extension.

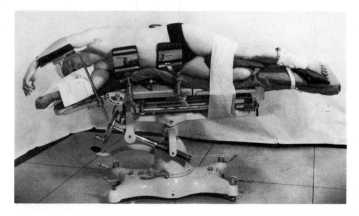

Figure 63   Lateral position of extension for kidney and chest surgery.

IMPORTANT POINTS

1. The upper arm is supported by a Carter Braine's arm support. The lower hand is placed at the side of the face and secured if necessary in the usual manner.

2. The underneath leg is flexed under the upper which is kept straight and secured to the table top with a padded bandage.

3. The patient is supported by pelvic and chest supports, which are well padded, and for additional security a bandage (padded strap or adhesive strapping) may be placed round the thighs and table top.

4. Pressure points to watch and protect are: the heels, between the legs, under the thigh retainer, upper and lower arms.

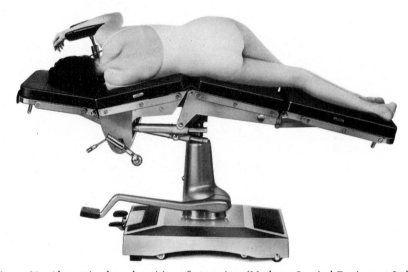

Figure 64   Alternative lateral position of extension. (Matburn Surgical Equipment Ltd.)

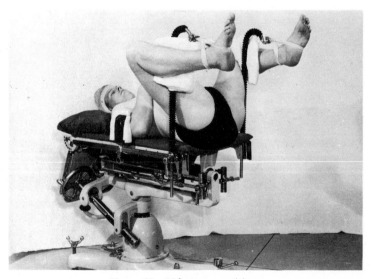

Figure 65   Lithotomy position.

Lithotomy position

This is used for operations on the external genital organs, perineum and anal region. The buttocks project well over the edge of the table at the junction of the centre and foot section which is lowered or removed. The legs are flexed at the hips and knees, and raised with the feet supported in webbing slings suspended from the lithotomy poles. A douching funnel may be fitted below the perineal area.

IMPORTANT POINTS

1. The arms are secured in the usual manner.

2. The patient is first placed supine on the table and is then lifted down until his buttocks are at the edge of the centre section (foot section lowered or removed). *Both* legs are then flexed at the same time, abducted and secured by the webbing slings outside the poles.

3. Pressure points to watch and protect are: the forearms, buttocks and inner aspects of the thighs, which must be protected from pressure by the poles with pads of gamgee or sponge rubber. Note that the lithotomy poles are padded with corrugated rubber to minimise still further any pressure on the patient's legs.

Breast and axilla position

This is the position for operations on the breast and axilla. It is a modified supine position, either with both arms extended and secured on arm tables, or one arm secured and the other on the affected side supported by a nurse (Chapter 5).

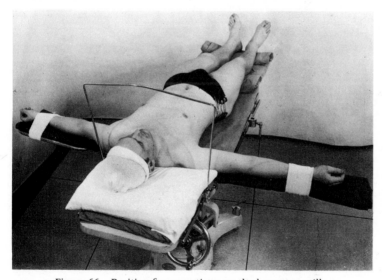

Figure 66   Position for operations on the breast or axilla.

IMPORTANT POINTS

1. The extended arms must not be abducted more than 90 degrees to the body.

2. Pressure points to watch and protect are: the heels, behind the knees and at the point where the arms are extended from the table.

Neck position

This position is used for operations on the neck, especially thyroidectomy and tracheostomy. The patient is placed in the supine position with a pillow or sandbag under the shoulder blades, and the head is held by a nurse or assistant with the neck well extended. Alternatively a padded horse-shoe provides a good support for the head in such operations. If local anaesthesia is being used, e.g., for tracheostomy, further restraint may be required and the patient is held by another assistant who immobilises him by the arms and thighs.

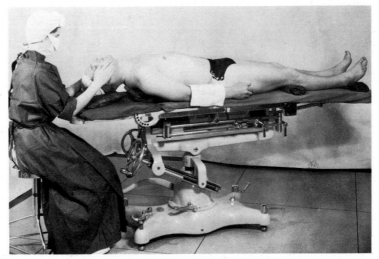

Figure 67   Positions for operations on the neck.

IMPORTANT POINTS

1. The head must be held exactly in the mid-line with the chin upwards and the neck extended.

2. The arms are secured in the usual manner unless being restrained by an assistant.

3. Pressure points to watch and protect are: the heels, behind the knees, the arms where they are secured, between the shoulder blades and the occiput if the operating time is lengthy.

Supine cranial position

This is used for frontal craniotomy and may be modified for parietal operations by rotating the head to one side. The patient's head is supported by a cranial support, and his thorax by the shoulder supports in conjunction with small pillows.

IMPORTANT POINTS

1. The degree of flexion or extension of the neck depends upon the surgeon's wishes and the most suitable position for maintenance of a clear airway.

2. The arms are secured in the usual manner (transfusions are generally administered via a vein in the foot during cranial operations).

3. Pressure points to watch and protect are: the heels, behind the knees, between the shoulder blades and the arms where they are secured.

Prone cranial position

This position is used for cerebellar operations and high cervical laminectomy. Some reverse Trendelenburg tilt is used and a padded strap placed round the thighs and the table top for additonal security. The shoulders and thorax are supported by shoulder supports in conjunction with small pillows.

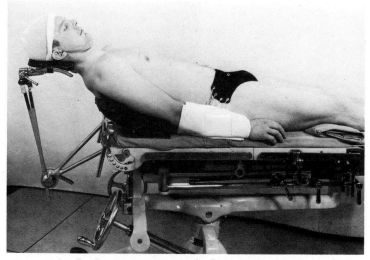

Figure 68   Frontal cranial position (modified supine).

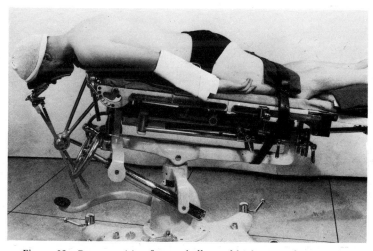

Figure 69   Prone position for cerebellar and high cervical operations.

IMPORTANT POINTS

1. The degree of flexion or extension of the neck depends upon the surgeon's wishes and the most suitable position for maintenance of a clear airway.

2. The arms are secured in the usual manner.

3. Pressure points to watch and protect are: the feet (the toes must project either over the foot end of the table or a soft pillow sufficiently large to prevent them being compressed against the table top), under the strap, the arms where they are secured, and the

shoulder supports which must be positioned to the points of the shoulders and not pressing on the root of the neck.

Sitting cranial position

This is a position for cerebellar cranial operations and high cervical laminectomy and is an alternative to that described in Figure 69. The patient is sitting and stabilised by the cranial support. The hands are placed in the lap and the body immobilised by securing the arms with body supports which are attached to the operation table at each side. These have been omitted in the illustration in order to show the position of the arms.

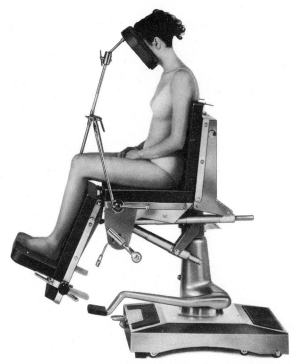

Figure 70   Sitting position in neurosurgical chair. Matburn 'break back' table. (Matburn Surgical Equipment Ltd.)

IMPORTANT POINTS

1. The weight of the patient must not be entirely supported by the cranial support. Body supports must be used to retain the patient in what would be a fairly comfortable position if he were conscious.

2. The degree of flexion of the neck depends upon the surgeon's wishes and the most suitable position for maintenance of a clear airway.

3. Pressure points to watch and protect are: the heels, behind the knees, the buttocks and the arms (which are protected by small pillows or folded towels).

Knee/elbow (rabbit) position

This is an alternative to lateral position (described under spinal puncture, Chapter 10) for lumbar laminectomy and removal of prolapsed intervertebral disc. The patient kneels with his head and arms supported on a pillow, and his body stabilised with body supports at each side of the table. For additional security a bandage or adhesive strapping may be placed round the thorax and table top.

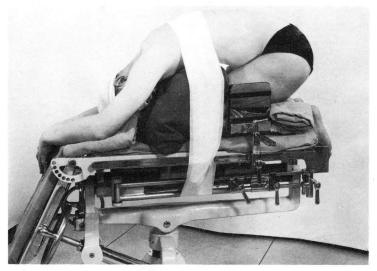

Figure 71   Knee/elbow (rabbit) position for laminectomy.

IMPORTANT POINTS

1. The pillow under the thorax and the retaining bandage may require adjustment in order that the patient's respiratory excursions are not impeded in any way. It may be necessary to use a pillow under the upper part of the chest and head only to leave the abdomen free for excursion.

2. The foot section of the table is lowered or removed, and the feet must project slightly beyond to avoid pressure on the toes.

3. Pressure points to watch and protect are: the insteps, between the thighs and the lower legs.

Jack knife position

One of the positions for rectal surgery or occasionally for lumbar laminectomy.

The patient should be placed in prone position with hips directly over the break in the foot section of the table. The arms should be flexed around the head of the patient and the lower part of the legs supported by a foot extension piece. The whole table is tilted into reverse Trendelenburg to the desired position.

IMPORTANT POINTS

1. A small pillow should be placed under the symphysis to avoid undue pressure and,
2. The patient's weight should be so balanced as to avoid pressure on the knees.

Supine hip position

This is used mainly for nailing a femoral neck fracture, but is suitable for osteotomy, slipped femoral epiphysis, etc. The patient is in a supine position, with his pelvis supported by a supplementary table top which is translucent to X-rays and incorporates a slot for introducing anterior position film cassettes under the pelvis. The lower section of the table is removed, the feet are secured to foot pieces and traction applied to both legs. Counter traction is obtained against a perineal post fitted at the pubis. Body supports, as illustrated, are needed only when lateral tilting of the table top is necessary in order to obtain greater exposure of the hip being operated on.

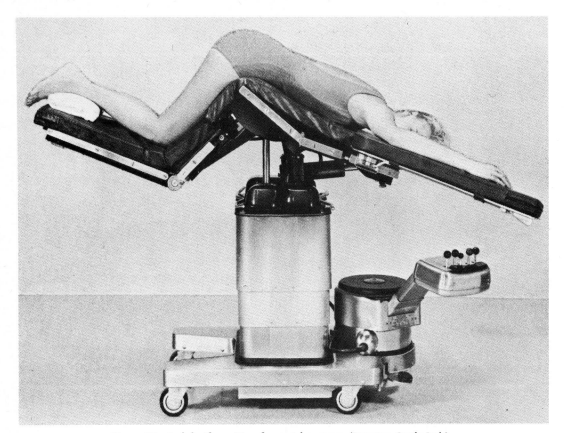

Figure 72   Jack knife position for rectal surgery. (Drayton Castle Ltd.)

Two X-ray machines are positioned to obtain anterior and lateral position X-rays. The lateral film cassette is fitted into the holder shown at the far side of the patient, corresponding to the hip being operated on. Note also that the lateral tilting is away from this side.

IMPORTANT POINTS

1. Both arms are placed across the chest or one is extended on an arm table for transfusion purposes.

2. The degree of abduction of the legs depends on the surgeon's wishes but must be adequate to allow positioning of the lateral X-ray machine. In the case of femoral neck fractures the foot on the affected side is usually internally rotated.

3. Pressure points to watch and protect are: where the feet are secured in the leather boot attachments, the buttocks (supported by a sponge rubber pad), the perineum, the arms and, if lateral tilting is used, at each body support.

Endoscopy position

This is a modification of supine position. The head is raised slightly and the endoscope introduced into the pharynx. The head is supported by an assistant and the upper part of the table lowered. The endoscope is introduced with the head held in the degree of flexion

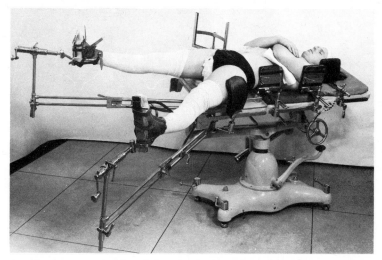

Figure 73   Femoral neck fracture, position for nailing procedures.

or extension required by the surgeon. In the case of an oesophagoscope the head is lowered so that the oesophagus, pharynx and mouth are in a straight line. In the case of a bronchoscope the head is turned to the side opposite to that of the bronchus being examined.

Some surgeons use a Haslinger head support which enables these extension and flexion manoeuvres to be accomplished by turning a hand wheel.

REFERENCES

HOUGHTON, M. and HUDD, J. (1967) *Aids to Theatre Technique,* 4th edn, chap. 4. London: Baillière, Tindall and Cassell.
JOLLY, J. D. (1950) *Operating Room Procedures for Nurses,* 3rd edn, London: Faber.
PEARCE, E. (1967) *Instruments, Appliances and Theatre Technique,* 5th edn. London: Faber.
YEAGER, M. E. (1966) *Operating Room Manual,* 2nd edn, chap. 3. New York: Putnam.

Preparation of the Operating Theatre and Sterile Supplies

Preparation of personnel

No one should enter the operating section without changing into suitable protective clothing and operating theatre footwear such as canvas shoes, rubber boots or sandals reserved exclusively for the purpose. This rule must apply equally when there are no operations in progress, for outside shoes and ordinary clothing will carry contamination by bacteria into the suite (Falk, 1942; Ministry of Health, 1959; Medical Research Council, 1968).

Personnel preparing for operations wear caps and masks in addition to suitable clothing and footwear. Ward staff and visitors are similarly attired during operations.

Research has proved that personnel should *not* take pre-operative showers. This apparently causes shedding of minute skin particles for a period of two hours afterwards, thereby increasing the risk of bacterial dissemination, particularly staphylococcus (Bethune *et al.*, 1965; Medical Research Council, 1968).

Surgeons, anaesthetists and male staff wear a poplin scrub suit which obviates the need for an additional gown when not assisting at operation. Although white is the traditional colour for this apparel, grey or blue is less tiring to the eyes. Green is acceptable also, but it does not provide any contrast between the clean and sterile fields. It is important to ensure that a person wearing a sterile gown is adequately covered. If the scrub suit is the same colour this makes it more difficult to observe.

Female personnel should wear a suit also, for it has been proved bacteriologically that suits minimise bacteriological dissemination compared with the standard dress in general use. Ideally the trousers and sleeves should have stockinette cuffs to restrain skin particles from axillae and perineum. The suit is best made from a closely woven poplin or fabric such as Ventile or Scotchguard (Speers *et al.*, 1965; Blowers and McCluskey, 1966). Alternatively, well-fitting dresses are better than gowns as they are less inclined to brush against sterile trolleys accidentally when passing.

The hair should be covered with a closely fitting cap. This can be made from a short length of stockinette, secured at one end with a rubber band and worn like a ski-ing cap. There are specially shaped caps such as the Johnson 'J' or 'M' cap or those of the disposable paper or non-woven fabric type.

Masks are probably the greatest potential source of infection. The traditional mask of four to six layers of muslin offers only limited protection. When first worn it may be reasonably efficient but soon becomes saturated with moisture vapour from the wearer's breath.

The most efficient mask is of the high filtration disposable type of which there are several varieties. These masks should be moulded to facial contours and actually filter the respirations as compared to deflection with paper or cellophane insert types. It is claimed that such masks achieve a 98 per cent efficient filtration as compared with only 40 per cent with the muslin mask (Ford *et al.*, 1967). Examples of these are the Bardic

(C. R. Bard International Ltd.), the Aseptex or Filtron (3M) and the Surgine (Johnson and Johnson).

When removing a mask, care should be taken to avoid touching that part which has acted as the filter, for the hands can easily become contaminated with bacteria. Muslin masks must be changed at least every two hours or preferably after each operation. Masks should *never* be worn 'around the neck'.

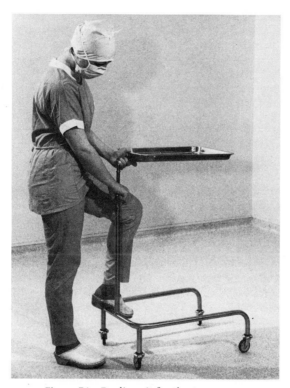

Figure 74   Poplin suit for theatre nurses.

Preparation of the operating theatre

Before an operating list, equipment is checked by the senior operating theatre nurse or the scrub nurse who also selects sterile packets, or may prepare instruments and special apparatus for sterilisation. Special attention is given to the operation table and accessories to ensure that these are correct and in working order. The shadowless light and other portable light fittings are inspected for illumination and focus. All electromedical apparatus such as the diathermy and suction machines or pipeline suction set are switched on and tested as described in the chapter on electricity.

Anaesthetic equipment is checked by the anaesthetic nurse or technician, under the ultimate supervision of the person in charge. Vital inspection includes gas cylinders, soda lime canisters, lamps and batteries of laryngoscopes, etc., and the replenishment of drugs required by the anaesthetist.

The junior staff or auxiliaries are responsible for damp dusting all equipment particularly the overhead shadowless light and ledges, etc., within the suite, followed by cleansing of the floor before sterile trolleys are prepared (Minter, 1952). They should check that steam pressure is adequate for instrument autoclaves, replenish supplies of sterile nail brushes, scrub solution, gown packets and supplementary items. Where individual bottles or flasks of sterile saline or water are in use for hand-lotion bowls, the necessary number of bottles are placed in the warming cupboard until the correct temperature has been reached. Replenishment of bandages, strapping, splints and lotions, etc., should be arranged before the operation list commences.

Preparation of instrument trolleys

Instrument trolleys should be prepared *immediately before* an operation. It is a bad practice to prepare all trolleys required for a list before the commencement of the first case, for even if they are covered carefully, it is impossible to guarantee sterility when required.

A comprehensive sterile packet system obviates the need to use Cheatle transfer forceps. If the chosen method includes sterile towels in cardboard or metal containers, the towels can be laid out on trolley surfaces by the gloved hands of the scrub nurse. There is no place in a modern operating suite for use of sterilised forceps stored half submerged in a container of disinfectant.

All surfaces of trolleys and tables which are to be used for setting out sterile instruments and apparatus should first be covered with a sterile impervious material before the application of sterile towels. This will prevent contamination of apparatus occurring should the sterile towels become soiled or wet. Suitable materials are disposable water-repellent paper sheets and proofed fabrics such as Ventile and Scotchguard.

After the instrument trays have been placed on the trolleys aseptically, the instruments are laid out by a nurse wearing sterile gown and gloves. It is a thoroughly bad practice for an 'unsterile' person to complete this arrangement using Cheatle transfer forceps, because of the great risk of contamination occurring when ungloved hands are moved to and fro over the sterile trolley.

Comprehensive sterile packets containing all the necessary equipment, and incorporating trolley drapes which fall into position as the packet is opened, will shorten the time taken for preparation and minimise bacterial contamination before operation (p. 102).

The scrub nurse

The nurse or technician acting as scrub nurse, scrubs up carefully, covers her operating theatre clothing with a sterile gown, and hands with sterile gloves. When scrubbing up, care must be taken to ensure that all parts of the hands and forearms are cleansed thoroughly, special attention being given to the nails and between the fingers.

Present-day opinion generally approves of a surgical scrub or wash which lasts no longer than five minutes. The conventional nail brush and soap technique is followed by a rinse containing 1 per cent Hibitane in methylated spirit. However, too much brushing tends to injure the surface of the skin and predisposes towards cross infection. It has been discovered that the use of nail brushes can be limited to the nails only, providing a hexachlorophane solution such as PHisoHex, Disfex, or a povidine solution such as Betadine is used as a presurgical wash. Alternatively, polyurethane sponges impregnated with dehydrated hexachlorophane are available (Smylie *et al.*, 1959; Lowbury *et al.*, 1964; Yeager, 1966). This wash is carried out for three minutes only and leaves the skin covered with a film of hexachlorophane which persists for some considerable time. Hexachlorophane is alcohol soluble so that the final spirit rinse to which most people are accustomed must be omitted. The hands must be dried with a sterilised towel before handling gown.

As it is impossible to render the hands completely sterile, they must not come into contact with any part of the outside of the gown or gloves. The correct method of putting on

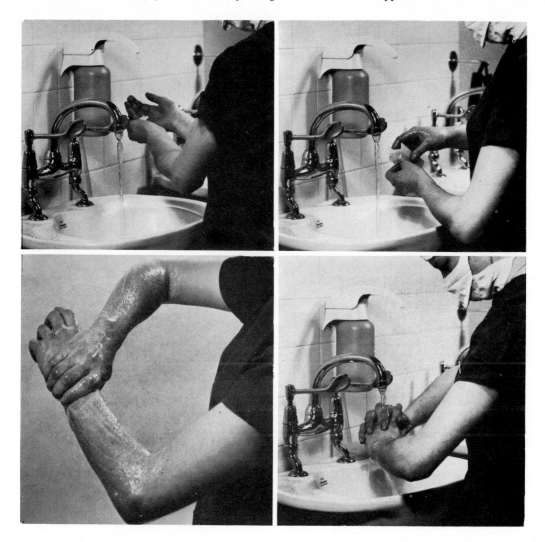

Figure 75 When using ordinary soap the scrub-up or presurgical wash should last at least five minutes under running water. Less time is required when a hexachlorophane-containing soap solution (e.g. PHisoHex) is used. With these the forearms and hands are washed for one minute with a small quantity of the solution and then rinsed.

Figure 76 Particular attention is then paid to the nails, utilising either a sterilised nail-brush or orange-stick which is then discarded.

Figure 77 The main wash should occupy a further full two minutes and consists of reasonably vigorous massage of the hands and forearms up to elbow level with a mixture of solution and water as shown. Care must be taken to ensure adequate cleansing between the digits and skin folds.

Figure 78 Finally the hands and forearms are rinsed thoroughly under running water. The taps are turned off with the elbows and the hands kept in an elevated position to prevent water running down from the elbows. The hands and forearms should then be dried with a sterile towel before assuming the sterile gown and gloves. The hands must not be rinsed in spirit following this technique.

gown and gloves in this way is illustrated. Nurses scrubbing up to assist at operations should keep their nails short and endeavour to avoid handling contaminated objects at all times, especially immediately before scrubbing up.

The scrub nurse is responsible for selecting, checking and arranging instruments required on the instrument table. She is responsible also for accounting for all instruments, needles and swabs or sponges at any stage of the operation, especially before any cavity is closed, and must inform the surgeon that these three items are correct, even though he may not ask. It is her duty also to prepare the ligatures and sutures, having them ready immediately when required.

A good scrub nurse will learn to anticipate a surgeon's needs, often having an instrument ready before being asked for it. Sometimes it may be necessary for the instrument nurse to act as surgeon's assistant in the absence of a house surgeon. The most advantageous way of placing the towels in position and assisting the surgeon are dealt with in a later chapter.

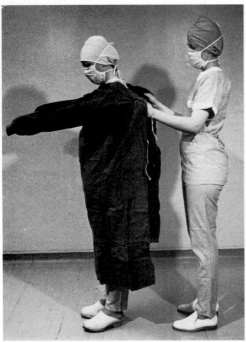 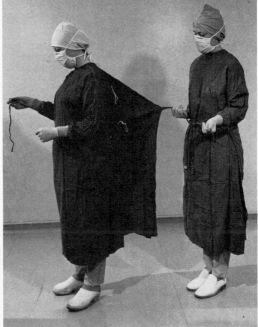

Figure 79   Showing the correct method of putting on a sterile gown, stage one.

Figure 80   Securing the 'back panel' which covers the unsterile tapes. This is carried out by another 'scrubbed' person.

The theatre runners or circulating nurses

In addition to the scrub nurse, one or two nurses or technicians are detailed to act as circulators. One nurse stays in the operating theatre, watching the scrub nurse and ready to bring anything she requires. Dispensing articles from sterile bags or packets, she replenishes sterile gowns and gloves on a sterile trolley or work top reserved for the purpose. It is incorrect for gowns and gloves to be removed from sterile containers by the hands of the operation team, even after the most thorough scrubbing.

The first circulating nurse also ties up the gowns, being careful to avoid touching any of the gown other than the tapes. She replenishes sterile warm or cold water in the lotion bowls and checks the swabs, displaying them on the counting rack in the required order.

The main duties of the second circulating nurse are to see that the instruments and trolleys are ready for the next case, and she should help in placing the patient on the operation table if a porter or technician is not available. She should also help the scrub nurse if the first circulating nurse has to leave the theatre, for on no account must it be left without one circulator.

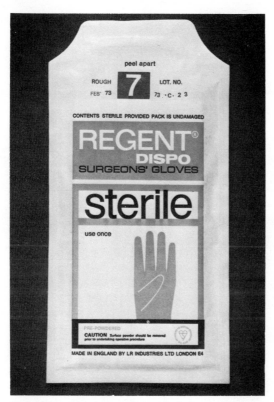

Figure 81   Peel pack containing sterile surgical gloves. (L.R. Industries Ltd.)

It is impossible to define in a textbook the exact duties of circulating nurses. These duties will, of course, depend on the layout and system of particular operating departments. Some operating departments prepare the instruments as packets and sterilise before the list. In this case the sterilising room circulating nurse could be utilised in the theatre for a greater period of time.

All notes and X-rays relating to the patient must be available and it is the duty of the operating theatre staff to ensure that these are easily at hand.

The ward staff

Case notes and X-rays should be brought to the operating department by the ward nurse accompanying the patient. She must be able to answer the questions of the theatre nurse or anaesthetist regarding the pre-operative preparation of the patient, especially the premedication, the nature of the drug, the time it was given, whether urine has been passed and the time the patient last ate. After changing into protective clothing, ideally she stays with her patient as the anaesthetic is being administered and afterwards assists in the removal of the gown and bandages. If possible the ward nurse should then accompany the patient into theatre and help in placing him in position on the operation table,

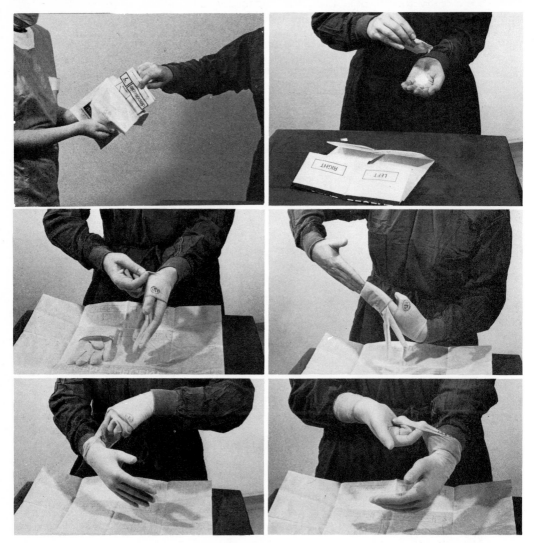

Figure 82   Showing correct method of putting on sterile gloves. The packet containing the gloves is first peeled open by the circulating nurse.

Figure 83   Powdering the hands – away from the sterile gloves.

Figure 84   Inserting first hand, holding by inside of cuff only.

Figure 85   Inserting second hand; glove on first hand in contact with *outside* of second glove only . . .

Figure 86   . . . the cuff of the second glove is pulled over the stockinette sleeve.

Figure 87   The remaining cuff is pulled over the stockinette sleeve.

removing ward preparation towels just before the surgeon is ready to apply the skin antiseptic. This may not always be possible in large operating departments, especially if there is a staff shortage on the ward. In this event, the ward nurse must convey all possible information regarding the patient to a member of the operating department staff at the point of check and transfer to the sterile area.

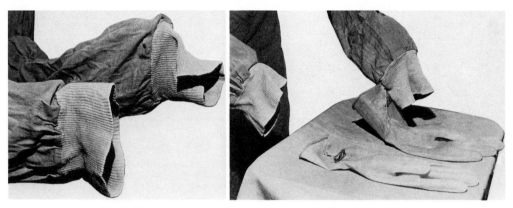

Figure 88   Closed glove technique; the hands are not pushed beyond the stockinette cuffs. (Pioneer Rubber Co., U.S.A.)

Figure 89   The left-hand glove is grasped *through* the left sleeve. (Pioneer Rubber Co., U.S.A.)

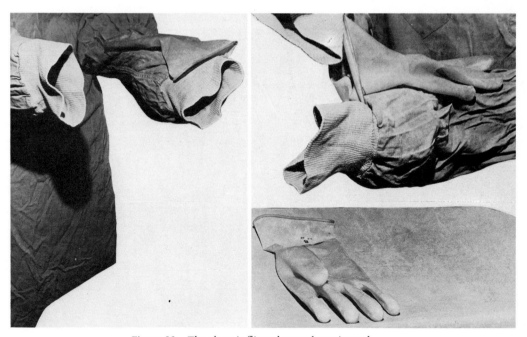

Figure 90   The glove is flipped over the wrist and . . .

Figure 91   . . . grasped by the second hand (through the gown sleeve).

Where the operation table is easily portable, and in a busy operating suite where two or more tables are available, the patient may be placed on the table in the anaesthetic room or in the transfer area. In this case the positioning may be accomplished in the anaesthetic room before entering the theatre, thus avoiding unnecessary disturbance in sterile areas. This system is applicable also with the Swedish Kifa operation table described in Chapter 4.

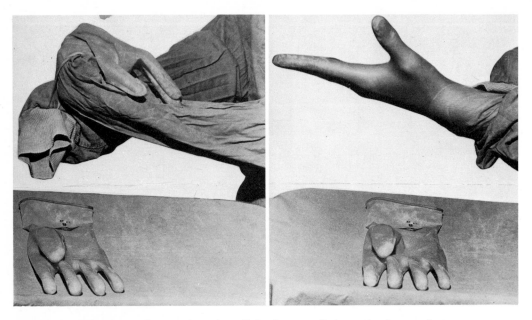

Figure 92   After stretching the cuff the glove is pulled over the sleeve and . . .

Figure 93   . . . the hand is forced through the stockinette cuff into the glove.
(All illustrations on pages 93-95 are by courtesy of Pioneer Rubber Co., U.S.A.)

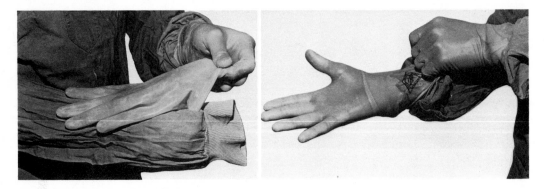

Figure 94   The second glove is put on in a similar manner except that one side of the cuff can be grasped with the already gloved hand and . . .

Figure 95   . . . the right hand is forced through the stockinette cuff into the glove.

An unconscious patient should remain in the recovery area at least until his reflexes return. If, for some reason, the anaesthetist authorises the return of a patient not fully conscious to the ward, he must be accompanied by a competent nurse and a tray, containing a mouth gag, tongue forceps, box-wood wedge, vomit bowl, swabs and a small towel. The patient's gown and blankets (preferably cotton) may be *slightly* warmed and ready to cover him when leaving the theatre. Handling the unconscious patient is dealt with in Chapter 10.

Details of the operation, together with any special instructions regarding the patient's post operative care, are conveyed to the ward sister either by the ward nurse who has stayed in theatre, or by the nurse designated to return with the patient after operation. These instructions should be written down to ensure accuracy. Increasingly patients are nursed by special staff in a recovery room adjacent to or in the operating suite and when recovered return to the main ward.

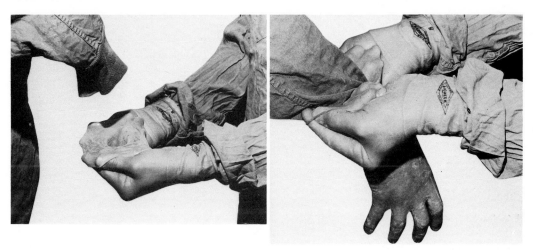

Figure 96   Method of gloving a second person; the cuff is stretched over the fingers of the helper, thumb of glove downwards . . .

Figure 97   . . . the hand is forced through the stockinette cuff and into the glove.

Swab checking and operation register

Whatever system of swab or sponge checking is in force, it is a very good practice to record the check in a register or on a record sheet attached to the patient's notes. The system, of course, will vary according to the method of checking, but it is necessary to state the total number of swabs used during an operation and to have the signatures of the scrub nurse and the circulating nurse, one of whom should be a registered nurse. Any mistakes made in this register must be rectified immediately by re-writing the whole entry before recording the next swab check. A sample register page is illustrated (Fig. 98).

All swab checking systems, however efficient, are dependent to a great extent on the human element, but certain precautions will help to avoid accidental discrepancies in the actual count.

No Loose Swabs should be allowed in the theatre, with the exception of those used by the anaesthetist which are dyed a distinctive colour. Swabs needed for dressings must be packed in fixed numbers in a dressing packet and are not introduced into the sterile area until required. Swabs used for operation are made into packets also and are checked very carefully both before and after they are used.

Date	Name	Hosp. No.	AGE	Ward	Operation	Surgeon Assistant	Anaesthetist Assistant	Swab/Instrument Check Instrument Nurse/ Assistant	Swab/Instrument Check Circulating Nurse/ Assistant	TOURNIQUET Time On	TOURNIQUET Signature	TOURNIQUET Time Off	TOURNIQUET Signature	Serial Number
1.3.73	John Brown	Z3265	22	A2	Laparotomy	Mr Jones Dr Stevens	Dr Green Dr Fells	S/N George ODA Smith	S/N Broad	—	—	—	—	1001
1.3.73	Mavis South	D2323	39	B3	Herniorraphy	Mr Jones Dr Stevens	Dr Fells	ODA Smith	S/N Brown	—	—	—	—	1002
1.3.73	Michael West	B5679	56	A2	Varicose Vein Stripping	Dr Stevens Dr Howe	Dr Fells	S/N George	S/N Broad	—	—	—	—	1003
2.3.73	Jack Dunn	C1212	62	E1	Arthroplasty of Hip	Mr Bones Dr Oseous	Dr Hard Dr Tims	S/N Ward S/N Evans	ODA Smith	—	—	—	—	1004
2.3.73	William White	A2215	20	E1	Menisectomy	Mr Bones Dr Oseous	Dr Hard	S/N Evans	ODA Smith	11.30	ODA Brown	11.50	ODA Brown	1005
														1006
														1007
														1008
														1009
														1010

A sample page from a swab and instrument check register which records application of tourniquets also.

Figure 98 Sample page from a swab check register.

A nurse should *never* bring an unsterile or loose swab into the operating theatre for any purpose. For wiping a surgeon's brow a small towel should be used, whereas for the mopping of a small area of bloodstained or soiled floor a clean mop or cloth is preferable. Similarly, a circulating nurse should *never* remove a swab from the theatre without permission of the scrub nurse. It is often the odd swab removed or introduced accidentally which is the cause for concern during a count.

Swab Location. This is very important and any swab which is packed into a wound and left in position for any period must have a suitable length of tape or thread attached to one corner e.g., tonsil swabs 15 cm by 2·5 cm (6 in by 1 in). This tape or thread is clipped with a haemostat and indicates the presence of a swab.

The swabs must be prepared from gauze which contains a continuous strand of barium (Raytec, Chex, etc.) and if there is any doubt regarding a missing swab, an X-ray can be taken before the wound is closed. The presence of a swab is indicated by the X-ray shadow of a barium strand. This is, of course, an additional safeguard and should not replace an efficient swab-checking system.

Large quantities of swabs may be used during a major procedure and even with the most careful swab count, with numbers reaching three figures, theoretically it is possible to lose a complete packet of swabs. There is a further safeguard, available commercially, which virtually eliminates this possible danger.

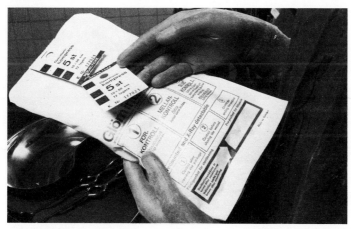

Figure 99   The Mölnlycke check system for swabs, showing the two-part check label.
(Mölnlycke Ltd.)

Mölnlycke of Sweden market pre-packed swabs incorporating a check mark on the outside of the packet. This check mark, which indicates the quantity of swabs contained within the packet can be torn into two halves. One half is retained by the scrub nurse and the other displayed in the swab check area. When the count is made, in addition to checking the number of swabs, the upper and lower halves of the check marks are compared to confirm the number of packets of swabs in use.

If Mölnlycke swabs are not available it is simple to modify the method to personal needs. Several colours of luggage type labels may be used and these are purchased with a perforation running across the centre. The number of swabs (i.e., fives) should be marked on each section together with a serial number. At operation it is simple to compare the serial numbers of each half during the swab check procedure.

Most operating departments have a special operation register into which details of the operations are entered each day. This book usually contains details of the patient, operation, surgeon and assistants, anaesthetist, anaesthetic and sometimes the name of the scrub nurse.

The preparation of dressings

At one time preparation of dressings or swabs was usually the duty of the theatre staff. Nowadays manufacturers' pre-prepared dressings are available in sizes to suit all requirements.

Swabs or sponges are prepared from gauze which may be cotton or rayon, both materials having excellent absorbency. The gauze must contain a continuous filament of X-ray opaque barium (Raytec, Chex, Mölnlycke). It is possible also to obtain sheets of foam cellulose which have a very high absorbency, and are very useful for abdominal packs and minute ophthalmic mops when cut to a suitable size.

Although the sizes of swabs vary enormously according to the type of operation and individual preference of the surgeon, there are some average types and sizes which are in common use.

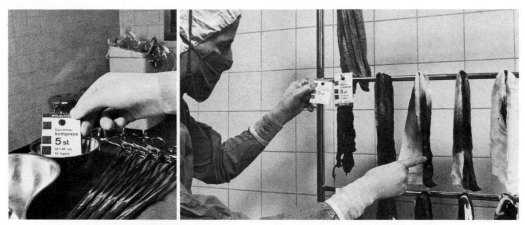

Figure 100   The empty package with attached upper half of check mark is handed to the circulating nurse. The lower half of the check label is retained in the sterile area, the empty package and upper half of the check label is handed to the circulating nurse. (Mölnlycke Ltd.)

Figure 101   When swabs are checked, the lower halves of the check marks are compared with the upper parts hanging with the swabs and a total count made of used and unused swabs. (Mölnlycke Ltd.)

Large Abdominal Packs. These can be made 45·5 cm (18 in) square, from about 36 layers of gauze. These should be stitched around the edges, and a short length of tape attached to one corner. A pair of haemostats is clipped to this tape which is left protruding when the packs are placed inside the abdomen. Soiled packs should not be washed for re-use. It has been proved that laundered packs predispose towards abdominal adhesions, probably due to detergent or soap residue.

Large Swabs or Sponges. These may be made as a pad 23 cm by 7·5 cm (9 in by 3 in) containing about 24 layers of gauze when folded, and 23 cm by 45·5 cm (9 in by 18 in) containing four layers when opened out. These sizes may be varied more or less as required but it is better to standardise to one size of large swab in a particular unit. Alternative sizes range from 15 cm by 10 cm to 23 cm by 23 cm (6 in by 4 in to 9 in by 9 in).

Small Swabs. These range from 5 cm square to 7·5 cm by 10 cm (2 in square to 3 in by 4 in), having about 16 layers. The important point is to ensure that there is sufficient difference of size between these and the larger types in use, to avoid any confusion during the swab checking procedure at operation.

Swabs and Packs. These should be bundled in fixed numbers (fives) by tying with thread, a narrow bandage, rubber bands or lightly stitching together. These bundles are checked by a second person before packing and are checked again by two persons before the operation commences. Manufacturers now supply swabs and packs already bundled in fives. (Medical Defence Council and Royal College of Nursing, 1963).

Anaesthetic Swabs. These must be made smaller than those in general use and coloured gauze prepared by the manufacturers is available for this purpose. The size of swabs required will vary according to individual preference but a 2·5 cm (1 in) square swab is usually adequate.

If the dyed gauze is not available it may be made simply by dyeing white gauze with a weak solution of brilliant green, gentian violet, Bonney's blue or proflavine. The gauze is then dried before making into swabs. Throat packs for the anesthetist should also be made from dyed gauze 5 cm (2 in) wide by 3m to 6 m (3 yd to 6 yd) long, depending on the thickness of gauze.

Rolls of gauze 7·6 cm or 11·4 cm (3 in or 4½ in) wide by 3 m or 4 m (3 yd or 4 yd) long made by folding 22·9 cm (9 in) wide gauze with a barium filament into three or two respectively are often used for packing off cavities, e.g., during gall-bladder operations or as a pack prior to the secondary suture of a septic wound. These may be used also for bandaging amputation stumps, to obtain even pressure over a skin graft although, for these purposes the gauze should not contain a radio-opaque filament.

Wool Balls, or Pieces of Gamgee. For the application of skin antiseptic, wool balls, or pieces of gamgee about 10 cm (4 in) square, are very useful. As these materials are not usually used in the operation area there is no need for them to be included in the swab count, and in addition they seem to hold the skin antiseptic better than the conventional gauze swab.

It is advisable to cover the wool balls with a thin layer of gauze or a short length of tubular bandage knotted upon itself. This is especially useful when adhesive substances such as gum mastic are being used which would otherwise cause wisps of wool to adhere to the skin. These firm compact pads held in a sponge forceps form an ideal sponge for cleansing contaminated wounds.

Alternatively, polyurethane sponge cubes 4 cm (1½ in) in size are very suitable for applying skin antiseptic and withstand sterilisation quite well.

Small Dissection Swabs, 'Bits', 'Pledgets' or 'Patties'. These are used during general surgery, thoracic surgery, neurosurgery and vascular surgery.

1. Compressed dental cotton-wool rolls 9 mm by 2·5 cm (⅛ in by 1 in) securely clamped in the jaws of a haemostat may be used as dissection swabs. These require very careful checking at operation as they conflict with the radio-opaque checking concept.

2. 'Bits' or 'pledgets' are prepared from pieces of Raytec, Chex, etc., gauze folded to form a mop about 1·25 cm (½ in) square.

3. 'Patties' are made from B.P.C. cotton-wool or lintine. A piece of cotton-wool about 2·5 cm (1 in) square is moistened and stitched with a length of strong black radio-opaque thread. After autoclaving these fluff out into a suitable size.

Lintine or 'Cottonoid' is supplied in sheets 30·5 cm by 7·6 cm (12 in by 3 in), which are cut into suitable sized 'patties'. These are stitched with a length of black thread, care being taken to avoid using actual knots to secure it in position. Knots and rough surfaces will damage delicate nerve tissue, and it is for this reason also that the 'patties' must be moistened slightly at operation.

All these small mops are made into bundles of 5 or 10 and are checked carefully before and after operation.

Wool Rolls. If required sterile these are cut to suitable size and re-rolled loosely before packing into the packets. If a high-vacuum/high-pressure autoclave is available they need not be rerolled.

Sterile Bandages of all materials, especially crêpe, are frequently required and may be packed into a separate dressings packet or container. A tightly wound bandage cannot be completely sterilised because the steam will not penetrate into the actual centre of the bandage, however the outer layers coming into contact with the dressings are sterile, and are therefore preferable to non-sterile bandages.

ENT and Ophthalmic Dressings. These are prepared and generally kept in separate packets containing suitable dressings for the eye and ear, including fast edge bandages, ribbon gauze, and eye pads made from best quality cotton-wool, covered each side with cotton bandage.

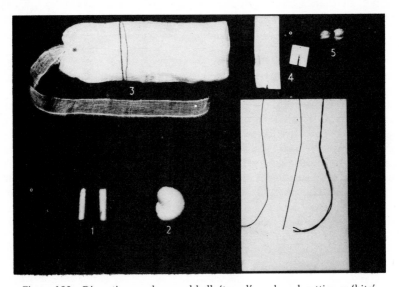

Figure 102   Dissection swabs, wool ball, 'taped' swab and patties or 'bits'.

1. Compressed cotton dental rolls for dissection swabs.
2. Wool ball covered with tubular gauze.
3. 'Taped' swab with barium strand.
4. Patties made from cottonoid.
5. Pattie or 'bit' made from ribbon gauze
   rolled into suitable size.

Operation linen

Operation towels, sheets and gowns are made from a strong close-weave material such as balloon fabric or repp, or a disposable non-woven fabric (paper), and may be white, although green, blue or grey is more restful to the eyes of the operation team.

It is better to minimise the number of towel sizes in an operating suite and generally three or four sizes and types will suffice. The average towel for covering a trolley should measure at least 121·9 cm (48 in) square, although a trolley measuring 121·9 cm (48 in) by 61 cm (24 in) will require an oblong towel measuring 182·9 cm by 52·4 cm (72 in by 60 in). This enables easier packet preparation by using one towel for the trolley drapes even if the trolley sizes are large.

For towelling lower limbs, these larger size towels 182·9 cm by 152·4 cm (72 in by 60 in) will be found useful also and will reduce the number of towels required to the minimum.

For abdominal surgery, there may be a preference for a large sheet measuring about

213·4 cm by 182·9 cm (84 in by 72 in) and having a longitudinal reinforced slit 30·5 cm (12 in) by 10·2 cm (4 in) placed centrally and slightly towards one end. This holed sheet or towel may be utilised also for operations in the lithotomy position, or a lateral thigh operation such as the insertion of a Smith-Peterson nail. The addition of two bag-shaped leg covers stitched to the edges of suitable holes, 30·5 cm (12 in) from each side of the central slit in a holed towel, obviates the need for extra towels to cover the legs in lithotomy position.

Gowns are made with long sleeves for the operation team and short sleeves for personnel who are not scrubbed up. They should be made with an overlap of material at the back which, when tied correctly, covers the unsterile tapes. This is especially useful if the surgeon turns his back to the operation area as may happen during intra-abdominal manipulations.

All linen materials should be kept in a good state of repair and examined for tears, etc., before packing in the packets or containers.

The preparation of packets

Most hospitals now use a sterile packet system. Separate linen or paper packets of sterile materials and instruments are prepared for individual operations, a fresh set of packets always being opened for each operation.

The outdated 'drum' system should now be condemned, for the risk of bacterial contamination due to ill-fitting shutters and lids is considerable. In addition, the use of a multi-item container for unwrapped items cannot guarantee sterility indefinitely especially if it remains open for a considerable period of time during an operation list. There is a version of the metal drum available called the Wessex Casket (see Chapter 6) which consists of a metal box incorporating high efficiency bacterial filters in the top and bottom panels. These filters are permeable to steam and the casket is suitable for sterilising trays of instruments. Even this is now of doubtful technique for the reasons given above.

Small items may be double wrapped and sterilised in a Bri-pac (Smith and Nephew) or Permapak (Luxan) box. The container then acts only as a dust cover until the inner packets are removed for use.

Small Towels. These are folded or rolled into a convenient size. A 'criss-cross' method of packing in boxes permits efficient air removal and steam penetration and is preferable to packing the articles in unbroken columns.

Large Towels or Abdominal Sheets. These are packed in a similar manner but it will be found advantageous to fold them in such a way that, when opened at operation, they are conveniently arranged for easy 'towelling up'.

This is accomplished (see illustrations) by folding the towels lengthways in sections about 22·9 cm (9 in) wide from each side to the centre. The 22·9 cm (9 in) wide finished folds are then folded again in 22·9 cm (9 in) sections equally from each end to the centre, making a folded towel about 22·9 cm (9 in) square which is a convenient size for packing. Towels folded in this way are less liable to become contaminated, especially in the centre, when opened out by two persons at operation.

Gowns. These are folded inside out in three or four folds, care being taken to contain all the tapes within the folds. The gowns are then rolled or folded equally from each end to the centre (see illustrations). This will ensure that when the gown is opened at operation, whichever end is grasped the gown will only unroll halfway and avoid touching the floor.

Macintoshes. In the operating theatre these have now been replaced either with a water-repellent disposable paper item or fabric such as Ventile and Scotchguard which can be laundered and re-proofed.

These items can be packed and sterilised in a similar manner to fabric towels or drapes.

Gloves. These are now supplied presterilised in peel-open packets. Alternatively, if reprocessing is unavoidable or special types of gloves are in use they may be put in individual packets which are placed in outer paper bags or Bripac/Permapak boxes.

Dressings and Bandages. These, including materials such as gauze and wool, are packed loosely and sterilised under the same conditions as towels and gowns.

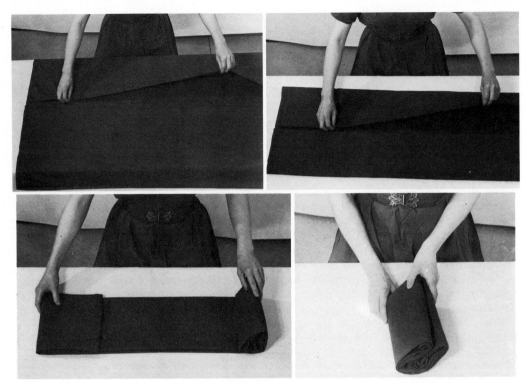

Figure 103   Folding a large towel, stage one.

Figure 104   Folding a large towel, stage two.

Figure 105   Folding a large towel, stage three.

Figure 106   Folding a large towel, completion.

Sterile packet systems

These methods have supplanted the use of drums and caskets. In principle they are quite simple and mean the preparation of sterile supplies either in parcels or sealed bags, the contents of which are used for one procedure only. Any supplies remaining are discarded for re-sterilisation and a fresh packet opened for the next procedure.

There are a number of different methods of packing sterile supplies, each has its advantages and disadvantages but basically all the items required for an operation are prepared together either in one or several packets, i.e., items required for an abdominal operation could be prepared as a comprehensive single set or divided into the various components as separate packets.

In the latter instance, one would contain the requisite number of gowns and small hand towels, a second rubber gloves, a third the requisite towels or drapes, swabs and gauze packs, etc., and a fourth the instruments and steam-sterilisable ligatures.

The packets are covered with a material which enables sterilisation to take place, acting also as a barrier to bacteria during the periods of storage before use. Amongst suitable wrapping materials are linen, crêpe paper and non-woven fabrics.

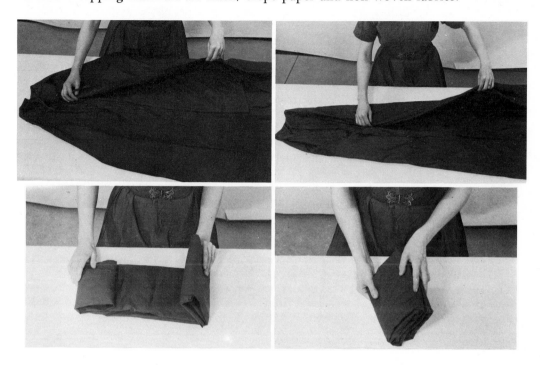

Figure 107   Folding a gown, stage one.

Figure 108   Folding a gown, stage two.

Figure 109   Folding a gown, stage three.

Figure 110   Folding a gown, completion.

No material is ideal for wrapping all items and although it is desirable to standardise to the most suitable, two or three types may need to be utilised according to requirements. The correct gauge of linen or paper must be selected for wrapping fabrics and instruments. Paper manufacturers in the United Kingdom now conform to a Department of Health specification in respect of sterilising wrapping papers. Items must always be double wrapped to prevent contamination after sterilisation or during opening of the packet (Allen, 1965; Speers and Shooter, 1966; Medical Research Council, 1968).

Irrespective of whether the packets are prepared in a Central Sterile Supply Department, Hospital Sterilising and Disinfection unit or the Operating Suite, basic techniques are similar. Space would not permit a description of all methods in use but there are several which are more generally approved, i.e., the comprehensive Edinburgh Pre-Set Tray system prepared in a Theatre Sterile Supply Unit; modified forms of the Pre-Set

Tray system; separate drape and instrument sets and supplementary items in paper and nylon.

The Edinburgh Pre-Set Tray system (in brief)

The most logical and time-saving method is to prepare all the requirements in one comprehensive packet. This is not a new idea for it has been in use for many years particularly in the United States but there are several problems associated with the method. Some difficulty may be experienced after sterilisation in completely drying out a packet containing a large number of instruments combined with drapes. This is especially so in the High-vacuum/High-pressure autoclave and is due to excessive condensate forming on the instruments during the steam phase.

Secondly, unless the correct packing procedure is carried out, instruments tend to become displaced during handling and transit and this is inconvenient when the packet is opened for use.

Research conducted by the Royal Infirmary at Edinburgh revealed that if instruments and drapes are packed and sterilised on solid aluminium trays of 12 s.w.g. or 14 s.w.g. weight, there is sufficient residual heat left to vaporise this excess condensate during the drying phase.

The trays are made to conform in width and depth to the British Standard High-vacuum/High-pressure rectangular autoclaves, i.e., 66 cm by 66 cm (26 in by 26 in). The size of the trays are such to allow setting out of instruments and drapes in the order of their use. The largest size 61 cm by 61 cm (2 ft by 2 ft) is adequate for a major surgery set, the medium 61 cm by 30·5 cm (2 ft by 1 ft) for smaller sets and the smallest 30·5 cm by 30·5 cm (1 ft by 1 ft) is designed for other supplementary items. Full details of tray specifications are given in the Appendix.

The Edinburgh trays are ideal, particularly when a considerable number of instruments are needed in a surgery set. However, they are not absolutely essential and smaller heavy-gauge aluminium pressed-out trays about 4 cm (1½ in) in depth may be utilised as an alternative.

Theatre Sterile Supply Unit

This can be part of the Central Sterile Supply Department, Hospital Sterilising and Disinfection Unit or built adjacent to the operating suite. It is basically the same layout as any CSSD which handles the processing of ward instruments and dressings. It should have a soiled truck unloading area; processing area for soiled instruments and which includes mechanical and ultrasonic washing machines; a tray assembly area; supplementary pack assembly area; soft goods supply storage area; prepared pack and tray holding area; sterilising area; processed stores area and administrative areas. Linen repair and inspection facilities may be incorporated in the unit or may form part of the hospital laundry services.

At Edinburgh a minimal amount of sterile instrument sets are stored in the operating suite. Each afternoon preceding elective surgical sessions, the operating department manager provides the service unit with a list which details surgical supplies required for each operation. General-use instrument sets are kept in the TSSU sterile store and delivered as required, while sets used in a specific theatre (e.g. cardiothoracic) are kept in the sterile storage area of the user theatre. The used sets are returned immediately to the Sterile Supply Unit, for processing and resterilisation. The operating suite does, of course, maintain a fixed stock of supplementary instrument packs for emergency use and linen packets including sterile gowns, swabs, dressings and other small items.

At the end of the operation, prior to folding over the linen covers of the trays used ready for removal from the operating theatre, the scrub nurse should dispose of any contents of gallipots, separate the used and unused instruments, collect used knife blades, broken glass vials, ligature packets and non-traumatic suture needles in a foil dish or other protective packet before placing in the paper disposal bag.

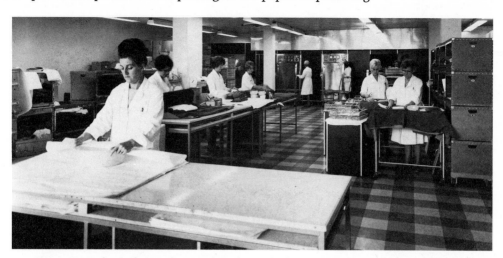

Figure 111　The work area of a central sterile supply department. Clean hoist to the operating theatres is in the background. (Northern General Hospital, Sheffield (Telegraph and Star Studios).)

The used trays, salvaged drapes and dressings, empty hand basins, plastic bag containing the soiled swabs and the stapled paper laundry bag are collected and returned to the Theatre Sterile Supply Unit. On arrival in the unit the laundry, swab and disposal bags are marked with a serial number designated for the operation so that the bags can be identified later if an instrument is found to be missing. These are placed in the laundry-holding section until the instruments have been processed and re-set on the tray or trays used during the operation. If the loss of an instrument is not detected at the off-loading bench it certainly will be detected while the instruments are being re-set. When the instruments have been re-set and it is clear that the numbers are correct the laundry bag, disposal and swab bags are disposed of in the appropriate manner.

Salvaged dressings and drapes are returned to the supply storage area and the tray with its linen covers is disassembled. Special instruments such as scissors, skin hooks and amputation knives are separated from the general instruments and washed separately. The remainder of the instruments are loaded into baskets for processing in the washing machine. Unused instruments are generally loaded into a separate basket and the used instruments into as many further baskets as may be required. Jointed instruments should be opened widely and those such as probes and nerve hooks which might drop out of the basket during washing can be clipped or thrust through plastic sponges to keep them within the basket.

There may be several instrument baskets per surgical operation and if the trays arrive at the service unit in rapid succession from different operating theatres it is important to be able to distinguish instruments used at one operation from those used at another. The Edinburgh Royal Infirmary have devised a labelling system to overcome this difficulty.

Above the tray off-loading bench there is a board on which hang groups of four metal discs (Fig. 112). The discs are marked with the operating theatre number and the serial number of the particular operation on the list. As each basket is loaded with instruments, an appropriate disc is hooked on to the rim of the basket and is left there till the instruments have been removed from the basket for re-setting at the end of the processing line. The tray checker removes the discs after checking the re-set tray. The discs are then returned to the board for further use.

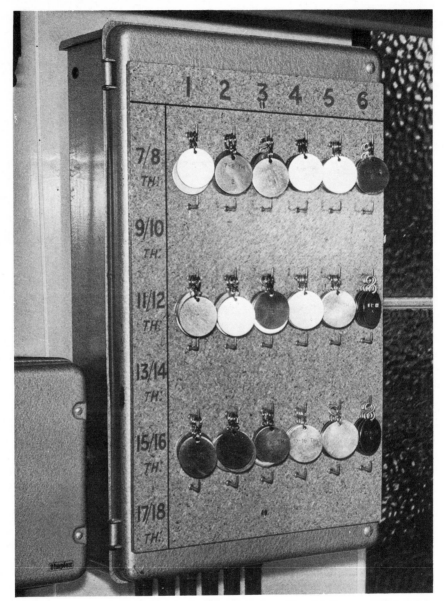

Figure 112   Identification discs for instrument baskets. (Royal Infirmary, Edinburgh.)

Whilst the instruments are being processed the large trays are cleansed with a suitable solution such as spiritous Hibitane 0·05 per cent and then transferred to the tray assembly area on to a 61 cm by 123 cm (2 ft by 4 ft) trolley. Two layers of fabric covers, one blue and one green are arranged over both the tray and the trolley. (The different colours are to differentiate between the cover handled by the circulating nurse and the cover handled by the scrub nurse wearing sterile gown and gloves.) These covers are pushed down into the tray by a wooden mould of appropriate size for the tray. A spring-retaining cord is stretched over the covers into the gutter round the upper aspect of the tray and the mould is then removed (Figs. 113 and 114).

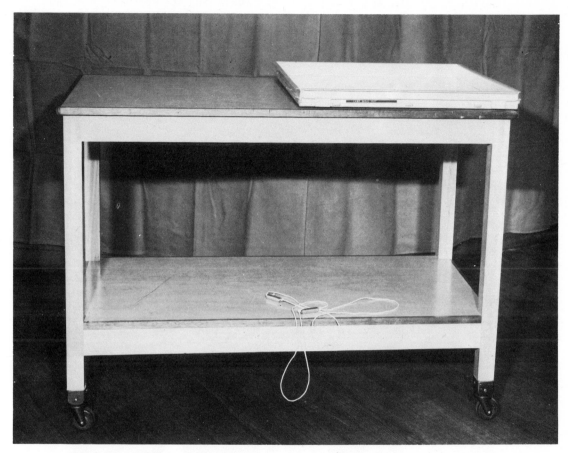

Figure 113   A full-size instrument tray positioned on the 121·9cm by 61cm (4ft by 2ft) trolley. The spring and retaining cord on the shelf below. (Royal Infirmary, Edinburgh.)

After the instruments have been washed, ultrasonically cleansed, dried and inspected they are set out according to the particular arrangement (Fig. 115). A set of swabs and fabric drapes are placed over the instruments to retain them in position during transit and sterilisation (Figs. 116, 117) and the covers are folded over as illustrated (Fig. 118). After sterilisation, the trays are held in the processed stores area until required. If prolonged storage is necessary after sterilisation an additional plastic dust cover is used.

A modified Pre-set Tray system

The 61 cm by 61 cm (2 ft by 2 ft) special tray is ideal, particularly when large instrument sets are needed, e.g. major laparotomy. As stated previously, if no T.S.S.U. is available the system is quite suitable for preparation and sterilisation within the operating suite. However, the autoclaves may be too small to take the large size tray and the alternative medium size, i.e., 61 cm by 30·5 cm (2 ft by 1 ft) may be inadequate for an average general set, or perhaps neither of these trays may be easily available. In these circumstances the Pre-set Tray system can be introduced utilising any convenient deep aluminium tray, providing it is of sufficient gauge to retain enough residual heat for drying the instrument set during the post-steam cycle. Alternatively, cardboard or polypropylene trays may be used although prolonged drying may be necessary.

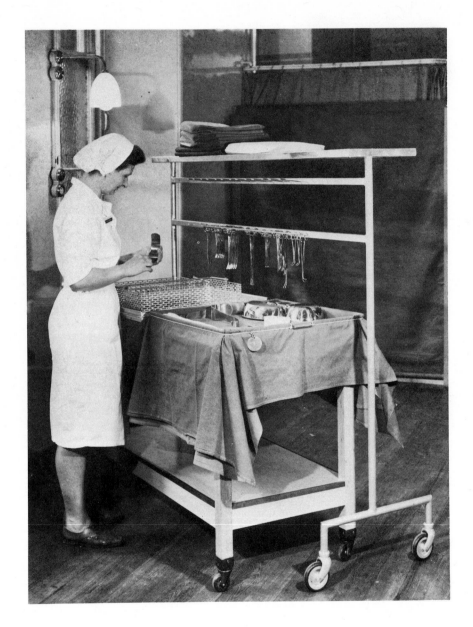

Figure 114   Tray assembler setting a full-size instrument tray. Note mobile instrument sorting frame. (Royal Infirmary, Edinburgh.)

Basically the method is similar to the Edinburgh system but as the trays generally do not have the special double gutter to accommodate the spring-retaining cord one layer of fabric cover is placed *outside* the aluminium tray (Figs. 120 to 129).

Separate drape and instrument sets

The Pre-set Tray system is only suitable when there are sufficient instruments to allow adequate time for processing and sterilisation. When this is impossible, the alternative is to sterilise the instruments separately and then add these to a suitable operation packet.

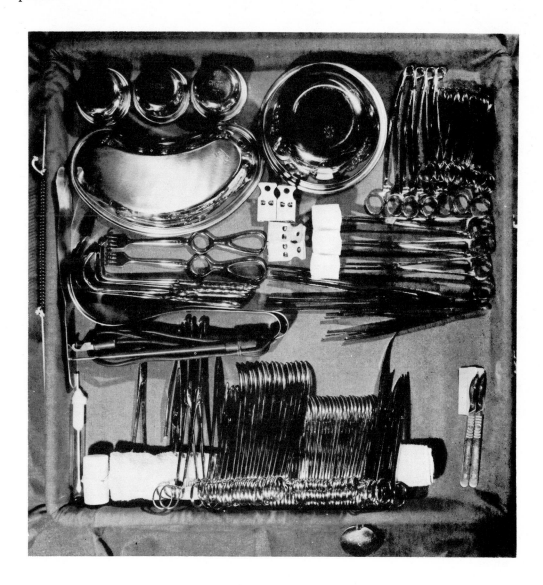

Figure 115   A large basic instrument set ready for linen drapes. Tray cover held in position by spring and cord. (Royal Infirmary, Edinburgh.)

All the swabs, and drapes, are prepared in a linen or paper packet. The method of folding is basically the same as that described under the modified tray system. Packet covers should consist of not less than two layers of fabric which act as a trolley drape also. Suitable fabrics include Repp, Ventile and Scotchguard (which are water-repellent and can be re-proofed in the hospital laundry (Brigden, 1964), see Appendix). In addition, there should be a plastic or paper dust cover if the packet is to be stored for longer than a few hours.

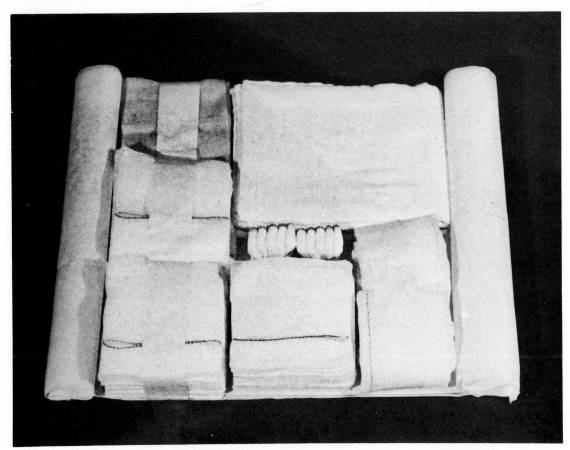

Figure 116   Linen drapes placed over set instruments, this helps to retain them in position during sterilisation and handling of pack afterwards. (Royal Infirmary, Edinburgh.)

Instrument trays can be wrapped as in Figure 130 or placed in a Wessex casket and this is preferable to open trays, which require the use of Cheatle transfer forceps.

Supplementary items

Single instruments and other supplementary items such as orthopaedic implants, additional packets of swabs, etc., can be packed into small packets or paper bags. Rigid containers can be used for some instruments and for steam sterilisation are made from cardboard or polypropylene. Except for Wessex caskets, metal containers are generally only suitable for the dry heat process.

Packets are prepared similar to those described previously utilising a diagonal method of folding the two layers.

Paper bags can either be heat-sealed or have a plain folded top. In the former case the Kraft bag incorporates a heat-sensitive adhesive band inside the open end (Thermotop). After the contents have been placed inside, the open end is sealed by squeezing between the heated jaws of a special heat-sealing machine. The bag generally has a small panel of heat-sensitive ink which changes colour after the packet has been sterilised. If this has

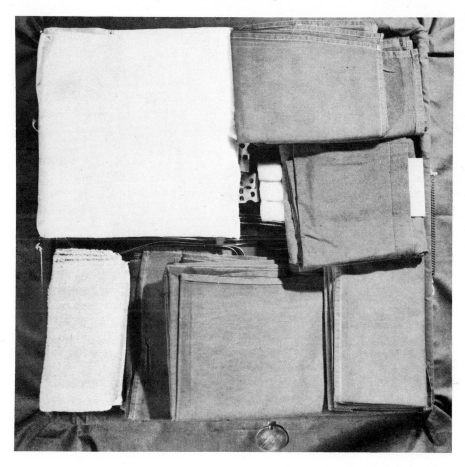

Figure 117   Swabs and dressings set for large basic tray. (Royal Infirmary, Edinburgh.)

not been provided a small piece of 3M indicator tape should be affixed to the bag for the same purpose. (3M indicator tape is in the form of dark stripes which appear on the surface of the tape if it has been through the sterilisation process. No 1222 is designed for steam sterilisation, No 1226 [Indair] is for dry heat and No 1224 [Indox] is for ethylene oxide.)

Folded top bags are prepared as illustrated and the folds held in position with a small piece of 3M indicator tape. The cardinal rule with paper bags is that two must always be used. The outer bag acts as a dust cover during storage so that when the inner is opened in the operation area the possible dissipation of dust is avoided.

Polypropylene Containers are tubular in form with a perforated lid. When the items have been packed inside the tube, the perforated lid retains a two-layer paper filter which permits passage of steam but acts as a barrier to dust and bacteria during storage. The lid is sealed on with a band of 3M indicator tape.

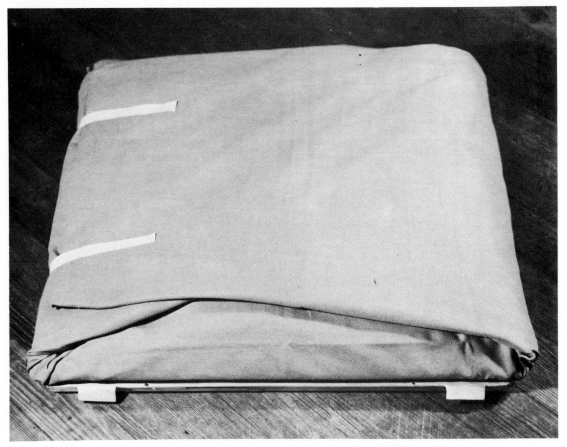

Figure 118   Large basic tray (packed). (Royal Infirmary, Edinburgh.)

Metal Containers are generally made from aluminium in the form of tubes or boxes. They are most suitable for dry heat sterilisable items such as osteotomes, special knives and syringes, etc., and as sterilisation is by conduction of heat the container can be sealed before processing.

Sterilisation and storage

Sterilisation of packets is dealt with at great length in the following chapter. After sterilisation a piece of cellulose tape imprinted STERILE may be applied to the packet and stamped with the date of autoclaving. Alternatively, the date can be marked on the 3M indicator tape used to secure packet folds. This date is a guide to turnover rather than sterility.

The packets should be stored in a clean dry environment until required. If this is in the

Theatre Sterile Supply Unit and the storage is likely to be prolonged for more than a few hours, the packets should have an outer dust cover made from plastic or paper. In a properly air-conditioned operating department normally it should be unnecessary to have dust covers but the packets must be stacked carefully in rotation of sterilisation date. This ensures that none are stored for too long a period.

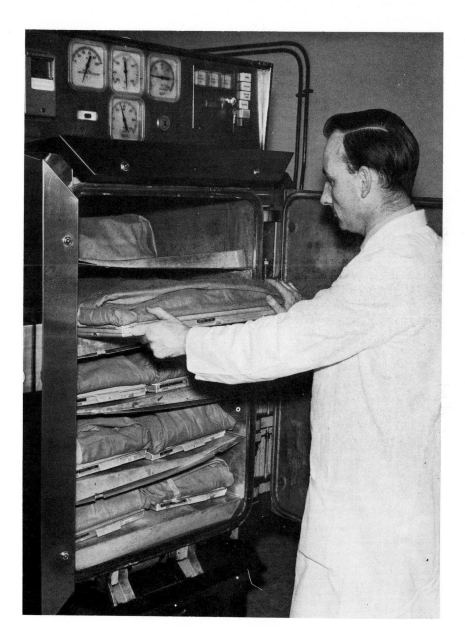

Figure 119   Sterilisation of trays (note condensation drain below each shelf) which is described in the following chapter. (Royal Infirmary, Edinburgh.)

Packets which usually require some form of dust cover within the operating suite are items such as orthopaedic implants or specialised instruments used infrequently. In this case, if the item is small enough, Bri-pac or Permapak boxes are very suitable and enable quite a number to be stored in a small area.

A high standard of cleanliness is necessary in packet storage areas. Shelving or cup-boards should be damp-dusted regularly with a suitable anti-bacterial agent (e.g., spiritous Hibitane 0·05 per cent).

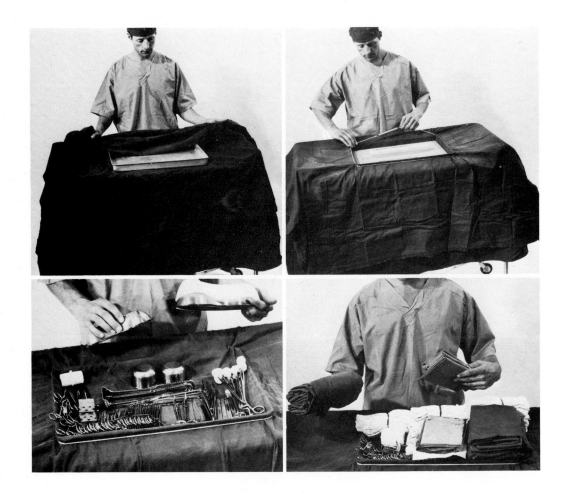

Figure 120   The modified pre-set tray system; aluminium tray placed on outer piece of blue Ventile.

Figure 121   Green trolley drape in position over aluminium tray, wooden former pushes drape flat, which is then held in position with a cord and spring.

Figure 122   Major basic instruments set out.

Figure 123   Swabs and drapes placed over instruments. This helps to retain them in position during sterilisation and handling afterwards.

Preparation for operation

The outer cover of the packet is opened by hand (Fig. 141), care being taken to avoid contamination of the inner packet which is opened by the scrub nurse as illustrated. With the Pre-Set tray very little additional preparation is needed with the exception of a few supplementary items (Fig. 154).

Where separate drape and instrument packets are in use these are opened aseptically and transferred to the main trolley by the scrub nurse. Items in rigid tubes or paper bags should, preferably, be removed with sterile forceps by the scrub nurse (Fig 154) although they can be dropped on to a sterile surface with care.

Gown packets should be opened only to the inner layers, which are left folded for opening by the instrument nurse just before gowning up. Gloves are dispensed from individual paper bags as required (Fig. 82, page 92).

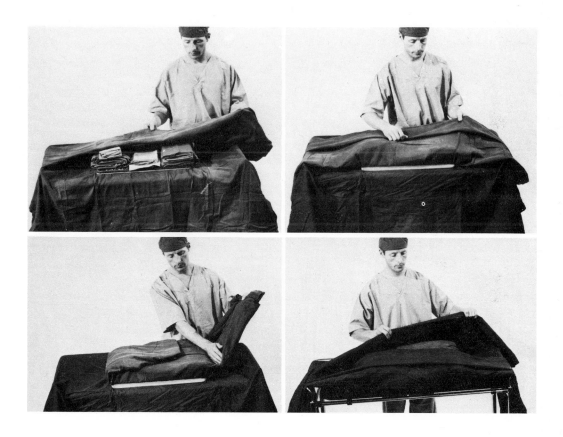

Figure 124   Rear part of green trolley drape folded to the front and then turned back on itself.

Figure 125   Front part of green trolley drape folded towards the back and then folded back on itself.

Figure 126   Second side fold of green trolley drape.

Figure 127   The outer blue piece of Ventile is folded as previously described.

Using this type of packet system, even during busy operation lists, the preparation time of trolleys is shortened considerably. Only one trolley need be prepared, the next instrument packet is opened as the next operation is ready to start. This ensures minimal bacterial contamination and reduces the rush or tension which previously tended to be present during preparations in the operating theatre.

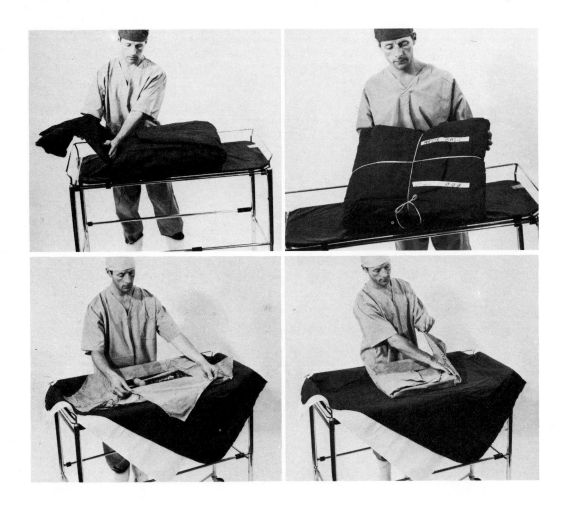

Figure 128   The final side folds of the blue Ventile.

Figure 129   The completed major basic instrument set ready for sterilisation. The contents, date packed and initials of tray assembler and checker are written on the 3M autoclave tape with felt pen magic marker).

Figure 130   Instruments packed separately to drapes; a fracture and bone set which is wrapped in three layers, fawn and blue Ventile and Sterilwrap crêpe paper. A diagonal method of folding is used with corners turned back for easy aseptic opening at operation. The first front fold, fawn Ventile.

Figure 131   The second side fold.

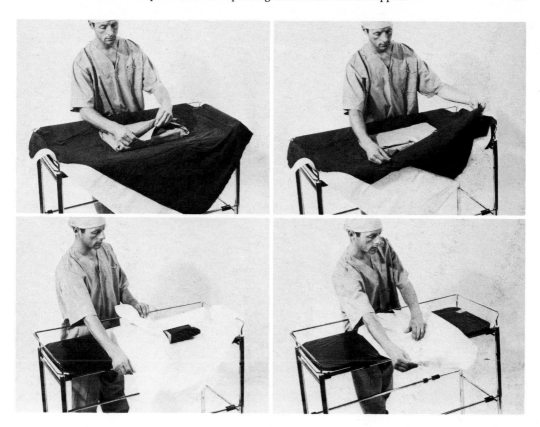

Figure 132   Tucking in the final fold, fawn Ventile.

Figure 133   The blue Ventile layer is folded in a similar manner.

Figure 134   The final paper layer folded diagonally as before, first side fold.

Figure 135   The front paper fold.

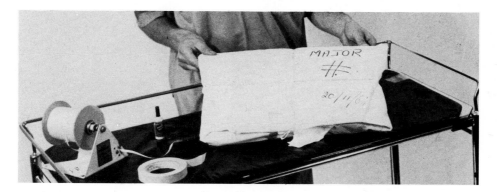

Figure 136   The completed packet ready for sterilisation. This paper layer is required only if the packet is being sterilised outside the operating suite. Note the packet is tied with cotton tape and a piece of 3M indicator autoclave tape has been applied.

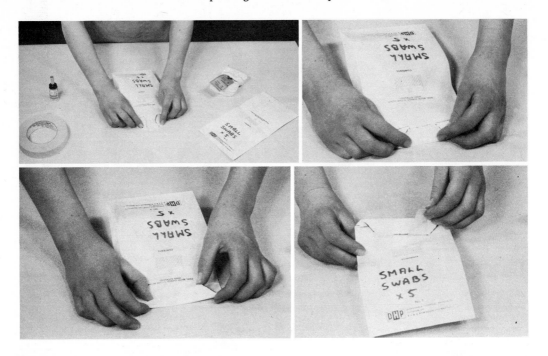

Figure 137   Supplementary items in Kraft paper bags, folded top – first diagonal folds.

Figure 138   Second fold.

Figure 139   Final fold . . . which is held in position with . . .

Figure 140   . . . a piece of 3M autoclave tape.

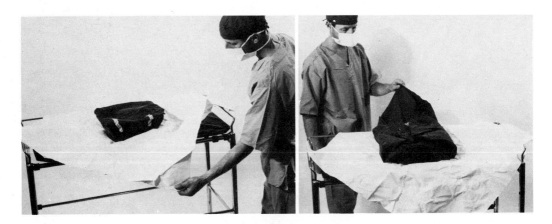

Figure 141   Opening sterile packets at operation; the outer crêpe paper layers are opened, utilising the turned-back diagonal corners.

Figure 142   The inner blue layer is also opened by the circulating nurse, fold one.

The care of instruments and apparatus

After use the instruments should be cleansed carefully with a stiff brush under running cold water. Alternatively, an ultrasonic cleanser or mechanical washing machine may be used combined with a suitable detergent solution, e.g., Pyroneg, Biotergic. The process should include a cycle of cold water followed by a detergent wash and finally a very hot rinse 83°C (180°F) (Fig. 155). Staff must be adequately protected by wearing aprons and rubber gloves.

If excessive contamination has occurred, e.g. following a septic operation, it is better to autoclave them for four minutes at 134°C (275°F) before processing. However, during subsequent cleansing the instruments must still be regarded as potentially infected due to the debris adhering.

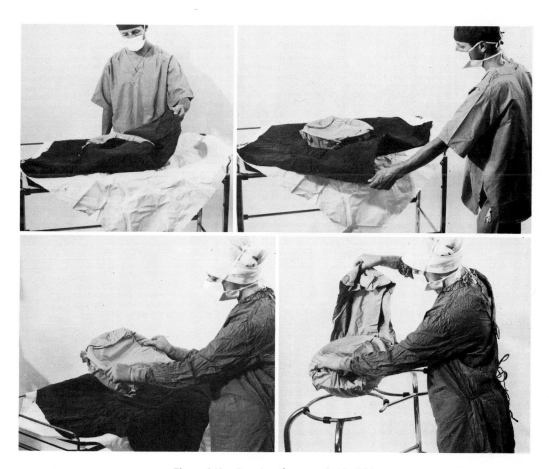

Figure 143   Opening the second side fold.

Figure 144   The final blue fold which exposes the innermost fawn wrapped package.

Figure 145   The scrub nurse lifts out the inner package (which contains a hand lotion bowl set complete with bowl stand drape).

Figure 146   Grasping the topmost part of the drape, the scrub nurse lowers the bowl and drape into the lotion bowl stand.

Instruments should be dried hot soon after removal from the washing machine, ultra-sonic cleaner or a hot detergent solution such as 0·5 per cent cetrimide or Pyroneg. After cleaning and drying they should always be examined carefully each time for defects, i.e., loose rivets and screws, cracking of forceps' jaws, lack of apposition between grooves and, in cutting instruments, blunt cutting edges, etc.

Debris inside joints may be removed by applying a little silicone solution such as M.S.A. 550 or instrument Lube, and 'working' the joint, which will create friction and express most dirt particles. If silicone is used the instrument must be re-washed before sterilisation.

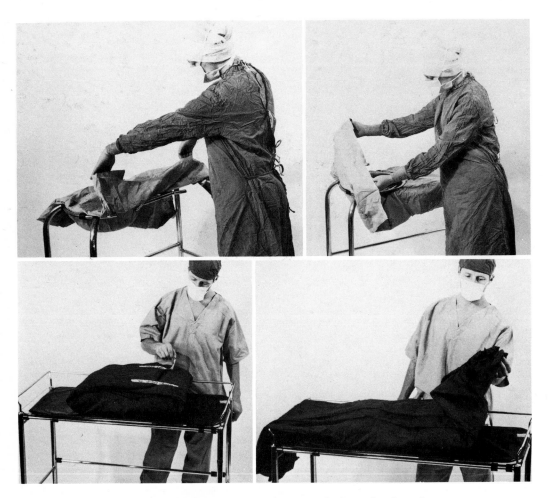

Figure 147   The drapes are opened to cover the lotion bowl stand . . .

Figure 148   . . . exposing the hand lotion bowl which is then filled with sterile water or saline. (Figure 19, page 30.)

Figure 149   Opening the pre-set tray of instruments; removing the autoclave tape after checking that it is the correct set and has been autoclaved.

Figure 150   The blue layers are opened by the circulating nurse.

Sharp Instruments. These should be handled with very great care. The cutting edges of fine cataract knives, scalpels, osteotomes and gouges, etc., must not be damaged. These instruments must be dried thoroughly after use to avoid rusting, as they are often manufactured from carbon steel.

The cutting edges of knives, etc., may be examined by viewing the edge under a strong light. A sharp knife edge will appear black, but if the edge appears as a broken or continuous white line, the knife is blunt and should be discarded for resharpening.

Scissors. These should have even edges and secure rivets. Good quality scissors require only occasional sharpening, in any case the scissors remain semi-closed during sterilisation, thereby protecting the edges.

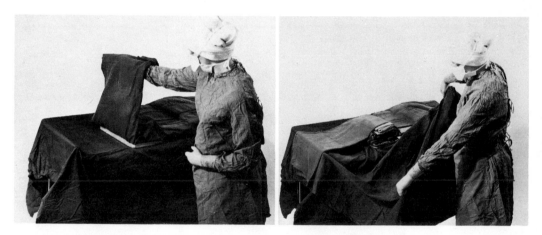

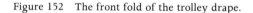

Figure 151   The inner green trolley drape is opened by the scrub nurse, the side folds.

Figure 152   The front fold of the trolley drape.

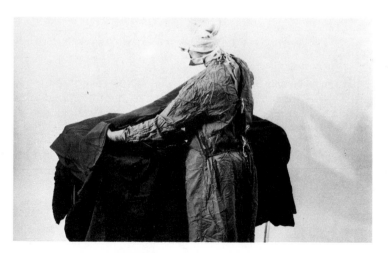

Figure 153   The rear fold is opened, note the front fold already opened protects the sterile gown of the scrub nurse as she stretched over the trolley.

Suture Needles. These are generally available now as disposable but, if for reasons of economy, re-use is necessary, they must be washed thoroughly after use, special attention being paid to the needle eye. Rust marks should be removed with fine steel wool and soap, following which the needles are carefully dried. They are sterilised by dry heat or autoclaving (utilising a piece of anti-rust paper) after packing in paper envelopes. Needles having blunt or rough edges should not be kept for further use and must be discarded.

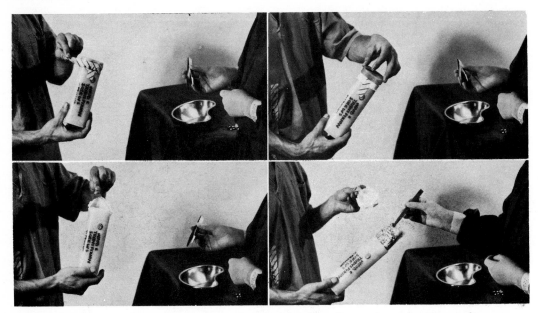

Figure 154   Supplementary items in a rigid autoclavable polypropylene tube; the autoclave tape is removed.

Figure 155   Removing the perforated lid, paper filters still in position.

Figure 156   Lifting off the paper filters, taking care not to touch the top sterile edge.

Figure 157   The contents of the tube are taken with sterile forceps by the scrub nurse.

Syringes and Hypodermic or Serum Needles (Non-disposable). These are rinsed thoroughly after use. Care must always be taken to remove blood from the inside of barrels and needles otherwise it will be impossible to sterilise them. An ultrasonic cleanser or good non-pyrogenic detergent such as Pyroneg, Biotergic, etc., should be used, and the needles checked for blockage by passing a stilette through.

Glass/metal special syringes are always dismantled before sterilisation; the different degrees of expansion between the metal and glass will cause cracking of the barrel. *All glass* syringes are sterilised assembled in the dry-heat oven or infra-red apparatus, and unassembled in the autoclave, as in the latter case it is possible that sufficient moist heat will not reach the piston of an assembled syringe.

With the exception of syringes having interchangeable barrels and pistons, care must be taken to avoid the exchange of components. Manufacturers generally engrave corresponding numbers or letters on the pistons and barrels to ensure correct assembly. Incorrect assembly may result in an ill-fitting piston.

If the syringes are to be sterilised by the dry-heat or pressure-steam method, after cleaning they should be carefully dried inside and out with acetone or ether before *very lightly* lubricating the piston with sterile liquid paraffin or silicone. solution. Silicone solution is preferable if the syringes are sterilised assembled as it obviates the risk of pistons becoming jammed in the barrel. They may then be wrapped individually in moisture permeable cellophane before being sterilised in packets, metal containers or glass tubes.

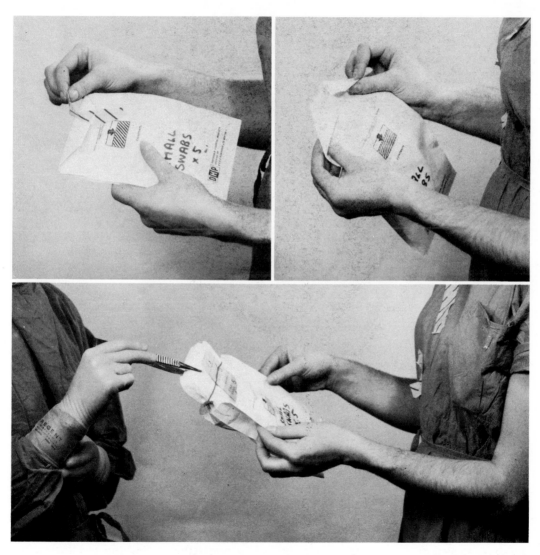

Figure 158   Supplementary items in folded top paper bags, 3M autoclave tape removed, opening first folds.

Figure 159   Utilising gusset to open remaining folds of bag.

Figure 160   Contents removed with sterile forceps.

Some special instruments such as cystoscopes, laryngoscopes and other endoscopic apparatus are made heat-sterilisable today, but manufacturers' instructions regarding sterilisation should be followed carefully. Endoscopes may be disinfected by 'pasteurisation' or by Formaldehyde at subatmospheric steam pressure, or in a chemical solution, e.g., Cidex, Hibitane 0·5 per cent. Ethylene oxide vapour can also be used if suitable apparatus and bacteriological control is available (Medical Research Council, 1968.

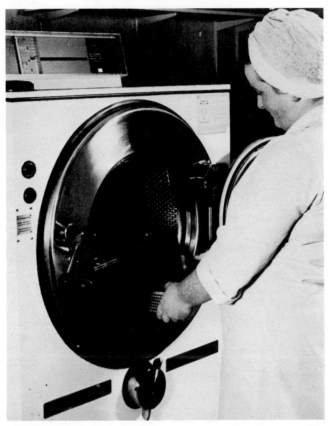

Figure 161   Helpex automatic washing machine for instruments and apparatus. The machine drum rotates in both directions, repeatedly plunging the moving items into a heated washing solution. Rinsing is accomplished by repeated immersion in hot water, cold water and, if desired, distilled water. Drying is accomplished by centrifuging to throw off water droplets, at the same time introducing a blast of hot (or cold) air. The cycle is controlled automatically by a punched card control system shown top left. (Sierex Ltd.)

After use, endoscopes are cleansed carefully, first under cold running water, and then in a hot detergent solution, special attention being given to the inside tube. A cotton-wool swab on a metal probe or a pipe cleaner will be found useful for cleaning and drying the inside of an endoscope. After drying, the instruments are lightly lubricated, inspected for general defects, including the lamps and lamp carriers which are tested before putting them away.

Non-disposable rubber drainage or suction tubing is washed through with cold water after use. The lumen of suction tubing can easily become blocked with hardened blood and debris caused by inefficient cleansing and repeated sterilisation. To avoid this, the tubing should be rolled between the hand and a board, or stretched in sections to dislodge any particles adherent to the lumen wall. The tubing is then flushed by attaching it to a pressure nozzle or tap and forcing cold water through it.

Following this, the tubing is washed with hot detergent solution and hung up to dry partially before sterilisation.

In most operating theatres a stock of assorted sterile drainage tubes is kept ready in nylon or paper packets. Special drains, such as Marian's suprapubic tubing for draining the bladder, are generally sterilised with the instruments when they are likely to be needed during an operation.

Non-disposable rubber catheters are cleansed as tubing, being rinsed through from the 'eye' end. After detergent washing and drying, the surface of a catheter must be examined for irregularities or deterioration and if found, the catheter should be discarded. A smooth surface is essential to avoid trauma to the delicate urethral mucosa.

Some catheters have an inflatable cuff or obturator bag which should always be tested before and after use.

Non-disposable Plastic Drainage Tubing and Catheters. Those made from vinyl resins (vinyl Portex), nylon, polythene, polypropylene, silicones and polycarbonates, are cleansed in a similar manner to rubber.

This type of tubing should be sterilised only when needed or stored dry in sterile packets. Many catheters are now supplied disposable and sterile in a packet.

Reusable Solution Rubber Gloves. These should be washed thoroughly in cold water before removing from the hands. They should be washed again in cold water to ensure complete removal of blood stains.

If the gloves have been used for a septic case they should be discarded. Following a clean case, they are scrubbed inside and out with a detergent solution.

The gloves are then dried either by hanging up until the outside is dry, turning, and then repeating the process, or rubbing each side with a towel whilst holding them on a warm surface.

Each glove is then tested for perforations by inflating with a foot pump, twisting the wristband so that the palm and fingers are under air pressure and plunging below the surface of a fluid (Williams *et al.*, 1966). Following this the sound gloves are finally dried and lightly powdered inside. Industrial methylated spirit may be used as the testing fluid to facilitate easy drying.

Gloves with perforations should be discarded as resistant tetanus spores may remain in the patch of a rubber glove.

Tests have shown that granulomata may form in wounds if a talcum glove powder is used. Talc deposition in the wound may occur if the surfaces of gloves are inadequately wiped before operation, or if a glove should become punctured during use.

Talc-free absorbable powders containing basically either starch or magnesium are less likely to cause this complication, although by 1965 the sixteenth case of starch granuloma had been reported (Bates, 1965). If this type of powder is used (Biosorb, K285, Diastol) only a minimum should be applied to the inside of the gloves only (British Medical Journal, 1973).

After powdering, the gloves are grouped in sizes, each cuff being folded over about 6·5 cm ($2\frac{1}{2}$ in). They are packed as pairs in separate paper or linen bags having two compartments, one for each glove. A small green or similarly dyed swab should be placed just inside the palm of each glove to ensure adequate penetration of the steam.

A small quantity of powder is required for use with each pair of gloves to lubricate the hands. This may be contained in small cellophane bags which are filled with about one teaspoonful of powder and placed *with the end open* in one compartment of the glove packet. Alternatively it is possible to purchase one brand of glove powder already packed in small sterilisable paper packets (Biosorb).

Regent, Velvex, Pioneer, etc. surgeon's disposable rubber gloves are also available. These are made from a latex rubber and are supplied presterilised together with a suitable glove powder. They are designed to be used only once for surgery but afterwards may be utilised in the wards and departments for non-sterile procedures.

Gum Elastic Catheters. These are now not often used as they are easily damaged and require very careful handling. They are cleansed in the usual manner, and after use *may* be submerged vertically in a suitable anti-bacterial agent such as Cidex or Hibitane 0·5 per cent. Ureteric catheters should be syringed through with a fine needle and syringe before resterilising and the lumen must be filled with the solution by means of a syringe and needle. Alternatively, formaldehyde at subatmospheric pressure may be used to sterilise these types of catheters.

Sterilisation by heat is always more reliable, and if this is difficult it may be advisable to consider using catheters made of a heat sterilisable material. It is for this reason that the latest forms of plastic are being found very useful for catheters and bougies.

REFERENCES

ALLEN, S. M. *et al.* (1965) *Lancet*, **ii**, 1343.
BATES, B. (1965) *Annals of Internal Medicine*, **62**, 335.
BRIGDEN, R. J. (1960) *The Nylon Packet System of Sterilisation*. London: Nursing Mirror.
BRIGDEN, R. J. (1964) *Nursing Times*, December 11.
BETHUNE, D. W., BLOWERS, R., PARKER, M. & PASK, E. A. (1965) *Lancet*, **ii**, 458.
BRITISH MEDICAL JOURNAL (1973) **ii**, 502.
FALK, H. C. (1942) *Operation Room Procedure for Nurses and Internes*, 3rd edn, pp. 24, 83. London: Putnam.
FORD, C. R., PETERSON, D. E. & MITCHELL, C. R. (1967) *American Journal of Surgery*, **6**, 787.
LOWBURY, E. J. L., LILLY, H. A. & BULL, J. P. (1964) *British Medical Journal*, **ii**, 531.
MEDICAL RESEARCH COUNCIL (1968) Aseptic methods in the operating suite. *Lancet*, **i**, 763.
MEDICAL DEFENCE COUNCIL AND ROYAL COLLEGE OF NURSING (1963) *Joint Memoranda on Safeguards to Remove Swabs*, etc.
MINISTRY OF HEALTH (1959) *Report on Subcommittee on Staphylococcal Infection in Hospitals*, p. 35. London: HMSO.
MINTER, S. (1952) *Theatre Technique for Nurses*, pp. 2, 10. London: Nursing Mirror.
SMYLIE, H. G., WEBSTER, C. V. & BRUCE, M. L. (1959) *British Medical Journal*, **ii**, 606.
SPEERS, R. & SHOOTER, R. A. (1966) *Lancet*, **ii**, 469.
WÄLLENBERG, E. & JÄRNHALL, B. (1956) *Svenska Läkartidningen*. **53**, 2578.
WILLIAMS, R. F. O., BLOWERS, R. & GARRARD, L. P. (1966) *Hospital Infection – Causes and Prevention*.
YEAGER, M. E. (1966) *Operating Room Manual*, 2nd edn, p. 18. London: Putnam.

6
Sterilisation

The sterilisation of materials used in an operating theatre is one of the most important aspects of theatre technique.

The main method of sterilisation (i.e. the destruction of all micro-organisms and spores) is by heat. However, gamma irradiation is being used for the sterilisation of catgut, catheters and bulk dressings, although at present the equipment required is too expensive for general hospital use (Jefferson, 1958; Darmady et al., 1961). Ultra-violet rays have a limited application for surface sterilisation providing the equipment is available for producing great intensities of light.

Disinfection (i.e. the destruction of all micro-organisms except spores) can be achieved by pasteurisation, sub-atmospheric steam and chemicals. The addition of formaldehyde to the sub-atmospheric steam process will effect sterilisation.

A great deal of research and many tests have been made regarding the minimal times and temperatures for sterilisation by a particular method. Times and temperatures quoted allow a margin of safety and are based upon bacteriologists' recommendations.

Bacteria and their destruction

We should recall our knowledge of the bacterial structure in order to appreciate fully its destruction.

A simple bacterium consists mainly of a cell wall surrounding protoplasm, which is a suspension of proteins in a solution of organic substances and salts.

One of the easiest ways of destroying bacteria is to upset the equilibrium of the proto-plasm. The simplest and surest way is to apply heat to cause some irreversible proto-plasmic change within the bacterial cell. This coagulation of protein depends to a great extent on the quantity of water contained by the bacteria. Vegetative bacteria contain about 80 per cent water, and as a result their protein coagulates readily at a relatively low temperature, and they are easily destroyed by five minutes' boiling (Perkins, 1956a). However, some bacteria contain within their protoplasm, oval or spherical bodies which will survive normal boiling. These bodies are called spores and our aim must be to destroy all bacteria and their spores during sterilisation.

The effect of moisture on the coagulation temperature of proteins bears a relationship to the temperatures at which bacteria are destroyed. Moist heat is a more efficient sterilising agent than dry heat, and when moisture is present bacteria are destroyed at much lower temperatures and shorter times than when moisture is absent.

When dry heat is used for sterilisation the process is primarily one of oxidation. Bacteria exposed to hot air may be dehydrated greatly before the temperature can rise sufficiently to cause death by coagulation. It is for this reason the death by dry heat is regarded as a slow burning up process or oxidation.

It is inadvisable to refer to the destruction of bacteria at a certain point (thermal death point) (McCulloch, 1945). A more accurate term refers to the combination of temperature and time (thermal death time); the higher the temperature the shorter the time. Generally speaking, a temperature of 121°C (250°F), at 15 lb per square inch (p.s.i.) of pressure steam for 15 minutes, will kill the most resistant spores. This timing commences only *when the correct temperature of steam has reached* **all** *parts of the materials being sterilised.* It is therefore considered necessary to allow a safety margin of time equivalent usually to about double the thermal death time to ensure adequate penetration of packets. However, *it is necessary to conduct individual tests to determine the penetration time with a particular type of autoclave and packet.*

Sterilisation by dry heat requires much higher thermal death times. As bacteria show a marked resistance to dry heat, a temperature in the region of 160°C (320°F) and an exposure of one hour are essential. This exposure period of one hour does not, of course, include the period of time necessary for all parts of the load to reach the temperature of 160°C (320°F).

Although dry heat is destructive to rubber and fabrics, it can be used for the sterilisation of glassware and instruments, such as fine knives, made from carbon steel which may otherwise rust if exposed to moist heat, and where sterilisation of surfaces only is required.

The effect of chemicals on bacteria is rather a complex action which varies with the nature of the chemicals used. A chemical reaction occurs between the bacteria and the chemical, being dependent on several factors including temperature, chemical strength, resistance of the organism and, most important, the duration of free contact between the two.

METHODS OF STERILISATION (GENERAL PRINCIPLES)

HEAT STERILISATION
1. Autoclaving (steam under pressure).
2. Dry heat.
3. Steam/formaldehyde (at Sub-atmospheric pressure).

HEAT DISINFECTION
3. Steam at sub-atmospheric pressure.
4. Pasteurisation.
5. Boiling.

COLD STERILISATION
6. Irradiation.
7. Ethylene Oxide.
8. Ultra-violet light radiation.

COLD DISINFECTION
9. Various chemical solutions.

Heat Sterilisation

1. Autoclaving

This is by far the most efficient method of sterilisation for materials that will stand up to heat and moisture (Medical Research Council, 1968).

The highest temperature which may be reached by boiling water in an open vessel is 100°C (212°F). With increased pressures, the water can be raised to much higher temperatures before it boils, e.g., at a pressure of 5 lb p.s.i. the temperature reaches 105·5°C (222°F); at 10 lb p.s.i. 115°C (239°F); and at 15 lb p.s.i. the temperature will reach 121°C (250°F), etc.

High pressures of steam, however, are not the only consideration for efficient sterilisation, as a pressure may be due to a mixture of air and steam with a relatively low temperature (McCulloch, 1945). It is the high temperatures which really matter but, in addition, the steam should be at a point where it has just changed from water into steam (phase boundary steam) (Walter, 1948). In this condition the steam not only has an increased temperature in relation to the pressure (sensible heat), but when it condenses on a cold surface (the materials being sterilised) a great deal of extra heat (latent heat) is given up. The latent heat absorbed by the materials being sterilised is more important for the destruction of bacteria than the sensible heat.

This steam heating of fabrics being sterilised by a process of condensation is relatively rapid (McCulloch, 1945), as compared with dry-heat sterilisation, which is slow, heat being conducted from one instrument to another and from one container to the next, etc.

The physical process of heating the fabrics to the sterilising temperature can be described as follows:

In a sterilising chamber (autoclave) which has been well exhausted of air the steam entering promptly fills the free spaces surrounding the load. As steam contacts the cool outer layers of the fabrics a film of steam condenses, leaving a minute quantity of moisture in the fibres of the fabrics. Air contained in the fabric interstices, being heavier than steam, is displaced by gravity in a downward direction, and the latent heat given off during the process of condensation is absorbed by that layer of the fabrics.

The next film of steam immediately fills the space created when the first film condensed into water, and it does not condense on the outer layer of the fabrics but penetrates into the second layer, condenses and heats it. This process continues until the whole load is heated through, and no further condensation occurs, the temperature within the packet or drum remaining at that of the surrounding steam.

If initial air elimination from the chamber is not good it will be difficult for the steam to displace air from the interstices of the fabrics, due to the small difference in density between the air pockets in the packets or drums, and the air which has gravitated below the load to the bottom of the chamber. This means that the pocketed air and steam may eventually mix, but it will be impossible to attain a sterilising temperature which is equivalent to that of the surrounding steam without prolonged exposure. A procedure involving a double- or multi-vacuum technique helps to extract this air and thoroughly heat the load before sterilisation commences. Exceptions to this rule are instruments, which require only one pre-vacuum as the air displacement from these loads is comparatively rapid if they are packed correctly.

In the Gravity Displacement Autoclave after a partial vacuum of about 20 in of mercury has been created, (an absolute pressure of 10 in of mercury, 250 mm Hg or 250 Torr), steam is admitted to the chamber and applied to the load until the selected temperature/pressure has been reached *in the chamber*. (Very low pressures are generally quoted with reference to the perfect vacuum. For this purpose a unit called the Torr is used; named after Evangelista Toricelli (1608–1647) who invented the mercury barometer. The Torr is equal to the pressure exerted by a column of mercury 1 mm high. Standard atmospheric pressure is 760 Torr on this scale – a perfect vacuum, 0 Torr.) Air from the interstices of the fabrics which has been displaced into the lower part of the chamber, but has not been discharged by the special thermostatic condensate release valve, is extracted by a second vacuum. A second application of steam displaces most of the remaining air pockets and thoroughly heats the load throughout to the surrounding steam temperature.

In the high-vacuum/high-pressure autoclave where an electric pump is used to obtain a vacuum, all air may be extracted in one operation or there may be a series of pre-vacuums and steam pulsations before the sterilising cycle. This breaks down any small airpockets and results in a final pre-vacuum of within 0·5 to 1·0 Torr.

It will be observed that the steam used for sterilisation of materials must have a certain temperature and pressure in order to be optimally effective. Furthermore, the steam must reach all parts of the load and unless packets or boxes are prepared very carefully, adequate penetration cannot be ensured. Materials should be packed with good spacing between the articles, with folds placed vertically to allow steam to pass easily in a downward direction through them, any tendency to force too many items in one packet or box being avoided. It should not be necessary to compress the box contents in order to close the lid, neither must a linen or paper packet be wrapped tightly to fit in an inade-quate size of cover.

Unless a pre-set tray is used, utilising heavy-gauge aluminium trays (p. 104) it is difficult to sterilise large quantities of instruments with bulky drapes. The unequal rate of condensation between the fabrics and instruments will require an extended drying cycle.

Arrangements for the correct supply of steam and maintenance of the apparatus is not a responsibility of the nurse, but if dressings are wet or damaged when removed from the autoclave there is something wrong with the apparatus or its operation and the engineer should be consulted.

Sterilisation by Autoclaving (application of methods)

Most hospitals use 'mains' steam (supplied from the boiler house) to operate autoclaves which are generally of two types, (1) the downward or gravity displacement type, and (2) the modern high-vacuum/high-pressure type. For hospitals without a mains steam supply, autoclaves are available which generate their own steam either by electricity or gas, and they are used in a very similar manner to the mains steam models.

The Gravity Displacement Autoclave

This works at a pressure of 18 to 30 lb p.s.i. producing a vacuum of between 380 to 250 Torr (15 to 20 in Hg, 380 to 508 mm Hg) via an ejector valve. It consists basically of a circular or rectangular metal chamber, surrounded by a hollow jacket of a similar material, being designed to withstand pressures of steam in excess of those in use. A suitable door, also designed to withstand high pressures of steam, and controlled by a single hand wheel, is fitted to one or both ends. The autoclave may be installed between two rooms, the materials to be sterilised being placed in the chamber from one room (the soiled side), and removed from the other (the clean side).

Steam reaching the autoclave from the boiler house is usually at a much higher pressure than required. A reducing valve reduces this pressure of from 50 or 80 lb p.s.i. to the level required and prevents any greater pressure of steam entering the autoclave than the maximum pressure at which it is designed to operate.

TO STERILISE

1. The inner chamber is loaded with packets or boxes which are placed in such a way that free passage of steam through the material is possible. This usually means placing the packets or boxes on their sides so that the steam passes through the folded layers. As steam is lighter than the air which is displaced it should enter the chamber at the top, pass through the load, and be discharged at the bottom through the thermostatic release valve.

2. The door is securely closed with the bolts 'well home' and must not be open again until the sterilisation is complete and the chamber pressure gauge reads zero.

There are two important gauges which are fitted to an autoclave, one recording the jacket pressure and one the chamber pressure. The pressure in the jacket may be kept on all day, but that in the chamber rises only when the appropriate valve is opened. Another essential accessory is the provision of a thermometer in the steam condensate release or discharge line, and when the correct temperature in relation to the pressure used has been reached by this thermometer the sterilisation cycle is commenced.

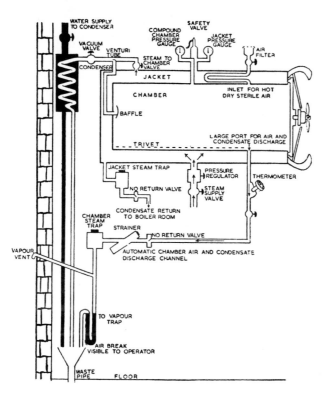

Figure 162   Diagram of a steam-pressure steriliser of the gravity air displacement type.
(J. M. Bowie – by kind permission.)

3. The first cycle is an initial vacuum, which is created and held for about 5 minutes, followed by the admittance of steam to the chamber. When the selected temperature/pressure has been reached *in the chamber*, a second vacuum is created and also held for 5 minutes (except for instruments). On the gravity displacement autoclave there is a limiting factor to the greatest degree of vacuum obtainable. With some types, fitted with a powerful ejector, this may be in the region of 300 to 250 Torr (18 in to 20 in Hg, 457 to 508 mm Hg) of mercury, but the average vacuum does not usually exceed 380 Torr (15 in Hg, 381 mm Hg).

4. In the second cycle the steam is admitted to the chamber again and raised to the selected temperature/pressure. For dressings, gowns and instruments, etc., in packets and boxes a temperature/pressure of 126°C (259°F) at 20 p.s.i. is maintained for 30 minutes.

Gloves and instruments on open trays should be sterilised at 130°C (266°F) at 25 lb p.s.i. for 6 minutes, and the former must be packed reasonably loosely to ensure good penetration of steam. This higher temperature of steam will not cause deterioration of the rubber, for it is the quantity of air left in the autoclave after the initial vacuum and the period of drying afterwards that really matters (Medical Research Council, 1959; Wells and Whitwell, 1960; Knox, 1961).

A vacuum of 250 Torr (20 in Hg, 508 mm Hg) means that only two-thirds of the air has been removed from the chamber. As steam enters it tends to rise rapidly, forcing the

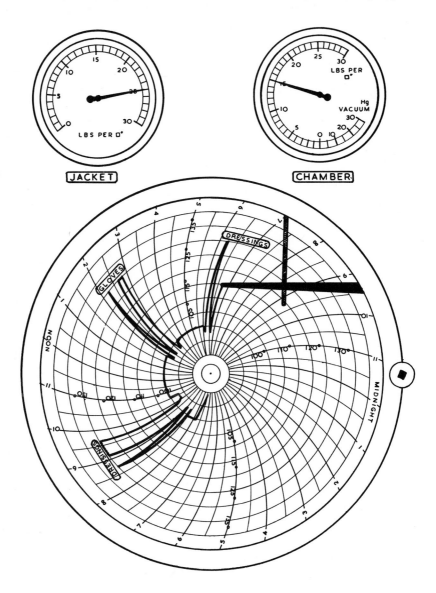

Figure 163 Autoclave jacket and chamber pressure gauges, time/temperature recorder chart, mounted on recessed panel. Dressings sterilisation cycle in progress, showing double-vacuum technique when the initial air elimination is a half to two-thirds of the chamber.

remaining air in a downward direction and through the thermostatic condensate release valve, and gloves should therefore be placed in the upper part of the chamber with their fingertips up or lying horizontally. In this position they will be exposed to practically pure steam for the greater period of sterilisation, sterility is assured and their life will be extended considerably.

If possible gloves should not be used until 24 hours after sterilisation, as the tensile strength will considerably improve, apparently due to the fact that rubber will give up excess moisture fairly quickly, but the last remaining amount of moisture comes off very slowly. If gloves are only slightly moist when put on, they are liable to become torn and this rest period seems to minimise the difficulty.

During this second steam cycle the holding time is correlated to the temperature indicated by the thermometer in the discharge line, which is always the coldest part of the chamber. During the period of sterilisation this thermometer must register one of the following temperatures and the holding time from this point must be *not less than the time period stated*:

130°C (275°F) for 3 minutes.
130°C (266°F) for 4 minutes.
125°C (259°F) for 8 minutes.
121°C (250°F) for 12 minutes.
115°C (240°F) for 18 minutes.

This is the temperature and time at which all parts of the load must be held and *it is advisable to increase the time by 50 per cent of that stated to ensure absolute safety*. The appropriate composite holding times and temperatures listed in Figure 170 allow this margin of safety.

5. The steam is released from the chamber, and the materials, with the exception of gloves, are dried in a vacuum for 40 minutes to one hour. Gloves need only 6 minutes drying from the time the vacuum reaches 450 Torr (12 in Hg, 305 mm Hg), providing the gloves are packed in individual *paper* bags before placing in the packets or boxes.

The moisture remaining finely distributed in the dressings, etc., during the period of sterilisation is at the same temperature as the surrounding steam. As soon as the pressure is reduced and the steam exhausted this moisture flashes into vapour by virtue of the residual heat in the fabrics and from the surrounding hot jacket, the temperatures of which are above boiling point. The real drying process therefore consists of getting rid of this steam vapour as fast as it forms.

This constitutes the final cycle of sterilisation, and with an efficient autoclave using steam at phase boundary point it should not be necessary to suck in air, which may be contaminated, except to break the vacuum. The air required for breaking the vacuum must be well-filtered, to avoid recontamination of the load, using a release valve incorporating a high efficiency filter such as one made from glass fibre or ceramic material. This filter may be disinfected during the steam cycle by allowing free steam to permeate through it.

6. After the correct period of drying the autoclave is switched off, the vacuum broken, *and when the chamber pressure gauge reads zero*, the door is opened. The operator should wash his hands and don a clean overall before unloading the chamber. The date of sterilisation and batch number should be applied to packets and boxes by means of a length of cellulose tape imprinted with the word STERILE at intervals throughout the roll.

STERILITY TESTS

It is a good practice to use some form of test material placed in the packets or boxes to indicate adequate sterilisation.

Chemical indicator tubes are reliable if stored properly and these should be placed in the centre of packets and boxes before sterilisation.

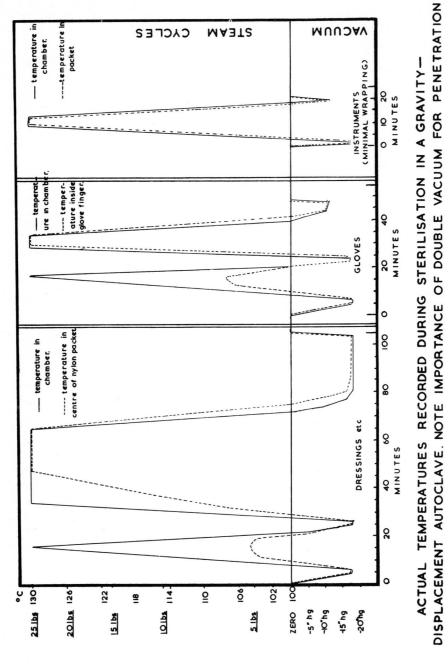

Figure 164　Record of sterilising temperature showing double-vacuum technique.

The fluid contained in these Browne's tubes changes colour when the correct sterilising procedure has been accomplished (Howie and Timbury, 1956). The change can be compared with that of the traffic signals, from red, through yellow to finally green, when the correct temperature and time have been attained. It is important to store these tubes at a temperature of less than 21°C (70°F), otherwise there may be a variable degree of premature chemical reaction, resulting in inaccurate readings when used for test purposes.

Browne's tubes are manufactured in four different types, covering the sterilisation of articles in gravity displacement autoclaves, high-vacuum/high-pressure autoclaves, dry-heat ovens and dry-heat conveyor ovens. These four types are:

Type One: Black Spot, for the sterilisation of dressings, gowns and gloves, etc., in the gravity displacement autoclave. Safety is indicated after 10 minutes at 125°C (259°F) or approximately 6 minutes at 130°C (266°F).

Type Two: Yellow Spot, for the sterilisation of all articles in the high-vacuum/high-pressure autoclave. Safety is indicated after 3·5 minutes at 130°C (266°F).

Type Three: Green Spot, for the sterilisation of syringes, glassware and instruments, etc., by the dry-heat process in a dry-oven. Safety is indicated after one hour at 160°C (320°F).

Type Four: Blue Spot, for sterilisation by the dry-heat process in an infra-red conveyor oven. Safety is indicated after 45 minutes at 160°C (320°F).

In all cases the tubes are operative over a range of temperatures and times. A lower temperature must be compensated by a longer exposure, and vice versa.

In some operating departments a separate box or packet is used, into which are placed some of the indicator tubes, and after being processed in the lower portion of the autoclave this is opened immediately. If the tubes have not changed colour correctly several other packets are opened aseptically, their tubes checked, and if the liquid is amber or red the batch is re-sterilised and a fresh tube used after the functioning of the autoclave has been checked.

Other chemical test indicators are available including Steamclox (a card with segments which change from pink to green according to time/temperature reached), and Diack controls, a tube containing a chemical tablet which changes colour in a similar manner.

Although these chemical test-tubes indicate the correct working of the autoclave they do not actually show the lethal effect of the sterilising procedure. Bacteriologists therefore prepare a test packet containing usually the spores of an organism of the thermophil group such as *Bacillus stearothermophilus*, which is extremely resistant to heat, and this may be placed in a packet or drum before sterilisation. After exposure to the sterilising process the packet is returned unopened to the bacteriologist for examination. However, bacteriological tests of an autoclave are not necessary for routine use and should be restricted to use as an occasional check on sterilising efficiency for the test takes up to three days to complete.

Another method of checking whether adequate temperatures are being attained by all parts of a load is by the use of thermocouples or electrical thermometers (Howie, 1961). These thermometers are placed in various positions within the packet or drum, and are connected to a control panel via wires which are contained in fibre-glass insulation. These wires pass either between the door gasket and its seating or for preference a special nipple in the chamber wall (especially applicable to high-vacuum/high-pressure autoclaves) and are placed in position before the door is closed. The temperatures may be checked at any time duing the period of sterilisation and rate of steam penetration to various parts of the load is clearly shown.

A very important addition to the autoclave is a time chart recording the sterilising procedures. This chart will indicate the vacuum, temperatures and relative times of each sterilising load, and is a reliable check for the operating theatre or service unit-supervisor, who is often unable to supervise every sterilising load. Once the correct temperatures and timings have been decided any variation by the autoclave operator is easily observed and the record chart is permanent for future reference. Recordings of pressure only are of no value as they do not indicate the temperatures attained, owing to the variable degree of mixture with air.

The High-vacuum/High-pressure autoclave

This works at a pressure in the region of 32 to 35 lb p.s.i. and a temperature of 134°C (275°F) to 136°C (280°F). A high-vacuum pump removes air from the chamber before sterilisation down to an almost complete vacuum of 0·5–1·0 Torr /0·5–1·0 mm Hg). The process is controlled automatically.

Although in earlier models of this apparatus attempts were made to obtain a high vacuum in one stage, it has been found that utilising a vacuum pump only will not achieve a vacuum much lower than 20 Torr (20 mm Hg). This was followed by steam at 134°C (275°F) for 3 minutes, a post vacuum of varying degree and admission of filtered air to the chamber. This type of cycle did not give consistent results for they often depended upon how the chamber was loaded and the kind of materials being sterilised.

Research has shown that a pre-vacuum/steam pulsation technique will achieve a much better removal of air from the autoclave chamber before sterilisation (Bolton, 1966; Knox and Pickerill, 1967). Basically, steam pulsation technique consists of allowing a charge of steam to enter the chamber after an initial high vacuum has been drawn, then following this by another vacuum draw and repeating the process to give two or more steam pulses. The logic is that any residual air is diluted each time and replaced with water vapour; each steam pulse and vacuum draw resulting in repeated reduction of air content without reducing the total pressure in the chamber. The high-vacuum/high-pressure autoclave relies upon a pre-vacuum stage which reduces the air content in the chamber to 1 mm Hg or less.

With negligible air in the chamber and some pre-heating of the load, penetration of steam into the items being sterilised is very rapid. High temperatures in the region of 134°C (275°F) are reached very quickly and an exposure to this temperature for 3·5 minutes will ensure sterility. It is important though, as mentioned previously, that all parts of the load must reach this temperature before timing commences. For automatic control of process a simple and accurate means of measuring the partial air pressure (pre-vacuum) and a load simulator which simulates the conditions within the packet or cardboard box are required. This obviates the need for a thermocouple within the load to control the process.

Depending on the size of autoclave chamber the total cycle in this type of autoclave is between 25 and 35 minutes. The chamber can be fully loaded with soft packets providing a few inches of space is allowed between the load and the chamber wall. An angled condensate plate should be fitted underneath each shelf on which pre-set trays are being sterilised. These slope downwards to one or other side of the chamber in order to prevent drips of condensate from the lower surface of a tray above wetting a tray below. (Fig. 119, p. 113).

THE CYCLE OF OPERATION

For a high-vacuum/high-pressure autoclave, this can be summarised as follows.

After loading the chamber and closing the door:

Stage 1. Pre-vacuum. The air is removed from the chamber by a vacuum pump and controlled steam pulsations. The vacuum achieved should be in the order of 0·5 to 1·0 Torr (0·5 to 1·0 mm Hg).

Stage 2. Sterilisation. Steam is admitted to the chamber and when all parts of the load have reached a temperature of 134°C (275°F) this is maintained for 3·5 minutes.

Stage 3. Drying. Achieved by an adequate post vacuum, checked periodically by a test packet of huckaback towels which when removed from the autoclave, unfolded and allowed to cool are not sensibly damp.

Stage 4. Breaking the Vacuum. This should be completed within 3 minutes, through a glass fibre or ceramic type filter having a methylene blue penetration of not more than 0·003 per cent.

The chamber is unloaded and the packets date stamped together if desired with the batch number of that particular load. Pre-set trays should have a plastic dust cover applied, especially if they are to be stored for more than a few hours. This cover should be applied only after the trays have cooled off.

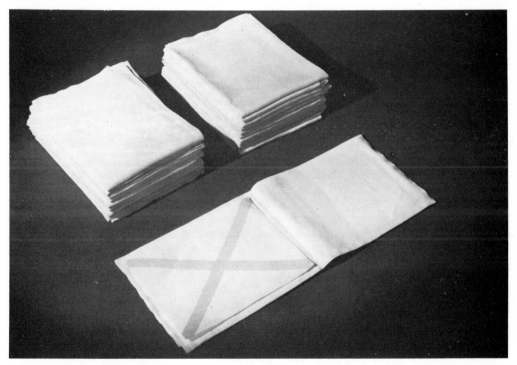

Figure 165   3M Autoclave Tape No 1222, crossed on the centre towel of a pile of 36 hucka-back towels, 36in by 36in folded to 12in by 12in and freshly laundered. This is tied up and placed in a Bripac box and then autoclaved *alone* in the autoclave. (3M Co. Ltd.)

STERILISER FUNCTION TESTS

These should be performed daily and the two most effective are the Bowie/Dick indicator tape test and the chamber vacuum leak test. The high-vacuum/high-pressure autoclave is a complex piece of machinery. Machines should have built-in safeguards which interrupt the sterilisation cycle if faults occur but this is not always so and the autoclave may appear to function correctly when in fact it is not.

A possible fault relates to inadequate extraction of air from the chamber during the pre-vacuum cycle. It may be due to a faulty pump but equally because air has leaked back through faulty door-seals or valves. This means that steam can penetrate the load only slowly and in an irregular way, which may result in unsterile packets.

The Bowie/Dick Indicator Tape Test. This test is a means of determining the efficiency of air removal from the steriliser chamber during the pre-vacuum cycle. It does not indicate directly that sterilisation is achieved, but that an adequate vacuum has been created to allow sterilisation to take place at 134°C (275°F) for 3·5 minutes or 126°C (259°F) for 12 minutes. In practice this is very simple. A standard test pack is made up con-

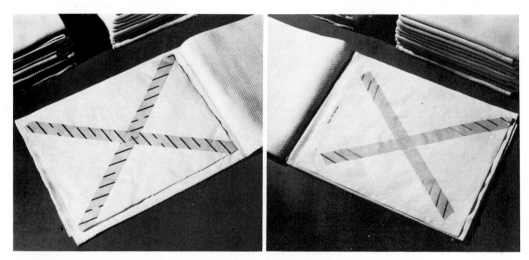

Figure 166   Tape showing a satisfactory result with uniform colour change.

Figure 167   This is an unsatisfactory result – the colour change is irregular and incomplete in the centre.

sisting of 36 huckaback towels, 6 square feet, (complying with B.S.I. 1781. TL. 5) folded and forming a stack 10 to 11 in (25 to 28 cm) high (Bowie, 1961; Bowie *et al.*, (1963). In the centre is placed a piece of paper 12 in (30 cm) square to which has been fixed a cross of 3M indicator tape No. 1222, such as is widely used for sealing packets, indicating they have been autoclaved. Alternatively, a sheet consisting entirely of the basic indicator tape material can be used. The towels should be washed initially before using and whenever they become soiled or discoloured. Between tests they are unfolded and hung out to air for at least one hour.

The test pack is placed in an autoclavable cardboard box (Bripac/Permapak) or wrapped in fabric or paper. It is now placed *by itself* in the autoclave and subjected to a standard sterilising cycle. Care must be taken to ensure that the 'Holding' or 'Sterilising' time does not exceed 3·5 minutes at 134°C (275°F) or 12 minutes at 126°C (259°F). If the automatic cycle is set for a longer holding time this must be cut short, for the purposes of the test, to 3·5 minutes, by using the manual control. Should there be any doubt about this the engineer should be asked for advice.

When the cycle is finished the pack is removed and the paper with the tape cross examined. After a satisfactory run the tape will show a colour change *which is the same at the centre as the edges*. If the tape at the centre is paler than it is at the edges it means there was a bubble of air there and the steriliser was not working correctly. If this happens the autoclave must be taken out of service immediately until the fault has been rectified.

Unless the test is carried out exactly as described it may not be truly reliable. In particular the following points should be noted.

1. The more air there is to remove, the more exacting will be the test, that is why the test pack is used by itself in an otherwise empty chamber.

2. The exact colour change shown by the processed tape may depend upon the storage conditions of that tape. The important thing is whether the *same colour change* occurs at the centre and the edges.

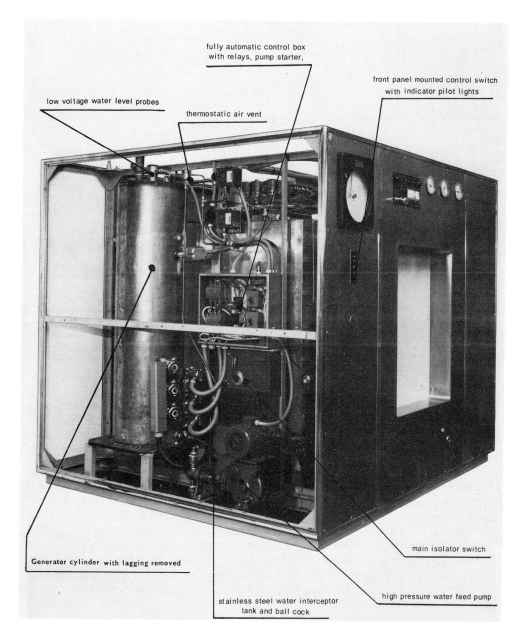

Figure 168   High-Vacuum/High-Pressure autoclave with steam generator. (British Steriliser Ltd.)

3. The contrast in colour change from centre to edge will be reduced to an unreadable level if long 'holding' periods are used. That is why the *'holding' period must not exceed 3·5 minutes at 134°C.* Even an extra minute or two may seriously affect a comparison of results.

4. *Because of this it is very important to realise that if an autoclave fails to pass the Bowie/Dick test as described, it cannot be made safe merely by increasing the 'holding' time until a uniform colour change is produced. Such a steriliser is in urgent need of skilled attention.*

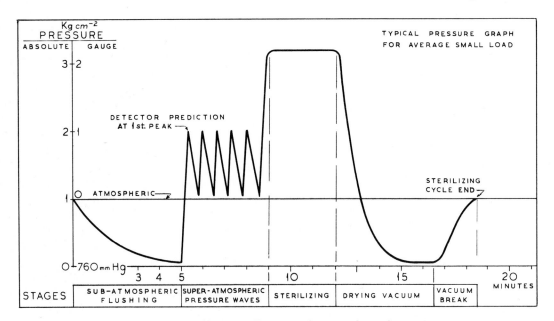

Figure 169   Graph showing hi-vac cycles. (British Steriliser Ltd.)

The Vacuum and Leak Test (instrumentation required). In order to carry out this test the autoclave requires additional instrumentation fitted, which is capable of measuring small variations in the degree of vacuum attainable within the chamber. Some autoclaves already incorporate the necessary instrumentation but modifications can be made to existing machines as follows:

1. The control camshift is modified so that a position can be obtained manually directly subsequent to the *'pre-vacuum'* position, when all valves on the camshaft are closed. This position should have a location cam and a significant reference mark on the camshaft position indicator, known as the *'leak test'* position.

2. A 0 to 100 mm Hg (0 to 100 Torr) absolute pressure gauge (tolerance ± one per cent F.S. reading) is mounted on the front panel, and connected via a manual valve directly beneath it in series with an electrical solenoid valve (normally closed) to the chamber by the shortest route in copper pipe of at least 0·25 in (0·6 cm) diameter, in such a way that the pipe will drain into the chamber.

The solenoid should be operated by a micro-switch actuated by the control camshaft so that the valve is opened only when the camshaft is in the 'pre-vacuum' and the 'leak test' positions.

3. A toggle switch is mounted on the front panel adjacent to the absolute pressure

gauge. This switch is wired in series with the coil of the vacuum pump motor contactor, so that the contactor may be de-energised and the motor stopped.

4. A Smith's or similar 0 to 30 minute timer is useful mounted on the front panel adjacent to the absolute pressure gauge.

5. An extra outlet may be fitted in parallel with, and adjacent to the absolute pressure gauge so that the gauge can be calibrated regularly against either a standard gauge or mercury column.

Note: Any other method may be used provided that the chamber is isolated by the valves which are normally used during a process, so that they are tested for leakage.

The recommended post-vacuum pressure should be less than 50 Torr (50 mm Hg absolute pressure) and it is possible to modify the camshaft in such a way that the solenoid valve to the leak test gauge can be opened and the post-vacuum pressure checked.

From this rather technical description of the instrumentation required the reader may imagine that the actual test is equally complex. This is not so for the vacuum and leak test can be conducted effectively by any supervisor of an operating suite or operating theatre service unit.

Method of performing the test (autoclave instrumentated as described):

1. Close and lock the door with the chamber empty. The steriliser must be on manual control.

2. Turn the control cam-shaft to *'pre-vacuum'* position and open manual valve beneath the absolute pressure gauge.

3. When the pressure indicated on the absolute pressure gauge is less than 20 Torr, turn the control camshaft to *'leak test'* position and wait 10 seconds for the vacuum valve to close.

4. Turn the toggle switch to the *'off'* position and wait until the needle on the absolute pressure gauge starts to return.

5. When the gauge needle starts to return, take a reading, set and start the timer for 10 minutes. When the times reaches zero take another reading on the absolute pressure gauge.

6. Close the manual valve beneath the absolute pressure gauge and turn the toggle switch to *'on'*.

7. Rotate the control camshaft to *'post-vacuum'* position and hold for 4 minutes. Note the reading on the absolute pressure gauge and rotate control camshaft once again to the *'break-vacuum'* or *'off'* position. Finally where applicable press the automatic *re-set* button and with the control camshaft in the *'off'* position, the door may be opened.

The test can be deemed a failure if the vacuum fails to reach 20 Torr, or the leak at stage 4 is greater than 10 Torr in 10 minutes. If this result is obtained skilled engineering assistance must be obtained and the cause of the fault investigated immediately.

The high-vacuum/high-pressure autoclave is a very effective method of steam sterilisation, providing regular efficiency tests and maintenance are instituted. It may not be possible to perform the vacuum and leak tests due to the appropriate instrumentation being non-existent. However, the Bowie/Dick Test must be carried out daily as described and will provide a reliable means of assessing the efficiency of the autoclave.

2. Dry Heat (in the Form of Hot Air)

This can be used for sterilising many items, but is destructive to linen and rubber or plastic articles, etc. (Perkins, 1956).

Certain articles can be sterilised easily and safely, including non-disposable syringes, glassware, needles, mechanical drills (especially the compressed air types), fine knives

MATERIALS BEING STERILISED	INITIAL VACUUM (Twice)		INITIAL STEAM CYCLE		STERILISING STEAM CYCLE			FINAL VACUUM (Drying)		TOTAL CYCLE (Approx.)
	Degree	Holding Time	Pressure	Temperature	Pressure	Temperature	Holding Time	Degree	Holding Time	
Gowns, towels, dressings, etc.; in PAPER, or LINEN PACKETS	300 to 250 Torr	5 min (each time)	20 lb 25 lb	125°C, 259°F 130°C, 266°F	20 lb 25 lb	125°C, 259°F 130°C, 266°F	30 min 25 min	300 to 250 Torr	40 min 30 min	90 min 75 min
Metal instruments on open trays, ligatures, etc.	Not needed		Not needed		25 lb	130°C, 266°F	6 min	Not needed		7 min
Metal instruments with minimal wrappings, ligatures, etc.	Not needed		Not needed		25 lb	130°C, 266°F	6 min	450 Torr	1 to 2 min	9 min
Metal instruments, ligatures, etc., in packets with normal wrappings	300 to 250 Torr	5 min (once only)	Not needed		25 lb	130°C, 266°F	15 min	300 to 250 Torr	7 to 10 min	27 to 30 min
Rubber gloves. (With gloves in upper part of chamber)	300 to 250 Torr	5 min (once only)	25 lb 32 lb	130°C, 266°F 134°C, 275°F	25 lb 32 lb	130°C, 266°F 134°C, 275°F	6 min 3 min	450 Torr 450 Torr	5 min 3 min	30 min 20 min
Intravenous fluids	Not needed		Not needed		10 lb 15 lb	116°C, 240°F 121°C, 250°F	60 min 45 min	Gradual exhaust of steam from chamber		...

Figure 170 Table of sterilisation by heat. A. Steam autoclave, gravity or downward displacement type.

Materials Being Sterilised	Initial Vacuum	Sterilising Steam Cycle	Final Vacuum (Drying)	Total Cycle
Gowns, towels, dressings, metal instruments etc., in packets or boxes	Approximately 0·5 to 1·0 Torr	$3\frac{1}{2}$ mins 134°C, (275°F)	5 to 10 min	Approximately 25 min

C. Dry-Heat Steriliser

Articles Being Sterilised	Period
Syringes, compressed air drills, some types of electric drills and saws, powders, osteotomes, etc.	With efficient circulation of hot air these should be exposed for a period of 60 minutes when the temperature has reached 160°C (320°F) in all parts of the load. This may mean a total cycle of between $1\frac{1}{2}$ to $2\frac{1}{2}$ hours, or more.

D. Boiling (disinfection)

Articles Being Disinfected	Period
All clean boilable metal instruments, glassware, etc.	Boil for 5 minutes, and ensure that they are completely covered.
Contaminated instruments, etc.	Boil for $\frac{1}{2}$ hour, allow to cool and boil for a further $\frac{1}{2}$ hour, precautions as above.

E. Pasteurisation

Articles Being Disinfected	Period
Non- boilable endoscopes (cystoscopes, etc.)	Maintain in a hot-water bath at 75°C (167°F) for 10 minutes (ensure they are completely covered and allow time for water to regain temperature when cool endoscope is added to the bath). Process in subatmospheric steam/formaldehyde autoclave at 82°C (180°F) for 90 minutes, total-cycle approximately $2\frac{1}{2}$ hours.

Figure 171 Table of sterilisation by heat. B. Steam autoclave, high-vacuum, high-pressure type.

and other delicate instruments which will withstand this dry heat but not the wet methods. Very suitable containers for sterilisation and storage can be made from aluminium tulle-gas boxes after they have been emptied. Larger items can be folded in sheets of aluminium foil, but care must be taken not to compress the packets unduly as puncture of the foil may occur.

A special electric oven is used, designed to achieve a uniform temperature in all parts of the apparatus. There are two types: (1) the gravity convection type, and (2) the mechanical convection type.

The Gravity Convection Type

This is limited to a small size, usually not exceeding about 1 ft^3 (0·027 m^3), has heaters in the base and sides, and relies upon air circulation according to the slight temperature differences of various parts of the chamber. Heated air rises and cooler air descends, being displaced by it. As the warm air ascends it gives off some of its heat to the load and at the same time the descending cool air is warmed as it passes over the heaters. The warm air now rises, the cool air descends again and the process is repeated, setting up gravity convection currents.

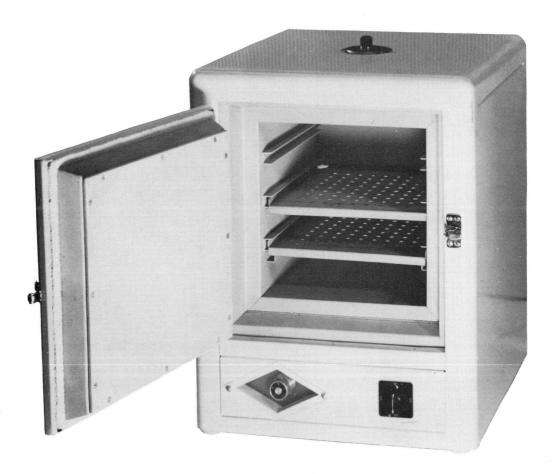

Figure 172   Dry-heat steriliser. (Laboratory Thermal Equipment Ltd.)

The Mechanical Convection Type

This utilises a motor blower to circulate the air.

The heater bank is contained in a chamber on one side, and separated from the working chamber by a perforated diffuser wall. An adjustable air inlet opens into the heater chamber directly in front of the heater bank and motor blower. Air is drawn through the air inlet over the heaters and is forced into the working chamber through another diffuser wall on the opposite side of the chamber. As the warm air gives off some of its heat to the load it passes back into the heater chamber, mixes with the incoming fresh air, and the process is repeated. This good circulation of warm air ensures even and rapid heating of the load being sterilised.

With both types of dry-heat sterilisers, *when all parts of the load* have attained the required temperature of 160°C (320°F), timing is commenced and should consist of at least one hour's exposure. The period necessary for even heating to be achieved varies considerably with the capacity of the oven, type of load and the containers in which the articles are packed. With the gravity convection steriliser, articles packed in aluminium boxes may require a total exposure of up to two and a half hours, and needles in glassine envelopes one and a half hours. With the mechanical convection steriliser this time can usually be reduced to one and a half hours and 80 minutes respectively. However, individual tests must be made with a particular oven using suitable Browne's tubes, green spot, stearothermophillus spore papers, and where possible a check by the engineer with thermocouples or electrical thermometers placed in the centre of the load.

Where disposable syringes are not in use some hospitals use the dry-heat method for their syringe service (Medical Research Council, 1945). The syringes are carefully cleansed, first with cold water, then Pyroneg, Biotergic, etc., or an ultrasonic cleaner, followed by acetone or ether to remove fat, etc., and the barrels are finally *very lightly* lubricated with a silicone solution. They are packed into containers which may be sealed before placing in the dry-heat steriliser. A useful container is one made as an aluminium tube, with a metal cap sealed in position over the open end. Alternatively glass tubes can be used and the open end occluded with a cotton-wool plug, although over-heating may lead to charring of it.

Infra-red ovens are more satisfactory for the sterilisation of syringes as better penetration of heat is achieved with a shorter exposure. The syringes are passed through the oven on a continuous conveyor-belt which is adjusted in speed to allow the correct period of exposure in the oven.

Powder used for powdering rubber gloves, etc., can be pre-sterilised by the dry-heat method. The powder is spread on to trays in a layer not greater than $\frac{1}{8}$ in (0·3 cm) depth before heating for the recommended time and temperature.

Heat Disinfection

3. Sub-atmospheric steam and formaldehyde pasteurisation

Whilst the two previous methods are practical and effective ways of sterilising most fabrics and instruments, there is still the problem of heat-sensitive articles such as plastics and optical devices. Previously there were only two cold methods which could be relied upon to kill spores, gamma irradiation (impracticable in the average hospital) and careful bacteriologically controlled ethylene oxide gas. Alder and Gillespie at the Bristol Royal Infirmary had been using steam at 90°C (194°F) to disinfect blankets for several years (Alder *et al.*, 1966). They were impressed with the minimal damage to most items which were disinfected. Further experiments resulted in a technique which is applicable to the pasteurisaton of heat-sensitive instruments.

In a modified autoclave, steam under sub-atmospheric pressure at temperatures below 90°C (194°F) will rapidly kill non-poring organisms after the air in the chamber has been removed by a high-vacuum pump. Most bacterial spores are killed also but a small proportion are very resistant. If formaldehyde vapour is added to the steam, it can destroy all spores and effect sterilisation. Low-temperature steam formaldehyde and high-temperature steam cycles can be incorporated in one and the same autoclave.

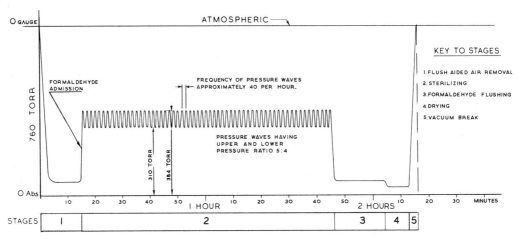

Figure 173   Graph of low temperature/formaldehyde method. (British Steriliser Ltd.)

THE CYCLE OF OPERATION

Low-temperature steam formaldehyde sterilisation can be summarised as follows:

After loading the chamber and closing the door:

Stage 1. Pre-vacuum. A flush of steam is drawn by the vacuum pump through the surrounding jacket and the chamber whilst the pressure is reduced to approximately 380 Torr (a vacuum of 15 in Hg, 38 mm Hg). At this point the jacket pressure is held steady and the pump continues to evacuate the chamber until a pressure of about 50 Torr (28 in Hg, 711 mm Hg) is reached. This is maintained for 10 minutes to effect complete air clearance from both the chamber and the load.

Stage 2. Sterilisation. A predetermined quantity of formalin is automatically delivered into the chamber from an externally fitted dispenser or container. The valves of the autoclave are so arranged as to admit about 55 ml of formalin per 100 litres (15 ml per ft^3) of autoclave chamber capacity. The formalin first enters a heated vapouriser where it is converted to steam and gaseous formaldehyde before passing into the chamber. At the same time there is a controlled injection of steam which allows the chamber pressure to rise into equilibrium with that of the jacket at about 380 Torr (15 in Hg, 381 mm Hg). Once this equilibrium pressure is reached (82°C or 180°F saturated steam temperature), continuous pressure waves of steam, followed by condensation are applied within the upper and lower absolute pressure limits of 384 and 310 Torr (15 to 17 in Hg, 381 to 432 mm Hg). These pressure waves occurring at approximately once every 90 seconds, promote penetration of the formaldehyde vapour into all parts of the load.

In order to maintain the formaldehyde concentration in a sub-atmospheric cycle, the chamber must remain virtually closed. This does produce a problem of the extraction of condensate which is formed during the decompression phase of each pressure wave. The removal of condensate is achieved through an automatic condensate release valve fitted in the chamber drain. Duration of the pasteurisation stage is normally in the order of 90 minutes and this is determined by bacteriological check of a standard load.

Stage 3. Flushing. The pressure is once more reduced in the chamber by means of the vacuum pump and a continuous flush of steam is applied. Pumping and steam flushing is carried out at an absolute pressure of about 50 Torr (28 in Hg, 711 mm Hg) and this ensures that most of the formaldehyde is removed from the chamber and the materials being pasteurised. This stage lasts for approximately 12 minutes.

Stage 4. Drying. A final reduction of pressure to 30 Torr (29 in Hg, 737 mm Hg) or less achieves drying of materials over a period of approximately eight minutes.

Stage 5. Breaking the vacuum. Filtered air is admitted until atmospheric pressure is reached in the chamber. This generally takes about two minutes.

Penetration tests. Lengths of narrow bore tubing form difficult test pieces; they are realistic, easy to prepare and to standardise and are readily included with any routine run. A useful method is to infect the lumen of a 2·7 m length of 3 mm bore plastic tubing with spores of *B. globigii* and *B. stearothermophilus*. These are processed in the laboratory in the normal manner and in some instances it has been found that the pasturisation cycle can be reduced to between 60 and 75 minutes and still maintain effective destruction of spores.

The following are some of the items suitable for disinfection by this method: nylon, Terylene, Acrilan and rayon fabrics; polyurethane; teflon tubing; perspex; silicone rubber; anaesthetic equipment such as endotracheal tubes, valves, connectors etc.; cystoscopes and other endoscopic instruments having electrical systems (low-voltage); catheters and tracheostomy tubes, etc.

4. Pasteurisation in water

Pasteurisation of endoscopes is carried out simply by immersion for 10 minutes in water at a temperature of between 75°C (167°F) and 85°C (185°F) (Francis, 1959). A thermostatically controlled water bath is used and even non-boilable instruments withstand this

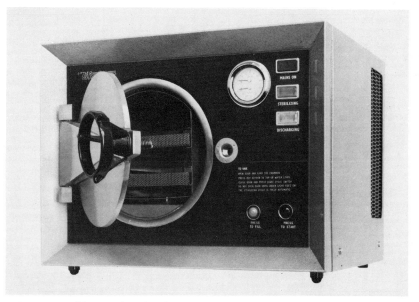

Figure 174   Portable autoclave (Little Sister) which can be operated from a standard 13A power socket. (Surgical Equipment Supplies Ltd.)

treatment very well. It is in practice as effective as boiling and will destroy vegetative bacteria very rapidly. Undoubtedly it is preferable to the use of chemicals if autoclaving is contraindicated and the sub-atmospheric steam method is unavailable (Medical Research Council, 1968).

5. Boiling

The boiling of instruments should be regarded as a means of disinfection only. This technique has no place in a modern hospital, nor indeed even under extremes of isolation. If a small portable autoclave is not available then an ordinary domestic pressure cooker will be an acceptable alternative.

Although most bacteria are killed by 5 minutes boiling some spore-forming organisms are not. This means that instruments cannot be guaranteed sterile if processed in this manner.

Cold Sterilisation

6. Radiation

Generally limited to sterilisation on a commercial scale there are two methods in general use, gamma irradiation from a Cobalt 60 source and electron bombardment from a linear accelerator (Mackenzie, 1966).

The usual dose is in the region of 2·5 M, rad. and the technique is highly successful for most disposable items which require sterilisation only once. Degradation and ageing does occur when sterilising some materials so care is taken to select those suitable for irradiation.

The Cobalt source is the most economical process if it can be kept running the full 24 hours. It has greater penetrating power than the linear accelerator which is more suitable for thin packets such a catgut, scalpel blades, needles, etc.

An irradiation sterilisation service provided by the Atomic Energy Authority at Wantage, Berkshire, England is available to hospitals. This service consists mainly of contract sterilisation although arrangements can be made to process a small number of items. The user is required to adhere to certain methods and sizes of packets. Full details are available from Irradiated Products Ltd., Denchworth Road, Wantage, Berks., England.

7. Ethylene Oxide

Ethylene oxide is suitable for sterilising heat labile articles. It is a method now well established in the United States, Germany, Switzerland and France; although in the United Kingdom until about 1965 ethylene oxide gas was limited to commercial processes. Use at hospital level has been minimal due to concern in respect of its toxicity and explosive characteristics and also the difficulty of controlling the efficiency of the process.

Ethylene oxide, known as a gas since 1859, has been used as an industrial disinfectant for over forty years and was introduced as a clinical sterilising agent in 1949 by Philip and Kays. The chemical acts by alkylating the proteins of micro-organisms thereby upsetting their equilibrium. If the process is applied correctly, this reaction is irreversible and reanimation of the alkylated germ is prevented.

The gas is an epoxide and unfortunately besides being an extremely efficient alkylating agent it has the ability to ignite with an exothermic reaction which has on a number of occasions blown whole factories into the air. This explosive polymerisation can be avoided, firstly by mixing ethylene oxide with an inert gas such as carbon dioxide, and secondly, by employing a sterilising process which extracts most of the air from the chamber before the introduction of ethylene oxide (Fischer, 1971). One process uses pure ethylene oxide under a constant vacuum so that it is impossible for the gas to leak out and mix with air (Weymes, 1966).

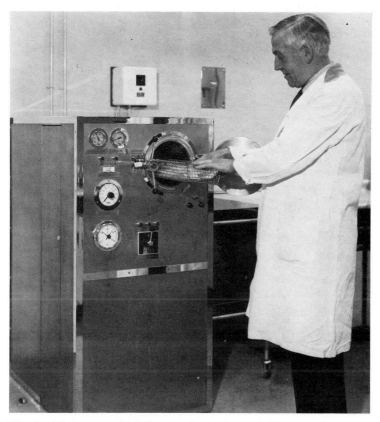

Figure 175   Sterivit Automated Ethylene Oxide Steriliser at Hallamshire Hospital, Sheffield. Applied for sterilising used cystoscope in rate volume.

A word of caution on safeguards to prevent explosions; cylinders of ethylene oxide stored in the liquid phase must be fitted within 2 to 2·5 metres (6 to 8 feet) of the steriliser served to avoid the possibility of separation. If separation and a leak in the line occurs, air may be drawn into the chamber with ethylene oxide to form a highly combustible mixture.

Initially care must be taken in cleansing instruments and apparatus that all visible protein material is removed; although a high pressure process (Sterivit) has been proved to have the ability to penetrate even salt encrusted spores e.g. when inactivating Statens Seruminstitut *B. subtilis* dried on pure quartz sand (Leo Pharmaceutical Products, Denmark, 1971, personal communication). The articles being sterilised must be dry, for if they are wrapped in polythene film whilst still wet, they will remain wet after sterilisation. The most suitable packing material is low density 300 gauge polyethylene or nylon film; used as one of two layers which are rapidly penetrated by ethylene oxide, moisture and heat under the appropriate controlled conditions.

An essential part of the sterilising process using ethylene oxide is the maintenance of adequate humidity (70–80 per cent) *with effective moisture distribution throughout the load.*

TABLE OF DISINFECTION BY CHEMICALS

ANTI-BACTERIAL AGENTS IN COMMON USE, DILUTIONS

(The minimum period of immersion unless otherwise stated is 10 minutes)

Chemical or proprietary preparation	CLEANSING AND DISINFECTION						DISINFECTION	
	Linen bowls, etc. (%)	Heavy contamination inanimate objects (%)	Burns, wounds, initial pre-surgical skin preparation (%)	Pre-surgical hand rinse (%)	Final pre-surgical skin preparation (%)	Anaesthetic apparatus (masks, tubes, etc.) (%)	Endoscopes electrodes, cables and lamps (%)	Metal instruments (osteotomes, etc.) (%)
Phenol (Carbolic acid) Aqueous	2·5	...	...	...	...	...	...	...
Cresol with soap solution (Lysol) Aqueous	2·5	...	...	...	...	...	...	...
Industrial methylated spirit	...	...	...	...	...	...	...	5
(Sudol) Aqueous	1	2	...	...	...	...	...	2
(Printol) Aqueous	1·25	3	...	...	...	...	...	3
(Printol D) Aqueous	1	2	...	...	...	...	...	2
(Hycolin) Aqueous	1	1·5	...	...	...	...	...	1·5
Chloroxylenol (Pure Detol) Aqueous	5	...	5	5	...	5	...	...
Chlorhexidine Gluconate (Hibitane, 5 per cent concentrate) Aqueous	0·5	...	1	...	...	0·5	10	...
Industrial methylated spirit	...	...	...	1	10	...	...	10
Cetrimide B.P. (CTAB Cetavlon) Aqueous	1	...	3	1	...	1	...	...
(Savlon Hospital concentrate) 15 per cent Cetavlon 1·5 per cent Hibitane Aqueous	0·5	...	3 to 1	...	...	0·5	10 (20 min)	10 (20 min)

TABLE OF DISINFECTION BY CHEMICALS—*continued*

Chemical or proprietary preparation	CLEANSING AND DISINFECTION					DISINFECTION		
	Linen, bowls, etc. (%)	Heavy contam- ination (%)	Burns, wounds, initial pre- surgical skin pre- (%)	Pre- surgical hands rinse (%)	Final pre- surgical skin pre- paration (%)	Anaes- thetic apparatus (masks, tubes, etc.) (%)	Endo- scopes, electrodes, cables and lamps (%)	Metal instru- ments (osteo- tomes, etc.) (%)
Industrial methylated spirit	...	...	...	3	...	...	10	...
Benzalkonium Chloride (Roccal, 10 per cent. concentrate) Aqueous	0·5	...	10 to 5	1	...	0·5	10	...
Benzalkonium Chloride—*cont.* Industrial methylated spirit	...	...	...	1	...	...	...	10
Domiphen Bromide (Bradosol, Dimittol, 5 per cent) Aqueous	...	...	10	10	...	0·5	10	...
Industrial methylated spirit	...	...	...	1	...	...	...	10
Thiomersalate (Merthiolate) Aqueous solution	...	...	...	...	...	...	0·1 (storage of bone)	
Activated Glutaraldehyde (Cidex) solution effective for 14 days after activation. 20 minute exposure to destroy pathogens	...	...	...	...	...	†	†	...
Iodine 2 per cent in industrial methylated spirit	...	...	...	...	Undiluted	...	...	...

TABLE OF DISINFECTION BY CHEMICALS—*continued*

Chemical or proprietary preparation	CLEANSING AND DISINFECTION					DISINFECTION		
	Linen, bowls, etc.	Heavy contam- ination	Burns, wounds, initial pre- surgical skin pre-	Pre- surgical hands rinse	Final pre- surgical skin pre- paration	Anaes- thetic apparatus (masks, tubes, etc.)	Endo- scopes, electrodes, cables and lamps	Metal instru- ments (osteo- tomes, etc.)
	(%)	(%)	(%)	(%)	(%)	(%)	(%)	(%)
(Betadine) antiseptic	...	...	...	Un- diluted	...	...	...	...
Surgical scrub	...	...	Undiluted	...	...	...	...	...
Proflavine Aqueous and emulsion	...	...	1:1000	...	...	...	...	...
Industrial methylated spirit	...	...	...	...	Saturated solution (approx. 1:1000)	...	...	...

Items marked thus † are suitable for disinfection by that particular method.

Figure 176   Table of disinfection by chemicals.

Humidification should be achieved automatically by the steriliser and there must be fail-safe mechanisms to monitor this and any other parameters of the process. Some authorities recommend that adequate humidity can be achieved by preconditioning the items to be sterilised, holding them in a room at 50–60 per cent humidity for several hours before sterilisation. This method is somewhat haphazard as compared to automatic humidification in the steriliser.

The Sterivit apparatus (Fig. 175) utilises a 15 per cent ethylene oxide, 85 per cent carbon dioxide mixture under pressure and with controlled humidity. There are a range of chamber sizes available between 25 litres and 2,000 litres, although one with a capacity of 100 to 500 litres (3·5 to 17·5 ft^3) will be adequate for most requirements of a hospital-based on CSSD or HSDU. The larger chambers are used mainly for sterilising bulky items of equipment such as complete ventillators or cardiovascular bypass machines. The sterilising process is automated as follows:

1. The steriliser is loaded, the door closed and start button activated.

2. The first stage consists of raising the temperature in the chamber to 55/60°C (131/140°F). A pre-vacuum is drawn and the chamber pressure reduced to approximately 70 Torr; at the same time steam is introduced to create a humidity of 70 to 80 per cent. This stage takes 20 to 25 minutes depending on the size of chamber.

3. Ethylene oxide 15 per cent with 85 per cent carbon dioxide is introduced from a gas cylinder directly into the chamber until a pressure of 55 lb per square inch (5·5 atmospheres) is reached. This achieves an ethylene oxide concentration of 1,200 mg per litre of chamber capacity, and exposure is maintained for 60 minutes.

4. A post vacuum of approximately 70 Torr is drawn and held for 25 to 50 minutes

depending upon the size of chamber. During this time air is drawn through a high efficiency filter and through the chamber to 'rinse' out ethylene oxide residues from the load. (Note: some other non-pressurised processes require extended periods of exposure for sterilisation; these may be between 1 and 4 hours. Under these circumstances elimination of toxic residues is proportionally more difficult, and takes a longer time. Residues extracted from the chamber must be vented to outside the building.

The total cycle of the Sterivit process depends on the size of chamber; at the lower end of the scale the 25 litre chamber steriliser takes 100 minutes, the largest chamber of 2,000 litres capacity takes 160 minutes for the whole process.

Practically all materials except metals absorb differing amounts of ethylene oxide. Under normal conditions the desorption of ethylene oxide is a slow process and for this reason many authorities recommend that, after sterilisation, goods should be stored on an open shelf for at least 24-hours and sometimes as long as four days before use. This is to allow elimination of the toxic residue by natural diffusion to atmosphere.

Using the high pressure method of sterilisation coupled with a short exposure and adequate post-vacuum the amount of depth of absorption of ethylene oxide can be reduced (Fischer, 1971). Furthermore, the high diffusion coefficient of the additive carbon dioxide, and the low concentration of a 15 per cent ethylene oxide mixture helps to reduce the problem still further. By an adequate post-vacuum, powerful filtered air-rinse under vacuum and elevated temperature, the ethylene oxide residues can be reduced to a negligible level. Under these circumstances a 24-hours shelf life before use should ensure desorption of any remaining residues.

A precaution worth taking following any ethylene oxide process is to take care that apparatus is not used with saline or blood products before it has been flushed with oxygen or sterile water. In these circumstances even a minute amount of ethylene oxide residue can react with the chlorine radicle to form chlorohydrates, the toxicity of which is not entirely understood at present. For similar reasons articles which have been sterilised by gamma irradiation should not subsequently be resterilised by ethylene oxide. This is the only instance when such precautions are necessary.

With ethylene oxide there are no means at present of adequately monitoring the actual ethylene oxide concentration at any given point during sterilisation. For this reason it is necessary to rely upon bacteriological controls. A method in common use is Oxoid prepared *B. stearothermophilus* on filter paper and *B. subtilis* (var globigii) 10^6 on aluminium strips prepared to the method of Beeby and Whitehouse (Cunliffe, 1966). Envelopes containing up to ten of these strips are placed at different points in the steriliser chamber and within all articles where it is considered that penetration could be a problem. The strips are incubated overnight and if no growth is apparent, the steriliser load is released for use after the 'airing' period.

Under careful preparation and control the spore test described is a good method of monitoring sterilisation. A simpler test utilising earth spores emanates from Denmark. The Danish State Serum Institute test consists of *B. subtilis*, first immersed in a solution of 0·9 per cent NaCl and then dried on pure quartz sand. The sand is then packed in a paper envelope which is used for test purposes in the normal manner. This is a very severe test due to the presence of salt (in contact with the spore) which tends to inactivate ethylene oxide. In practice it could be regarded as more appropriate to the working situation desmay not be adequately precleansed.

A chemical indicator can be included with each packet to indicate to the user that it has been through the ethylene oxide process; it is not a direct indication of sterility. A gas indicator tape with green stripes is available which changes shade after exposure to ethylene oxide. Chemical sachets or impregnated filter papers can be prepared in the laboratory and these change colour after being exposed to the gas (Colquhoun, 1969).

Examples of heat-labile equipment suitable for sterilisation by ethylene oxide are: cardiac catheters, endoscopes (including cystoscopes), cryoprobes, aortic grafts, ophthalmic instruments, plastic and rubber tubing, senoran evacuator, Sengstaken tubes, Birds respirator.

8. Ultra-Violet Light Radiation

This is a form of surface radiation with light having a wavelength of 2537 Ångstrom units. It is only suitable for sterilising surfaces as its penetration is poor. Amongst its uses is the sterilisation of small items such as bone chips, grafts and blades.

Ozone liberated by the process may prove objectionable, especially during sterilisation of air. High intensities of light are required and unless care is taken by personnel, over-exposure to ultra-violet radiation may result.

Cold Disinfection

9. Chemical solutions

We now emphasise the term *disinfection* in preference to *sterilisation* because under normal conditions chemicals cannot be relied upon to kill spores. It is a method which is used only when sterilisation by heat is impracticable and is ineffective unless the chemicals can reach all parts of the articles, which *must* be free from debris, blood and pus, i.e., as in ethylene oxide sterilisation (McCulloch, 1945; Perkins, 1956b; Sykes, 1958).

It must be realised that although fairly short periods of contact with certain chemicals will ensure the destruction of bacteria these short periods refer only to articles which have smooth surfaces, such as solid scalpels. If an instrument has rather intricate parts or joints some time will be required for the chemical to penetrate into the indentations or joint surfaces.

If the chemical is used in combination with heat the period for disinfection will be reduced. The importance of using heat for sterilisation whenever possible cannot be over-emphasised.

Many new chemicals are now in use in the operating theatre, but the lists on pages 150–152 include also some of the older and well-established ones. In all cases the instrument must be thoroughly rinsed before use to remove chemical traces which at high concentrations may prove irritant to body tissues.

The phenol and coal-tar derivative group

CARBOLIC ACID (PHENOL)

At a dilution of 5 per cent this will kill most bacteria in 10 minutes, but cannot be relied upon to destroy spores. Even at a dilution of 5 per cent it is corrosive and should not come into contact with body tissues or serious burns may result. It may be used for the pre-surgical disinfection of heat-labile instruments, such as cystoscopes, etc., but is largely being replaced by less toxic chemicals. Liquid carbolic acid or liquified phenol, which is a clear solution, should be dyed a distinctive colour to avoid confusion with other chemicals, and most usual colours in common use are blue, red or green. Carbolic acid solution must always be thoroughly rinsed off instruments before use.

CRESOL WITH SOAP SOLUTION OR LYSOL

This is also a very corrosive chemical except in dilute solutions below 2·5 per cent. It may be used at a dilution of 5 per cent for general disinfectant purposes, such as disinfection of soiled linen and floors, etc., but is very largely obsolete, and has been replaced with one of the less corrosive derivatives, e.g., Sudol.

SUDOL

This is a clear soluble disinfectant of the lysol type with somewhat reduced corrosive hazards and a germicidal potency generally twice that of Lysol B.P. For general disinfectant purposes in potentially heavily contaminated situations, e.g., infected linen and floors, the dilution is 2 per cent. For surface disinfection when the contamination is light, e.g., walls, tables, trolleys, etc., the dilution is 1 per cent, which falls within the range of 'in-use' dilutions recommended by Kelsey and Maurer in 1967. Rubber gloves must be worn.

PRINTOL

This is a clear soluble disinfectant with a phenolic base but rather less corrosive than the lysol type. Its dilution in heavily contaminated situations is 3 per cent but for routine surface disinfection this can be reduced to 1·25 per cent (Kelsey and Maurer, 1967).

PRINTOL D

This is similar to Printol except that it incorporates a detergent system which increases its capacity to reach the source of infection through dirt and organic contamination. Dilutions of 2·5 per cent for heavy contamination and 0·75 per cent for routine surface disinfection (Kelsey and Maurer, 1967).

For the disinfection of infected linen the manufacturers recommend a dilution of 0·5 per cent for four hours with both Printol and Printol D.

HYCOLIN

This is a balanced combination of synthetic phenols which are less corrosive than lysol. It is used for general purposes at a dilution of 1 per cent and this should be increased to 2 per cent for heavy contamination.

These four synthetic phenolic disinfectants are effective against all common grampositive and gram-negative organisms including *Pseudomonas aeruginosa* (*pyocyanea*). They are compatible with anionic and non-ionic substances such as soaps, anionic detergents, etc.

CHLOROXYLENOL (DETTOL)

This is a relatively non-toxic non-irritant antibacterial agent which is active against most organisms, including the streptococcus, but rather less active against certain gramnegative organisms. The destruction of spores is somewhat doubtful.

Dettol antiseptic contains 4·8 per cent chloroxylenol and 9 per cent terpineol, and is used at a dilution of 5 per cent for general disinfection purposes, 10 minutes being the minimal period of immersion recommended for disinfection.

It is not advisable to bring chloroxylenol preparations, especially strong solutions, into contact with plastics as they tend to cause deterioration of the material.

CHLORHEXIDINE (HIBITANE)

This is a well established antibacterial agent which is proving to be of great use. Single or infrequent applications to the intact skin of any strength solution will not cause irritation, but repeated applications of a 1 per cent solution may eventually give rise to erythema. The dilutions in common use should not give rise to any irritation of the user's skin (Rose and Swaine, 1956).

Hibitane Hospital Concentrate 5 per cent is a solution of 5 per cent chlorhexidine gluconate and an aqueous dilution of 0·5 per cent of the concentrate is used for the surface disinfection of inanimate objects, such as bowls, tables, etc. This dilution of Hibitane concentrate is equivalent to 0·025 per cent effective concentration of the antibacterial agent, chlorhexidine gluconate.

For the prophylactic treatment of wounds a Hibitane concentrate dilution of 1 per cent in water (0·05 per cent effective concentration) is used; for pre-surgical skin disinfection, 10 per cent dilution in 70 per cent industrial methylated spirit (0·5 per cent) with an added dye such as geranine or methylene blue (Lowbury, 1961); for the *emergency* pre-surgical disinfection of heat-labile instruments which are immersed for a minimum of 10 minutes before use a dilution of 10 per cent of Hibitane concentrate in 70 per cent industrial methylated spirit (0·5 per cent); and for the final pre-surgical rinse of hands (unless pHisoHex is being used), 1 per cent dilution of Hibitane concentrate in 70 per cent industrial methylated spirit (0·05 per cent). *Dilutions given in brackets always refer to the effective concentration of the antibacterial agent.*

The Hibitane concentrate is generally supplied coloured a distinctive red, and is effective against a wide range of gram-positive and gram-negative organisms. Although as with other antibacterial agents, blood slows down the bacterial activity of Hibitane it is claimed that at a dilution of 0·4 per cent (0·02 per cent) in 50 per cent blood, considerable bactericidal effect is retained. At the dilutions in common use Hibitane cannot be relied upon to kill spores, but it appears quite comparable with other similar antibacterial chemicals. Except in the greater dilutions it is not compatible with soaps and should not intentionally be combined with these.

HEXACHLOROPHANE

This is an antibacterial agent which can be combined with soap in a proportion of usually 2 per cent (Gould *et al.*, 1957; Lowbury, 1961). Pre-surgical washes called pHisoHex and Disfex are available and enable the scrub-up time to be reduced to three minutes. The method of use has already been described in the previous chapter.

Hexachlorophane is more effective against gram-positive than gram-negative organisms, but its main value lies in the regular use of a solution or soap containing the chemical. If the surgeons and theatre staff use pHisoHex, Disfex or hexachlorophane soap regularly it has been shown that the bacterial flora of the skin is reduced, and it is quite possible to rely upon a three-minute pre-surgical wash under these conditions (Smylie *et al.*, 1959). However, as the effect is cumulative, it may require repeated applications before its action is effective. But care must be taken not to use hexachlorophane preparations for regular total body bathing; there is a possible risk of absorption of hexachlorophane into the blood stream (Scowen, 1972).

The quaternary ammonium compounds

(Effective against gram-positive organisms but not against gram-negative organisms.)

CETRIMIDE B.P. (C.T.A.B. CETAVLON)

This is in effect an antibacterial detergent. It is not compatible with soap, but used in a dilution of not less than 0·5 per cent possesses very useful detergent properties which may be applied to the cleansing of contaminated wounds.

Although the higher concentrations are necessary for detergency, its antibacterial properties extend down to 0·2 per cent and at this dilution cetrimide may be used for the general washing of equipment such as bowls, etc.

Cetrimide has been combined with chlorhexidine to increase its antibacterial action against gram-negative bacteria and this preparation is available, known as Savlon Hospital concentrate, which is supplied as a concentrated solution containing 1·5 per cent chlorhexidine gluconate and 15 per cent cetrimide.

The dilutions of Savlon Hospital concentrate are as follows:

For general antibacterial purposes, such as washing equipment an aqueous dilution of 0·5 per cent Savlon Hospital concentrate is used; pre-surgical rinsing of hands or the preliminary treatment of burns and clean wounds, 1 per cent aqueous dilution of the concentrate; for contaminated or dirty wounds, 3 per cent aqueous dilution of the concentrate; for the *emergency* disinfection of heat-labile instruments which are immersed for a minimum of 10 minutes before use a dilution of 10 per cent of the concentrate in 70 per cent industrial methylated spirit may be used.

BENZALKONIUM CHLORIDE (ROCCAL, ZEPHIRAN)

This is similar in action to the other quaternary ammonium compounds. The B.P. solution contains 50 per cent w/v of benzalkonium chloride; Roccal (Bayer) contains 1 per cent benzalkonium chloride and Roccal concentrate (Roccal 10X) contains 10 per cent. If used at a dilution of not less than 0·5 per cent it has very useful detergent properties which may be utilised for the cleansing of contaminated wounds (Spalton, 1951). Its antibacterial properties extend down to 0·025 per cent for irrigation of the bladder, but for general purposes the greatest dilution is not less than 0·5 per cent.

For pre-surgical skin preparation and the cleansing of contaminated wounds the aqueous dilutions should be between 1 and 0·5 per cent effective concentration respectively. A 70 per cent industrial methylated spirit may be substituted as the dilutent for pre-surgical skin preparation when a more rapid action is desired. When full detergency is not required, a dilution of 0·5 per cent aqueous (0·05 per cent) is quite adequate for antibacterial purposes, and this dilution should be used for the general disinfection of inanimate objects such as bowls or linen etc.

For the final pre-surgical rinse of hands a dilution of 1 per cent (0·1 per cent) aqueous or in 70 per cent industrial methylated spirit should be used, and at this concentration there should not be any undue irritation to the user's hands.

Roccal or Zephiran can be used for bladder or urethral irrigation in the dilution of 0·05 per cent (0·005 per cent), but for retention lavage this dilution must be increased to 0·025 per cent (0·0025 per cent).

DOMIPHEN BROMIDE (BRADOSOL)

This is another antibacterial agent similar to the previous two. It is supplied as a concentrate of 5 per cent and is incompatible with soap and proflavine, except in the greatest dilutions (Eisman and Mayer, 1947).

Where full detergency is required the dilution should be in 10 per cent (0·5 per cent); for general disinfection, 0·4 per cent (0·02 per cent).

It must be remembered that the quaternary ammonium compounds are relatively inactive against certain gram-negative bacilli, especially Pseudomonas pyocyanea.

Mercurial preparations

THIOMERSALATE (MERTHIOLATE)

This is an organic percurial preparation, which although the pure substance contains about 50 per cent of mercury it is relatively non-toxic when used at the recommended dilutions of the commercial preparations.

The aqueous and stainless solution is prepared mainly for the storage of homogenous bone grafts in the 'Merthiolate Bone Bank'. The dilutions vary according to the technique, and full details are given in the chapter on Orthopaedic Surgery.

Formaldehyde

Although formaldehyde is a very powerful and effective disinfectant, its use for pre-surgical disinfection is largely falling into disrepute unless combined with sub-atmospheric steam. Disinfection failures in formalin cabinets have been described for many years and it is doubtful whether the formalin vapour penetrates the lumen of catheters even with control of the humidity in the cabinet. The use of formalin combined with sub-atmospheric steam, has been described on page 145.

ACTIVATED GLUTARALDEHYDE

This is a 2 per cent aqueous solution buffered to a pH 7·5–8·5 by the addition of 0·3 per cent sodium bicarbonate.

Cidex is a commercial preparation of glutaraldehyde containing an anti-rust agent. Vegetative bacteria and tubercle bacilli are killed in 20 minutes and some spore-forming species are killed in three hours (Spalding, 1963; Stonehill *et al.*, 1963; Medical Research Council, 1968).

The solution is suitable for disinfecting lensed instruments such as cystoscopes and other types of endoscopes providing the instrument is clean and partially dismantled. It is also suitable for anaesthetic masks etc.

The in-use dilution is slightly irritant to skin and mucous membranes and severely irritant to the eye. All instruments should be rinsed thoroughly in sterile water before use in surgery.

Once activated the solution is effective for a maximum of two weeks.

Other antibacterial agents in use

PROFLAVINE

This is used as three preparations, aqueous 1 per cent solution, paraffin and flavine emulsion 0·1 per cent, or as a saturated solution in industrial methylated spirit, which is used for pre-surgical skin preparation.

The aqueous preparation can be used as a dressing for wounds or burns; the emulsion is especially suitable for applying as a pack to a contaminated wound or over a skin graft in addition to the routine treatment of wounds and burns. For a pack the emulsion is applied in a saturated gauze roll, but for skin graft pressure pads it is preferable to use gamgee tissue, which should be wrung out fairly dry and autoclaved before use.

IODINE

As a 2 per cent solution in industrial methylated spirit, this is still regarded by many as the ideal pre-surgical skin preparation. It is certainly the most lethal to bacteria of all preparations used for this purpose, but unfortunately it does produce an occasional skin irritation which is disturbing for the patient. If a wound is very heavily contaminated and there has been a lengthy delay of the patient's admission to hospital the use of an iodine pre-surgical skin preparation may be indicated.

POVIDONE-IODINE (BETADINE)

This is a non-stinging, non-staining, film-forming, water-soluble iodine complex (Marr and Saggers, 1964). It is not irritating to skin and mucous membranes and unlike iodine tincture can be safely bandaged or applied as a compress. It is a topical disinfectant that retains the unique, non-selective microbiocidal activity of iodine, without the undesirable side effects mentioned above. It kills all organisms including spores and has a more prolonged action than ordinary iodine. Its brown colour can easily be washed off skin as well as cotton, wool and silk and its action is unimpaired by blood, serum, pus or soap.

Betadine is available as an aqueous antiseptic solution which is used undiluted for pre-operative skin preparation and as a surgical scrub. The latter contains a suitable detergent and forms a rich lather which is non-staining and non-irritating.

Note: Bacterial contamination of dilute solutions such as cetrimide and chlorhexidine can occur under certain circumstances. For this reason cork enclosures or cork liners in screw-cap bottles should not be used as cork appears to nourish and protect organisms. Contamination can occur also with the practice of 'topping up' half-empty bottles or of refilling stock bottles without resterilisation. Another cause may be due to the use of unsterile solutions or glass-ware or the transfer of bacteria to bottles during use (e.g., from the fingers of nurses con-taminated while handling infected articles or patients).

Bottles of disinfectant solutions should be date-stamped and used in rotation. Stocks must be kept at a minimum, and the points made above observed. (Medical Research Council, 1968).

Many hospital authorities have established a policy to limit the number, variety and variations in dilutions of disinfectants in general use. Such a policy ensures that the most effective chemical is chosen and lends itself also to economy.

APPLICATION OF METHODS

It is important to remember that the easiest and most effective method of sterilisation is by moist heat, and whenever possible is the method of choice. If an antibacterial agent is used, a thorough pre-cleansing is as vital as the application of the chemical which should always be given sufficient time to penetrate to all parts of the instrument.

Anaesthetic Apparatus. After careful cleansing, inside and out with soap and water or a chemical detergent such as Pyroneg or cetrimide, rubber face masks, rebreathing bags, corrugated tubes, airways, endotracheal or bronchial tubes should be immersed in 0·5 per cent aqueous Hibitane or Savlon for a minimum period of 10 minutes. Alternatively they should be immersed in Cidex solution for a similar period of time. A rebreathing bag or corrugated tubes should be hung up to dry, care being taken to ensure that the inside of the bag and corrugations are thoroughly dried. The airways and endotracheal or endobronchial tubes may be dried by placing them on a towel covering a warm surface.

Ideally corrugated tubes, 'Y' pieces, Heidbrink valves and some rubber airways and endotracheal tubes, etc., should be autoclaved after a thorough cleansing, but it is inadvisable to treat the vinyl plastic variety in a similar manner as they tend to become opaque. Before autoclaving a 'cuffed tube' the cuff or obturator bag must be empty. A method of disinfecting ventilators is described in Chapter 10, page 251.

Bougies, Catheters, etc. These are dealt with under the appropriate headings, e.g., metal, plastic and rubber.

Electrical Apparatus. Quite a large proportion of electrical apparatus used in surgery is now manufactured suitable for sterilisation by heat. Care must always be taken to observe the manufacturers' instructions regarding a particular instrument as it is possible for some parts to be heat sterilisable and others not.

A large proportion of electrical leads and illuminated retractors are now made auto-clavable, but after use they should be dried very thoroughly to minimise corrosion.

Those not sterilisable by high temperatures should be immersed in a 10 per cent aqueous solution of Hibitane (0·5 per cent), for a minimal period of 30 minutes, sterilised by ethylene oxide or alternatively subjected to the sub-atmospheric steam/formalin process.

Diathermy or cautery electrodes may generally be autoclaved. If heat sterilisation is contraindicated *emergency* disinfection may be effected by immersing them in a 10 per cent aqueous solution of Hibitane (0·5 per cent) or Cidex for a minimal period of 10 minutes.

Several of the more modern electric bone drills and saws may be autoclaved complete; in most cases, however, only the outer motor cover or the flexible drive is sterilisable in this way. The cable must be covered with a sterilised cotton sleeve before use and care taken to ensure that no moisture has collected on or near electrical contacts.

Generally speaking, electric lamps are damaged by heat and should therefore be sterilised ideally by ethylene oxide, or immersed in a chemical antibacterial agent such as 10 per cent aqueous solution of Hibitane (0·5 per cent) or Cidex.

Endoscopes. The same rules apply to endoscopes, including cystocopes, bronchoscopes, oesophagoscopes, etc., but extra care must be taken with optical attachments such as telescopes, lenses and lighting attachments.

A rapid increase of pressure of steam may cause cracking of the optical attachments, although in practice with modern apparatus this complication is minimised. Similarly breakage may occur if a hot endoscope is cooled too rapidly in cold water before use. Sometimes only the sheath of an endoscope is heat sterilisable, and if the optical and lighting system is required sterile it must be processed by sub-atmospheric steam/formalin, ethylene oxide, or immersed in a 10 per cent aqueous solution of Hibitane (0·5 per cent) vertically for a minimal period of 10 minutes. On no account must instruments containing lenses come into contact with any alcohol-based solutions; it will dissolve the lens-mounting cement.

Pasteurisation of endoscopes is carried out simply by immersion for 10 minutes in a boiler thermostatically controlled at 75°C (167°F)–85°C (185°F) instead of 100°C (212°F), and it is enough to destroy vegetative bacteria very rapidly. Undoubtedly this is preferable to the use of chemicals when higher temperatures are contraindicated.

Metal Ware. This is sterilised by autoclaving at 134°C (275°F)/32 lb p.s.i. for six minutes, little or no drying being necessary. Alternatively the articles are contained within a packet and sterilised with the drapes (p. 104).

Glassware. Generally all glassware may be autoclaved if certain precautions are taken and steam can reach all surfaces of the glass. To avoid breakage it is advisable to pre-heat the articles being sterilised by placing them in the autoclave chamber beforehand.

After sterilisation glassware should be allowed to cool slowly, thereby avoiding cracking which may occur if the articles are cooled too rapidly. Glassware should not be sterilised together with metal instruments as the latter can cause unnecessary breakages. Dry-heat sterilisation is the method of choice for all glassware.

Gloves (re-processable solution type). These are lightly powdered inside with a talc-free absorbable glove powder and packed as pairs in individual packets. They are autoclaved for six minutes at 130°C (266°F)/25 lb p.s.i. using the standard autoclave cycle followed by a short period of drying or 134°C (275°F)/32 lb p.s.i. for three and a half minutes.

Linen. Gowns, caps, masks and operation drapes are packed into linen, paper or nylon packets or Bripac/Permapak boxes. These are sterilised at 126°C (259°F)/20 lb p.s.i. for 30 minutes or 134°C (275°)/32 lb p.s.i. for three and a half minutes.

Lotions. Normal saline and sterile water for hand lotion use should be prepared as individual glass bottles of ½ or 1 litre capacity, which are autoclaved so that the temperature of each container is maintained at 115°C (240°F)/10 lb p.s.i. for 30 minutes. (British Pharmaceopoeia, 1963).

The holding period of sterilisation depends upon a number of factors which include type of autoclave, capacity and load, i.e., $\frac{1}{2}$ or 1 litre bottles. This period should be determined initially by a thermocouple recording the temperature reached inside a bottle of water at the centre of the load. Subsequently the temperature/holding period is checked either by an integrated thermocouple or a black spot Browne's tube suspended in one of the filled bottles. The holding period selected for a load of mixed $\frac{1}{2}$ and 1 litre bottles must be that suitable for the latter.

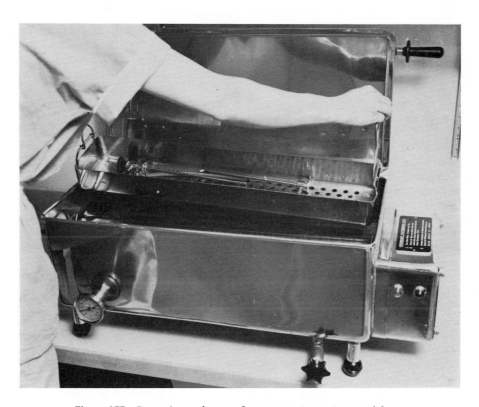

Figure 177   Removing endoscope from pasteuriser using tray lifters.

When sterilising bottles of liquid in an autoclave certain precautions must be taken. The metal caps must have a well-fitting rubber washer which is renewed regularly; a pre-vacuum is drawn and steam admitted to the chamber gradually; and after sterilisation the steam pressure must be reduced over a period of about 30 minutes otherwise the liquid may boil violently and the bottles burst. *A post-vacuum must not be drawn.* At this stage some autoclaves incorporate a special fluid cycle with spray cooling after sterilisation whilst (Howie and Timbury, 1956) maintaining pressure of air in the autoclave chamber. This avoids bursting of bottles.

After sterilisation the caps of the bottles are sealed with *sterile* cellulose tape or a plastic seal. Once a seal on a sterile bottle has been broken, the stopper removed and the contents exposed to the air a *sterile* label does not indicate sterility of the contents. Saline or water from a sterile bottle or flask must not be used for injection, infusion or washing of sterile instruments unless the seal of the bottle is unbroken at the time of use.

Once opened and not used such bottles should be regarded as contaminated and must be discarded. Bottles such as the Matbick type incorporate their own seal.

Metal Instruments. These are divided into the heat sterilisable and non-heat sterilisable types.

The heat sterilisable metal instruments are made generally of stainless steel which will not rust if the instruments are dried after use. Such instruments, including scissors, dissecting and artery forceps, metal bougies and catheters, etc., may be sterilised on open trays in an autoclave for six minutes at 130°C (266°F)/25 lb p.s.i.

Non-autoclavable instruments made from carbon steel, such as solid scalpels, twist drills and osteotomes, etc., are better sterilised by dry heat or ethylene oxide.

In the dry-heat process of sterilisation the instruments are exposed to a temperature of 160°C (320°F) for one hour *plus* additional time necessary to allow heat penetration to all parts of the load. This additional period ranges between a half and one and a half hours.

In an emergency a 10 per cent Hibitane (0·5 per cent) solution in industrial methylated spirit will disinfect metal instruments in a *minimum* period of ten minutes, providing that the chemical has access to all parts.

Nail Brushes. These should be autoclaved at 130°C (266°F)/25 lb p.s.i. for six minutes, or 134°C (275°F)/32 lb p.s.i. for three and a half minutes. The most satisfactory method is to autoclave the brushes in a metal brush dispenser and keep them in the dry state until needed. A separate clean brush is then used for each person.

Needles. Hypodermic needles, after a thorough syringing through, should be autoclaved, or dry-heat sterilised at the recommeded time for instruments.

The best method for reprocessable suture needles is to prepare the needles as sets in paper bags and sterilise by the dry-heat method or autoclaving. Using the latter method, a small piece of vapour phase inhibitor anti-rust paper should be included with the needles when packing; this applies also to steam sterilisation.

It is very important to ensure that no debris is lodged in the eye of a suture needle or at any point along the shaft before sterilisation. Suture needles are difficult to clean; ideally pre-sterilised disposable suture needles should be used.

Rubber Goods. Some of these, including non-disposable tubing, drainage sheeting, catheters and certain endotracheal and endobronchial tubes can be autoclaved providing the drying cycle is not prolonged.

Macintoshes are treated with an antibacterial agent such as 0·5 per cent aqueous Hibitane, and if heavily contaminated should be autoclaved.

Powders. The only satisfactory method of sterilising powders to avoid clumping is by dry heat. Dusting powders, etc., should be distributed in their final containers in small quantities of no more than 15 g and sterilised in a hot-air oven for 90 minutes at 150°C (320°F). After sterilisation they should be packed into sterile containers, observing aseptic precautions.

Plastics. Most non-disposable plastics in common use in the operating theatre may be sterilised by wet heat, but care must be taken as at boiling-point and above they become softened and easily damaged.

Polyvinyl chloride (vinyl Portex, both translucent and ivory Magill variety) and polythene tubing, etc., should be sterilised in ethylene oxide, pasteurised in sub-atmospheric steam/formalin or in a pasteuriser as previously described on p. 147 being wrapped in lint, gauze or placed on a removable perforated tray covered with a similar material. They may also be coiled and loosely tied with a cotton bandage which is grasped with Cheatle transfer forceps when removing the tubing from the pasteuriser. These precautions should prevent indentations, etc., occurring whilst the plastic is at the softened stage. Most polyvinyl tubing can now be purchased ready sterilised.

Nylon tubing can be sterilised by this method also, but due to its high melting-point

200°C (328°F) steam sterilisation as recommended for metal instruments can be employed.

Plastic tubing should never be shaken upon removal from the pasteuriser as it is then very brittle and may break at the point where it is secured with bandage.

It is important to ensure that there are no kinks or air bubbles in the tubing during pasteurisation and it is preferable to fill the tubing with water beforehand. Kinks in the tubing will result in flattened sections and air bubbles with inefficient disinfection of the lumen. Plastic tubing which has flattened sections or irregularities following sterilisation can often be returned to its original shape and section by re-heating and then cooling rapidly whilst maintaining the desired position.

The use of other items of plastic equipment in the theatre is rather questionable due to the danger of static electricity formation (Chapter 3), but all inanimate objects such as arm supports and translucent X-ray cassette holders for fracture tables, etc., are disinfected with a 1 per cent aqueous solution of Hibitane or Savlon before and after use. Other antibacterial agents which may be used for this purpose are Roccal and Bradosol at their recommended dilutions. The usual type of materials used for these articles are perspex and fibre glass.

Suture Materials. Most ligatures and sutures available in foil or plastic sachets are presented as sterile peel-open overwrap packets. Unopened inner sachets can be disinfected by immersion in a suitable fluid recommeneded by the manufacturer for a minimum period of 30 minutes before use.

Plastic envelopes containing sterile non-boilable catgut are stored in a fluid supplied by the catgut manufacturers which consists basically of isopropyl alcohol.

Monofilament Nylon and Silkworm Gut. These are generally sterilised with the instrument sets but can be autoclaved separately in packets at standard autoclave temperatures and times.

Braided, Twisted, Plaited, and Floss Silk, Nylon, or Linen Thread, etc. These are wound on to metal, nylon or glass ligature reels and are autoclaved. Sterile peel-open packets containing various sizes of nylon, silk and linen thread.

Metal Wire, Mesh and Suture Clips. All are autoclavable before use as described under metal instruments. They may be stored in dry sterilised boxes or packets, but in the case of Cushing's or McKenzie's ligature clips these may be included in the set of instruments.

REFERENCES

ADAMS, I. (1970) *Hospital Administration and Construction*, **12**, 10, p. 74.
ALDER, V. G., BROWN, A. M. and GILLESPIE, W. A. (1966) *Journal of Clinical Pathology*, 19, 83.
BOLTON, J. (1966) *British Hospital Journal*, May 13, 867.
BOWIE, J. H. (1961) *Sterilisation of Surgical Materials. Symposium.* London: Pharmaceutical Press.
BOWIE, J. H., KELSEY, J. C. and THOMPSON, C. R. (1963) *Lancet*, i, 586.
British Pharmacopoeia (1963) p. 396.
COLQUHOUN, J. (1969) *British Hospital Journal*, July.
CUNLIFFE, A. C. (1966) *Proceedings Central Sterilising Club*, April 29–30th.
DARMADY, E. M., HUGHES, K. E. A., MURT, M. M., FREEMAN, B. M. and POWELL, D. B. (1961) *Journal of Clinical Pathology*, 14, 55.
EISMAN, P. C. and MAYER, R. L. (1947) *Journal of Bacteriology*, **54**, 668.
FISCHER, E. (1971) Meeting on ethylene oxide sterilisation, University of Wales, September 6th.
FRANCIS, A. E. (1959) *Proceedings of the Royal Society of Medicine*, **52**, 998.
GOULD, B. S., FRIGERIO, N. A. and HOVANESIEN, J. (1957) *Antibiotics*, 7, 457.
HOWIE, J. W. (1961) *Journal of Clinical Pathology*, **14**, 49.
HOWIE, J. W. and TIMBURY, M. C. (1956) *Lancet*, ii, 669.
JEFFERSON, S. (1958) *Radioisotopes*, p. 278. London: Newnes.
KELSEY, J. C. (1970) *British Hospital Journal*, March 20th.

KELSEY, J. C. and MAURER, I. M. (1967) *Public Health Laboratory Service Bulletin,* **26**, June.

KNOX, R. (1961) *Journal of Clinical Pathology,* **14**, 13.

KNOX, R. and PICKERILL, J. K. (1967) *British Hospital Journal,* December 15th.

LOWBURY, E. J. (1961) *Journal of Clinical Pathology,* **14**, 85, 88, 89.

McCULLOCK, E. C. (1945) *Disinfection and Sterilisation,* 2nd edn. London: Kimpton.

MACKENZIE, S. (1966) *British Hospital Journal,* September 16, 1733.

MARR, M. S. and SAGGERS, B. (1964) *Nursing Times,* June 12.

MEDICAL RESEARCH COUNCIL (1945) *The Sterilisation, Use and Care of Syringes.* War Memo. No 15. London: HMSO.

MEDICAL RESEARCH COUNCIL (1959) Working Party. *Lancet,* **i**, 425.

MEDICAL RESEARCH COUNCIL (1968) Aseptic methods in the operating theatre. *Lancet,* **i**, 763.

PERKINS, J. J. (1956a) Bacteriological and surgical sterilisation by heat. In *Antiseptics, Disinfectants, Fungicides, Chemical and Physical Sterilisation.* Edited by C. F. Reddish. New York: Lea and Febiger.

PERKINS, J. J. (1956b) *Principles and Methods of Sterilisation,* p. 163. Springfield, Ill.: Thomas.

RENDELL-BAKER, L. (1970) *Hospitals,* October.

RENDELL-BAKER, L. and ROBERTS, R. B. (1970) *Current Researches in Anesthesia and Analgesia,* November.

ROSE, F. L. and SWAINE, G. (1956) *Journal of the Chemical Society,* **4**, 4422.

SCOWEN, PROF. (1972) *Report of U.K. Committee on the Safety of Medicines, 'Hexachlorophane',* February.

SMYLIE, H. G., WEBSTER, C. V. and BRUCE, M. L. (1959) *British Medical Journal,* **ii**, 606.

SPALTON, L. M. (1951) *Chemist and Druggist,* November 24.

SPALDING, E. H. (1963) *Association of Operating Room Nurses' Journal, U.S.A.,* May/June.

SYKES, G. (1968) In *Disinfection and Sterilisation,* pp. 170–339. Edited by McCulloch. London: Kimpton.

STONEHILL, A., KROP, S. and BORICK, P. M. (1963) *American Journal of Hospital Pharmacy,* 20, 458.

WALTER, C. W. (1948) *The Aseptic Treatment of Wounds.* New York: Macmillan.

WELLS, C. and WHITWELL, F. R. (1960) *Lancet,* **ii**, 643.

WESSEX INSTRUMENT CASKET, Feature article. *British Hospital Journal,* March.

WEYMES, C. (1966) *British Hospital Journal,* September, 1745.

7

Ligature and Suture Materials

A suture is a stitch used in surgery to approximate living tissues or structures until the normal process of healing is complete.

A ligature is a suture used to encircle a blood-vessel to arrest or control bleeding.

Ligatures and sutures are divided into two main groups: the absorbable and the non-absorbable. The absorbable are digested and absorbed during the process of healing. This group includes surgical catgut, polyglycolic acid, collagen tape and living sutures fashioned from tendons or fascia. The non-absorbable group remain permanently in the tissues after the process of healing is complete. This is especially useful when the tissues are weakened and require reinforcement for some considerable time after operation, as in the case of herniorrhaphy. This group includes natural materials, such as silkworm gut, and man-made fibres of the nylon or polyester type.

ABSORBABLE LIGATURES AND SUTURES

Catgut

The most generally used material in this group is surgical catgut, which is substantially pure collagen prepared from the submucosal layer or attached peritoneum of milk lambs' intestine.

The preparation of surgical catgut is controlled by the Department of Health. All manufacturers must reach very high pharmaceutical standards laid down by law before their product can be marketed.

THE PREPARATION OF SURGICAL CATGUT

Before export to this country the intestines of freshly killed New Zealand milk lambs are cleansed and frozen within three hours of death.

On arrival at the catgut laboratories the intestines are rapidly thawed and slit longitudinally into three or four ribbons. Batches of ribbons are then thoroughly scraped under a water spray to remove muscle and fatty material. The process is called sliming.

The ribbons of gut may be treated also in several baths of an alkaline solution to remove the fat by saponification.

According to the diameter of the gut required, two or more ribbons may be spun together into strands before drying under tension followed by polishing the surface of the strands.

This dried catgut is now known technically as raw *plain* catgut. After sterilisation this catgut would be absorbed in muscle tissue in approximately 5 to 10 days, or about a quarter of that time in the peritoneum or serous membrane.

In order to prolong the time of absorption in the tissues the raw catgut can be hardened or chromicised by immersing the strands in a chromic salt solution bath. As chromic salts are normally colourless, it is usual to add colour to this bath to indicate visually the difference between *plain* and *chromic* catgut.

The degree of hardness depends upon how long the catgut is immersed in the chromic salts. The most generally accepted degree to day is medium chromic catgut which, under normal conditions, will persist in the tissues from 15 to 20 days, or a quarter of that time in the peritoneum and serous membrane.

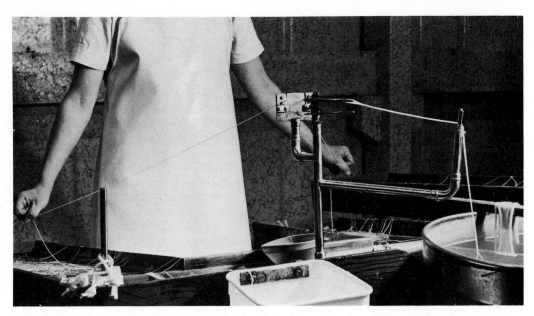

Figure 178   Splitting New Zealand milk lamb intestines into ribbon. (Ethicon.)

Each of the strands is then graded carefully into about eight standard metric sizes ranging from 0·75 to 5 (6/0 to size 2). (*The ligature or suture sizes quoted first refer always to BPC metric gauge, the sizes in brackets are the old equivalents. The metric size approximates the diameter of the strand in millimetres × 10.*) The full range from thinnest to thickest is 0·75 (6/0), 1 (5/0), 1·5 (4/0), 2 (3/0), 2·5 (2/0), 3 (0), 4 (1), 5 (2). These strands also undergo a tensile strength test over a surgeon's knot, and must reach a minimum BPC breaking load.

Size	BPC minimum breaking load tensile strength	Typical tensile strength supplied
0·75 (6/0)	0·07 kgf*	0·34 kgf
1 (5/0)	0·15 kgf	0·64 kgf
1·5 (4/0)	0·35 kgf	1·04 kgf
2 (3/0)	0·65 kgf	1·72 kgf
2·5 (2/0)	0·85 kgf	2·58 kgf
3 (0)	1·25 kgf	3·54 kgf
4 (1)	2·20 kgf	4·53 kgf
5 (2)	3·0 kgf	5·55 kgf

* kilogram force

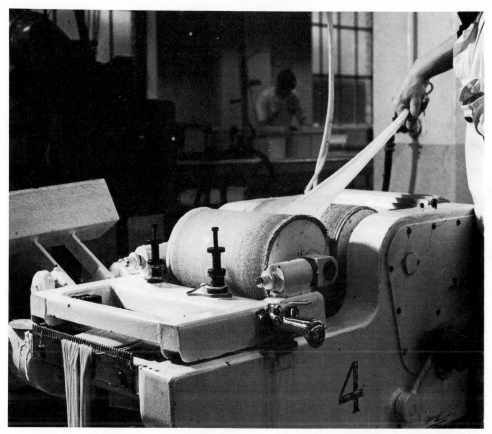

Figure 179   Machine sliming to remove fatty material from milk lamb's intestine. (Ethicon.)

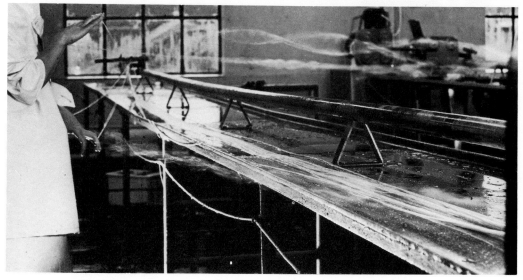

Figure 180   Spinning multiples of ribbon into raw surgical catgut. (Ethicon.)

After dividing the finished catgut into convenient lengths of 76 cm (30 in) or 1·52 m (5 ft), it is either wound on to card formers, plastic formers or coiled into a suitable size for the container. Sterilisation is effected by exposing the catgut to gamma irradiation or electron bombardment after it has been packed and sealed.

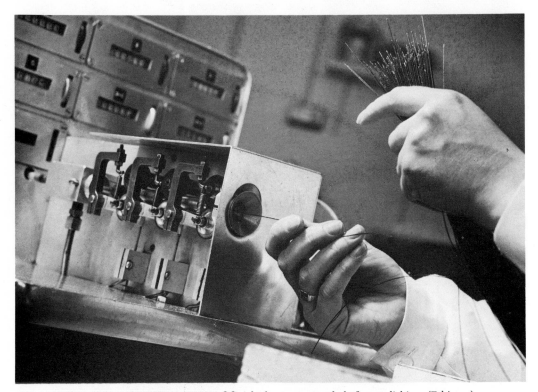

Figure 181   Electronic gauging of finished catgut strands before polishing. (Ethicon.)

Before this process of sterilisation, which is carefully controlled by laboratory tests, the catgut is packed either in plastic envelopes or aluminium foil packets containing a solution similar to purified industrial methylated spirit. The plastic packets are heat sealed, and the aluminium foil packets sealed with a special process. This is done under clean conditions as sterilisation follows afterwards.

Packets of catgut are generally presented in a sterile peel-open overwrap outer cover.

THE SIZES OF CATGUT IN GENERAL USE

This will depend a great deal upon the requirements of a particular surgeon. The tendency, however, is for the finest possible size to be used in all cases, and with the continual improvement of tensile strength the sizes in common use are much finer than those used in previous years.

For the ligation of small blood-vessels 2 or 2·5 (3/0 or 2/0) *plain* catgut is generally sufficient. Large blood-vessels and pedicles, such as those requiring ligation in gynaecological surgery, require a stouter *chromic* catgut, size 4 (1) or thicker.

The suture of stomach or bowel in the adult necessitates using size 2·5 or 3 (2/0 or 0) *chromic* catgut, whereas a child needs 2 (3/0) for these tissues.

In an adult the peritoneum and muscle can be sutured with *chromic* sizes 4 or 5 (1 or 2), a child will require at least a size smaller, 3 (0).

If subcutaneous tissue is sutured a size 2 or 2·5 (3/0 or 2/0) *plain* catgut is preferable, especially in the case of a subcutaneous suture for thyroidectomy.

Some surgeons will use *chromic* catgut throughout an operation, but if *plain* catgut is used it is important that this is not introduced as a suture (or ligature) into the peritoneum due to rapid absorption, except in very special circumstances decided by the surgeon, e.g., in the urinary tract.

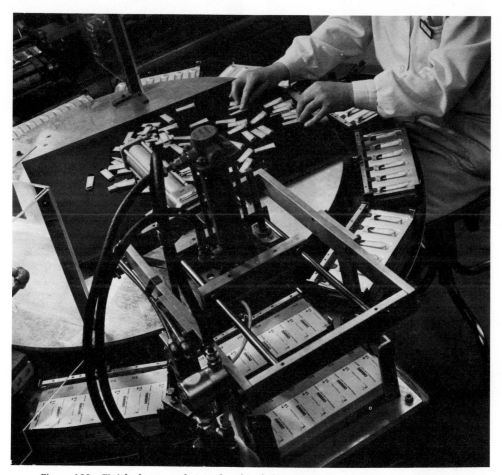

Figure 182   Finished sutures being placed in foil packets before sterilisation. (Ethicon.)

THE HANDLING OF SURGICAL CATGUT

At operation the circulating nurse peels open the outer overwrap cover. The inner packet is taken by the scrub nurse using long sterile forceps.

A plastic envelope is opened first by shaking the contents to one end of the packet and then tearing across from the 'V' cut or cutting across the other end whilst holding over a kidney dish to catch the fluid contained.

An aluminium foil packet is opened by tearing across the V-cut at one side of the

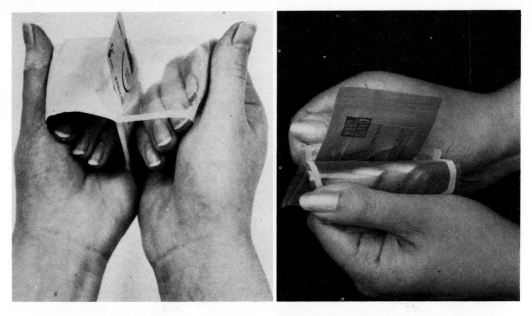

Figure 183   The peel-open overwrap packet which contains the suture packet. (Ethicon.)

Figure 184   Plastic peel-open overwrap packet. (Davis & Geck.)

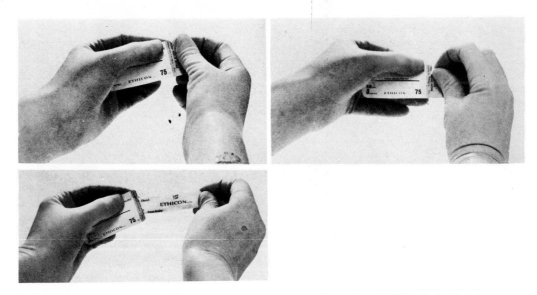

Figure 185   Opening an aluminium foil catgut pack. The packet is held with the thumbs together on either side of the notch. (Ethicon.)

Figure 186   Tearing open along the dotted line. (Ethicon.)

Figure 187   Removing the suture. (Ethicon.)

packet. Care must be taken not to squeeze the packet as this is done, for fluid may be sprayed out under pressure and may cause damage to the user's eyes.

1. The catgut is removed from the tube or packet with sterile forceps, together with the size label which is useful for reference, especially when several sizes are in use.

2. In general surgery the catgut is removed from the packet and each end of the strand grasped with the gloved hands being stretched slightly to remove the kinks. In orthopaedic surgery this operation *may* have to be performed using forceps, care being taken to ensure that the catgut is not crushed with the forceps except at the end of a strand. A crush mark in the centre of a ligature or suture may cause it to break during handling.

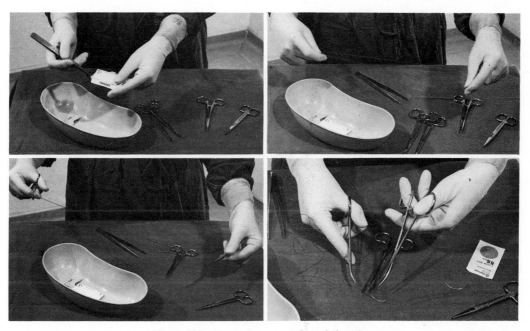

Figure 188   Removing catgut from foil packet.

Figure 189   Stretching catgut by hand to remove kinks.

Figure 190   Stretching catgut with forceps to remove kinks.

Figure 191   Threading a suture needle with forceps.

3. The material is then cut up into suitable strands for ligatures or sutures which are threaded on to needles either by hand, or for orthopaedic operations by using a non-touch technique. The material should be threaded from within the curve of the needle outwards, leaving one end about 5 to 10 cm (2 to 4 in) long. The material may be locked in the eye of the needle either by passing through a second time in the same direction or by tying a single knot. If it is frequently necessary to have a locked suture, it is preferable to use a special needle such as the Paterson or spring-eye needle, which locks the catgut without passing it through the eye a second time or tying a knot.

Even with Paterson eye or spring-eye needles two strands of catgut always pass through the tissues. This creates unnecessary trauma, especially when suturing delicate tissue.

The use of non-traumatic sutures is now well established and this obviates the disadvantages of doubling the suture when using a needle having an eye.

Non-traumatic sutures are manufactured by fusing the suture material into a needle designed with one end hollowed.

Catgut is very suitable for use in non-traumatic needles, and is supplied as prepared general closure intestinal or plastic sutures, sizes 4 to 1 (1 to 5/0) on various shapes and sizes of needles.

Catgut ligatures and sutures must not be left exposed for any length of time. Ideally the ligature or suture is only removed from the tube or packet just before required, but if prepared previously it must be kept covered with a small sterile towel.

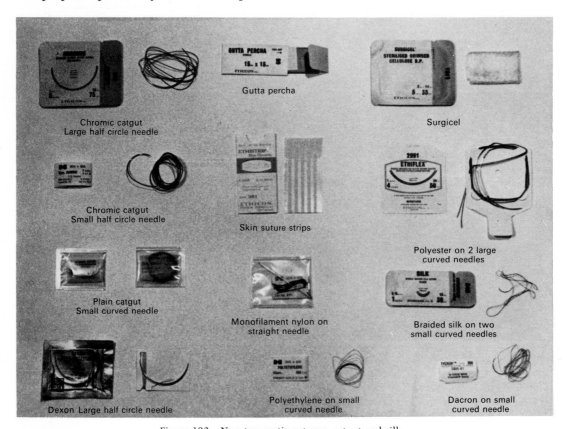

Figure 192   Non-traumatic sutures, catgut and silk.

It is very important to ensure that catgut is *not* soaked before use as this causes the material to swell and increases the speed of digestion in the tissues. Passage once through the tissues will lubricate the suture sufficiently for use. If the surgeon insists on pre-moistening the catgut, it may be drawn *very gently* through a moistened glove or swab.

Care must be exercised when handling catgut to avoid fraying, as this will weaken the strand considerably and may cause the breaking of a suture line post-operatively.

Dexon

For many decades the only absorbable suture in general use was catgut. In 1970, a synthetic absorbable material became available for the first time under the trade name Dexon and this product is now well established as an alternative to catgut

Dexon is a synthetic polymer of glycolic acid, a naturally-occurring substance. It is absorbed in tissues essentially by hydrolysis and not digested by proteolysis as are gut and collagen. The material is developed by extrusion as fine strands which are then braided to form a uniform gauge thread. Tests have shown a minimal absorption in tissue at 15 days, maximum absorption at 30 days and essentially complete resorption after 60 to 90 days after operation.

A polyglycolic acid suture is extremely inert and causes minimal tissue reaction. Size for size with catgut it is stronger, is fray resistant and does not become slippery in use. The BPC gradings of breaking load in kgf over a surgeon's knot can be summarised as follows:

0·75 metric	(6/0)	0·44
1	,,	(5/0)	0·82
1·5	,,	(4/0)	1·3
2	,,	(3/0)	1·8
2·5	,,	(2/0)	2·8
3	,,	(0)	4·5
4	,,	(1)	5·9

The material is handled in precisely the same manner as catgut. The main contra-indication is that it should not be used where extended approximation of tissues must be maintained; a non-absorbable material is more suitable for this purpose. As with all sutures care must be taken with respect to drainage and closure of infected wounds. Dexon requires special care in placing the first knot; it will not slip and 'snug' down under additional throws. The first throw is always placed exactly where required and knots tied in this way remain secure. Dexon is not suitable for resterilisation at hospital level.

Although Dexon is used mainly for deep sutures it can be used as a conventional skin suture or as a subcuticular closure. This technique is particularly suitable for cosmetic surgery where minimal tissue reaction is essential.

Living sutures

These are tissue sutures obtained from the patient himself.

The most usual are strips of fascia lata used in Gallie's herniorrhaphy and obtained from the lateral aspect of the thigh. In one method the strips of fascia 0·5 cm by 18 cm ($\frac{1}{4}$ in by 7 in) approximately are obtained through a long thigh incision, following which the fascial defect and skin are sutured. It is possible also to remove these strips via two small incisions using a fasciatome, but in this case the fascial defect is not sutured.

The fascial strips are secured on a large-eye Gallie's needle either by locking the fascia through itself or stitching with separate silk sutures before being darned into position over the hernial defect.

Tendons may be used in a similar manner also, the plantaris tendon of the leg being suitable as its removal results in minimal interference with function.

Collagen tape

Reconstituted chromic collagen tape (Ethicon) is intended as a substitute for auto-logenous and homologenous fascia used in various repair operations.

Its advantages over the patient's own fascia, or over beef fascia are that it avoids an operation on the leg to obtain fascia lata; it ties easily without the need of secondary sutures; it is stronger than fascia of similar mass; and it contains no extraneous tendinous material as that found in beef fascia.

In ophthalmic surgery collagen tape can be used as a frontal muscle sling for the correction of blepharotosis or ptosis. Ptosis may be congenital or senile but generally it is acquired by accident which severs either the levator muscle or the third cranial nerve, or by the invasion of the muscle by a tumour.

The frontalis sling operation is normally used if there is no demonstrable levator muscle action, or if a previous levator shortening operation has failed to give the desired results. The general principle is to use two loops of fascia approximately 30·5 cm (12 in) in length as slings to raise the eyelid. These slings are carefully buried in order to achieve the best cosmetic results.

In other branches of surgery it can be substituted where fascia would normally have been used. In repair of lacerations of the liver for example or in nephropexy the breadth of the suture is an advantage with these extremely soft tissues. Collagen tape can be insetted with a suitable needle such as Gallie's or Wright's.

Collagen tape is supplied in lengths of 60 cm (24 in) by 3 mm ($\frac{1}{8}$ in) in width.

NON-ABSORBABLE LIGATURES AND SUTURES

Materials in this category may be divided into two classes, those manufactured from natural raw materials and those which are entirely synthetic, being prepared in the laboratory. Non-absorbable sutures are not generally used in an infected wound as they may cause sinus formation.

Natural Materials

Silkworm gut

This is obtained from the glands of the silkworm, and is drawn out into monofilament (one strand) threads of varying diameters, measuring about 25·4 to 35·6 cm (10 to 14 in) in length and of a slightly roughened surface.

The four main sizes are: fine, medium, strong and extra strong, and may be dyed various colours from white or pink to purple or black, according to the size. The strands of gut are kept together by threading them through a metal H-piece of short lengths of rubber tubing.

Silkworm gut is used mainly for skin sutures, deep 'through-and-through' tension sutures for the abdominal wall or to retain a dressing in position by suturing it over the wound. This latter method is particularly suitable where it is difficult to retain a dressing in place, as following excision of pilonoidal sinus. The use of this material is now largely superceded by the introduction of the synthetics.

Silk thread

A material which may be either twisted or braided from numerous gossamer strands, supplied on spools of 25, 50 or 100 metres. It is white or black generally, but can be obtained in various other colours to special order. It should always be rewound on to metal, nylon or polypropylene spools before sterilisation, for if left on wooden spools the expansion of the wood will stretch and weaken the material.

Armour Suture Laboratories supply braided silk already wound on a spool contained in an autoclavable ligature egg.

The sizes vary from very fine 0·75 to 6 (6/0 to 4) or even stronger. These sizes must comply with the minimum BPC breaking load.

The minimum breaking load in kg force, over a surgeon's knot, braided silk are as follows:

Size		BPC minimum breaking load	Typical tensile strength supplied
0·75	(6/0)	0·20 kgf	0·30 kgf
1	(5/0)	0·40 kgf	0·64 kgf
1·5	(4/0)	0·75 kgf	0·95 kgf
2	(3/0)	1·3 kgf	1·54 kgf
2·5	(2/0)	2·0 kgf	2·3 kgf
3	(0)	3·0 kgf	3·27 kgf
4	(1)	4·5 kgf	4·58 kgf
5	(2)	6·0 kgf	6·40 kgf
5·5	(3)	7·0 kgf	—
6	(4)	8·0 kgf	—

The very fine sizes from 0·75 to 2 (6/0 to 3/0) are useful in vascular and nerve anastomosis, plastic surgery and intestinal suturing; 2 to 4 (3/0 to 1) are very suitable for ophthalmic surgery; 2·5 to 4 or 5 (2/0 to 1 or 2) for general ligatures or sutures; and up to size 6 (4) or more for large pedicles such as haemorrhoids, etc.

It is important to use serum-proofed silk to reduce capillary attraction, which is the peculiarity of a plaited or braided material. The capillary attraction which a non-serum proofed material has is rather dangerous as bacteria may lodge in the minute spaces of the braiding, becoming a permanent source of irritation and wound infection.

Where many silk sutures are required during the operation either non-traumatic, ready-needled sutures are used or alternatively it is advantageous to thread the needles beforehand and autoclave ready for use. The appropriate needles are threaded with various sizes of silk and are stitched loosely on to a pad before sterilisation. In this method very great care must be taken to check the total number of needles both before and after operation.

Linen thread

A ligature or suture which is prepared from linen flax and is used in a similar manner to catgut. Many surgeons use it for ligatures and sutures of the viscera, muscle and skin.

Some manufacturers dye the thread in various colours, although the standard colours are cream/white or black. Linen thread is obtained on wooden spools containing 25 to 100 m (25 to 100 yds) and should be rewound on to ligature spools before sterilisation. The thread is available also ready sterilised in packets containing up to 50 cut strands (Ethicon) and wound on autoclave spools (Armour).

The tensile strength of linen must comply with the minimum BPC breaking load over a surgeon's knot.

Size		BPC minimum breaking load
0·75	(6/0)	0·30 kgf
1	(5/0)	0·60 kgf
1·5	(4/0)	1·25 kgf
2	(3/0)	1·9 kgf
2·5	(2/0)	3·0 kgf
3	(0)	4·0 kgf
4	(1)	6·3 kgf
5	(2)	8·2 kgf

Cotton thread

Originating from cotton plants the fibres are usually twisted rather than braided. It has a limited use, mainly for fine ligatures, for the tensile strength of cotton is the least of all sutures available. It does, however, gain about 10 per cent in strength during sterilisation at the expense of some shrinkage. For this reason cotton should be prepared as cut lengths and not wound on to spools.

A combination of cotton and polyester fibre in black or white is available under the trade name of Ethicot (Ethicon).

It is supplied in sizes 3/0 to 1, with a minimum breaking load in kg force over a surgeon's knot of:

Size		Breaking load
2	(3/0)	0·79 kgf
2·5	(2/0)	1·7 kgf
3	(0)	2·6 kgf
4	(1)	3·4 kgf

Ethicot is serum-proofed and non-capillary.

Synthetic Materials

Nylon

This was the first synthetic plastic suture material which was developed during the last war and it is obtainable in two main categories – monofilament and multifilament or braided.

THE MONOFILAMENT VARIETY

This is a single strand of nylon, generally blue in colour, which is similar to silkworm gut and may be used as such, but has a smoother surface.

It is supplied in sizes ranging from 0·75 to 5 (6/0 to 2) which must comply with the minimum BPC breaking load in kg force over a surgeon's knot.

Size		BPC minimum breaking load (tensile strength)	Typical tensile strength supplied
0·75	(6/0)	0·25 kgf	0·37 kgf
1	(5/0)	0·50 kgf	0·73 kgf
1·5	(4/0)	1·0 kgf	1·13 kgf
2	(3/0)	1·6 kgf	1·63 kgf
2·5	(2/0)	2·7 kgf	2·77 kgf
3	(0)	3·5 kgf	3·67 kgf
4	(1)	5·5 kgf	5·58 kgf
5	(2)	7·0 kgf	7·43 kgf

The material can be obtained in several lengths, from 36 to 102 cm (14 to 40 in), the shorter length for skin sutures and the longer length for the nylon darn in herniorrhaphy, or for suturing muscle.

The finest sizes are suitable for plastic face sutures, whereas the strongest are more applicable for 'through-and-through' abdominal tension sutures. A monofilament nylon suture must be cut at least 10 mm ($\frac{3}{8}$ in) long, as slight slipping of the knot may occur under certain conditions.

Nylon as a single strand is relatively inert and may be left in the tissues with very little unfavourable reaction occurring.

THE BRAIDED VARIETY

This can be compared to braided silk and is used in a similar manner. The sizes available range from 1·5 to 6 (4/0 to 4) and the same tensile strengths as braided silk apply. There are generally only three colours available: white, black and green, which do not refer to a particular size but are only preferential colour choices. It is supplied on spools containing 25 to 100 m and is rewound in a similar manner to silk or linen thread unless the spools are autoclavable (Armour).

The material is available also ready sterile in packets and as sterile non-traumatic sutures. Braided nylon, like monofilament, is often used for hernia repair and may be prepared as a nylon mesh which is stitched over the hernial defect.

Sizes 1·5 to 2·5 (4/0 to 2/0) are used for plastic surgery, skin sutures or fine intestinal sutures, 2·5 to 4 (2/0 to 1) for ligatures and general muscle sutures, and 5 to 6 (2 to 4) for herniorrhaphy or large pedicle ligatures.

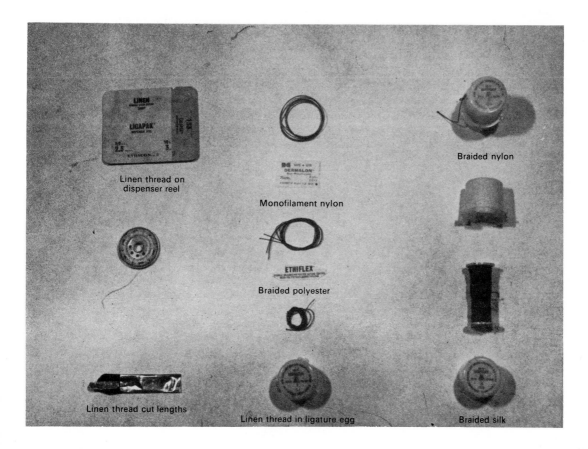

Figure 193   Linen thread and braided materials, mersilene, nylon and silk; monofilament nylon.

Polyester yarn or terylene

This is supplied as a braided material and is marketed surgically under several trade names, including Ethiflex (Ethicon), Dacron (Davis and Geck) and Arbralene (Armour). Ethiflex (green in colour) is coated with polytetra fluoroethylene to ensure smoothness and handling with no risk of flaking or fraying. Dacron is available in white or blue thread and Arbralene in white or black.

Sizes in common use are 1 to 2·5 (5/0 to 2/0) for plastic, skin, ophthalmic, or intestinal sutures and ligation of small vessels; 3 to 5 (0 to 2) for muscle sutures and stout ligatures. The materials available are serum proofed and are handled in a similar manner to braided silk, braided nylon, or linen thread.

Linear polyethylene

Under the trade name Dermalene (Davis and Geck), linear polyethylene is available as a monofilament suture. It has excellent tissue tolerance and foreign body reactions are considerably reduced.

Dermalene is blue in colour and has a low elasticity with a soft pliable feel and minimum stretch. It knots firmly with a double knot and has a reduced tendency to slip. Its main use is in vascular anastomoses, plastic surgery and other procedures which require exceptionally inert sutures.

Sizes available are 1 to 2 (5/0 to 3/0) either with or without needle attached.

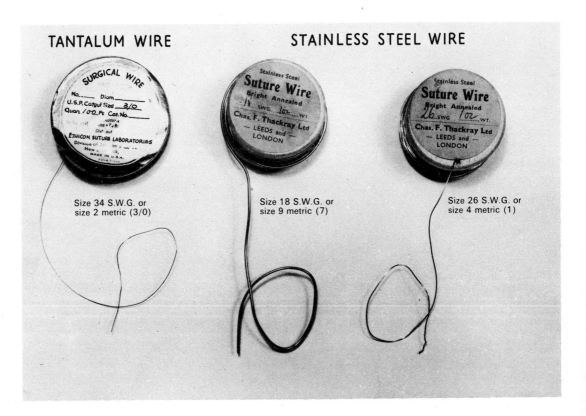

Figure 194   Monofilament suture wire.

Polypropylene

Monofilament polypropylene, coloured deep blue, is available under the trade name Prolene (Ethicon). The material is extremely inert, stronger than monofilament nylon in most sizes and very malleable; it will crush and deform easily upon knotting. This knot-holding characteristic is superior to other synthetic suture materials.

Care must be taken not to resterilise Prolene more than three times by standard autoclaving, otherwise loss of strength will occur.

The material is available in sizes 0·5 to 5 (7/0 to 2), with or without needles. Prolene is suitable for any instance where a non-absorbable suture is required.

Metal wire

Suture wire is prepared mainly from three metals – non toxic 18/8 stainless steel SMO or EN 58 J, the alloy tantalum and silver.

All these may be obtained as a single-strand suture and the first two as several strands, either twisted or braided, known as multifilament wire.

The multifilament wire is more flexible and less likely to kink during handling. The sizes are graded either as BPC metric or S.W.G. (Standard Wire Gauge). The former vary from 0·5 to 9 (7/0 to 7), and the latter gauge from fine 40 S.W.G. to stout 18 S.W.G.

Surgical suture wire is used mainly today in orthopaedics and thoracic surgery. For tendon sutures sizes 0·5 to 2 (7/0 to 3/0) or 40 S.W.G. to 30 S.W.G. are suitable, whereas a stouter wire of sizes 3 to 9 (0 to 7) or 29 S.W.G. to 18 S.W.G. would be needed for wiring fragments of bone in apposition.

It may be used also for closing an abdominal incision in the obese or carcinomatous patient, for oesophageal anastomosis, closure of a chest incision or as a mesh in the repair of hernial defects.

It is very important that wires made from different metals are not used in contact with each other in the tissues, as a reaction may occur resulting in corrosion (Chapter 23).

Fine wire is used for threading tonsil, nasal and aural snares.

Metal clips (ligature)

Ligatures of flattened silver wire are used in neurosurgery and chest surgery for arresting haemorrhage from small vessels or compressing nerve endings by clipping them. One variety is known as Cushing's or McKenzie's clips and are V-shaped, being prepared with a special cutting clamp which bends and cuts the wire in one operation.

The small V-shaped clips, each arm being about 0·45 cm ($\frac{3}{16}$ in) long, are stored on a stand or galley, and are removed with special forceps, being handed in the forceps to the surgeon. The wire, clamp, galley and insertion forceps are sterilised together by autoclaving.

The clips are very useful for ligating small vessels which are too small or inaccessible for hand ligatures.

Metal clips (suture)

These are metal clips, having two sharp points which, when the clip is closed, grip the edges of a skin incision. They are generally used to approximate a wound which heals quickly, e.g., in the region of the neck. They may be used also to close an abdominal incision or thigh incision in conjunction with tension sutures.

The two main types in use are Michel and Kifa. Both are loaded on to special insertion forceps, but the Kifa has two projecting lips on its upper surface which allow easy removal after healing has taken place. When these lips are squeezed with forceps the clip open quite easily.

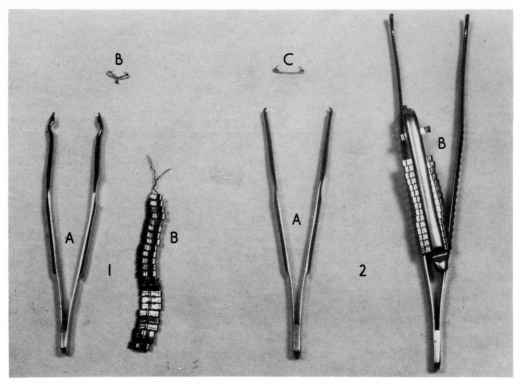

Figure 195   Michel and Kifa skin suture clips.
1A. Insertion and removal forceps (Kifa).
1B. Suture clips (Kifa).
2A. Insertion forceps (Michel).
2B. Clip galley loaded with clips (Michel).
2C. Suture clip (Michel).

8
Storage and Handling of
Ligature Materials and Associated Instruments

As a continuation of the previous chapter, we must now consider the storage and handling of ligature materials and associated instruments. Formerly, these would have been described as part of the 'ligature trolley', which consisted mainly of metal and glass dishes for the storage of sterilised instruments in an antibacterial solution. Nowadays, the use of such 'solution' storage techniques is outdated; emphasis has already been given in Chapter 6 to the importance of heat sterilisation and the dry storage of sterilised items.

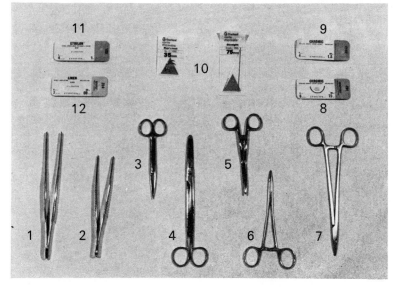

Figure 196   A selection of ligature and suture requirements.

1. & 2. Dissecting forceps, non-toothed.
3. Scissors, stitch.
4. Carless suture scissors.
5. Kilner needle holder.
6. Fine needle holder.
7. Mayo needle holder.
8. Catgut suture – general closure with needle attached.
9. Catgut ligature.
10. Suture needles of appropriate size and shape (see Figure 200).
11. Nylon – monofilament.
12. Linen thread.

Virtually all sizes and types of ligatures, sutures, scalpel blades and needles etc, can be purchased presterilised. Those items which are more convenient to process at hospital level can easily be presented in sterile packets or boxes (Brigden, 1962). All such sterile supplementary items are stored in dispensers or other suitable containers on trolleys, shelves or in cupboards in the sterile preparation room.

If ligature materials, e.g. braided materials such as silk and polyester, are sterilised at hospital level, they should be prepared as cut lengths or wound onto cards or metal or nylon spools before sterilisation, either with the set of instruments or in packets. (Wooden spools swell during sterilisation and cause damage to the material by stretching it.) The spools may be contained in ligature eggs which are marked with the size of material; one manufacturer supplies ligature material already prepared in this way (Armours).

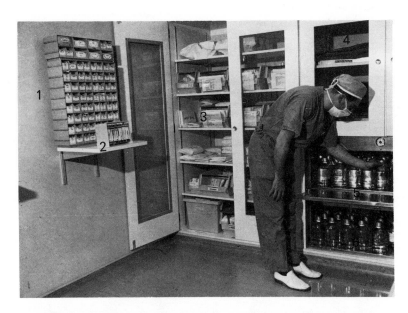

Figure 197   Storage of sterile requisites in clean utility or sterile preparation room.
1. Boxes of ligature and suture requirements stored in dispenser.
2. Sterile scalpel blades in dispenser.
3. Supplementary sterile instruments in packets.
4. Preset trays of sterile instruments.
5. Heated cabinet for lotions.
6. Lotions stored at room temperature.

Wire may be stored on metal spools also, but if possible these should be of a larger size to avoid rather small loops of wire which would otherwise tend to kink during the preparation of sutures. Manufacturers also prepare wire lengths and sutures, packed in sterile packets, and these are of special use in tendon repair. A Pulvertaft wire suture for tendon repair is available wound on a card, but this must be sterilised before use.

In many operating theatres, scalpel handles, probes, fine dissecting forceps, Michel and Kifa suture clips, suction nozzles etc. are sterilised in packets as supplementary items. These are used in conjunction with ligature requirements and are stored as described previously.

Date rotation of sterile packets is a good practice. Under clean, dry, storage conditions an intact packet will keep the contents sterile. However, freshly sterilised items should always be positioned behind those already in store and by doing this the use of outdated products is avoided.

The ligature storage trolley, shelves or cupboards should be given a thorough clean each week. Packets must be inspected for integrity and replaced if there is any doubt in respect to seals or surface.

General ligature requisites

SUTURE NEEDLES

These are made from plated carbon steel or martensitic stainless steel and occasionally austenitic stainless steel (Chapter 23). The stainless steel needles are to be preferred as they do not rust or snap easily as may the carbon steel variety. The small extra cost is amply compensated for by these two advantages.

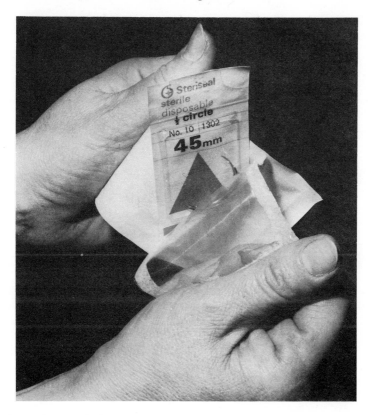

Figure 198   Sterile disposable suture needles in peel-open packet (Steriseal).

All needles fall into two principal classes: cutting needles and round-bodied needles.

1. *Cutting Needles* have sharp edges, are often triangular in section, and cut a track as they pass through the tissues. They are only used on strong tissue which will not be unduly damaged, such as fascia, muscle tendon and skin. The edge of cutting needles must be sharp, and they must be examined regularly for wear, being discarded when worn as the cost of resharpening would exceed the cost of replacement.

2. *Round-bodied Needles* cause less damage and do not actually cut the tissues, but make a puncture which closes very easily afterwards. They are used for suturing delicate tissue such as mucous membrane, fat and intestine.

Almost any style or shape of suture needle may be obtained as a non-traumatic variety; needles into which the catgut or other suture material is fused. This avoids the double thickness of material which is always present when it has been threaded through a needle eye. Round-bodied, non-traumatic needles are used for the closure of intestine, stomach, the ducts of glands, blood-vessels, and for the suture of nerves or any delicate tissue which may become traumatised during suture with conventional needles. Cutting, non-traumatic needles are used in plastic surgery for the suture of the face and other areas of skin, to minimise scar formation. They are used sometimes also for tendon suture, or for conjunctival and corneal suture in ophthalmic surgery.

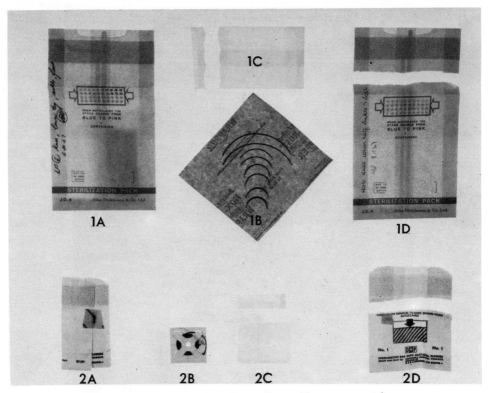

Figure 199   Heat seal bags for needles and ligature materials.

1A. Heat seal bag containing needle set.	2A. Heat seal bag containing ligature material.
1B. Set of needles which are wrapped in a piece of Non-Rust paper.	2B. Braided nylon on card former.
1C. Inner glassine bag.	2C. Inner glassine bag.
1D. Outer heat seal bag showing torn top.	2D. Outer heat seal bag showing torn top.

Suture needles are further subdivided into straight, curved, half-circle, five-eighths circle, and special shapes or types.

Straight Cutting Needles. Size 6·5 to 10 cm ($2\frac{1}{2}$ to 4 in) in length, are used for skin sutures. The most common type are called Simm's abdominal needles.

Straight Round-bodied Needles. These are usually the fine intestinal type. Sizes 5 to 7 are used for intestinal suture or as a fixation needle during nerve and tendon suture. In the latter case, the degree of pull required (upon the proximal and distal segment of the nerve or tendon) to allow approximation of the cut ends, is maintained by passing a round-bodied needle through each segment, and this prevents retraction during suture. (An alternative would be to use silk 'stay' sutures for this required pull.)

Curved Cutting Needles. These are used mainly for the suture of skin. Sizes 10 (small) to 20 (fine) are used on a needle holder, and those 2/0 (large) to 9 (medium) are used by hand (hand needles).

These needles may be obtained in normal or fine gauge, depending upon the wishes of the surgeon, but needles used in the region of the face should always be the very finest possible.

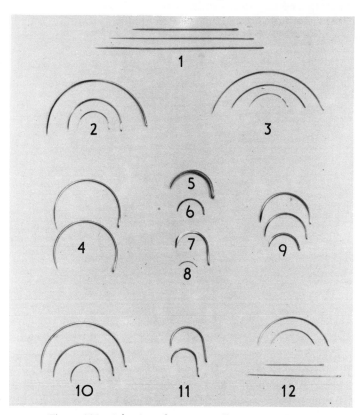

Figure 200   Selection of suture needles in general use.

1. Straight triangular cutting needles (Simm, skin).
2. Half-circle triangular cutting needles (muscle tendon, fascia, etc.).
3. Curved triangular cutting needles (skin).
4. Five-eighth-circle round-bodied and lance-point needles (Moynihan, for peritoneum and muscle respectively).
5. Fascia needle (Gallie).
6. Half-circle triangular cutting needle (fistula).
7. Reversed cutting-edge needle (Hagedorn).
8. Curved triangular cutting needle (non-traumatic, for eye and plastic surgery).
9. Trocar-point needles (Mayo, for muscle and pedicles, etc.).
10. Half-circle round-bodied needles (peritoneum, fat, etc.).
11. Round-bodied fish-hook needles (Symond, for hernia repair, etc.).
12. (*Top*) Curved round-bodied needles (peritoneum, intestine, fat, etc.).
12. (*Bottom*) Straight round-bodied needles (intestine, transfixion ligatures).

Amongst special curved cutting needles the ophthalmic types deserve individual description. These are very fine needles ranging from size 1, which is about the size of a 16 curved cutting needle, to size 6, which is a quarter of that size. There are, of course, special needles such as the Stallards which is a flattened section corneal needle and others which have reversed cutting edges, etc.

Some surgeons use ordinary cutting needles for the suture of tendons, but most express a preference for the non-traumatic type, such as the Pulvertaft, or multi-filament wire suture. The Pulvertaft is a single strand, fine 40 S.W.G. stainless steel wire, (0·5 metric/7/0) fused into a size 18 curved or straight cutting needle, and is supplied wound on a card which can be sterilised by autoclaving, or dry heat. The multifilament wire suture is welded in to one end of a similar size needle and packed ready sterilised in a plastic or foil packet. Both of these sutures are available as a single-armed (one needle) or double-armed (two needles) assembly.

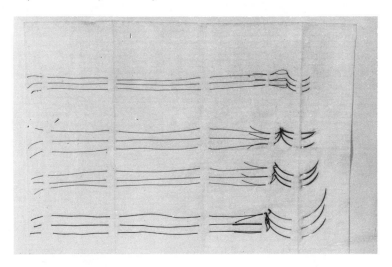

Figure 201   An autoclaved suture pack, opened out for use.

Half-circle Cutting Needles. These are used mainly for the suture of fascia and muscle tendon. Sizes 10 (small) to 20 (fine) are used on a needle holder and sizes 2/0 (large) to 9 (medium) are generally held in the surgeon's hand. Special needles of this type are: for fistula, which are coarse, strong needles; and Lane's which have rather a large eye in comparison to the gauge, which is very useful for threading silk up to size 2/0.

The fistula needles range from size 3/0 (large) to 4 (small), and the Lane's from size 1 (small) to 4 (fine), the larger size being equivalent to a size 17 ordinary half-circle needle.

The Five-eighths Circle or Fully Curved Needle. This is generally of the Moynihan variety. These needles resemble a five-eighths circle as their name implies, and are based upon the idea that nearly every surgical stitch when tied, approximates a circle very closely. In consequence, the more closely the track of the needle follows this, the more evenly will the tension be applied to the tissues.

These Moynihan needles may be round-bodied or cutting edge, which are used for suturing peritoneum or fat, and muscle tendon respectively. The round-bodied type is conventional, but the cutting needle has a flattened lance point, which is rather spear-shaped.

There are three sizes, small 8·2 cm ($3\frac{1}{4}$ in), medium 10 cm (4 in) and large 11·4 cm ($4\frac{1}{2}$ in), with a smaller round-bodied size about 3·8 cm ($1\frac{1}{2}$ in), for intestinal suturing.

Special Shapes and Types. Mayo, Symond's round-bodied fish hook, Hagedorn's reversed, and Gallie's fascia needles are the most popular, all of which are held in a needle holder for use.

The Mayo Suture Needle. This needle (for catgut), having a large square eye, is a very strong needle used extensively in gynaecology and obstetrics, or where excessive leverage may occur, e.g. during the repair of a hernia.

There are two varieties, the round-bodied and the trocar point (cutting), sizes ranging from 1 (medium) to 4 (small).

Symond's Fish Hook and Hagedorn's Reversed. These are both fish-hook in shape and are used for inaccessible suturing. The Symond's needle is round-bodied and the Hagedorn's has a reverse flattened point.

Sizes vary from 1 (large) to 10 (small), size 6 being useful for hernia repairs.

Gallie's Fascia Needle is a very broad, flattened needle, with a large eye and a lance point. A strip of fascia lata may be threaded on to this needle and used in hernia repair operations.

There are only three sizes, the most commonly used being small 3·8 cm (1½ in); the other two sizes are medium 4·5 cm (1¾ in) and large 5·7 cm (2¼ in), all of which are half-circle in shape.

It should be pointed out that the sizes of general needles, i.e., curved cutting needles, etc., vary only a little from one size to the other. The nurse will find that many surgeons use alternate size needles in which the difference of size is easily discernible, e.g., 2, 4, 6, 8, 10, etc.

Bonney Reverdin Needles are special needles which in effect incorporate their own needle holder.

These needles have an eye near to the point which is open on one side. A small, slender shutter may be slid along the handle to close this eye after the suture material has been inserted into it. The closed needle is passed through the tissues first; then the eye is opened; the suture material gripped; the eye closed, and the needle is withdrawn, pulling the suture material through the tissues to complete the stitch.

The finer varieties are used by plastic surgeons, e.g., for the repair of a cleft palate, but the most commonly used are the coarser varieties, favoured by gynaecologists, e.g., for uterine suturing (see instrument appendix).

Scalpel blades and handles

The Bard Parker scalpel handle permits the fitting of various sizes and shapes of scalpel blades according to the wishes of the surgeon.

There are six sizes of scalpel handles on the market at present; they are, sizes 3, 4, 5, 9, 3L and 4L. Of these the nurse will find that sizes 3, 4 and 5 are the most generally used.

Sizes 3 and 4 are the general purpose handle of medium length; size 5 is a long fine handle, useful during laminectomy, etc.; size 9 is a short fine handle of special use in plastic surgery; sizes 3L and 4L are long general purpose handles of application for deep cavities. The latter three sizes are only recent additions to the range.

Of the Paragon, Swann Morton, Gillette and similar ranges, the most popular sizes of scalpel blades are 10, 11, and 15, which fit handles 3, 3L, 5 and 9; sizes 20, 22, 23 and 24 which fit handles 4 and 4L.

Of the Gillette range, sizes A, B and C fit handles 4 and 4L; size D fits handles 3, 3L, 5 and 9.

Most manufacturers are now packing their scalpel blades in grease-free packets, such as the Vapour Phase Inhibitor or metal foil pack. The packet is designed as a sterile peel-open type with the blade ready for use. Individual packets of blades are presented in dispenser boxes which can be stored in a suitable rack.

Most skin-graft knives now incorporate disposable blades available in a sterile peel-open packet. If they are supplied unsterilised these may be coated with a light oil before wrapping in their protective paper cover. This oil should be removed before sterilisation, by soaking in a little trilene or ether, after which the blades should be lifted out and dried carefully. This should not be done in a confined space owing to the vapour liberated.

Skin graft blades can be sterilised by dry heat or alternatively by steam providing they are wrapped in vapour phase inhibitor anti-rust paper.

Solid scalpels

Most of these instruments are made from carbon steel because of the difficulty of obtaining a really good edge with stainless steel.

Under this heading come orthopaedic scalpels, cartilage knives, tenotomy knives, bistouries, etc.

ORTHOPAEDIC SCALPELS

These vary in size from a small 2·5 cm (1 in) blade to a 23 cm (9 in) amputation knife and are either straight or bellied in shape. The edges of these should be inspected regularly after use for bluntness, as described in Chapter 5. They are used where there is a risk of breaking a detachable blade, e.g., excising fibrous tissue at a fracture site.

Swann Morton have produced a disposable solid type blade and handle, which is similar to the Bard Parker knives but does not snap easily and may be used in all cases where a solid scalpel is required.

CARTILAGE KNIVES

These are rather a small type of solid knife, the three most popular being the Munro, Smillie and Fairbank.

The Munro has a long handle, with a short blade and a slender stem between the blade and the handle. The Smillie knives have a chisel-type point and are made as a set of three; two with concave edges, one curved for the right and one for the left, and a straight chisel blade for use with a special retractor. The Fairbank knives are made as a set of two; one curved for cutting to the right, and one curved for the left. They have a small blunt probe point with the cutting edge at one side only and are used mainly for meniscotomy as opposed to meniscectomy (Chapter 23, Fig. 348).

TENOTOMY KNIVES

These are long and slender, being used for dividing a tendon through a small puncture wound. They either have one or two cutting edges, generally with a sharp point. Amongst the most popular are the Parker's double cutting-edge spear-type point, the Jones' single cutting edge and the Adam's set of seven shapes, including blunt and sharp-pointed varieties. There are too many types for individual description, as many surgeons arrange the sharpening of their knives to suit individual tastes.

BISTOURIES

These are knives which are generally used in conjunction with a special probe or guard for the division of ligaments or fibrous bands of tissue, etc., e.g., during a strangulated hernia operation.

Although there are bistouries with sharp points, the most generally used are those having a probe point which ensures that the cutting is only with the side edge of the knife.

All these knives can be sterilised by dry heat.

Scissors

Although it is better to sterilise those scissors in common use together with the general instruments, it is common practice to store at least the special types of scissors in autoclaved packets.

Scissors may have both points sharp, both blunt, or one sharp and one blunt. They are made from martensitic stainless steel or plated carbon steel, although the latter are not often used in the operating theatre, except perhaps for cutting dressings.

Scissors having both points sharp are generally used for removing sutures, or are of a special type such as fine iridectomy scissors. They may be straight, curved on flat or angled on flat and are mostly of the fulcrum lever principle, although some special iris scissors such as the De Wecker's have a special spring cross action, enabling the surgeon to use them between his forefinger and thumb. It is very useful to reserve ordinary stitch scissors for use on the ligature trolley during the preparation of ligatures and sutures, so that they do not become mixed with the scissors reserved for the surgeon. Scissors having both points sharp and with serrated edges are available for cutting cartilage, used almost exclusively by the plastic surgeons. Stitch scissors are useful also for cutting fine wire sutures not stouter than 30 S.W.G.

The majority of scissors used for dissection have both points blunt or rounded and are available straight, curved on flat or angled on flat. The most popular are the Mayo scissors or modifications of this pattern, the most usual sizes being from 13 to 20 cm (5 to 8 in) in length. In addition to dissection, these scissors are often used for cutting ligatures and sutures, although it is better to reserve a separate pair for this purpose, to give the surgeon the advantage of scissors used exclusively for dissection.

Although Mayo scissors may be obtained in lengths up to 23 cm (9 in), when a long fine pair is required, the surgeon will often prefer a pattern such as the Metzenbaum, McIndoe 18 cm (7 in) or similar. If he requires a heavier pair, his choice may include Nelson's or Mile's which are made in lengths up to 28 cm (11 in), and as straight or curved on flat blades. These longer scissors are of special use in thoracic surgery.

A short fine pair of scissors for use in plastic surgery, peripheral nerve or tendon surgery would be the 13 cm (5 in) Kilner or Strabismus scissors, both available as straight or curved on flat blades. The Kilner's scissors have flattened, fine points, which made them very adaptable for skin dissection.

Scissors having one sharp and one blunt point are useful for cutting dressings although they may be reserved for use by the assistant when he is cutting ligatures and sutures. Some dressing scissors are made with a blunt platform extending from the tip of the lower blade. This facilitates the introduction of the lower blade under a dressing or bandage, and prevents injury to the patient's skin.

In orthopaedic theatres it may be necessary to store a variety of probes, drills, osteotomes, and gouges, etc., in sterile boxes or packets. The difference between the various types is described in Chapter 23.

Suture clips

These are generally loaded on to a special galley which also forms part of an approximation forceps (Fig. 195). The insertion forceps are grooved for the Michel-type skin clips, but are, in addition, bowed for the Kifa type to accommodate the projecting lips.

Drainage tubes, catheters, syringes, and hypodermic needles

A selection of these may be stored in autoclaved packets or purchased ready sterile from the manufacturer.

The handling of ligature and suture materials

It is very bad practice to prepare ligatures and sutures for several operations at the beginning of an operation list. Materials so prepared have to be stored on a 'stock' trolley and even with the greatest care it is impossible to guarantee sterility.

A separate, small, sterile trolley may be used as an operation ligature trolley for each case, but it is a more convenient procedure to use a corner of the instrument trolley, placing the prepared materials between two small sterile towels. It is preferable that these towels be of a different colour to the general drapes so that they serve to isolate the ligatures, etc., from the rest of the trolley.

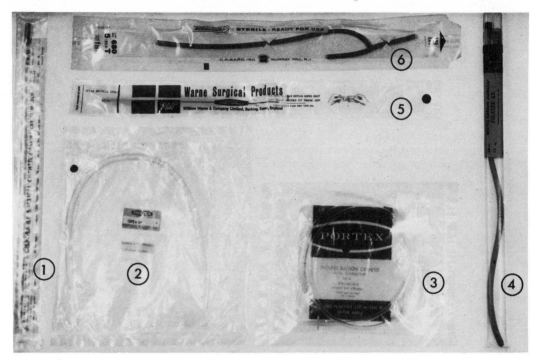

Figure 202

1. Endotracheal suction catheter.
2. Short polyvinyl suction drain.
3. Long polyvinyl suction drain with connector.

4. Foley type catheter in rigid container.
5. Foley type catheter in peel-open plastic pack.
6. 'T' tube drain in peel-open pack.

The scrub nurse collects her requirements with long handled forceps from the packets opened by the circulating nurse, placing them into a kidney dish.

The scrub nurse may prepare several ligatures and sutures at the commencement of the operation but should avoid having too many exposed, especially if the operation is a long one. The length of a ligature should not generally exceed 30·5 cm (12 in); a continuous suture length ranges between 45·7 and 61 cm (18 and 24 in), and an interrupted suture length should be between 30·5 and 45·7 cm (12 and 18 in).

If the surgeon insists upon a non-touch technique being used, the scrub nurse must handle all ligatures and sutures with forceps, taking great care to avoid crushing the material, especially catgut.

The handling of catgut has been dealt with in Chapter 7. If the surgeon is using a braided material such as silk or polyester, and he requires the suture locked in the eye of the needle, the material will have to be knotted once upon itself. Doubling braided materials through the needle eye is not satisfactory as they tend to slip. Ideally, of course, a non-traumatic suture or a Paterson eye needle should be used.

When tension sutures are being prepared, using thin rubber or plastic tubing to prevent 'cutting in' of the suture after tying, the needle is threaded and a 2·5 cm (1 in) length of tubing passed over the needle point and slid into position overlying the material in the eye. This will prevent the suture material (especially monofilament nylon) from becoming unthreaded, and will simplify positioning the tubing before the suture is tied. The surgeon will require two pairs of artery forceps for each tension suture to secure the ends until he is ready to tie them, after the musle has been sutured.

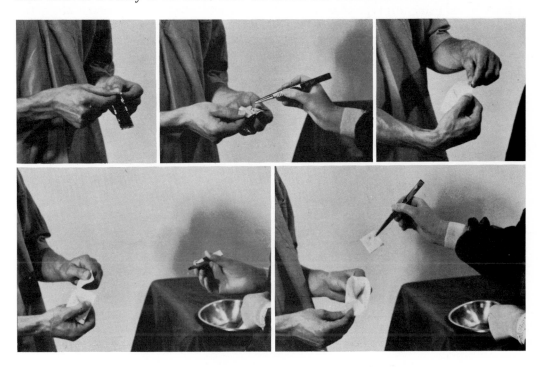

Figure 203   Peeling open a sterile scalpel blade foil packet.

Figure 204   Scrub nurse removing sterile scalpel blade from peeled-open packet.

Figure 205   Ligature packet in heat-sealed Kraft paper bag. First the bag is nicked, then . . .

Figure 206   . . . torn across without touching the torn edge . . .

Figure 207   . . . the packet is opened utilising the side gussets and the scrub nurse removes the inner sterile packet with forceps.

Only the end of a needle holder's jaws must be used to grip a needle which is held at a point one-third from the eye and two-thirds from the needle point, the only exception being a fish hook and Gallie's fascia needle. These are gripped at a point about one-quarter from the eye.

Gripping the needle in the one-third/two-thirds position ensures that the surgeon can pass the needle the maximum possible distance through the tissues without further adjustments and with the least possible risk of it snapping at its weakest point, which is near the eye.

When preparing a needle and holder for a right-handed surgeon, the nurse holds the instrument in her right hand and grips the needle with its point facing her left hand. The procedure is reversed for a left-handed surgeon and when the needle is to be used vice versa.

Some needle holders have a cranked handle, and when viewed sideways it will appear that the jaws are at a lower level than the handle. The needle should be gripped so that when it is in the correct position for use the cranked handle is above the level of the jaws and not vice versa when viewed sideways. Suturing of fairly superficial tissues and skin is easier when using this type of needle holder, as the cranked handle remains above the level of the skin even if the jaws are below. This means that the surgeon is able to hold his hand parallel to the skin instead of at an angle, and so avoids obscuring his view of the suture line.

REFERENCE

BRIGDEN, R. J. (1962). Sterile Packets for Implants and Special Instruments. *Nursing Mirror*, March 30.

9

Draping Operation Areas and Assisting the Surgeon

Although it is the ultimate responsibility of the surgeon to ensure that the operation area is correctly draped following skin preparation, this is frequently left to an experienced member of the operating theatre staff.

Furthermore, another doctor usually acts as the surgeon's first assistant, but there are occasions when a theatre nurse has to act in this capacity. This is especially so in the smaller hospital, where the medical staff is limited in number, but it must be fully understood that the duties of theatre staff do not normally include those of first assistant.

Preparing the operation area

1. ELECTIVE PROCEDURES

In most cases the first pre-surgical skin preparation is performed in the ward. This generally consists of cleansing the operation site and surrounding area, followed by shaving. The first preparation may also include the application of a non-irritant skin antiseptic and sterile towels. This only applies, of course, to cases where there are no open wounds, for these generally require surgical toilet under anaesthesia.

In theatre, the sterile towels are removed and the operation area is painted with the antibacterial agent of choice, i.e., alcoholic Hibitane 0·5 per cent, alcoholic iodine 2 per cent, or Povidone iodine, etc. Application of this antiseptic should commence first at the site of incision, continuing in ever widening circles or squares, until a sufficient area has been covered. A second application of antiseptic, using fresh swabs, is made after the first has dried (Public Health Laboratory Report, 1965; Medical Research Council, 1968).

It is essential to paint a much larger area than required for the purpose of operation (Falk, 1942; Gainsbert et al., 1967; Hamilton Bailey, 1967). This should extend at least 15·2 cm (6 in) beyond the area isolated by the sterile towels or drapes, to allow manipulations or readjustment of towels during operation.

When the operation site is near the genitals or anus, the application of a skin antiseptic should be towards this area which is painted last. The swab used for this purpose must always be discarded after passing over the anus.

The suggested minimal areas of preparation for various operations are listed in Figure 208.

2. CONTAMINATED WOUNDS

Any open wound must have a thorough toilet under anaesthesia before applying the usual skin antiseptic.

Sterilised nylon bristle nail brushes and an antiseptic detergent such as aqueous Savlon 3 per cent are ideal for this purpose. To assist efficient cleansing of a limb, a large, sterile, shallow tray is placed under the wound area and used as a douche tray.

At least two brushes must be available for this procedure, the first being used for the initial cleansing of skin for a wide area surrounding the wound, and the second in a separate bowl of solution for the wound itself. During initial cleansing, the wound is covered with a sterile swab or towel and it is at this stage that any hairs are shaved away.

AREAS OF SKIN PREPARATION IN WARD AND THEATRE

AREA OF OPERATION	AREA OF PREPARATION
Skull	Entire skull, forehead, ears and neck.
Face	Entire face and neck and if necessary including the ears. For eye operations the eyebrows *may* be shaved off, and the lashes are cut with petroleum jelly smeared scissors.
Chest—	
Supine	From mid-abdomen to shoulders and neck, extending laterally round loins and thorax, on both sides.
Lateral	From mid-abdomen to shoulders; including the lateral aspects of the thorax and loins on the affected side and extending over the spine.
Abdomen	From the nipples to the upper part of the thighs, extending laterally round abdominal wall and pelvis, on both sides; including the genital region.
Genital region	From the umbilicus to mid-thighs, extending laterally round the pelvis and including the genital and anal regions.
Anal region	The upper part of both thighs, the buttocks, genital region and lower part of the abdomen.
Spine	From the shoulders to the upper part of the thighs, including the anal region and extending laterally round the loins and thorax.
Hand, forearm and upper arm	From the finger tips to the elbow (or shoulder for upper arm).
Foot and ankle	From the toes to knee level for full circumference of the limb.
Lower leg and knee	From the toes to mid-thigh for full circumference of the limb.
Hip and thigh	Whole of the leg, buttocks, and genital region; extending up to the level of the ribs; and over the lateral aspect of the abdomen on the affected side.

Figure 208

Although a certain amount of care should be exercised when cleansing a wound, to avoid damage to exposed nerves, etc., it is very important to remove as much debris as possible. The sterile nylon brushes will be found useful for this, but large fragments of foreign materials or damaged tissue and blood clots which cannot be removed by gentle brushing should be left for removal by the surgeon.

After a thorough toilet, the area is dried with a sterile swab or towel, and skin antiseptic applied before placing the drapes in position.

When a general anaesthetic is not practicable, the surgeon will administer local or regional anaesthesia following minimal cleansing and before wound toilet is commenced.

Draping the operation area

The operation area must be draped to allow free access for the surgeon, but the towels should be so arranged that manipulations do not expose any unprepared skin areas.

A sterile water repellent sheet (e.g., Ventile fabric or disposable paper) should be placed in position first, to prevent contamination should the sterile drapes become damp or soiled.

Methods of towelling or draping are essentially practical procedures, depending upon the wishes of the surgeon, the area, and sizes of towels available. In this chapter we must therefore confine ourselves to general observations, and use these as a basis for practice.

ABDOMINAL OPERATIONS

The sterile water repellent sheet should extend from knee level to the chest with a central aperture about 30·5 cm (12 in) long by 10·2 cm (4 in) wide, but may be omitted in operations on children to avoid overheating.

Alternatively, four pieces of Ventile fabric may be draped to surround the incision area. One piece of fabric should always be placed in position over the pubic area first, followed by a piece on each side and another one over the chest.

However thorough the preparation is, the skin surface will not remain surgically clean indefinitely. If the operation lasts for more than half an hour or so, the patient will begin to perspire resulting in surface contamination from organisms within the sweat pores. In order to minimise this contamination the skin may be covered with a piece of self-adhesive polyvinyl sheet (Vi-Drape, Steridrape or OpSite).

This polyvinyl sheet is applied immediately following the initial water repellent towels. A piece of self-adhesive Vi-Drape, Steridrape or OpSite is stretched over the area and with a sterile swab is smoothed flat from the centre to the periphery. This ensures positive adhesion and avoids air bubbles being trapped beneath the sheet.

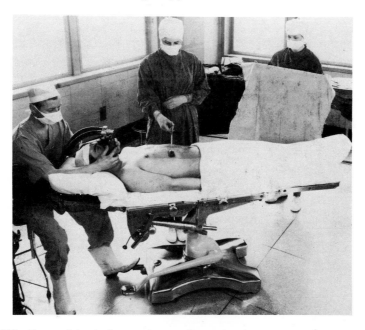

Figure 209   Upper abdominal operation, applying the skin antiseptic in ever-widening squares.

The incision is made through the plastic sheet and underlying skin.

The entire area may then be draped with a large abdominal sheet having a central

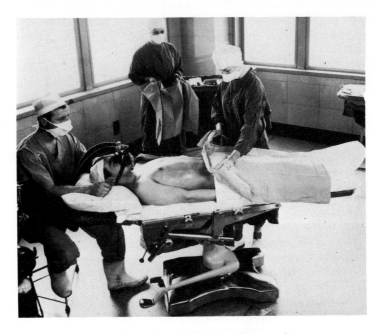

Figure 210   Piece of ventile positioned over pubic area.

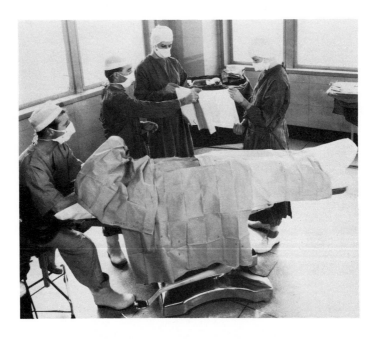

Figure 211   Four pieces of Ventile in position, application of polyvinyl sheet. The protective backing is removed from the self-adhesive Vi-Drape, Steridrape, or OpSite as shown, taking care to ensure the sheet is kept under tension to avoid creases.

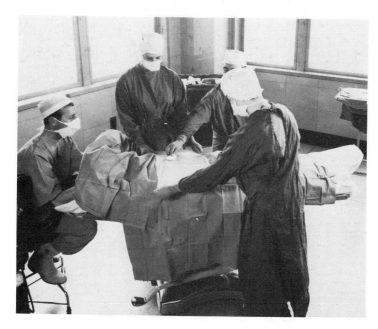

Figure 212   The polyvinyl sheet applied to the abdomen and smoothed into position with a swab from the centre to the periphery, to avoid air bubbles being trapped underneath. (The incision is made through the plastic sheet on attached skin.)

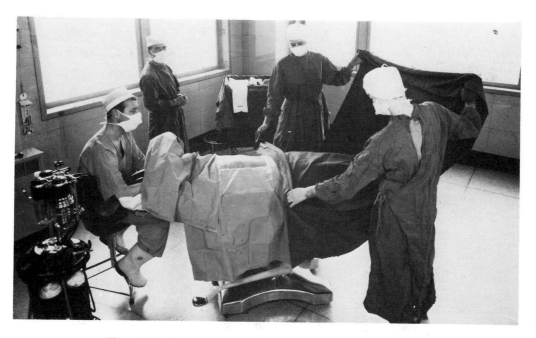

Figure 213   The lower extremities are covered with a large drape.

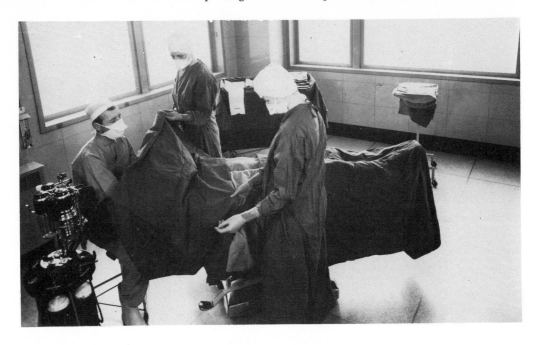

Figure 214   A second large drape is placed over the chest and head (a wire screen may be
used to isolate the anaesthetist and provide clear access to the patient's airway).

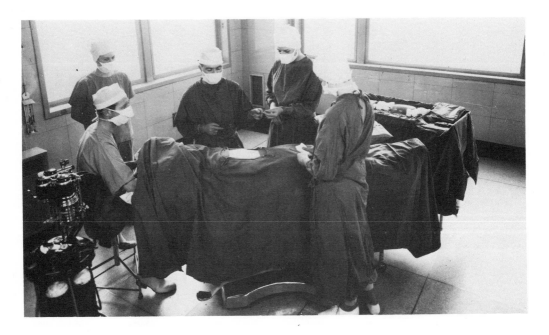

Figure 215   'Holed' abdominal sheet positioned over previous drapes, towel clips applied.

aperture, or four/five towels positioned as previously described. This arrangement appears the neatest, and prevents the side towels from slipping down.

The patient's arm or arms abducted on an arm table or support for transfusion or other purposes, should be covered with small towels before commencing the abdominal draping.

A metal wire frame fitted to the operation table head, and draped with the upper part of the abdominal sheet, may be used to isolate the anaesthetist from the sterile areas. It also prevents the drapes from covering the patient's face and obscuring a clear observance of his appearance. The frame is of special use when the patient is conscious and a local or spinal anaesthetic has been administered. Care must be taken, however, to avoid the patient's arm coming into contact with the metal frame, especially if diathermy is being used as this could result in accidental burns (Fig. 216).

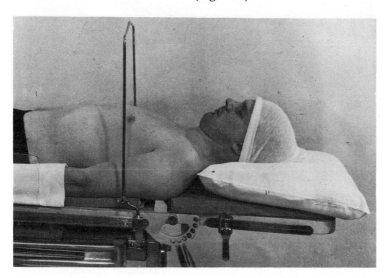

Figure 216   Anaesthetic screen at operation table head. (If the patient is broad, soft pads will be required between the patient's arms and screen uprights.)

If a polyvinyl barrier sheet has not been applied to the skin during draping, after the incision has been made, small skin or 'tetra' towels may be clipped to the skin edges. It is however an inferior technique, for the 'tetra' towels soon become soaked with blood unless they are formed from small pieces of polyvinyl sheet.

THORACIC AND KIDNEY OPERATIONS

Several small pieces of water repellent fabric and standard towels are draped similarly to abdominal operations, leaving the area of incision exposed.

LIMB OPERATIONS

It is important that the drapes are secured to withstand any manipulations of a limb during operation.

In addition to small towels, some larger, about 152·4 cm (5 ft) square, should be available – two for a lower limb, and one for an upper limb.

Only the incision area of the limb should be exposed during operation, unless of course multiple incisions are necessary as for the ligation of varicose veins. Towels may be used to cover the unrequired skin areas, but a sterile stocking made from stockinette or calico stitched at one end is less bulky.

It is very important that all parts of a limb (including the foot) which will be subject to handling by the surgeon must be painted with skin antiseptic.

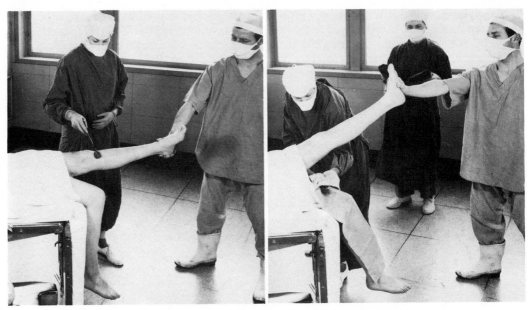

Figure 217   Draping the lower limb; application of skin antiseptic.

Figure 218   Piece of Ventile positioned over other leg.

In orthopaedic surgery, Vi-Drape, Steridrape or OpSite are generally applied to the skin thereby providing a skin towel through which the surgeon makes his incision.

A sterile water repellent sheet must be placed under the limb before the towels and should extend well about the operation site. For operations on the lower extremities, this means from the foot end of the operation table to mid-thigh, or higher if necessary. When one leg is involved, the water repellent sheet covers the other completely. In the case of of upper limb operations, it should cover the arm table and extend well up to the axilla. With the arm across the chest, the water repellent sheet is placed, extending from lower abdomen to axilla.

After covering and overlapping the water repellent sheet with towels, a 'shut off' towel is used to isolate the prepared from the unprepared areas of the limb. This towel is placed under the limb and crossed over on the opposite side, to be secured with a towel clip or clips.

EAR, NOSE AND THROAT OPERATIONS

In all cases the upper part of the head and hair may be draped in almost the same way.

Two opened towels and a water repellent sheet are placed under the patient's head, the upper towel is crossed over a point above the operation area and secured with a towel clip, i.e., for operations on the eyes, at a point in the centre of the forehead; for operations on the mouth or nose, at a point over the nose bridge after covering the closed eyelids with a sterile swab, etc.; and for operations on the ear, just superior to the ear on the affected side.

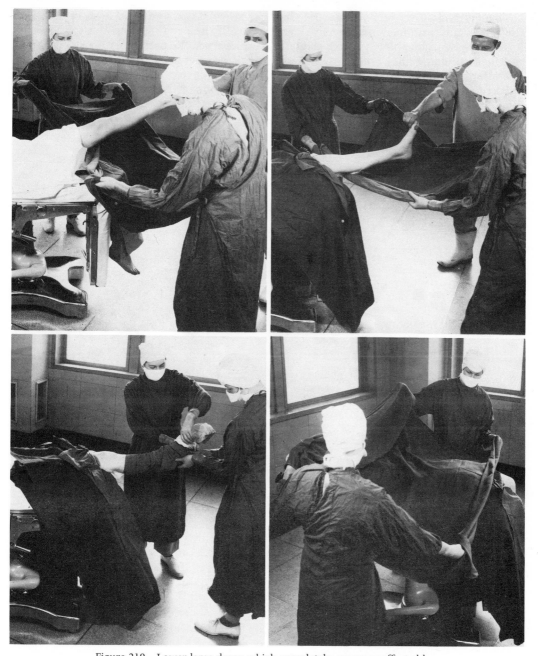

Figure 219   Lower large drape which completely covers unaffected leg.

Figure 220   After application of a small piece of Vi-Drape, Steridrape or OpSite to the incision area the lower part of the leg is wrapped in a sterile towel.

Figure 221   A calico bag is placed over the wrapped leg to retain towel in position, this may be bandaged or clipped.

Figure 222   Draping is completed with another large sheet placed over the upper part of the patient. This procedure is suitable for a meniscectomy or similar operation on the knee.

This method of draping will ensure that the hair is always covered and, in addition, the sterile towel underlying, cover the area beneath the head.

The draping is completed by covering the lower part of the patient with a sterile water repellent sheet and one or more towels extending from just below the operation area. For operations on the eyes or ears, the lower half of the face, including the nose, should be covered; for those on the mouth or nose, the lower part of the drapes extends from the chin.

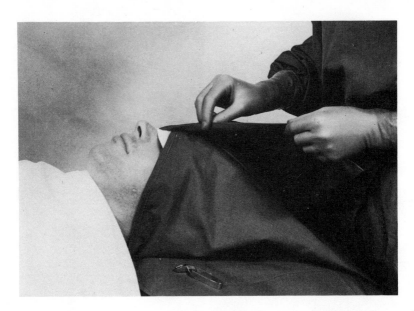

Figure 223   Draping head for E.N.T. operation. Showing two-towel technique for covering hair.

OPERATIONS ON THE NECK

The head is covered as for ENT operations, but the towel is crossed over at the centre of the chin.

A pad of sterile wool should be tucked in at each side of the neck to absorb any blood which may trickle down during operation. This is followed by a sterile water repellent sheet across the chest and one or more towels to cover this and the lower extremities.

The use of towel clips to secure towels in this region is often avoided by surgeons, due to the difficulty of applying towel clips to the chin without risking scarring. Not only is this a serious consideration, but it is very irritating to find that these clips frequently pull away during the course of operation. The alternative is to use three or four monofilament nylon sutures at each point and these cause very little trauma. The sutures are cut out before removing the drapes.

CRANIAL OPERATIONS

These often last a long time and it is important that the drapes remain secure and sterile throughout the whole period. Furthermore, unless great care is taken, soiling of the towels after incision involves the risk of contamination from the underlying skin. It is for this reason that many surgeons prefer an antibacterial barrier placed in position before the final drapes.

Supine or Prone Position. This requires a sterile water repellent sheet to be placed under the head first.

Three small towels are then submerged in an antibacterial agent, e.g., aqueous Savlon 1 per cent, and wrung until almost dry. These are placed as a triangle, surrounding the incision area and are clipped into position on the scalp. Alternatively, polyvinyl sheet (Vi-Drape, Steridrape or OpSite) may be applied to cover the whole scalp. The closed eyelids must always be covered with a sterile swab or eyepads.

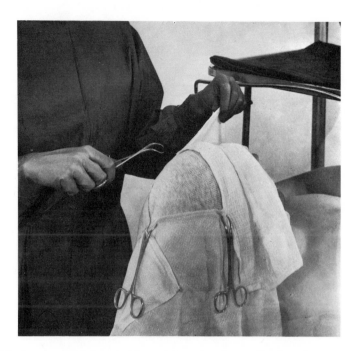

Figure 224   Draping head for cranial operation. Showing application of antiseptic towels.

The anaesthetist must have access to the patient's airway during operation and further drapes should always be placed with this in mind. A sterile water repellent sheet extending from the antiseptic towels and across the chest is draped over a large instrument table or wire screen placed about 30·5 cm (12 in) above the patient and at shoulder level.

The final towel is placed around the head, first draped over the water repellent sheet (covering the instrument table or wire screen), and then over transfusion stands at each side of the operation table (Fig. 225).

This method of draping will ensure complete isolation of the anaesthetist from the operation area, and by forming a tent over the patient provides good access to the patient's airway and lower extremities.

The Neurosurgical Sitting Position. This position with the head flexed and immobilised by a cranial support, requires first a sterile water repellent sheet and towel placed across the shoulders extending from neck level to cover the chair back.

The draping is then completed as previously described, but the towels are draped first over an instrument table positioned just in front of the patient's forehead, and then over transfusion stands at each side of the operation table.

SPINAL OPERATIONS (INCLUDING LAMINECTOMY, SYMPATHECTOMY, DECOMPRESSION, EXCISION OF PILONOIDAL SINUS, ETC.)

The Prone Position. A patient placed in the prone position (or the knee/elbow flexed rabbit position), for lumbar, sacral, or mid-thoracic approach, may be draped as for abdominal operations, utilising the 'holed' water repellent sheet and towel.

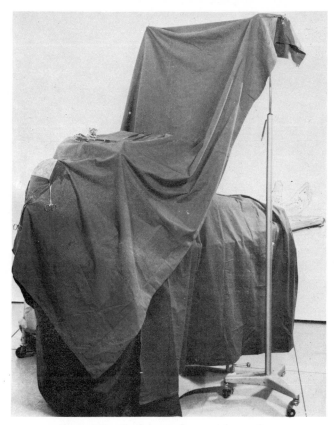

Figure 225   Final drapes for cranial operation.

High Cervical Areas. These can be draped similarly, but in addition the head should either be isolated with antiseptic barrier towels, or covered first by using the two-towel technique described for ENT operations. The cross-over point of the towels should be at the occiput.

Pieces of sterile cotton-wool tucked in at each side of the neck will prevent soiling due to blood trickling down during operation.

Lateral Position. These should be draped similarly to thoracic procedures, using four separate water repellent sheets and towels.

In all cases, Vi-Drape, Steridrape or OpSite can be applied as for an orthopaedic operation.

PERINIAL OPERATIONS (VAGINAL, RECTAL, CYSTOSCOPY, URETHAL OPERATIONS, ETC.) IN THE LITHOTOMY POSITION

The first stage is placing a sterile water repellent sheet under the buttocks. This is important, as it prevents contamination from the lower part of the operation table which would otherwise become rather wet during the course of the operation.

A 'holed' water repellent sheet or plastic adhesive drape is used to isolate the operation area from surrounding unprepared skin and this is followed by a special drape having two lateral leg 'bags' stitched to either side of a central slit. The central slit is adjusted around the operation area and the 'bags' cover both legs and operation table stirrups. The upper and lower ends of the 'holed' towel cover the abdomen and lower end of the operation table respectively.

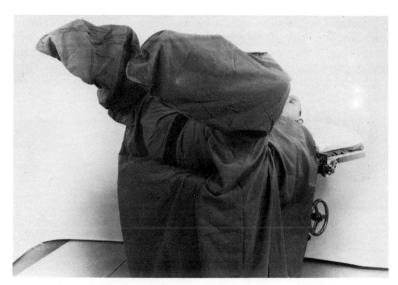

Figure 226   Lithotomy drapes, showing special 'holed' towel with bag-shaped leg covers.

Alternatively, a small towel may be placed over each leg and stirrup, followed by a standard 'holed' towel with its slit over the operation area, and sides secured around each leg and stirrup.

A sterile douche tray may be added after the drapes have been positioned correctly.

Synchronous combined excision of the rectum performed simultaneously from the abdominal and perineal route by two surgeons, requires complete draping of the two areas. This is achieved by using a drape as previously described, but having a slit which will extend from the anus to the umbilicus. A small towel is placed to cover and isolate the genitals.

Many surgeons operating in the perineal region appreciate a towel draped as a trough between the patient and themselves. One edge of this towel is secured just below the operation area and to the towel covering the leg and stirrup on each side, the other edge being clipped to the surgeon's gown. This method will prevent dropped instruments from slipping to the floor and will provide the surgeon with a 'shelf' for his swabs, etc., if he should so desire. Alternatively a narrow table placed transversely may be used and is placed in position before draping.

Assisting the surgeon

It would be very presumptous to even suggest that the technique, of assisting the surgeon either as first assistant, second assistant or scrub nurse, can be learned from a book. This, like draping the operation area, can be perfected only by careful practical study under the experienced surgeon or theatre superintendent. There are, however, certain basic points which are fairly universal and common to assisting in general.

THE SCRUB NURSE

The development of logical thinking plus a silent technique, whereby metal instruments may be picked up or put down with minimal noise, cannot be over-emphasised (Ginsberg *et al.*, 1967; Willingham, 1971).

The instrument or Mayo trolley is prepared by laying out only those instruments which will be required in the early stages of the operation. These instruments are replaced with others when necessary and as the operation progresses. The instrument trolley should not be crowded as this only leads to confusion, especially at a later stage of the operation.

It is important that the instruments should always be laid out in the same order, not only for tidiness, but because many valuable seconds can be lost searching for a vital instrument. A standard method of preparation of this and other trolleys used in the operation area will reduce delays, especially during critical periods.

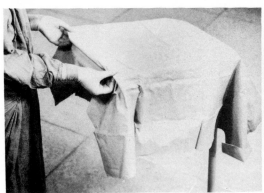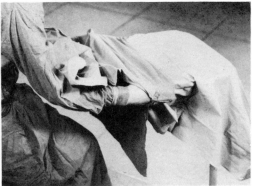

Figure 227   Preparing the Mayo trolley, first a piece of water repellent Ventile, tucked under the tray edge to secure.

Figure 228   The fabric bag is slid over the tray. This ensures a sterile surface underneath and in the vicinity of the upright as well as the upper surface of the tray.

The majority of surgeons appear to prefer the order of instruments whereby those required first are placed on the right-hand side of the instrument trolley facing them. This is, of course, a very flexible rule and must be adapted to suit the needs of a particular surgeon, but once established should be strictly adhered to.

The suggested order of instruments would be: at the front of the trolley from right to left, scalpels, dissecting forceps, scissors, artery forceps; at the back of the trolley, retractors, tissue forceps, etc., and any special instruments which may be required at that particular time. If the trolley has a raised edge, the handles of the instruments should project slightly over this edge. Accidental contamination of these projecting instruments is unlikely as the Mayo trolley should be positioned well within the sterile operation area. Many people will disagree with this statement, but it is much easier to pick up an instrument, silently and correctly, when placed in such a manner.

Instruments having sharp points, such as scissors and scalpels, etc., must be placed with their cutting edges or points away from the surgeon.

Soiled instruments should be cleansed before replacing them on the instrument trolley. A small wire basket clipped to the front of this trolley is useful but is more applicable to thoracic and vascular surgery, where it is essential to remove blood clots from instruments before re-use.

Sharp instruments (indeed any instruments) must not be left lying on drapes covering the patient. If the surgeon requires the scalpel conveniently at hand, it should be placed in a small kidney dish and may be held by an assistant.

When passing instruments, they are placed firmly into the surgeon's hand, and it should not be necessary for him to reach for them. Most instruments such as artery forceps, tissue forceps, towel clips, scissors, etc., are always handed in the closed position, on the first ratchet when that is applicable. An instrument should always enter the surgeon's hand so that it may be used without further adjustment. With artery forceps, especially of the curved type, this means the point at the correct angle required by the surgeon, viz., generally upwards.

Self-retaining retractors are also handed for use in the closed position; but self-retaining bone clamps, dissecting forceps, and multiple joint cutting forceps should generally be open when handed to the surgeon.

These are, of course, only a few of the many instruments which the nurse will handle, but it is her duty to determine the correct way to handle a particular instrument *before* operation (Falk, 1942).

Naturally, the method of passing instruments will depend upon the way in which the surgeon is accustomed to taking them, i.e., if a surgeon extends his hand for a scalpel with the palm uppermost, the scalpel is placed with the blade horizontal, pointing towards the instrument nurse and with its cutting edge facing in the same direction as the extended finger tips. As he closes his fingers on the handle, the cutting edge will be in the correct position for use.

The non-touch technique of passing instruments is now virtually obsolete for it is logical that as the surgeon handles the instruments with his gloved hands there seems no reason why the scrub nurse should not do likewise. However, in orthopaedic surgery care should be taken to avoid touching sterile implants or the points of instruments with the gloved hands.

The preparation and threading of suture needles has been dealt with in the previous chapter, but we must now consider the correct way of handing the prepared suture to the surgeon.

If the needle has been mounted on to a needle holder, this instrument should be handed to the surgeon so that as he takes it, the needle is facing in the correct direction for immediate use. A right-handed person will require the needle facing his left hand, and a left-handed person vice versa. The long end of the suture material is held by the nurse either with her fingers or with a forcep, whichever is applicable, until the assistant takes over or the surgeon has completed his first suture.

A hand or large curved needle is held by its mid-shaft, between the index finger and thumb, with the eye facing the nurse and the point towards the surgeon. A straight needle is held between the index finger and thumb but with the eye facing the surgeon and the point towards the nurse. Presenting the needle in this way will allow the surgeon to complete his first suture without further readjustment.

Ligatures may be handed to the surgeon in ligature eggs, grasped between forceps or the fingers. In the first case, the surgeon will lift the ligature egg from the nurse's extended palm. Care must be taken to ensure that there is sufficient ligature material protruding from the egg, for if it is too short it may slip back through the hole and require re-threading. After use, the egg is returned to the instrument nurse by dropping it back into her hand.

In the second case, a length of ligature material grasped between forceps should not exceed 30·5 cm (12 in) the surgeon using the 'instrument tie' with forceps in each hand.

When ligatures are tied by hand, the nurse must ascertain with which hand the surgeon is accustomed to tying. If he uses a left-hand tie, the nurse should face the surgeon, holding the ligature taut, with one end in her right hand and the centre in her left. He will generally take the ligature with his right hand, so that the short end is ready for grasping with his left. This procedure is, of course, reversed for a right-hand tie.

The most important point regarding *all* instruments is that they must be given a rapid final check before handing to the surgeon or his assistant. Special attention is paid to adjustable screws, ratchets, scalpel blades, their edges, and any moving parts on a particular instrument. Although instruments are always checked by a responsible person before sterilisation, this rapid final check should *never* be overlooked.

The position of the scrub nurse in relation to the surgeon is dependent upon his wishes, and also the area and type of operation. The most logical place is that facing him, for in this position she can follow the surgeon's movements, anticipating he requirements. Some surgeons, however, prefer, the scrub nurse a little to the side and behind their operating hand which is extended back as the instruments are required.

It is very difficult to make hard and fast rules regarding this, but readers will find the following to be of general application.

For operations on the face, neck, chest, abdomen or thighs, with the surgeon standing at the right-hand side of the operation table, the nurse should be opposite his right hand and with the instrument trolley at her left. A surgeon standing at the left-hand side of the operation table will require the scrub nurse opposite his left hand and her trolley at the right.

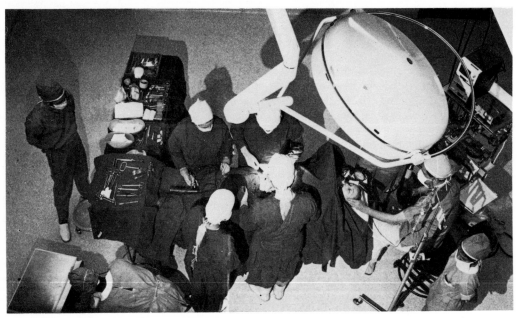

Figure 229   An abdominal operation correctly draped, showing relative positions of surgeons and instrument nurse, etc.

During operations on the lower limbs the nurse may adopt a similar position as above, or stand at the foot of the operation table facing the surgeon, and with the instrument trolley in front of her.

When a surgeon is at the operation table head, i.e., during craniotomy, the best position for the scrub nurse is opposite his right hand with her instrument trolley or neurosurgical table placed over the patient. If the surgeon is left handed the position may be reversed.

A similar position is adopted at the other end of the table when the knee is flexed over the foot end of the table which is lowered or removed, as during excision of torn meniscus.

An operation performed on the arm table is best served by the nurse standing behind her instrument trolley, facing the patient, and with the surgeon at her right or left, with his assistant opposite.

Occasionally the nurse will be compelled to stand behind and a little to the side of the surgeon owing to the nature of the operation. This is often necessary, for example, during Smith Petersen pinning for fractured neck of femur, where X-ray apparatus occupies considerable space normally required by the instrument nurse.

Whichever position is adopted, the nurse should always be able to observe the surgeon's movements and be capable of handing him his instruments with the minimum of inconvenience (Pearce, 1967).

Finally, it is the duty of the scrub nurse to keep a very careful check on the instruments, needles and swabs or packs, etc., used in the operation, and she should be able to account for *all* at any stage of the operation. She should always inform the surgeon of their correctness before being asked, and must obtain acknowledgment in every case.

THE SURGEON'S FIRST ASSISTANT

Occasionally it becomes necessary for a member of the nursing staff to act as first assistant.

The purpose of an assistant is to help the surgeon as required, and it is only he who can decide to what extent this assistance is necessary. As the practical knowledge of his assistant increases, so the surgeon will permit him or her to assist more fully. It must be understood that the assistant's duties are to follow the surgeon's wishes exactly, and to perform only those actions which the surgeon expects or are duly requested.

This obvious statement is, of course, only a repetition of that made at the beginning of this chapter, for we must realise that a good assistant is trained in a particular surgeon's ways and methods by practical guidance, and certainly not from a book. The following suggestions are meant as a basis for the embryo assistant, but will be of some help to those who may be called upon suddenly to assist the surgeon.

The assistant either faces the surgeon, standing at the opposite side of the operation table, or is placed at the surgeon's side opposite to the place occupied by the instrument nurse or second assistant.

The main duties of a first assistant are to keep the operation field unobscured and free from blood, either with a suction tube or gauze swabs, using with the latter a 'dabbing' action rather than wiping which may disturb minute blood clots and increase bleeding. Where excessive bleeding is anticipated from the incision, the surgeon may require pressure to be applied at each side of the wound as the incision is made. This applies particularly to operations on the cranium, due to the vascularity of the scalp.

If the assistant is permitted to apply haemostats to severed vessels, care should be taken to grasp only the vessel and a minimum of surrounding tissue with the forceps tip. Excessive tissue clamped with a vessel will require an unnecessarily stout ligature with consequent risk of slipping, and furthermore, resultant necrosis of the tissue may affect healing.

Whenever possible the surgeon will apply forceps to vessels after dissection from surrounding tissue and before division. He will apply his forceps across the vessel first, followed by the assistant who places his in close proximity. The vessel will be divided by scissors or if the forceps are very close, with a scalpel.

During ligation of a vessel the forceps are held by the assistant in such a manner that they may be re-applied immediately should the ligature slip. After the ligature has been placed around the forceps, the handle is depressed, and the points elevated towards the surgeon, avoiding excessive leverage. It should not be released until he indicates (usually by saying 'off') and care must be taken to do this comparatively slowly in order that the first hitch of the ligature may be tightened on the vessel.

Deep vessels do not generally permit the elevation of forcep points, but they should always be directed towards the surgeon unless he indicates to the contrary.

When cutting a ligature the scissors are held by the thumb and third finger, with the index finger extending along the shanks to the joint, thereby steadying the instrument. As far as possible, the scissor points only are used for cutting, for if the whole length of the blades is used, more than the ligature may be divided, possibly with disastrous results. Ligatures should be cut fairly short, about 1·5 mm ($\frac{1}{4}$ in), except for the larger vessels which the surgeon will indicate.

In order to avoid the contamination of clean instruments the used instruments should always be returned to the instrument nurse, and not dropped on the drapes covering the patient or on the instrument trolley.

Skin or tetra towels may be applied in various ways but the following will be found to be universal. The surgeon places the edge of one towel along the opposite side of the incision, with the main part of the towel lying over the wound. The assistant applies

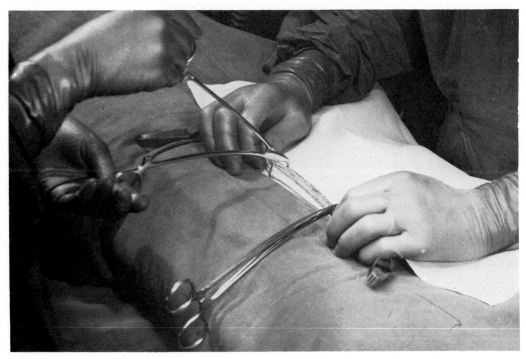

Figure 230   Application of skin towels, stage one.

several Tetra towel clips along this edge to include the towel and skin, with their handles lying away from the wound. The process is repeated along the opposite edge of the incision, and both towels turned back over the skin and forceps. A clip at top and bottom of the wound completes the process, the skin edges thereby being covered and isolated from the underlying tissues.

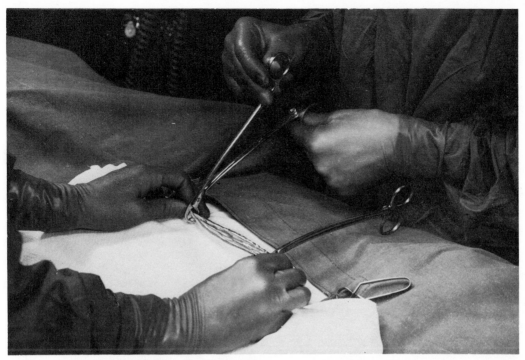

Figure 231   Application of skin towels, stage two.

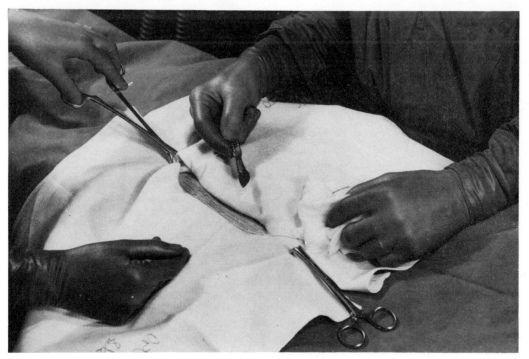

Figure 232   Application of skin towels, stage three.

If polyvinyl sheet (Vi-Drape, Steridrape or OpSite) is being used instead of skin towels the following points must be noted:

1. After applying the skin antiseptic and allowing sufficient time of contact, the skin must be thoroughly dried with a sterile swab or towel.

2. Two persons stretch the plastic sheet which is then smoothed over the adhesive and by a third person using a sterile swab or towel, working from the incision site outwards to expel trapped air bubbles.

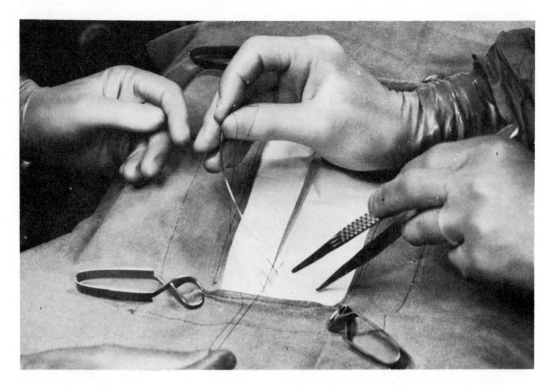

Figure 233   Following the surgeon's suture. Simple continuous suture, 'touch' technique.

Deep retractors are placed by the surgeon and should *not* be removed by the assistant unless he or she is requested to do so. Superficial retractors, on the other hand, require some alteration of position during the initial dissection and a good assistant will, if the surgeon permits, learn to follow him in this respect without any effort on the surgeon's part. The retractors will be moved to provide the surgeon with the greatest possible access in the particular area which he is working but this is dependent on the degree of retraction permissible.

The care with which a retractor must be used cannot be over-emphasised and undue force must be avoided owing to the trauma which can result. The surgeon will decide the degree of retraction possible and this must not be exceeded, the tendency being for the retractor to be *held* and not *pulled*.

Any form of retractor used in the location of a delicate organ such as the liver or lungs, requires some form of pack or swab between it and the organ concerned. A pack should never be obscured by a retractor without the knowledge of the surgeon and instrument nurse, and the assistant should ensure that used packs and swabs are returned to the scrub nurse rather than dropped on to the floor, to assist her in the location of packs and swabs after the operation.

Small swabs or sponges should not be removed from sponge-holding forceps by the assistant, owing to the danger of these swabs being mislaid, especially when large quantities are being used. It is the duty of the scrub nurse to change these swabs when necessary so that a very careful check can be made of the total in circulation.

Any swabs or sponges used as packs must have a tape attached which is always visible and must have a haemostat clipped to it.

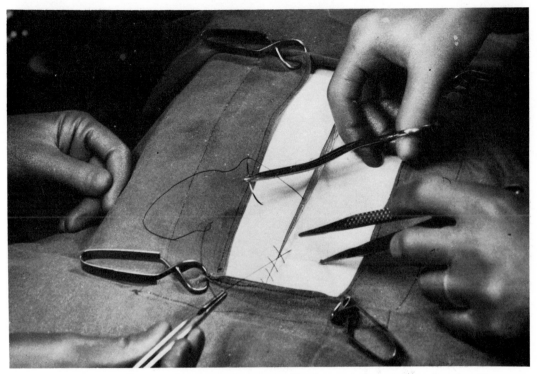

Figure 234   Following the surgeon's suture. Simple continuous suture, 'non-touch' technique.

Soiling of the drapes which can occur when opening the bowel, etc., is avoided by using additional towels or packs just before the incision is made. These may be a distinctive colour, often red, and are placed to isolate the bowel from the general drapes. Instruments used for the procedure should remain on these towels or in a separate kidney dish, and are discarded with the towels when the bowel closure is complete (Falk, 1942).

The surgeon and his assistant change their gloves before concluding the operation and whilst the soiled drapes are being removed.

Hot saline packs prepared by the scrub nurse are replenished when necessary, unless the surgeon indicates that a particular pack should remain in position. This maintenance of moisture and warmth is particularly applicable to exposed bowel which should be kept covered whenever possible.

Sutures are cut in a similar manner to ligatures, but a continuous suture requires the assistant to follow the surgeon, keeping each loop taut as it is made.

After the first knot has been tied, the continuous suture should be held about 7·6 cm

(3 in) from the first loop, pulling the strand a little towards the side of the incision. As the surgeon passes his needle through the tissues and makes each loop, the strand is released. It is then grasped again and the loop held taut, the process being repeated until the surgeon has sutured the entire length of the wound. The degree of tension varies but should be sufficient to prevent each loop slipping, without drawing the tissues together tighter than required by the surgeon.

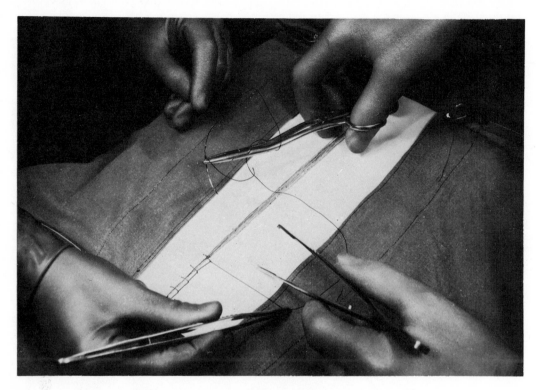

Figure 235   Following the surgeon's suture. Continuous blanket suture, 'non-touch' technique.

Where a non-touch technique is operable, this procedure must be performed with forceps, preferably of the non-toothed variety or those specially designed for the purpose. Care must be taken to avoid crushing the material, for if this occurs in the middle of a strand, it may break during suturing or at some stage post-operatively.

Certain continuous sutures, such as the blanket type, require the assistant to hold the material in the correct position for the surgeon to catch each loop with minimum delay. Various methods are illustrated.

Skin sutures are cut at least $1 \cdot 3$ cm ($\frac{1}{2}$ in) long for subsequent removal. Tension sutures, or those retaining drainage tubes are always left longer than those used for general closure, for easy identification. A different colour of suture material is also very useful for these special sutures which are often removed at different intervals to the skin sutures.

The correct application of dressings may be supervised by the first assistant, although this task is completed by the scrub nurse, except in special circumstances.

THE SURGEON'S SECOND ASSISTANT

This duty is frequently delegated either to a nurse or dresser who requires experience before assisting in the capacity of instrument nurse or first assistant. During major operations it may be essential to have a fully experienced person in this position.

Generally the second assistant helps the first by holding extra retractors and performing the duties which the surgeon may indicate.

If a member of the nursing staff is delegated this task, she will assist the instrument nurse when not required by the surgeon. The duty forms a valuable basis in the training of future scrub nurses.

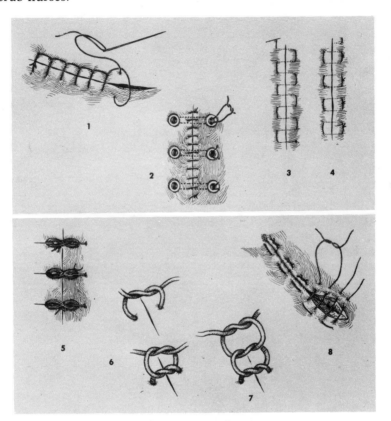

Figure 236 Types of sutures.

1. The blanket or continuous locked suture.
2. Continuous suture and method of using perforated buttons to support tension sutures.
3. Continuous mattress suture.
4. Interrupted mattress suture.
5. Figure-of-eight sutures around pins.
6. Method of placing first and second half-hitches in the square or true knot.
7. The square knot reinforced by third half-hitch.
8. The Halsted interrupted mattress suture.

(From *Manual of Operative Procedure*.   Ethicon Sutures Ltd.)

The infected case

Extreme care must be taken to avoid cross infection following an infected operation (Medical Research Council, 1968). Precautions can be instituted very easily when it is known from the start that the operation is potentially contaminated with pathogenic bacteria. However, the greatest danger lies when halfway through an operation it becomes apparent that infection is present.

There are various routines for dealing with this situation but fundamentally the purpose is to *minimise bacterial contamination of clean objects within the theatre* and so simplify cleaning of the room after operation.

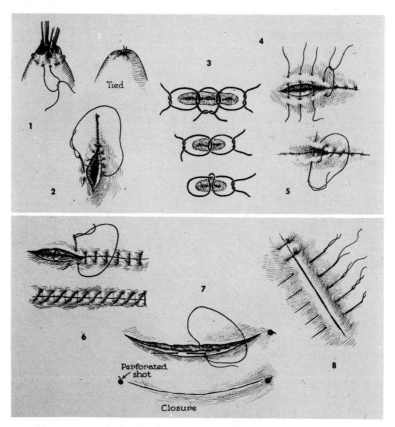

Figure 237   Types of sutures.

1. Purse-string suture around open stump.
2. Closing stump by Cushing stitch.
3. Methods for ligation of pedicles with anchored ligatures.
4. Interrupted Lembert inverting stitch.
5. Continuous Lembert stitch.
6. Two methods of continuous over-and-over closing sutures.
7. Subcuticular suture for closure of skin incision. Perforated buckshot used to anchor suture.
8. Interrupted skin sutures – multiple needle technique.

(From *Manual of Operative Procedure*.   Ethicon Sutures Ltd.)

The most important principle is to make all present realise that special care must be taken, and some visible warning can be used which makes this obvious to anyone entering the room during operation. If this warning contributes towards decontamination measures then so much for the better. The following is a routine which can be modified to suit local requirements.

Let us assume the operation was thought to be relatively clean at commencement and at some stage during the procedure it is decided that infection is present.

Suitable sizes of folded towels are placed at each entrance door and soaked with a disinfectant, e.g., Lysol, Printol, Hycolin, etc. Persons entering or leaving must walk over the moist pads and in addition to the disinfectant action of the pads this is the visible warning of potential contamination.

Any cupboards in the theatre containing clean supplementary items are sealed with a

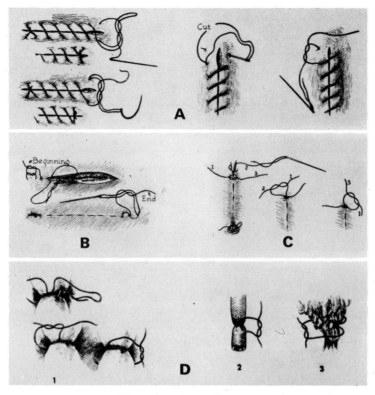

Figure 238   Types of sutures.
A. Variety of methods for securing the ends of completed continuous sutures. Technique for securing ends of both double and single sutures demonstrated. Note method of dividing suture to avoid double thickness of knot.
B. Method of beginning subcuticular suture by placing square knot lateral to incision. Method of ending suture at opposite end of incision.
C. Alternate method for the completion of subcuticular continuous suture by placing a holding knot around end of subcuticular suture.
D. Methods of placing transfixing ligatures to prevent slipping.

    1. Transfixing ligature of pedicle.
    2. Method of placing transfixing ligature in vessel.
    3. Tying transfixing ligature of omentum or of hernial sac.
      (From *Manual of Operative Procedure*.   Ethicon Sutures Ltd.)

piece of adhesive tape. The circulating nurse brings in paper or plastic disposal bags for used swabs and soiled linen.

The scrub nurse should keep all soiled instruments separate from the clean items on her trolley. These may be placed either in a large kidney dish or a suitable hand lotion bowl. Swabs or towels must not be dropped on to the floor but must be placed directly into the disposal containers.

If a swab check is in progress, the soiled swabs are placed on a sheet of water repellent paper which after checking is completed should be folded over and placed in the disposal bag. The circulating nurse should wear rubber gloves for this task, alternatively it can be left for the scrub nurse to complete at the end of the operation.

After application of the dressing, the scrub nurse, still wearing her gown and gloves, carefully bundles up the soiled linen, swabs and dressings, and places them in their respective disposal containers. Any adhesive strapping brought into close proximity to the operation area should be discarded. The surgeon and his assistants dispose of their gowns and gloves in a similar manner, taking care not to contaminate their hands. It is advisable for them to change their scrub suits before continuing other operations.

Used suture needles, unused ligatures and sutures, together with the scalpel blades should be disposed of. Ideally the soiled instruments in the kidney dish or hand lotion bowl are wrapped up in towels and sent for terminal disinfection by autoclaving. The outer layers of these towels (which should be clean) are wrapped over after the scrub nurse has removed her gloves. Trolley contents, even though they are unused are dealt with in a similar manner.

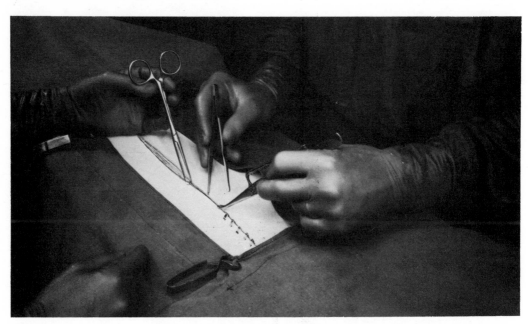

Figure 239   Insertion of Michel suture clips.

The scrub nurse should ensure that any potentially contaminated item within the theatre is disposed of by her before removing gown and gloves.

If it is impossible to send bulky bundles for autoclaving the instruments can be dealt with separately. With this technique the scrub nurse carries (still wearing gown and gloves) the bowl of instruments into the dirty utility toom. The bowl is filled with a strong solution of disinfectant by the circulating nurse. After the scrub nurse has completed her clearing of the theatres, the instruments are cleansed with a brush (which is discarded afterwards) and then placed on a suitable tray for terminal disinfection in the steriliser. Linen is soaked in a suitable disinfectant (Chapter 6) for 12 hours before being sent to the laundry. Unused dressings must either be autoclaved or discarded, unused linen is better soaked with the soiled in case it has been accidentally contaminated.

The scrub nurse then removes her gown and gloves taking care not to contaminate her hands. The theatre is thoroughly cleaned and the floor treated with a disinfectant before further use. All personnel involved in cleaning the contaminated room should wear masks throughout the procedure and change into clean theatre clothing afterwards. Shoes should be left soaking in a disinfectant solution for the recommended period.

REFERENCES

FALK, H. C. (1942) *Operating Room Procedure for Nurses and Internes,* 3rd edn. London: Putnam.

GINSBERG, F., BRONNER, L. S. & CANTLIN, V. L. (1967) *A Manual of Operating Room Technology.* Philadelphia: Lippincott.

HAMILTON BAILEY (1967) *Demonstrations of Operative Surgery,* 3rd edn. Edinburgh: Livingstone.

MEDICAL RESEARCH COUNCIL (1968) Aseptic Methods in the Operating Suite. *Lancet,* i, 763.

PEARCE, E. (1967) *Instruments, Appliances and Theatre Technique,* 5th edn. London: Faber.

PUBLIC HEALTH LABORATORY REPORT (1965) *British Medical Journal,* i, 1251.

WILLINGHAM, J. (1971) *Operating Theatre Techniques.* English Edition.

10
Anaesthetics and the Anaesthetic Room

Anaesthesia is a complex, highly developed science.

So vast it this clinical field that it would be quite impossible to describe in this chapter all the equipment and techniques which are available to-day. For further information the reader is advised to consult a textbook dealing specifically with anaesthesia.

The anaesthetic nurse, assistant or technician must familiarise themselves with the basic principles of apparatus and the use of drugs in the particular theatre in which they work. It would be wrong to suggest that it is necessary to know all the mechanisms of anaesthetic apparatus, or all the effects and complications of certain drugs, but an intelligent and sensible understanding of the basic principles involved is essential in order to give efficient assistance to the anaesthetist.

The maintenance of anaesthetic apparatus is the task of an expert, and the anaesthetic assistant should not tamper with complicated mechanisms about which he or she knows nothing, for it is the anaesthetist's ultimate responsibility to ensure that the apparatus is working correctly before use. However, minor servicing described in this chapter can easily be accomplished by the experienced anaesthetic assistant in co-operation with the anaesthetist. The anaesthetic nurse or technician who has a natural aptitude for dealing with things mechanical may obtain further information from the technical booklets applicable to a particular anaesthetic machine.

The anaesthetic room, general layout

In Chapter 1 we learned that the anaesthetic room should be of the same hygienic construction as the theatre and sterilising room. Where there are several anaesthetic rooms in a multiple theatre suite, the construction, equipment, and layout of each should be identical whenever possible. Equipment should not be interchanged between rooms, and to avoid this it is important to ensure that adequate replacements are available.

All anaesthetic rooms should contain dust-proof cupboards, having an adequate number of wide shelves with an impervious surface and, if possible, glazed doors. Equipment stored in these cupboards is laid neatly on the shelves, labelled and in order. All items must be clearly visible and *always* kept in the same place. Items such as laryngoscopes should be duplicated as they are known to fail at crucial moments. Unless absolutely essential, the cupboards should not be used as a store for general replacements. Various sizes of endotracheal tubes, etc., may be kept separate by storing them, complete with their connectors, in individual paper bags. These plus laryngoscopes and other equipment are conveniently stored in a dispenser (Fig. 242) which also has provision for holding anaesthetic masks on pegs. This prevents damage to the mask cushion. In this way, equipment can be arranged ready for immediate use, and the preparation of special trolleys is simplified.

Separate locked cupboards should be reserved for scheduled and DDA drugs, and the keys carried by the anaesthetic nurse or theatre sister on duty. These cupboards may also contain the register used for recording dangerous drugs administered to the patient in theatre. It is the legal obligation of the anaesthetist to enter all use made of dangerous drugs, the name of the patient and quantity used. Drugs for immediate use may be stored in a locked drawer fitted to the anaesthetic machine. Provision should be made to secure the anaesthetic machine to a wall when left unattended.

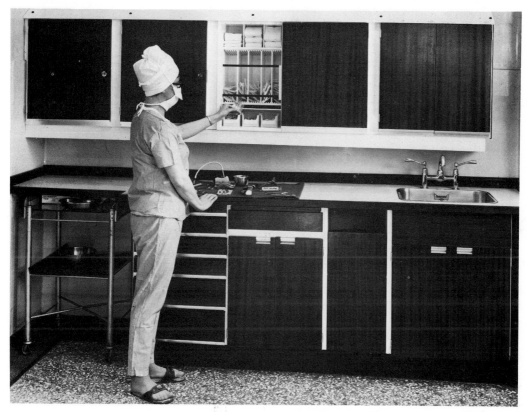

Figure 240   Anaesthetic room storage units at the Royal National Orthopaedic Hospital, London.   (Cuxson Gerrard Ltd.)

A small wash basin with elbow-operated mixing taps and requisites for 'scrubbing up' should be provided in the anaesthetic room. This basin should be positioned away from areas in which sterile trolleys are being used.

An adequate suction machine or pipe line suction device must be available, together with a suction tube and selection of suction nozzles and catheters with connectors of proper size. This should be in addition to the general theatre suction machine and unless being used by the anaesthetist in theatre, is always kept ready in the anaesthetic room, as the timely use of suction machine can be life-saving on occasions. (A suction device working off the oxygen cylinders on the anaesthetic machine is to be deplored. There is the danger that the oxygen may be used up very quickly and result in anoxia from lack of oxygen in inspired gases unless the device is connected exclusively to its own cylinder. This danger is obviated if piped gases are in use).

A dispenser should be provided containing a selection of disposable sterile syringes in sizes ranging from 2 ml to 20 ml, hypodermic and intravenous needles.

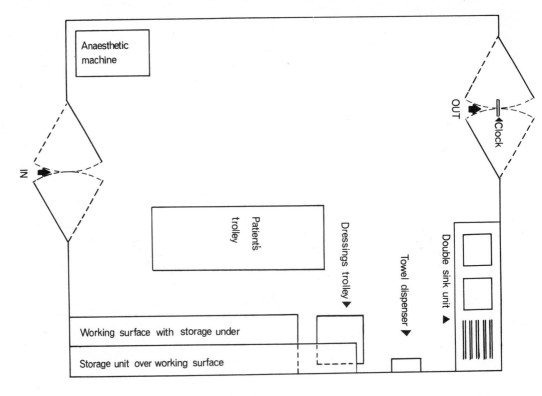

Figure 241   Floor plan of a typical anaesthetic room, similar to that depicted in Fig. 240.
(Cuxson Gerrard Ltd.)

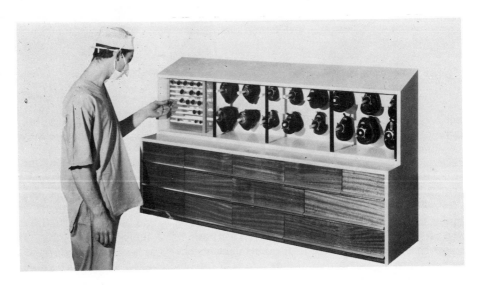

Figure 242   The Gerrard-Reading anaesthetic equipment dispenser for airways, face masks,
endotracheal tubes, connections, laryngoscopes, etc.   (Cuxson Gerrard Ltd.)

In addition to general diffused lighting, a small manoeuvrable spotlight, wall or ceiling mounted, is useful during intravenous procedures.

Two trolleys about 45·7 cm (18 in) square are necessary for the exclusive use of the anaesthetist for transfusions and local anaesthetic techniques.

At least two transfusion stands should be available; a Martin transfusion pump (Fig. 243) to enable rapid transfusion of blood should be fitted to one, or ideally to each of the stands, to supplement the pumping device of plastic recipient sets.

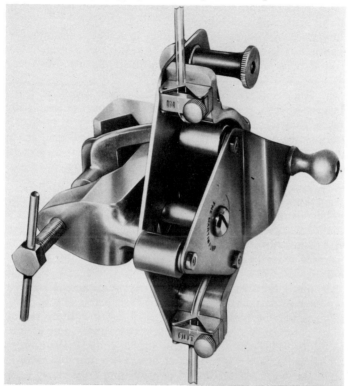

Figure 243   The Martin transfusion pump.   (Eschmann Bros & Walsh Ltd.)

Essential equipment always ready for use should include a sphygmomanometer, stethoscopes, tracheostomy set, cardiac arrest set and transfusion sets. Access to a defibrillator and monitoring apparatus is essential (Chapter 3).

All movable equipment is positioned suitably for the anaesthetist's convenience and when the most advantageous arrangement has been made, should remain unchanged to avoid confusion.

Types of anaesthesia

Although methods of anaesthesia can broadly be grouped into several main types, it is important to realise that they are not separate entities, for each may be and often is used in conjunction with the others.

The main types are given below. (Note. The names of drugs when given first time refer to the *British Pharmocopoeia* nomenclature, those following in brackets refer to the brand names).

1.   General anaesthesia induced by inhalation of gases or the vapour of volatile liquids which vaporise readily at normal room temperatures. These include:

Nitrous oxide. Stored in cylinders in a liquid form, under pressure, often referred to simply as 'gas'. Nitrous oxide is a weak agent of which high concentrations (50–60 per cent) are used in conjunction with other anaesthetics and oxygen.

Cyclopropane. A potent gas stored in cylinders in a liquid form and used only in low concentrations (15 per cent). It is flammable and explosive and therefore must not be used in the presence of cautery or diathermy.

Ether. A volatile liquid which has a wide margin of safety in use although prolonged inhalation can cause post-operative vomiting and depression has an unpleasant, irritant smell, is inflammable and explosive when mixed with oxygen.

Halothane (Fluothane). A volatile liquid which is neither inflammable nor explosive. Its characteristics include lack of irritation of the respiratory tract; effectiveness in low concentration; rapid recovery after administration; absence of side effects such as vomiting.

Methoxyfluorane (Penthrane). Similar to halothane but vaporises less readily; induction and recovery are slower has analgesic properties in low concentration.

Trichloroethylene (Trilene). A blue coloured liquid with a relatively slow rate of vaporisation. Trilene has a predominantly analgesic effect and is used to supplement other gaseous anaesthetics. Used alone as a 0·5 per cent mixture in air it can be administered in small amounts in childbirth to relieve pain without loss of consciousness, cannot be used in a closed circuit in the presence of soda lime, which is incompatible with Trilene.

2. General anaesthesia induced by the intravenous administration of drugs such as the short acting barbiturates. The most commonly used in this class are thiopentone sodium (Pentothal, Intraval), methohexitone sodium (Brietal); and non-barbiturates such as propanidid (Epontol), a very short acting agent, ketamine hydrochloride (Ketalar) and Althesin, a steroid anaesthetic agent. Epontol is very suitable for use in accident and dental departments.

Other drugs, although they may not necessarily be anaesthetics in themselves, are often used intravenously in combination with those listed above. Drugs in this class include analgesics such as pethidine, phenoperidine (Operidine), pentazocine (Fortral) and papaveretum; 'competitive blocker' muscle relaxants such as curare (Tubarine), gallamine triethiodide (Flaxedil), pancuronium bromide (Pavulon) and toxiferine (Alloferin); depolarising muscle relaxants such as suxamethonium (Scoline); hypotensive agents such as trimetaphan (Arfonad) and pentolinium (Ansolysen). In addition there are antidotes and stimulants which are discussed on page 253.

3. Local anaesthesia induced by surface application, local infiltration, regional nerve block and epidural or subdural spinal injection of drugs such as procaine (Novocaine), lignocaine (Xylocaine), amethocaine (Decicaine), prilocaine (Citanest), bupivacaine (Marcaine) and cinchocaine (Nupercaine). Cocaine is used for surface application only, e.g., ophthalmic surgery.

4. Induced hypothermia is a state of lowered body temperature produced by physical cooling of patients who are under the effect of a general anaesthetic, and the so-called lytic cocktail of which the most important element is chlorpromazine (Largactil, Megaphen).

5. Neuroleptanalgesia is a state of indifference and insensitivity to pain induced by the intravenous administration of a potent analgesic drug combined with a tranquilliser, e.g. phenoperidine (Operidine) or fentanyl (Sublimaze) combined with a butyrophenone tranquilliser such as droperidol (Droleptan) or haloperidol.

The patient is easily rousable with a normal blood pressure and when awakened remains quiet. He is in a state of apathy and mental detachment in which he is mildly sedated and uncaring about his surroundings.

Preparation for anaesthesia

1. The gas cylinders and soda lime canister, etc., on the anaesthetic machine are checked by an experienced anaesthetic nurse or technician (if permitted to do so), and reserves of these, together with bottles of halothane (Fluothane), trilene and ether are kept nearby.

2. The anaesthetic nurse also sets out instruments and apparatus required by the anaesthetist. She or he prepares trolleys and trays when necessary for open ether, intravenous anaesthesia, endotracheal intubation, and local, regional or spinal analgesia.

The anaesthetic machines

Although there are many varieties of anaesthetic machines, the principles involve the supply of anaesthetic gases to the patient, either alone or in conjunction with the vapour of volatile anaesthetic agents. Most operating theatres are now supplied with piped gases, but nevertheless each machine must be fitted with oxygen and nitrous oxide cylinders for emergency use in case of failure of piped gas supplies.

Anaesthetic Gas Cylinders are coloured in accordance with a British Standards Institute code. Oxygen cylinders are painted black with a white top and O_2 printed in black; nitrous oxide are blue with N_2O printed in black; cyclopropane are orange, with C_3H_6 printed in black; and carbon dioxide are painted grey with CO_2 also in black.

These colour codings, together with some others which are *not* generally used on anaesthetic machines, but may be found in hospitals, are described in the Appendix.

Regulators are attached to each cylinder to reduce the high-pressure gases, thereby making delivery easily adjustable through individual rotameters which control the amount of gases flowing into the machine and to the patient. There is a cylinder contents gauge either for each cylinder or fitted between two cylinders of the same gas.

Before connecting a new cylinder, after the protective cap has been removed, the valve should be opened momentarily to expel any dust which may have lodged in the valve seating. Failure to observe this may cause grave damage to the delicate gauges on the machine. The procedure is known as 'cracking the cylinder'.

Modern anaesthetic machines incorporate cylinders which have valves of the 'pin index type', which cannot be connected to the incorrect regulator. The fibre washer between the cylinder and cylinder yoke or regulator yoke must be changed regularly, as it becomes worn.

The cylinder valve must be centred correctly with the cylinder yoke or regulator yoke, and the holding screw turned carefully into its location on the back of the valve, using *hand pressure* only. A leak at this point when the valve is opened usually indicates a worn or absent washer or the gas cylinder being connected to the wrong pin index yoke (Fig. 255).

With the male fitting type of valve, used for large oxygen and compressed air cylinders, the bullnose regulator or reducing valve is screwed into the valve seating by hand, and is further tightened with a spanner unless it carries an 'O' ring seal in which case it should be tightened by hand only. If a leak is apparent which cannot be cured by tightening the hexagon nut, the regulator should be replaced at the earliest opportunity, after trying another cylinder. Sometimes a leak may be due to a damaged cylinder valve seating.

Important. On no account must *any* grease be used on cylinders, regulators or connections, for the friction produced by the gas may ignite the grease and cause an explosion.

Cylinder capacities and pressures are listed in the Appendix.

Varieties of anaesthetic machines

There are many different types of anaesthetic machines manufactured. Fundamentally, these machines consist of three main groups: (1) a semi-closed circuit Boyle's type to which can be added a closed circuit; (2) similar to (1) but incorporating a ventilator; (3) a self-contained carbon dioxide absorption circle (closed) circuit. For purposes of clarity the basic characteristics of a Boyle's type anaesthetic machine will be described followed by specific reference to particular models.

1 AND 2. BASIC BOYLE'S TYPE ANAESTHETIC MACHINE

These machines are designed to use pipeline gas supplies; plus reserve cylinders or just cylinder gas supplies. For pipeline gas supplies the machine is connected to the pipeline outlet by flexible rubber hoses incorporating self sealing Schrader connectors. In addition the machines are generally fitted with two nitrous oxide cylinders, two oxygen cylinders and one carbon dioxide cylinder. The extra gas and oxygen cylinders are reserves. There may also be provision for cyclopropane (C_3H_6), but the gas cylinder should be removed from the machine when not in use to eliminate the fire/explosion hazard due to its explosive properties.

The high-pressure gases pass through regulators or reducing valves to the rotameters and thence into a common supply tube either direct to the patient, or are diverted through the halothane (Fluothane) trilene or ether vaporiser, and thence to the reservoir bag. From this bag the gases are carried via the corrugated rubber tube, angle piece and face mask or endotracheal tube to the patient (Fig. 244). Adjustment of an expiratory valve situated between the corrugated tube and the face mask enables expiration and excess gases to escape.

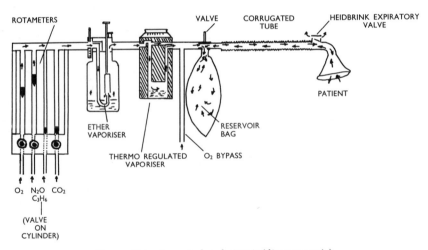

Figure 244   A semi-closed circuit (diagrammatic).

Regulators or reducing valves on anaesthetic machines are usually of the Adam's or endurance type, and they reduce the high gas pressures to 5 or 10 p.s.i.
This enables easy delivery of the gases through individual high-pressure rubber tubes or soldered metal tubes to the control flowmeters (rotameters).

A separate regulator is used for each gas cylinder. An aneroid gauge attached to the regulator indicates the pressure of the cylinder contents.

Rotameters have now superseded other forms of flowmeters for anaesthetic use, due to their greater accuracy.

A rotameter is an accurately made conical glass tube containing a 'float' or 'bobbin' which rises and rotates as the flow of gas increases. The flowmeter must be set perfectly vertical, otherwise the float will not spin round. If not vertical, friction will be caused between the float and the glass wall, and the reading will be inaccurate. A non-spinning float usually requires the flowmeter to be realigned and cleaned by the maintenance engineer.

Rotameters are individually calibrated according to the type and quantity of gas used. These calibrations are shown in the Appendix.

With the exception of cyclopropane, the flow of gases is controlled by a fine adjustment needle valve on the rotameter. Cyclopropane is generally controlled directly from the cylinder by a special key, circular being the safest to avoid accidental jarring when in use.

The three or four rotameters are grouped together, feeding gases into the machine. The oxygen flowmeter is always placed at the extreme left of the 'flowmeter bank', followed by the cyclopropane, carbon dioxide and nitrous oxide on the extreme right. An oxygen bypass lever supplies emergency oxygen when an increased flow of pure oxygen is required.

Vaporisers are of two types:

(A) The standard Boyle type with an unknown percentage of vapour delivered which changes with time of use and many other factors too numerous to control.

(B) The thermo-compensated type with a known percentage of vapour delivered within various ranges of temperature and gas flows.

The Boyle type. This incorporates a valve or slotted drum which allows the anaesthetist to divert a portion or all of the fresh gases above the surface or through the volatile anaesthetic agent before passing to the patient. The proportion of gases not diverted into the vaporisers passes directly to the patient.

The gases enter the vaporiser via a U-shaped tube over which there is positioned a plunger holding a cylindrical hood. This plunger may be lowered over the open end of the U-tube to increase the vapour concentration. When preparing the machines this plunger must be kept up, except when filling the bottles with anaesthetic agent. It is then lowered to cover the U-tube to prevent liquid entering this tube, which would lead to a dangerously high concentration of vapour.

Both the ether and trilene vaporisers on the Boyle's machine are practically identical, the only difference being that the trilene bottle is smaller and sometimes of coloured glass.

The vaporisers are situated outside closed circuit – this is known as V.O.C. (vaporiser outside circuit) and in no circumstances do the patient's respirations pass through it.

The vaporisers are filled with anaesthetic agent through the filler cap, a small plastic funnel being found very useful for the purpose. The trilene bottle should not be filled above the 100 ml (4 oz) level and the ether above the 150 ml (6 oz) level. Ether or *any* anaesthetic must be put into the bottle either by the anaesthetist *only* or *directly under his supervision.*

Trilene is dyed blue, ether is colourless and with the advent of halothane (Fluothane) which is also colourless very great care must be taken to avoid mistakes.

Before the anesthesia is commenced, the control levers of the vaporisers are placed in the closed position and the plungers set at their highest level.

The thermo-compensated type. This type, e.g., Fluotec, has replaced the standard vaporiser for the modern tendency is to use vaporisers producing known concentrations. With these vaporisers known percentages of halothane can be added to the fresh gases of any standard continuous flow anaesthetic apparatus. The patient's respirations are not diverted through halothane as dangerously high concentrations would result.

With the Fluotec Mark 3 any concentration of halothane (Fluothane) between 0·5 per cent and 5 per cent can be chosen by rotating a calibrated control dial to the appropriate setting. The delivered concentration of the anaesthetic is almost independent of the following factors which have an important effect on the performance of a Boyle's vaporiser.

1. Room temperature variation
2. Cooling of the liquid by evaporation
3. Duration of use
4. Level of the liquid
5. Variation in the total flow of fresh gases
6. The effect of shaking
7. Pressure fluctuations due to use of ventilators.

Variable factors 1, 2 and 3 are compensated for by a thermostat (bi-metallic strip) fitted in the vaporising chamber. This corrects for these variables within a range of 18°C–35°C (65°F–95°F).

The vaporising chamber is designed so that the calibration is constant from full to almost empty, i.e., while there is still just a trace of liquid visible through the level window (factor 4).

Factors 5 and 7 are considered by a special type of gas control which ensures accurate results at fresh gas flows as low as 250 ml per minute to 10 litres per minute. (Channel F, Fig. 246.)

Factor 6 is compensated for by a series of wicks which ensures complete saturation of the gas in the vaporising chamber and so the effect of shaking is eliminated although the vaporiser must be kept upright when charged with halothane (Fluothane).

The liquid capacity of the Fluotec Mark 3 is 135 ml when filled completely, the wicks retain 25 ml. The principle of use can be described as follows.

Fig. 245 shows diagrammatically the Fluotec Mark 3 in the 'Off' position and Fig. 246 in a calibrated 'On' position. In the 'Off' position, gas from the rotameters enters inlet A and as shown by the arrows passes to the channel B in the rotary valve C. The gas continues through the main cover D, thermostat E and along the channel to outlet G and thence to the patient via the corrugated tube and the face mask or endotracheal tube. No vapour is picked up during this journey as the inlets and outlets to the vaporising chamber are closed.

As the control knob K is turned to a calibrated position the 'On' position in Fig. 246 is reached. In this position the metered gas in channel B splits into two streams. One stream passes through port H into the vaporising chamber where it comes into very close contact with the wicks, which are soaked with halothane (Fluothane). The gas becomes saturated with halothane vapour and leaves the chamber through port J. From here it enters the channel F and then joins up with the other stream in the main cover D and the mixed streams pass out of the vaporiser at G and thence to the patient.

The concentration of halothane is controlled by the restrictions of the temperature sensitive thermostat E and the control channel F. The restriction of the thermostat E alters according to the operating temperature. Changes in the dial position alter the restriction of control channel F.

A Penthrane thermo-compensated vaporiser is available for the administration of methoxyflurane (Penthrane). This vaporiser, (Pentec 2) operates in a similar manner to the Fluotec. Methoxyflurane concentrations between 0·2 and 2 per cent can be delivered in gas flows as low as 250 ml per minute.

Pin safety system. As mentioned previously (page 227), great care must be taken to ensure only the correct anaesthetic agent is added to the vaporiser. Cyprane/Fraser Sweatman Incorporated have introduced a safety pin system for use with thermo-compensated vaporisers. This consists essentially of non-interchangeable bottle units which fit the combined filler and drain of the vaporiser.

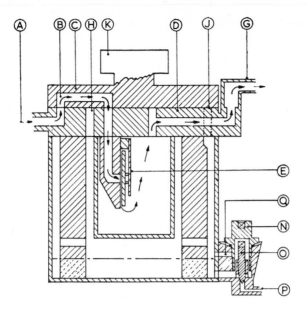

Figure 245   The 'Off' position of the Fluotec vaporiser shown diagrammatically.

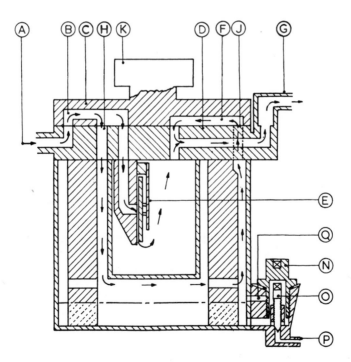

Figure 246   Showing the Fluotec vaporiser in the 'On' or any calibrated position.

The bottle adaptor incorporates a cap which will fit only the correct anaesthetic liquid bottle. Attached to this cap are two flexible tubes. On the delivery end of these tubes is attached a plug which fits into a socket in the filler drain unit. This filler socket is normally sealed by a blank plug P (Fig. 247). The plug on the bottle unit is inserted in

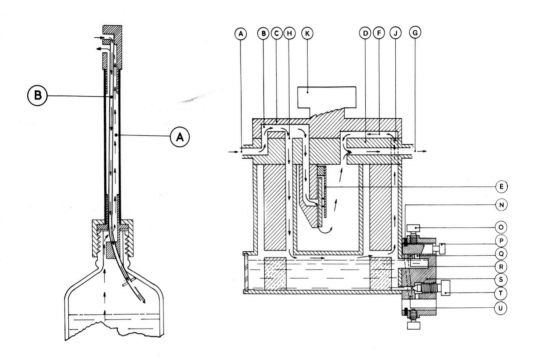

Figure 247   Pin safety system for anaesthetic volatile liquids. Diagram of system fitted to Fluotec vaporiser. (Cyprane/Fraser Sweatman Incorporated).

Key: A Outer tube, pin safety unit.
B Inner tube, pin safety unit.
P Blank plug in filler socket on vaporiser.
O Retaining screw.
Q Channel to vaporiser.

R Displaced air channel when filling.
S Combined filler/drain unit on vaporiser.
T Drain tap.
U Drain socket and displaced air channel when draining.

place of the blank plug (Fig. 249). With the holes down, the retaining screw is tightened and the bottle raised to a level higher than the level of the filler (Fig. 250). Liquid flows down the outer tube A and enters the vaporiser at Q. The displaced air passes out of the vaporiser at R and up the inner tube B. (Fig. 247). When the liquid level has risen to the level of the outlet hole R, which corresponds to the full mark on the filler window, the flow will automatically stop because no more air can be displaced.

For draining purposes the adaptor/plug on the bottle unit is fitted into the drain socket U with the holes in the adaptor/plug uppermost. The retaining screw is tightened and drain tap T opened. The anaesthetic liquid flows out of the vaporiser and down the outer tube A. The displaced air in the bottle passes up to inner tube B and is vented to atmosphere via the channel U.

All these vaporisers are positioned as 'vaporiser out of circuit', i.e., only fresh gases pass through the chamber allowing very accurate percentages to be selected. In contradistinction to the above arrangement, the vaporiser on the Marrett head is 'in circuit',

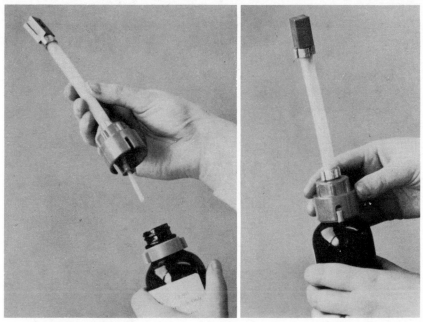

Figure 248   Fitting the pin safety cap and unit to bottle of anaesthetic liquid.

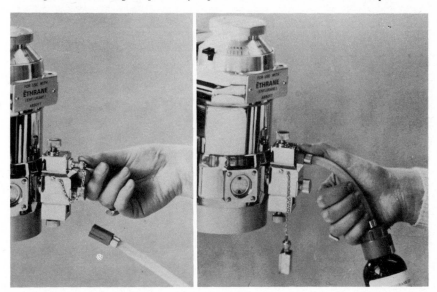

Figure 249   The pin safety system adaptor/plug is fitted into the filler socket (after removing a blank plug P) making sure the flow holes in the plug are downwards.

with the patient's respirations passing through the chamber. In the latter instance, great care and skill is needed to ensure safe concentrations.

The reservoir bag made of thin anti-static rubber is generally of a 1 gal (4·5 litre) capacity. The anaesthetic gases enter this bag via a drum valve, which is generally a permanently-open 'T' junction.

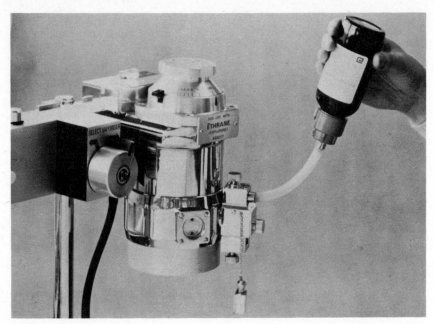

Figure 250   Pin safety system raising the bottle to fill the vaporiser.

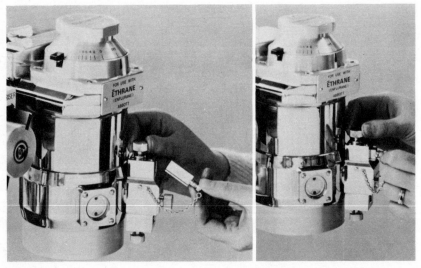

Figure 251   Replacing the pin safety system blank filler plug and securing with the retaining screw before the vaporiser is used.

This bag should be tested regularly for leaks by inflating and submerging in water. There is a tendency for cracks to appear in the folds.

After prolonged use, the reservoir bag is removed from its mount and inverted to drain off condensed moisture vapour, prior to cleaning and sterilisation.

The corrugated tube, made of anti-static rubber and having a wide bore, is joined to the machine at one end and the angle piece at the other by slightly conical metal or hard rubber unions. The union at the angle piece incorporates an expiratory valve.

The tube must be checked regularly for punctures as there is a tendency for deteriora-

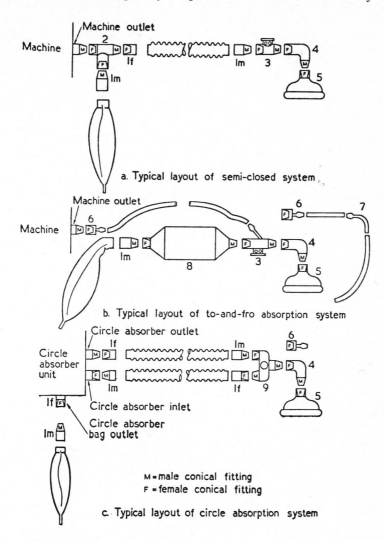

a. Typical layout of semi-closed system

b. Typical layout of to-and-fro absorption system

M = male conical fitting
F = female conical fitting

c. Typical layout of circle absorption system

Figure 252   Typical layouts for breathing attachments of anaesthetic apparatus BSI 3849.

tion to occur in the corrugations. After use it should be stretched and suspended straight for a period, to release condensed moisture which is often lodged in the corrugations and then sterilised at least at the end of a list if not after each operation.

British Standard 3849 (1965) specifies certain sizes of joint fittings on anaesthetic machines. Basically it requires that the delivery end of the anaesthetic machine shall have a male conical fitting, and the face mask a female conical fitting. The conical fittings on all components of adult size from the male delivery end of the anaesthetic machine shall be in the sequence male-female in the direction of gas flow (Fig. 252).

The nominal size of adult cone and socket joints is 22 mm diameter. For paediatric use the size is reduced to a nominal 15 mm diameter except that the female connector to the machine outlet, the male conical fitting leading to the mask and the female conical fitting of the face mask should be of adult size (22 mm).

The expiratory valve on modern apparatus is usually of the Heidbrink type. This is a spring-loaded valve upon which tension may be adjusted to create a slight resistance against the patient's expirations. When closed circuit is used the valve is completely closed and it is necessary to cut the gas flow down to basic oxygen requirements.

Other expiratory valves such as the Coxeter or Magill type may be in use, but basically they are also a spring-loaded valve which acts in a similar manner.

The metal angle piece connects to the face mask, made from anti-static rubber manufactured in a modified funnel shape which, when applied to the patient's face, moulds with the facial contours forming an airtight fit.

The two basic types are (*a*) those having a solid or moulded lip of suitable design and (*b*) those having an inflatable cushion.

Although the cushion type (*b*) must not be over-inflated, even when not in use it should contain a proportion of air to avoid deterioration of the inner surface of the rubber. A small plug blocks the air inlet after inflation, and the mask should be stored on the connecting flange with the cushion upwards or on horizontal pegs as in the Gerrard-Reading dispenser (Fig. 242).

The trilene inter-lock unit is mounted in the circuit between the trilene vaporiser and the reservoir bag. This drum valve is so designed that the trilene vaporiser control cannot be moved from the 'Off' position unless the drum is set at open 'circuit'. The interlock device also incorporates an emergency oxygen level which enables the administration of a plentiful supply of oxygen to the patient if the need arises.

The danger of using trilene in a circle circuit is that it reacts with heated-up soda lime to form a highly toxic agent di-chloracetylene, which in susceptible patients may cause palsy of various cranial nerves or fatal encephalitis and necrosis of the liver.

An anti-static rubber harness may be used by the anaesthetist to maintain the face mask in position.

The Clausen and Connell head harness are the two in common use. Both are attached by two or three hooks, either fixed to the face mask or on a ring which fits over it. The Clausen harness has three limbs with several perforations, which may be suitably attached to the three hooks. The Connell has only two specially designed loops which are adjustable and maintain a friction hold on the two limbs.

All rubber items used on anaesthetic apparatus with the exception of endotracheal tubes and some airways have anti-static properties (see chapter 3).

An endotracheal tube and connection may be attached directly to an expiratory valve and the corrugated tube by substituting a Magill catheter connection for the angle piece and the face mask. In this case the corrugated tube and expiratory valve are supported carefully, to avoid pulling on the endotracheal tube after insertion. This is achieved by using adhesive strapping, Sellotape, or a specially designed head harness such as the Connell, after placing a pad of gauze or sponge rubber between the expiratory valve mount and the patient's face. Under BSI standard the Magill or similar connection must have an internal diameter of not less than 11 mm. This also applies to the machine end of the endotracheal tube connections.

An airway may be used in the patient's mouth to prevent the tongue from falling back, (impeding or obstructing respirations) and also prevent teeth clenching an endotracheal tube. There are many varieties, but all are of a curved moulded shape which fits comfortably in the pharynx, holding the base of the tongue forward. A metal insert prevents compression of the airway by the teeth if it has been manufactured from a soft material. They may be made from rubber, thermoplastics (Portex vinyl) or less commonly from metal. The most generally used are the Phillips rubber type in six sizes, and the Guedel rubber or plastic in four sizes plus two extra small sizes for infants.

The Heirsch airway is similar to the Phillips, but has an oxygen feed tube fitted to the metal insert, which is of special use in children.

Where the Phillips metal insert has side perforations, it is intended that these perforations remain above the level of the rubber or plastic moulding. This is a safety arrangement whereby the patient's airway would not become obstructed should the main aperture become accidentally blocked, e.g., with the edge of the sheet or blanket.

THE CARBON DIOXIDE ABSORPTION CIRCLE CLOSED CIRCUIT ADDED TO THE BASIC BOYLE'S MACHINE

In the circle apparatus two corrugated tubes are used, one for the delivery of gases to the patient through a one-way inspiration valve, and another through which the expiratory gases are directed into the rebreathing bag via another one-way expiration valve.

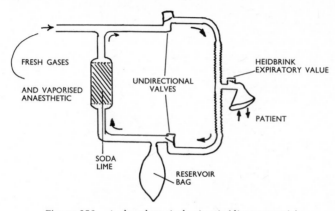

Figure 253   A closed or circle circuit (diagrammatic).

The patient's expirations, from the reservoir bag, pass through the soda lime canister and a selected proportion of carbon dioxide is removed. The expirations then mix with fresh gases from the rotameters which may have been passed through the vaporiser. It is possible also to pass the patient's expirations through a special vaporiser although this is not common practice. (This is then termed vaporiser in circuit.) This gas mixture is directed through the inspiration valve and along the corrugated tube back to the patient, thereby completing the circuit (Fig. 253).

The soda lime will only absorb a certain amount of carbon dioxide before it becomes exhausted, but modern methods of manufacture have produced a substance which will allow several hours of use before exhaustion is apparent.

The Boyle circle type absorber, Mark 3. This consists of a double-chamber, reversible soda lime canister, capacity – 1·8 kg (4 lb), fitted to a control head by means of a central tube which is screwed into the head with a large plastic hand nut. The canister is made of transparent acrylic material to enable the colour change of indicating soda lime to be seen easily. A condensation trap fitted to the base of the central tube prevents an accumulation of moisture in the soda lime. Unidirectional inspiratory and expiratory valves are incorporated in the control head in addition to an adjustable spill valve and a

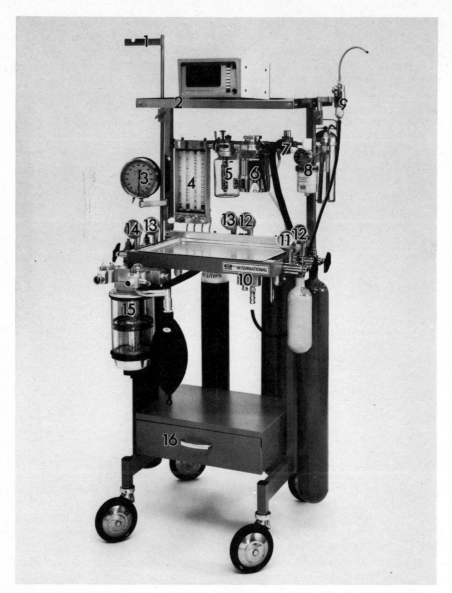

Figure 254   Anaesthetic Machine (Boyle International Specification Model) (The British Oxygen Co. Ltd.).

1. Transfusion hook.
2. Shelf for accessories such as monitoring apparatus.
3. Sphygmomanometer.
4. Bank of four rotameters: oxygen, cyclopropane, carbon dioxide and nitrous oxide.
5. Boyle type ether vaporiser.
6. Fluotec halothane vaporiser.
7. Gas outlet with flexible tube for connection to CO₂ absorption unit 14.
8. Suction unit for connection to pipeline.
9. Oxycaine spray for local topical anaesthesia, operated from oxygen supply (10).
10. Oxygen supply (to operate 3 and 9).
11. Cyclopropane cylinder contents gauge.
12. Nitrous oxide cylinder contents gauges.
13. Oxygen cylinder contents gauges.
14. Carbon dioxide cylinder contents gauge.
15. Carbon dioxide circle circuit absorption unit.
16. Accessories storage drawer.

lever which allows the soda lime canister to be excluded from the gas circuit when not required or during filling. A manometer can be fitted which screws into the control head.

The transparent canister is divided centrally by a perforated metal baffle which effectively reduces 'channelling' of gases (bypassing the soda lime). In use, the gases are routed down through the central tube and up through the soda lime, so that the soda lime in the lower chamber becomes exhausted first. When the colour change in the lower chamber is complete, the soda lime in the chamber may be replaced and the canister refitted with the freshly filled chamber uppermost. When used in conjunction

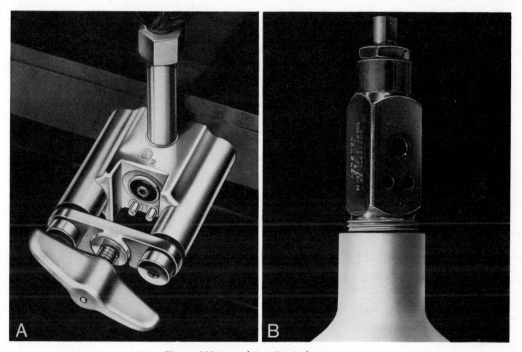

Figure 255 A. and B.   Pin index system.
A. Pin index cylinder yoke, retaining clamp rotated hooked in position. Note fibre washer surrounding gas inlet and two projecting pins just below. These pins correspond to the position of the two holes in the cylinder valve C. The distance between the pins varies according to the type of gas in use, i.e., oxygen, nitrous oxide, carbon dioxide or cyclopropane. This prevents incorrect coupling of cylinders to the machine.
B. Oxygen cylinder with pin index (flush type) valve. The upper hole is the gas outlet which fits over the inlet on the cylinder yoke. A gas-tight union between the two is accomplished by applying *hand pressure* only to the screw on the retaining clamp shown in B which is rotated to hold the cylinder in position.

with the Boyle's anaesthetic machine, the absorber is mounted on a support bracket fitted to either front leg of the table frame, and the fresh gas supply tube is plugged into the anaesthetic gas outlet on the manifold panel. Fresh gases are supplied from the main part of the Boyle's machine and enter the absorber through an inlet at the back.

Soda lime of 4/8 mesh having little or no dust should be used. After refilling the canister, it should be blown through if possible with oxygen, to remove any dust which may have accumulated in the packing.

Modern soda lime preparations such as Calona (B.O.C.) or Durasorb (M.I.E.) contain a coloured indicator, which retains its colour so long as the soda lime remains active.

After four to six hours' use, Durasorb changes from a pink to a cream colour and should be replaced. Calona indicates exhaustion by a change from green to brown. Many machines are now fitted with transparent absorber canisters which permit the colour of the soda lime to be easily observed.

The canister should always be filled to the top with soda lime to utilise the full effect of carbon dioxide absorption.

The Waters' canister 'to and fro' method of carbon dioxide absorption consists of a

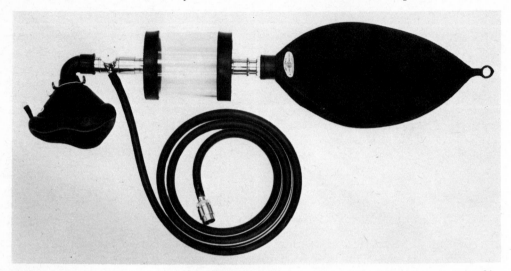

Figure 256   Waters' 'to and fro' carbon dioxide absorption canister. (The British Oxygen Co. Ltd.)

cylindrical metal or plastic canister containing soda lime, a reservoir bag, conical mount/ expiratory valve with side tube for fresh gases and angled mount for face mask, or Magill mount for endotracheal tube.

The canister is placed as close to the patient as possible. The patient's respirations pass through the canister twice and it is an efficient method of carbon dioxide absorption, although the heavy canister is rather difficult to secure in position.

2. ANAESTHETIC MACHINE WITH VENTILATOR

It is possible to utilise almost any type of ventilator with the basic Boyle's apparatus. An example of an anaesthetic machine which has a permanently fitted ventilator designed as part of the apparatus is the Blease Northwick Park Anaesthetic Trolley.

This machine has the characteristics of a Boyle apparatus but incorporates a variable frequency, variable phase, time cycled pressure or volume limited ventilator of the Manley type. The ventilator is operated entirely by the gas delivered through the anaesthetic unit to the patient. A sensitive manometer, recording both positive and negative pressures, is fitted to the unit. The machine incorporates a closed circle circuit carbon dioxide absorption unit.

3. THE MARRETT CIRCLE CIRCUIT MACHINE

This is a compact apparatus which is used in many hospitals and has the virtue that it is easily transportable when a suitable cylinder stand is incorporated.

The machine consists of two main parts – the head and the cylinder stand or table. The head is supplied with gases in the usual manner from cylinders and regulators fitted to a circular stand or anaesthetic table similar to the Boyle's apparatus.

Four moderately high-pressure rubber or soldered metal tubes convey the anaesthetic gases from the regulators to the bank of four rotameters on the anaesthetic head. The head has two vaporisers – one for ether or halothane (Fluothane) and one for trilene – together with a soda lime canister, all of which are controlled by three separate circular knobs which actuate complicated drum valves.

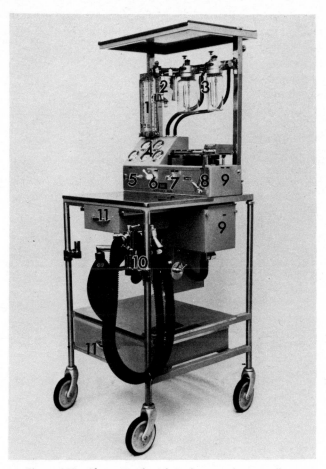

Figure 257 Blease Northwick Park Anaesthetic Trolley.

1. Bank of four rotameters: oxygen, cyclopropane, carbon dioxide and nitrous oxide.
2. Fluotec halothane vaporiser.
3. Boyle type ether and trilene vaporisers.
4. Oxygen and nitrous oxide cylinder contents gauges; patient circuit pressure gauge.
5. Negative pressure control arm and weight.
6. Emergency oxygen lever.
7. Ventilator on/off tap.
8. Tidal volume scale.
9. Manley ventilator.
10. Carbon dioxide circle circuit absorption unit.
11. Accessories storage drawer.

The ether vaporiser uses special copper baffle plates, four to six in number, which conduct the heat from the rest of the apparatus and surrounding atmosphere, thereby aiding the vaporisation of the ether or halothane (Fluothane).

The fractional knob control enables the anaesthetist to divert proportions of the anaesthetic gases and patient's expirations through selected baffles, thereby adjusting the concentration of vapour.

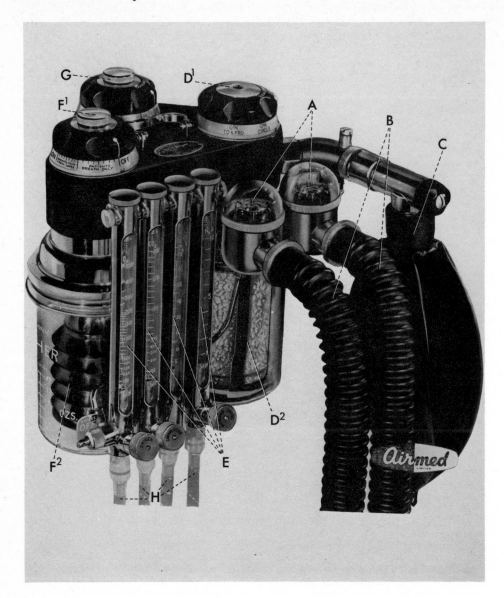

Figure 258   Circle circuit anaesthetic head (Marrett).

A. One-way inspiratory and expiratory valves.
B. Corrugated tubes to patient.
C. Reservoir bag and control valve.
D¹. Soda lime canister control valve (closed circuit).
D². Soda lime canister (Perspex).
E. Rotameters.

F¹. Ether or halothane vaporiser control valve.
F². Ether or halothane vaporiser; note baffles.
G. Trilene vaporiser control valve.
H. Non-interchangeable connections to gas-reducing valves.

Great skill is needed when using this type of vaporiser with halothane (Fluothane), for being 'in circuit', not thermoregulated, the concentration of vapour is difficult to maintain at a constant level. It is used *only* with spontaneous breathing.

The trilene vaporiser has a smaller bottle than the ether, and consists of a single perforated tube terminating below the level of the liquid. The concentration is controlled by a drum valve very similar to the ether vaporiser, but incorporating a device interlocking with the soda lime canister. Refilling is accomplished as for the ether vaporiser.

An interlocking device is provided to prevent trilene being used when the soda lime has been turned on and vice versa.

A circle or closed circuit has many advantages, including the conservance of expensive anaesthetic vapours or gases such as cyclopropane and halothane (Fluothane); the very accurate control of anaesthetic agents and degree of anaesthesia using minimal anaesthetic (especially useful with the poor risk patient and long operations); the conservance of body moisture and heat.

The reader is reminded again that little detail has been given regarding the maintenance of these anaesthetic machines. It is the grave responsibility of the anaesthetist to ensure that the machines are in good working order, and the degree of simple maintenance by the anaesthetic nurse or technician depends upon his or her experience, mechanical ability and, above all, the anaesthetist's orders in this matter. There should be a routine planned maintenance either by the manufacturer or a specially trained service engineer.

Ventilators

It is now commonplace to use controlled respiration during anaesthesia or following traumatic conditions such as head injuries. This may be accomplished simply by rhythmically squeezing the anaesthetic reservoir bag or by mechanical ventilators.

Many types of ventilators have been developed; some are specifically for use during anaesthesia, whereas others are suitable for mechanically assisted artificial ventilation. There are others which can be used for both purposes, utilising air or a mixture of air and oxygen.

Basically ventilators could be divided into three main groups:

1. *Flow generators.* A *fixed volume* of gases (taken from a constant flow) is delivered into the lungs. A wide *variation in the pressures* reached at the end of inspiration (or inflation) may be observed on the manometer gauge, e.g., when a patient tries to breathe against the machine, irregular patterns result with high and low values at random.

Fibrosed and stiff or congested lungs, airway obstruction including excessive secretion, foreign body, broncho-spasm, etc. (low compliance), all will require high-pressure values. Should this pressure reach a certain level, usually 40 to 70 cm of water, a safety valve blows off a proportion of the given volume.

Any leak will deprive the patient of the comparable proportion of the original delivered volume and therefore the pressure (manometer) gauge will register a suspiciously low value.

2. *Pressure generators.* With these the ventilator produces a selected pressure within the limits of time imposed by the respiratory rate. The amount of gases required for this pressure depends upon the compliance of the lungs and chest; and will need a variable volume of gases to achieve this. The ventilator will compensate for all but the gross leaks by delivering a larger volume of gases.

3. *Ventilators providing a choice of volume or pressure.* Some ventilators are electrically driven (with a manual control for emergency), others convert a continuous flow of

oxygen or compressed air from a cylinder or pipeline, into an intermittent flow to the patient. It would be impossible to mention all the ventilators available and we will therefore confine ourselves to a few observations on three, the Cape Bristol Ventilator, the Barnet Ventilator Mark 3 and the Bird Respirator.

THE CAPE BRISTOL APPARATUS

This is a two stage constant volume flow generator, electrically driven, which can be used for long term ventilation of the lungs post-operatively or in the treatment of respiratory insufficiency.

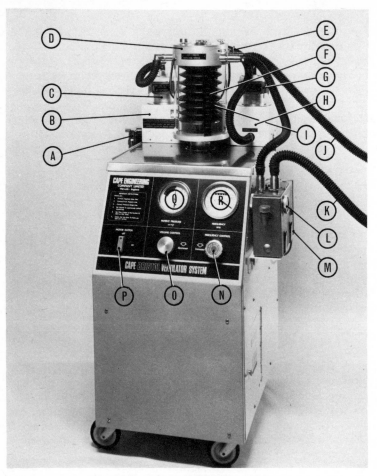

Figure 259   The Cape Bristol Ventilator.

A. Air/Oxygen mixing valve.
B. Hinged filter console.
C. Inspired air filter.
D. Ventilating head.
E. Safety clips (tubing).
F. Calibrated scale (volume).
G. Expired air filter.
H. Heater mantle.
I. Bellows.
J. Expiratory tubing.

K. Inspiratory tubing.
L. Humidifier water tank.
M. Humidifier electrics.
N. Respiratory rate control.
O. Volume control.
P. On/Off switch.
Q. Pressure gauge.
R. Respiratory rate indicator (with 'Hours Run' recorder).

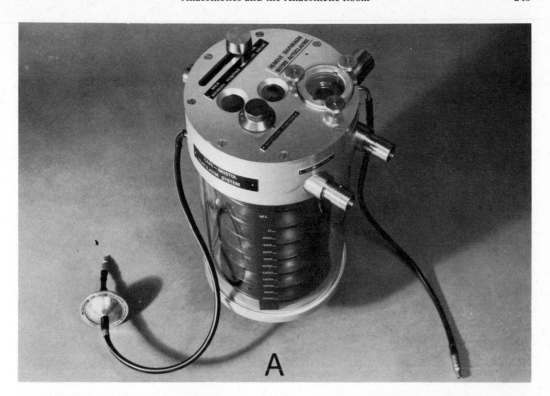

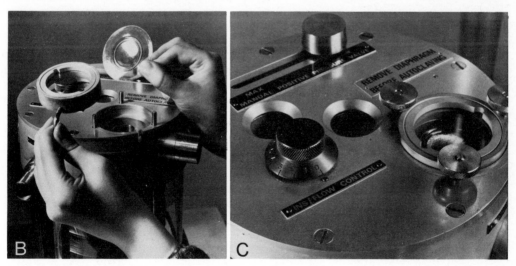

Figure 260A   The Cape Bristol ventilating head rests on top of the pump unit and is located by a single large diameter cone. It is easy to lift off without the use of tools and there is no dismantling other than the disconnection of tubing. The head can be positioned so that the patient tubing can be led off from either the left or right hand side of the ventilator.

B.   The uni-directional valves in the head are easily accessible for cleaning. The expiratory valve is pressure operated; the diaphragm is disposable and cannot be autoclaved. The ventilating head can be autoclaved at 134°C (275°F).

C.   The inspiratory flow control and deadweight valve adjustment.

Figure 261A   The two filters are mounted in a console on the top of the cabinet. Each of the two filter casings contains an identical disposable filter cartridge (B). This cartridge is in accordance with BS.3928 with a penetration of less than 0·001 per cent against a sodium chloride test cloud with a mean particle size distribution of 0·5 micron diameter.

B.   The expiratory filter rests on a heated mantle which vaporises the moisture content of expired air and thus prevents any build-up of expiratory resistance. The casings can be autoclaved.

C.   A small line filter is interposed between the pressure gauge and the ventilating head to keep the pressure gauge 'clean'.

The volume of gas delivered by the machine can be adjusted between 0–2,000 ml, with a frequency range of 10–50 respirations per minute. The inspiratory/expiratory timing is fixed at a ratio of 1–2 and is mechanically controlled. A negative or sub-atmospheric phase can be introduced to assist expiration and this is shown on a manometer. There is a safety deadweight valve which limits the pressure which can be applied to a patient's lungs (maximum 70 cm H_2O).

During long-term ventilation, i.e., via a tracheostomy, a water bath humidifier or ultrasonic nebuliser should be fitted between the machine and the patient on the inspiratory side of the circuit. The water bath humidifier heats the water contained to 50°C (122°F) which gives an air temperature of approximately 37°C (98°F) at the patient connection.

The main feature of this apparatus is the ease with which the patient circuits can be sterilised. The ventilating head and humidifier can be autoclaved and there is a bacteriological filter system on both the inspiratory and expiratory sides (Figs. 260, 261).

THE BARNET VENTILATOR MARK 3

This provides electronically controlled time cycling of a volume or pressure generator incorporating either negative phase or patient triggering. The selection of any one cycling system automatically switches the remaining systems out of circuit and therefore the machine can be regarded as three independent ventilators in one unit. Operation of the ventilator is simplified by grouping and colour coding all controls specific to each mode of operation.

Time cycling (colour coded yellow) allows a range of respiratory rates between 6 and 60 per minute with an independent adjustment of inspiratory and expiratory phase times between 0·5 and 5 seconds.

Volume cycling (colour coded orange) is achieved by monitoring the expired tidal volume on the respirometer and adjusting the flow rate control, tidal volume selector and negative pressure control.

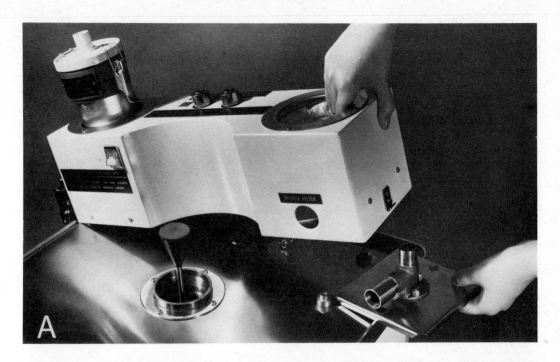

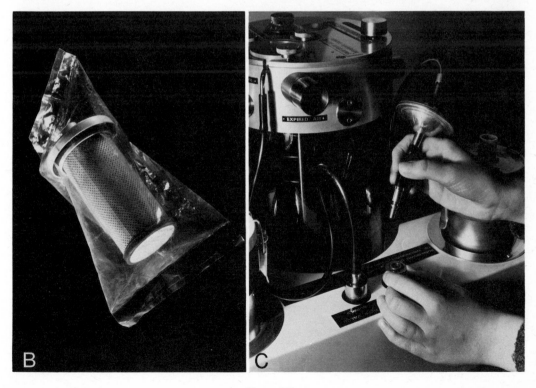

Figure 261

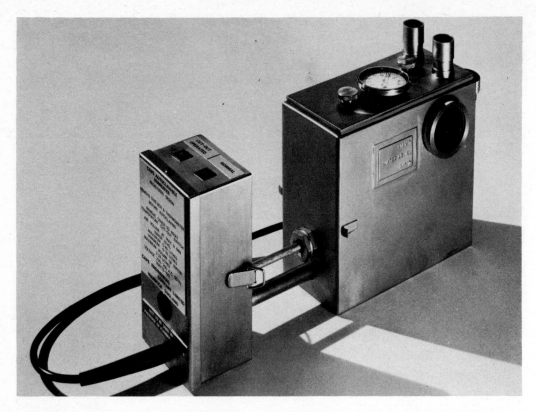

Figure 262   The Cape Bristol humidifier is a thermostatically controlled heated water bath. The water tank can be detached from the electrical control box and after removing the thermometer can then be autoclaved.

Pressure cycling (colour coded green) at required level is selected by setting a calibrated control marked 0–45 cm H_2O.

In operation, volumes between 30 ml and 1,400 ml may be achieved. The positive pressure exerted within the lungs is monitored by a pressure gauge 0–50 cm H_2O; a safety valve limits the maximum positive airway pressure. In expiration, a sub-atmospheric negative phase may be introduced between 0 and minus 12 cm H_2O.

The patient trigger facilities are sensitive to minus 1 cm H_2O, which is equivalent to only 5 ml tidal exchange. If the patient fails to trigger the ventilator, respiration continues automatically at the rate previously selected.

The Barnet ventilator operates electronically through a low voltage battery which is charged by a trickle charger built into the machine. In the event of power failure, the ventilator can be used for periods up to 24 hours away from the mains supply.

Ancillary equipment which can be added includes a humidifier, CO_2 circle absorption unit and alarm unit.

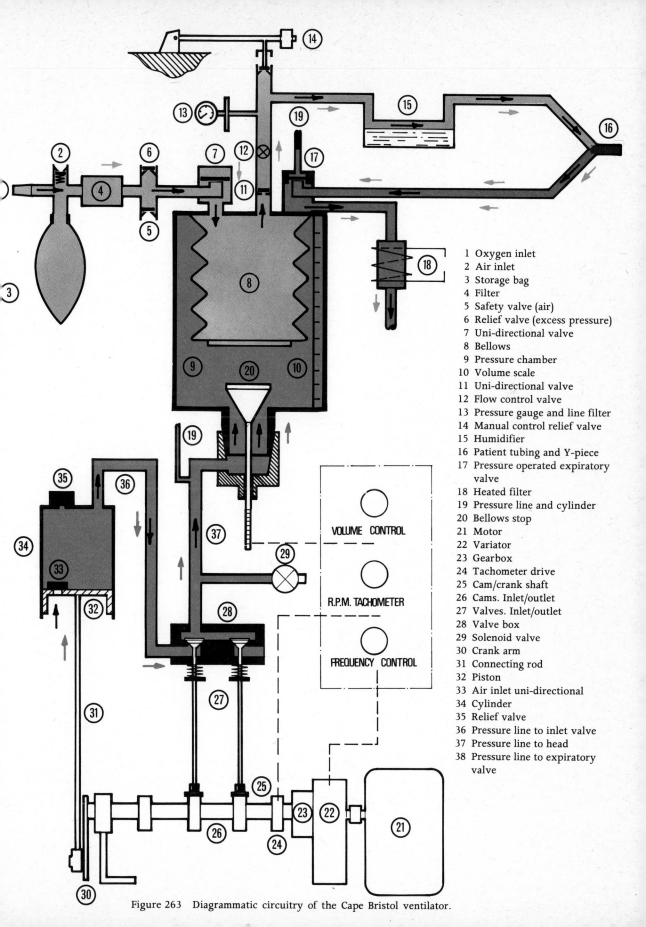

Figure 263 Diagrammatic circuitry of the Cape Bristol ventilator.

1 Oxygen inlet
2 Air inlet
3 Storage bag
4 Filter
5 Safety valve (air)
6 Relief valve (excess pressure)
7 Uni-directional valve
8 Bellows
9 Pressure chamber
10 Volume scale
11 Uni-directional valve
12 Flow control valve
13 Pressure gauge and line filter
14 Manual control relief valve
15 Humidifier
16 Patient tubing and Y-piece
17 Pressure operated expiratory valve
18 Heated filter
19 Pressure line and cylinder
20 Bellows stop
21 Motor
22 Variator
23 Gearbox
24 Tachometer drive
25 Cam/crank shaft
26 Cams. Inlet/outlet
27 Valves. Inlet/outlet
28 Valve box
29 Solenoid valve
30 Crank arm
31 Connecting rod
32 Piston
33 Air inlet uni-directional
34 Cylinder
35 Relief valve
36 Pressure line to inlet valve
37 Pressure line to head
38 Pressure line to expiratory valve

VOLUME CONTROL

R.P.M. TACHOMETER

FREQUENCY CONTROL

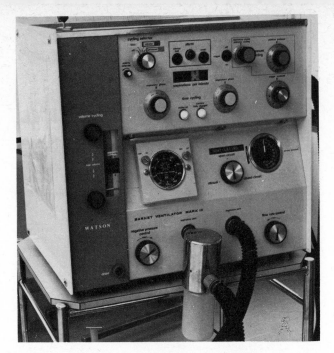

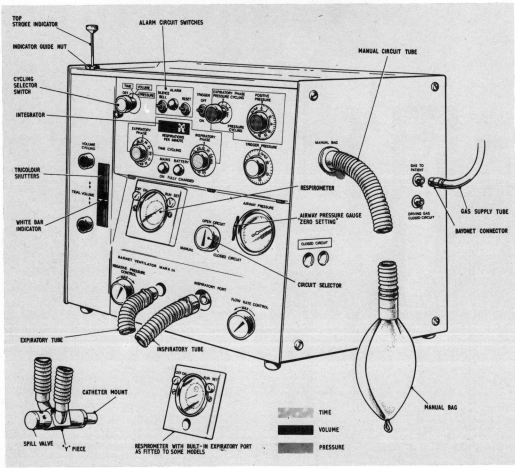

Figure 264 Barnet Mark 3 ventilator.

THE BIRD RESPIRATOR

This is a patient-triggered pressure generator operated from an oxygen or compressed air supply.

Basically the respirator consists of a transparent box-like structure divided into two chambers by a diaphragm. As gas flows into one chamber the diaphragm moves valves which allow gas into the second chamber and thence into the patient's lungs, during the inspiratory phase. The expiration is generally passive with the lungs deflating normally by their own elasticity, during this phase fresh gas flows into the respirator ready for the next inspiratory phase.

The sensitivity dial can be adjusted so that either the patient's weakest effort at inspiration will trigger the machine into adequate ventilation, or the patient must make a larger effort in order to do this. The respirator can provide complete controlled ventilation when the sensitivity control is set at zero. A sub atmospheric pressure can be introduced at the expiratory phase if required.

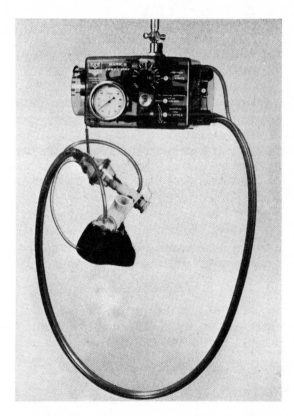

Figure 265   The Bird respirator. (Bird Corp. U.S.A.)

The Bird respirator is very useful for re-educating the patient to breathe on his own account following conditions which have necessitated prolonged artificial ventilation. In America, where it originates, the machine is used a great deal for inhalation therapy utilising various medicaments and nebulisers.

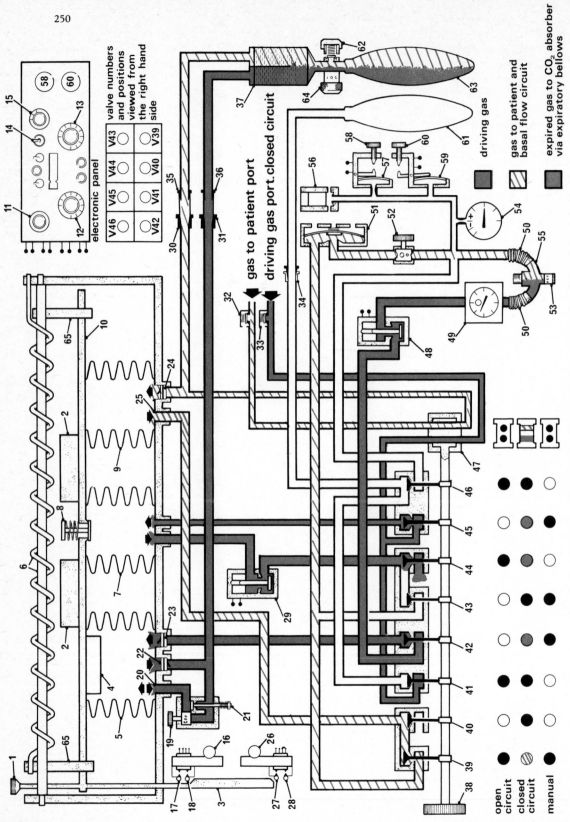

Figure 266 Barnet Ventilator Mark 3 diagrammatic representation of closed circuit (see key). (Reproduced from Automatic Ventilation of the Lungs by Mushin et al., by kind permission of the publishers Blackwell Scientific Publications Ltd.)

Terminal disinfection of ventilators presents a number of problems, for with the exception of the Cape Bristol ventilator and corrugated tubes, external valves and connections, many of the components cannot be sterilised by heat. In the case of the electrically driven ventilators it may be unwise to utilise ethylene oxide gas due to the danger of an explosion if traces remain after sterilisation.

For these reasons, no one perfect technique of disinfection has yet been devised. A method has been devised for disinfecting the Cape ventilator and all types of ventilators and this involves the use of formalin (Sykes, 1964). Liq. Formaldehyde B.P. 100 ml is added to the water in the humidifier (5 per cent solution). A 2-litre reservoir bag and Y piece is then connected between the expiratory port and inspiratory port. A further 2-litre bag is fitted over the air inlet. The machine is run for four to eight hours to circulate the formalin vapour after which all tubing, traps and the humidifier are washed with tap water. The humidifier is then refilled with a 0·06 per cent solution of ammonia and the machine is allowed to ventilate for eight or more hours until there is no trace of formalin vapour detectable. The humidifier is finally rinsed well with tap water.

Another method consists of disinfection of the ventilator circuit by ultrasonic nebulisation (Judd *et al.*, 1968). An ultrasonic nebuliser, such as the DeVilbiss or LKB,NB 100, is used to produce a mist of hydrogen peroxide (20 vols) which is circulated through the machine in a similar manner to that described for formalin. This is carried out for a period of 60 minutes followed by ventilation of air for 1–4 hours depending on the type of ventilator. (See Appendix for method applicable particularly to Cape ventilator.)

In the absence of a heat sterilisable or component replaceable ventilator such as the Cape Bristol, this method is relatively rapid, bacteriologically effective, technically convenient, safe, and does not interfere with the function of the machine. Any hydrogen peroxide left in the machine will quickly break down into oxygen and water. When using hydrogen peroxide it is wise to protect the hands with rubber gloves to prevent cutaneous desquamation caused by contact with the hydrogen peroxide mist.

The Bird respirator can be stripped down to the actual respirator box and the accessories cleansed in Savlon 10 per cent followed by immersion in two baths of 14 per cent hypochlorite solution for at least 15 minutes each. The respirator itself can be disinfected only in ethylene oxide gas without the use of heat.

Open ether

Even with the advent of the newest and complicated anaesthetic techniques, the administration of open ether is still used occasionally and might well be valuable in the event of a major disaster.

Induction of anaesthesia is accomplished by the patient breathing through a gauze pad on to which is dropped a quantity of ether. Initially, ethyl chloride is commonly used to induce unconsciousness, because it is less unpleasant to breathe than the ether vapour.

The thickness of gauze should be adequate to prevent the drops of ether from falling on

Key to Figure 266

Gas circuit relevant references

1 Top stroke indicator	19 Negative pressure control	47 Gas switch valve
2 Weights	20 Open connector	48 Expiratory solenoid valve
3 Microswitch actuating plunger	21 Negative pressure limiting valve	49 Wright's respirometer
4 'Inverted top hat'	22 to 24 Non-return valves	50 Breathing tubes
5 Expiratory bellows	25 Open connector	51 Diaphragm valve
6 Rod with helical spring	26 Lower volume cycling tidal volume control	52 Flow rate control valve
7 Centre bellows	27 Volume cycling microswitch contact	53 Expiratory spill valve
8 Centre bellows blow-off valve	28 Alarm microswitch contact	54 Airway pressure gauge
9 Closed circuit bellows	29 Inspiratory solenoid valve	55 Patient Y-piece
10 Beam	30 Rear closed circuit port	56 Pressure relief valve
11 Cycling selector	31 Front closed circuit port and exhaust to	57 Pressure cycling diaphragm
12 Time cycling expiratory phase control	atmosphere	58 Positive pressure cycling control
13 Time cycling inspiratory phase control	32 Gas supply to patient port	59 Trigger pressure diaphragm
14 Trigger on/off switch	33 Driving gas, closed circuit port	60 Trigger pressure control
15 Pressure cycling expiratory phase control	34 Manual bag port	61 Manual bag
16 Upper volume cycling tidal volume control	35 Outlet tube from CO$_2$ absorber	62 Reservoir bag spill valve
17 Alarm microswitch contact	36 Inlet tube to CO$_2$ absorber	63 Closed circuit reservoir bag
18 Volume cycling microswitch contacts	37 Partitioned soda lime canister	64 Air entraining valve
	38 Circuit selector control	65 Levers exerting spring pressure on
	39 to 46 Poppet valves	beam (10)

to the patient's face. Twelve to sixteen layers of gauze are usually adequate and these are 'tented' away from the face by a wire frame called a Schimmelbusch mask. As the outer edges of the gauze can become moistened with ether during a long period of anaesthesia, it is preferable to cut this gauze pad to the mask shape (as indicated in Fig. 268) to prevent the gauze from actually coming into contact with the skin.

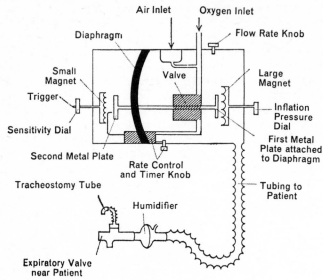

Figure 267   Diagrammatic circuitry of the Bird respirator, Mark 8. (By courtesy of the *Nursing Times*, London.)

A piece of gamagee measuring about 23·5 cm by 35·6 cm (9 in by 14 in), and having a central slit exposing the nose and mouth, is placed to protect the face. A similar piece is placed over the mask and ether dropped through the slit on to the underlying gauze. These pads also prevent the patient from obtaining air round the edges of the mask.

In order to minimise the risk of burns from liquid anaesthetic, the anaesthetist may require petroleum jelly for the lips, and sterile castor oil drops for the eyes after the ether has been administered. These should always be available when open ether is being administered.

Intravenous anaesthesia

A selection of intravenous anaesthetic agents, relaxants, stimulants and antidotes should be clearly labelled and available for the anaesthetist.

The intravenous barbiturates in common use are thiopentone sodium (Pentothal) 2·5 per cent, methohexitone sodium (Brietal) 1 per cent, and the hypnotic propanidid (Epontol) 5 per cent (supplied as a solution) and Ketamine hydrochloride (Ketalar). A 2·5 per cent solution is prepared by dissolving 0·5 g in 20 ml of sterile pyrogen-free distilled water respectively.

Phenoperidine (Operidine), pethidine and pentazocine (Fortral) are used extensively. Pethidine is often diluted to a 1 per cent solution containing 10 mg per ml.

Relaxants in common use include the 'competitive blocker' muscle relaxants such as curare (Tubarine), gallamine triethiodide (Flaxedil), pancuronium bromide (Pavulon) and alcuronium toxiferine (Alloferin); and depolarising muscle relaxants such as suxamethonium (Scoline).

Stimulants available should include nikethamide (Coramine), aminophylline, methedrine, methoxamine (Vasoxyl, Vasoxine), metaraminol (Aramine), megimide, daptazol, isoprenaline (Insuprel), noradrenaline (Levophed) and adrenaline. Antidotes commonly needed include atropine, prostigmine, nalorphine (Lethidrone) and levallorphan (Lorfan).

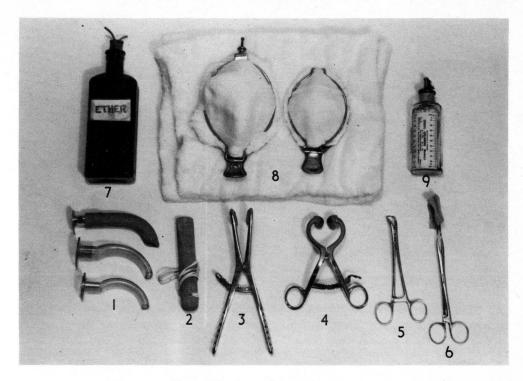

Figure 268   Open ether requirements.

1. Airways (Phillip and Guedel).
2. Boxwood wedge.
3. Mouth gag (Mason).
4. Mouth gag (Doyen).
5. Tongue forceps.
6. Pharyngeal swab-holding forceps.

7. Ether bottle with dropper (Bellamy Gardner).
8. Open inhalers, adult and child (Schimmelbusch).
9. Ethyl chloride.

It is the anaesthetist's responsibility to prepare these solutions, but if the anaesthetic nurse is permitted to do so, she should check the preparation with a second person and show the anaesthetist the ampoules or bottle from which the injection has been prepared.

A 10 ml or 20 ml disposable sterile syringe is used for barbiturates, and a 2 ml or 5 ml disposable sterile syringe for other drugs, including pethidine, relaxants, antidotes, etc. The integrity of the sterile packet containing the syringe should be checked by trying to squeeze the air from the inside.

The sizes of needles used vary with individual choice but for general purposes a size 12 or 14 hypodermic needle is usual, with perhaps a size 18 for small or delicate veins. The anaesthetist will require a number of 'filling' needles (plastic quills) to aspirate drugs from the ampoules, and larger bore serum needles size 1 for rubber-cap bottles.

For continuous or intermittent intravenous injections, either the syringe and needle are left in position so that small quantities may be injected as required, or a special needle such as the butterfly Gordh or Mitchell is left in the vein and the syringe attached to the needle each time injection is necessary.

Continuous intravenous anaesthesia can be maintained by using a very weak intravenous solution, which is administered via a saline transfusion, or small quantities of the drug can be injected into the rubber transfusion tube, as required.

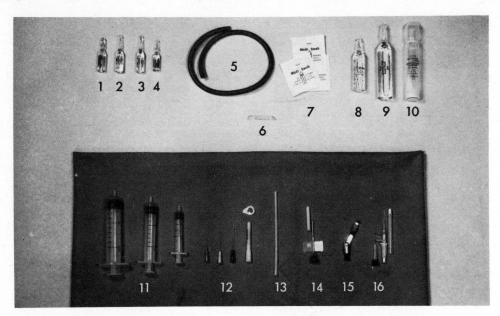

Figure 269   Requirements for the intravenous induction of anaesthesia.

1. Succinyl choline (Scoline).
2. Curare (Tubarine).
3. Pethidine (DDA).
4. Atropine.
5. Rubber tubing for tourniquet.
6. File.
7. Spirit-impregnated Mediswabs.
8. Propanidid (Epontol).
9. Water for injection.
10. Thiopentone Sodium (Pentothal).

11. Disposable syringes 20 ml, 10 ml and 2 ml.
12. Hypodermic needles Nos. 20, 12 and 1 with needle case.
13. Disposable filling cannula (Kwills).
14. Disposable Gordh needle (Armoven).
15. Mitchell needle.
16. Disposable needle (Plextrocan).
Not illustrated: disposable butterfly needles.

Where it is the habit of the anaesthetist to prepare a few different solutions at once, he should label syringes to aid identification.

It is only the anaesthetist who is responsible for the right drug being injected. Accidents have occurred, and so a nurse should never be offended if the anaesthetist does not appear to trust her spoken word. He must be absolutely certain; where life is concerned, personal considerations are of no account. It is not sufficient to check the name on the outside of the ampoule box. The inscription on the ampoule itself is the *only* proof that the correct drug is being given.

Endotracheal and endobronchial intubation

Apparatus for passing an endotracheal tube must be ready before the commencement of any anaesthetic induction, even if the anaesthetist has not requested its preparation. In resuscitation this procedure will be one of the first performed by the anaesthetist, unless a tube is already in position. Laryngoscopes used when introducing an endotracheal tube include the Magill straight-blade and the anatomical shaped blade Mackintosh types which are illustrated.

There are four basic types of endotracheal tubes, the nasal type and the oral type, both cuffed and non-cuffed. Although each is identical in diameter, the nasal tube is *slightly* softer when pressed between the fingers, and this allows it to comply with the configuration of the nasal space. Some endotracheal tubes are armoured by incorporating a

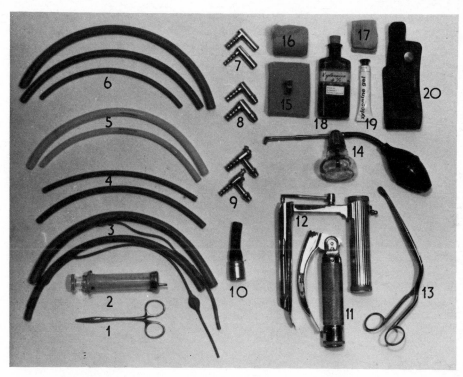

Figure 270   Requirements for endotracheal intubation.

1. Artery forceps (Spencer Wells).
2. 10-ml syringe.
3. Endotracheal tubes, cuffed (Magill).
4. Endotracheal tubes, nasal (Magill).
5. Endotracheal tubes, oral, plastic (Magill).
6. Endotracheal tubes, oral, rubber (Magill).
7. Endotracheal tube connections (Rowbotham).
8. Endotracheal tube connections (Cobb, plain type).
9. Endotracheal tube connection (Cobb, with suction access).

10. Endotracheal catheter mount (Magill).
11. Laryngoscope (Mackintosh).
12. Laryngoscope (Magill).
13. Endotracheal tube forceps (Magill).
14. Atomiser for topical local anaesthetic.
15. Catheter mount clip.
16. Gauze roll for pharyngeal pack.
17. Anaesthetic swabs.
18. Local anaesthetic for topical application, e.g., 4 per cent lignocaine (Xylocaine).
19. Tube lubricant, e.g., lignocaine (Xylocaine) gel.
20. Endotracheal head harness (Hudson).

Note. Sellotape, or similar, should be available.

metal or nylon spiral within the tube wall. These tubes have less tendency to become kinked or compressed and are of special use during operations on the skull and chest.

The endotracheal tube is used:

1. When in the opinion of the anaesthetist the airway is liable to be obstructed.

2. For operations in which it is necessary because of surgical technique, e.g., head and chest operations.

3. For upper abdominal operations and artificial ventilation.

4. When the towelling and position of the patient prevents the anaesthetist gaining easy access to the patient's head, and thus guaranteeing a free airway, e.g., craniotomies.

5. To prevent the inhalation of blood or vomit, e.g., emergencies.

6. In the treatment of cardiac arrest.

The anaesthetist generally is likely to use an endotracheal tube which has a terminal cuff which, when inflated with air, impinges upon the tracheal mucosa, thereby sealing the lungs from the upper respiratory passages to prevent the inhalation of blood or vomit. It is important to realise that there is not a fixed volume of air necessary to secure air-tight fitting of the tube within the trachea. The amount may vary between 2 ml and 10 ml of air and this can be tested by the anaesthetist when inflating the lungs.

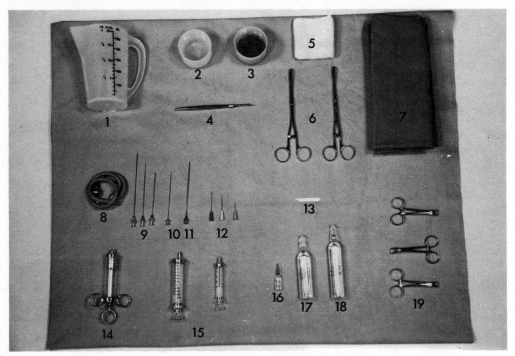

Figure 271   Requirements for local or regional analgesia.

1. 0·5 litre measuring jug.
2. Skin antiseptic.
3. Bonney's blue for marking infiltrated area.
4. Skin pen and nib.
5. Green swabs.
6. Sponge holding forceps, Rampley (2).
7. Sterile towels.
8. Self-filling attachment (Pidkin), for Labet syringe.
9. Locking needles (Labet).
10. Brachial plexus needle (Short point).
11. Filling needle.
12. Hypodermic needles (18, 12 and 1).
13. File.
14. Syringes (Labet).
15. Syringes, 10 ml and 2 ml.
16. Adrenaline 1 in 1000.
17. Lignocaine (Xylocaine) 1·5 per cent.
18. Sterile distilled water.
19. Towel clips.

A nurse may be asked to clip off the pilot tube when the anaesthetist has inflated the cuff so that it just fits the lumen of the trachea. If a pair of artery forceps is applied, only the tips are used, and as near the syringe as possible; this saves wear and tear of the pilot tube. Endotracheal tubes are now available with pilot tubes which incorporate a self-sealing valve thereby obviating the need to use forceps.

Nasal tube sizes range from 3 mm to 5 mm for a child; 5 mm to 6·5 mm for an adolescent; and 6·5 mm to 9 mm for an adult. Oral tubes range from 3·5 mm to 6·5 mm for a child; 7 mm to 8 mm for an adolescent; and 9 mm to 12 mm for an adult.

The experienced anaesthetic nurse or technician will learn to select the sizes and type of endotracheal tubes required, but where cuffed tubes are to be used, they must always be tested by inflating the cuff before handing to the anaesthetist. All the apparatus should be laid out in the order required, giving special attention to the provision of correct size

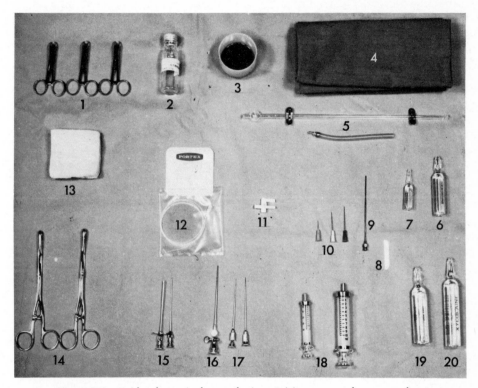

Figure 272 Epidural or spinal anaesthetic requisites prepared as one packet.

1. Towel clips.
2. Sterile CSF specimen bottle.
3. Aqueous skin antiseptic.
4. Sterile towels.
5. Spinal manometer and connecting tube.
6. Bupivacaine (Marcaine) with 1 in 200,000 adrenaline.
7. Cinchocaine (Heavy Nupercaine).
8. File.
9. Filling needle.
10. Hypodermic needles, size 20, 12 and 1.
11. Three-way tap.
12. Epidural plastic cannula.
13. Green swabs.
14. Sponge holding forceps, Rampley (2).
15. Epidural needles.
16. Spinal needle.
17. Spinal needles.
18. Syringes, 2 ml and 10 ml.
19. Sterile distilled water.
20. Lignocaine (Xylocaine) 1·5 per cent.

tube connections, and laryngoscopes in good working order. The electric lamp on the latter must illuminate brightly and if necessary the battery should be changed before use. A second laryngoscope must always be available in case of lamp failure during use. The care of electrical endoscopes has been dealt with in Chapter 2. A tube of lubricant is usually required and this may be combined with a local anaesthetic such as 2 per cent lignocaine (Xylocaine). An example of a non-anaesthetic lubricant is K-Y jelly. A suction machine with long suction catheters is prepared, together with a small bowl of clean water for rinsing the catheters. A surface anaesthetic e.g., 4 per cent lignocaine (Xylocaine) and laryngeal spray may be required. A selection of apparatus is shown in Fig. 270.

The endobronchial tube is in effect an extended cuffed endotracheal tube of smaller dimensions, which is passed into the left or right bronchus. Formerly during chest operations, the anaesthetist utilised two tubes, one in the unaffected lung for the purpose of anaesthesia, and one in the other for the purpose of aspiration during operation. Endobronchial tubes have an inflatable cuff to isolate the intubated lung. It is now common practice to use a divided airway or doubled lumen cuffed tube such as the Carlens: this achieves the same purpose. The anaesthetist will require a bronchoscope of suitable type, in addition to the standard laryngoscope, etc., and may also need a long bronchial spray with a surface anaesthetic, e.g., lignocaine (Xylocaine).

All endotracheal and endobronchial tubes must be cleaned thoroughly with a brush and warm antibacterial detergent solution after use. Those having inflatable cuffs are checked before being stored away, care being taken to avoid water entering the cuff or pilot tube. The tubes are always sterilised after use although absolute sterility cannot be guaranteed during intubation.

After use, laryngoscope blades should be dismantled from the battery handle, cleaned and sterilised by autoclaving. Most modern instruments have nylon insulation and gold-plated electrical contacts which will withstand autoclaving. If they are the older type either ethylene oxide sterilising or pasteurising will have to be resorted to.

Local or regional anaesthesia

This may range from a simple injection for infiltrating a small area, to an extensive nerve block.

Whereas a 10 ml or 20 ml syringe is adequate for a minor procedure, involving the injection of a few millilitres of anaesthetic agent, it is preferable to use a self-filling syringe for larger quantities. The alternative is to leave the needle in position and prepare several syringes filled with anaesthetic agent, using these consecutively.

A fine hypodermic needle of size 18 or 20 will be required for the initial 'weal', followed by a longer one of wider bore. A selection of needles should be availble, ranging from 2 to 4 in (5·1 cm to 10·2 cm) in length, and 20 to 26 B.W.G. in gauge.

Anaesthetists require exploring needles having long points and others having short points. A short point needle is essential for nerve blocks, especially the brachial plexus block, where a long point needle may increase the risk of pleural puncture or perforation of a blood-vessel.

Amongst the anaesthetic agents most commonly used are lignocaine (Xylocaine) bupivacaine (Marcaine) and procaine.

A 1·5 or 2 per cent lignocaine is used for the initial infiltration or when only a small quantity is required. Where a larger quantity is necessary, the strength of solution is reduced to 1 per cent or 0·5 per cent and the amount injected limited to the maximum dose of the agent (e.g., the maximum dose of plain lignocaine (Xylocaine) in a normal healthy adult is 13 to 15 ml of a 1·5 per cent solution, 23 ml of a 1 per cent solution or 46 ml of a 0·5 per cent solution). Dosage must be reduced in the ill and elderly.

In order to produce vasoconstriction, and thereby lessen capillary haemorrhage, adrenaline may be added in the proportion of 1 in 400,000 to 1 in 100,000 according to the total amount of solution being injected. A 1 in 400,000 solution may be prepared by adding 1 ml of 1 in 1000 adrenaline to 399 ml of local anaesthetic agent. A 1 in 100,000 solution may be prepared by adding 1 ml of 1 in 1000 adrenaline to 99 ml of anaesthetic agent. A 1 in 100,000 addition of adrenaline also prolongs the action of the local anaesthetic by delaying absorption up to six hours and thereby increases the safety margin for larger doses. In the case of lignocaine the maximum dosage becomes approximately twice that of the plain solution.

An easy way of preparing a small quantity of 1 in 400,000 adrenaline is to add the contents of a 1 ml ampoule of 1 in 1000 adrenaline to a 20 ml ampoule of saline solution from which 1 ml has been withdrawn, leaving 19 ml; 1 ml of this mixture is added to a second 19 ml ampoule containing anaesthetic solution. Should this be done by the anaesthetist, the nurse's watchful eye would make sure that the first ampoule containing the saline is safely discarded after removing 1 ml, so as to avoid accidents.

It should be pointed out that on occasions the surgeon requires only the effect of the adrenaline and 1 in 100,000 or 1 in 400,000 adrenaline solution is prepared with saline only.

The computation of local anaesthetic solutions, with or without adrenaline, is entirely the anaesthetist's responsibility, although selected strengths may be prepared by the pharmacist before they are required. If the anaesthetic nurse is permitted to prepare injections, she should *always* check the preparation with the anaesthetist, retaining all containers for his inspection.

Following operation, when a local anaesthetic has been administered, great care must be taken to avoid injury to areas which may remain analgesic for several hours. This applies especially to the use of hot-water bottles and electric blankets as a post-operative measure.

The topical application of anaesthetic agents such as cocaine to the eyes and lignocaine, etc., to the mucosa of the mouth, pharynx or respiratory tract, requires special after-care. The eyes must always be covered for several hours, as foreign bodies may impinge upon the cornea without the patient feeling their presence. Even with a minor operation, a patient who has had an application of local anaesthetic to the mucosa of the respiratory tract is not permitted to eat or drink for at least four hours following operation and can cough effectively, as the resultant paralysis of the soft palate and epiglottis would allow foreign matter to enter the trachea. Watch also for possible reactions to the local anaesthetic including convulsions. If there is the slightest doubt or history of previous sensitivity a small test dose should be given first.

Spinal and epidural anaesthesia

Requirements for spinal anaesthesia should always be autoclaved before use in a special spinal packet.

Spinal anaesthesia is produced by making a spinal intrathecal injection of a heavy or light solution (in relation to the specific gravity of CSF) of anaesthetic agent such as cinchocaine (Nupercaine), lignocaine (Xylocaine) and bupivacaine (Marcaine). In spinal anaesthetic the drug mixes with the cerebrospinal fluid and bathes a portion of the spinal cord and nerve roots, thereby rendering part of the body analgesic as well as paralysing the muscles. The extent of its desired action is determined by the anaesthetist and depends upon the volume of solution, the specific gravity of the solution and the position of the patient during and immediately after injection.

Epidural analgesia is produced by the slow injection of a larger volume of local anaesthetic agent into the epidural space between the ligamentum flavum and the dura. A special needle or cannula is used to facilitate the introduction of an indwelling nylon catheter through which the anaesthetic agent is injected.

For injection, the patient may either be sitting up with his legs over the side of the operation table, and head and shoulders bent forwards; or lying on the side with his legs drawn up, the head and shoulders being bent towards his knees.

Storage of equipment

Rubber equipment, e.g., endotracheal tubes deteriorate and soften with time, therefore overstocking should be avoided. Rubber should be stored at temperatures below 21°C (70°F). No lubricant based on liquid paraffin should be used; it ruins rubber.

Drugs should also be stored at relatively low temperatures. The reserve stock and those particularly sensitive to heat such as scoline and heparin should be kept in a refrigerator.

The patient

So far we have dealt with the apparatus and drugs necessary for the induction of anaesthesia and we must now consider the patient himself.

A patient comes to the theatre with a certain amount of apprehension, even although he may be the last person to admit this. The manner in which he is treated may seriously affect the induction of anaesthesia and his subsequent recovery. He should be made to think that he is the centre of attention, and that all possible skill is being used for his welfare.

In Chapter 1 we stated that the patient should always be accompanied to the theatre by a ward nurse, and if possible this nurse should remain with him until the induction of anaesthesia is complete. The psychological effect of this is very good, for the patient feels reassured by the presence of a ward nurse who is often the person responsible for his nursing after the operation.

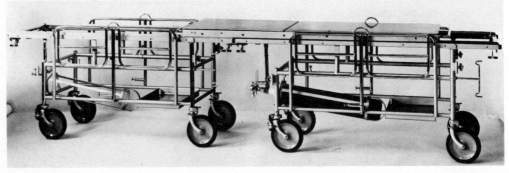

Figure 273   Transfer trolley system which avoids taking the ward trolley into the sterile areas. (A. C. Daniels & Co. Ltd.)

Some or all of the duties described for the assistance of the anaesthetist may equally well be performed by the anaesthetic nurse, theatre technician or ward nurse, whichever is most suitable and convenient.

The patient must be accompanied by X-rays, case notes, signed consent for anaesthetic and operation, pathological reports and drug sheet and any other relevant information which will be of use to the surgeon or the anaesthetist. The ward nurse should know the preparation which the patient has had, the time at which food or drink was last taken, the type and amount of pre-operative drugs administered, and the time at which they were given. She is responsible for seeing that any dentures have been removed, and must know whether the patient has passed urine or has been catheterised, and the time and amount passed, together with any abnormalities detected in routine ward tests.

A practice used increasingly is to transport the patient to the operating department on his bed. The patient is then transferred to a theatre trolley before entering the sterile zone. Alternatively a transfer trolley top system may be utilised (Fig. 273). The patient is anaesthetised on the trolley or may be transferred on the underlying canvas stretcher to the operation table in the anaesthetic room.

A patient must *never* be left alone in the anaesthetic room or theatre for he may be confused following the administration of the pre-operative drugs or sedative, and this may lead to accidental personal injury, like a fall from the trolley or operation table. Identification of the patient, his correct operation and correct site is of paramount importance. This procedure starts in the ward where some identification of the patient's name and case number must be attached to him before he is transferred to theatre. The house surgeon must mark the operation site with an indelible marker indicating the correct side or digit. This is especially important with the unconscious patient, aged or child. The identification can either be in the form of a bracelet (only removable by cutting it off) or details written on the patient by means of a skin pen.

On arrival at the theatre the patient's identification is checked against the case notes and operation list. If conscious, he is further asked his name. The anaesthetic and operation consent form must also be checked.

The surgeon should see the patient before anaesthesia is induced and confirm it is the correct patient, operation and site. This is of vital importance if a limb or digit is to be amputated.

There is no reason why the patient should not be made as comfortable as possible whilst awaiting the anaesthetist. Unless the patient is unconscious with the attendant dangers of an obstructed airway, it is a simple matter to remove excess pillows just before induction is commenced. The nurse should see that the patient is kept as quiet as possible, and should not encourage conversation unless it is obvious that the patient feels more relaxed doing so.

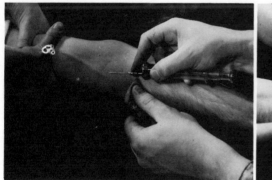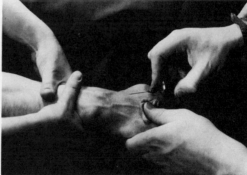

Figure 274   Method of holding upper arm for an intravenous injection, as an alternative to a tourniquet.

Figure 275   Method of holding wrist for an intravenous injection, as an alternative to a tourniquet.

During induction the nurse stands by in case the patient becomes restless, but if he does she must not attempt to wrestle with him but must apply gentle restraint, with one arm across the legs just above the knees, using the other arm to prevent any wild flinging about of the patient's arms. She should not hesitate to ask for further assistance in dealing with the obstreperous patient and wild alcoholics.

For intravenous injection, the selected arm is extended towards the anaesthetist and either a quick-release tourniquet applied to the upper arm, or the nurse constricts the venous return by encircling the upper arm with her hands. The patient clenches his fist to make the veins prominent, and after the anaesthetist has aspirated blood into the syringe which probably indicates that the needle is in a vein, the compression of the upper arm veins is released at the anaesthetist's request. The nurse stands at the head of the trolley or operation table to support the patient's jaw when relaxation is complete. The anaesthetist will then apply pressure over the area of injection, which is continued by the nurse when the inhalation anaesthetic is commenced.

Providing the anaesthetist inserts the needle into a vessel on the lateral aspect of the antecubital fossa or the back of the hand, the tragedy of intra-arterial injection is minimised.

Too many nurses regard the maintenance of a good airway in the unconscious patient as just 'holding' up the jaw. Although this *may* suffice in some cases, the nurses must realise the principles behind any method chosen.

When unconscious, the muscles supporting the lower jaw relax, allowing it to sag. The tongue is also paralysed, allowing it to fall backwards, thereby obstructing the patient's airway.

The basis of keeping an airway clear is supporting the jaw and extending the head.

The nurse should place her fingers behind the angle of the jaw on each side, lifting it slightly forwards. This will pull upon the muscle attachments of the tongue, preventing it from falling backwards and thereby maintaining an unobstructed channel between the mouth and larynx. The same effect may be accomplished by lifting the chin forwards in a similar manner.

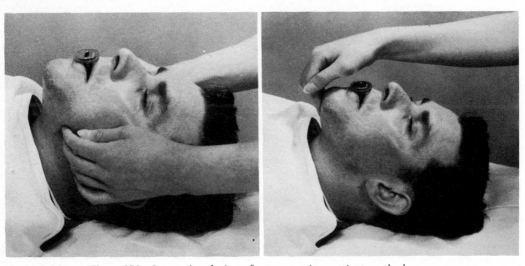

Figure 276   Supporting the jaw of an unconscious patient, method one.

Figure 277   Supporting the jaw of an unconscious patient, method two.

An unobstructed airway is indicated by quiet respirations, as noisy breathing is obstructed breathing. The position of the head or lower jaw may require adjustment to achieve this object – so the nurse should use her hands, sense of hearing and observe the patient's colour and respiration.

As the patient loses consciousness, following the i.v. injection of a barbiturate and relaxant, especially in emergency situations it is possible for regurgitation of stomach contents to occur before the anaesthetist has inserted the endotracheal tube. The nurse or anaesthetic assistant may be required to perform the Sellick manoeuvre as soon as unconsciousness intervenes.

The Sellick manoeuvre (Sellick, 1961) consists of temporary occlusion of the upper end of the oesophagus by backward pressure of the cricoid cartilage against the bodies of cervical vertebrae. This prevents regurgitation of oesophageal or stomach contents during induction of anaesthesia, and also prevents gastric distension from positive pressure ventilation administered by face mask (or mouth to mouth resuscitation).

Before induction, the cricoid is palpated and lightly held between the thumb and second finger. As anaesthesia begins, moderate pressure is exerted on the cricoid cartilage mainly by the index finger. As soon as unconsciousness intervenes, firm pressure can be applied without obstructing the airway and this is maintained until the endotracheal tube has been inserted and the cuff inflated.

The nurse should not speak during the initial stages of anaesthesia, as it is possible for the patient's hearing to become acute, hearing being the last sense to go, and is accentuated as unconsciousness supervenes. She should not begin to remove the bandages or covers until the patient is completely unconscious.

The anaesthetic nurse or technician will hand instruments, etc., to the anaesthetist as required and like the instrument nurse in theatre, will try to anticipate his requirements.

The anaesthetist has many things to watch during the course of anaesthesia, including the colour of the patient, the pulse, respiration, blood pressure, cardiac activity (sometimes by means of an electro-cardiogram), in addition to keeping the general condition of the patient under observation. He *may* assign certain duties to the anaesthetic nurse or technician in this respect, and may require him or her to keep a record of the patient's pulse, and if sufficiently experienced, blood pressure also. He or she will adjust the rate of flow of transfusions, indicated by the anaesthetist, and replace transfusion solutions under his directions.

Guedal describes four stages of anaesthesia which are demonstrable with ether and cyclopropane. However, with the short-acting barbiturates, the patient falls rapidly asleep and excitement is rarely seen.

The first stage is one of analgesia when peripheral sensation is lost, but the nervous system is under control. In the first stage of induction there are frequently swallowing movements, followed by regular respiration and analgesia.

The second stage is one of excitement, with movements of the limbs followed by tonic spasms of the muscles, dilated pupils and roving eyeballs. Quite often this stage is very short and almost absent, especially when anaesthetising the deeply sedated patient.

The third stage is the stage of surgical anaesthesia which may range from moderate to deep according to the type of operation. During this stage, the anaesthetist is on his guard against:

The fourth stage which is respiratory and cardiac arrest.

If the patient collapses on the operation table with acute cardio-circulatory arrest his recovery may well depend upon prompt action by all the theatre staff. Without treatment, irreversible damage may occur in three minutes and a lasting recovery of the brain, and thus the whole body, is impossible after eight minutes.

As the anaesthetist and anaesthetic nurse have a vital part to play, the catastrophe is being dealt with in this chapter.

The following is an outline of the type of scheme most prevalent today.

CARDIOCIRCULATORY ARREST

If this has occurred immediate steps are taken to restore adequate ventilation and circulation. The anaesthetic nurse will be required to keep a record of the time from the first warning, calling out this time, initially, at 15 second intervals with particular emphasis at each minute.

The anaesthetist, having given warning and noted the time, tilts the operation table head downwards, stops the anaesthetic, ensures that the airway is clear, and administers oxygen under pressure. He may later pass an endotracheal tube if one is not already inserted; time is precious.

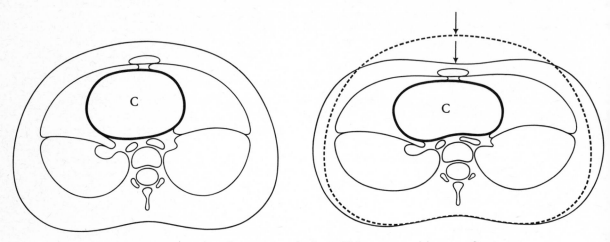

Figure 278   In external cardiac massage, the heart (C) is compressed between the sternum and the spinal column by depressing the sternum with the hands by about 3–4 cm (by kind permission Roche Products Ltd.).

At the same time the surgeon commences external cardiac massage. (It is now accepted that circulation can generally be maintained in cardiac arrest without thoracotomy and by rhythmic external manual compression of the sternum which in turn compresses the heart between it and the spine, forcing out blood into the aorta. Relaxation of the thoracic cage releases the pressure on the heart and allows it to fill with blood. Thus must be done on a rigid surface similar to the operation table, boards under a mattress or on the floor.). The compression on the lower half of the sternum must be by the heels of the hands (not the fingers), one on top of the other, aided by the weight of the body. This pressure should not be exerted on the ribs or epigastrium otherwise fracture of the ribs or rupture of the liver or spleen may occur.

Depression of the sternum should be at least 3 to 4 cm with each stroke, with a frequency of between 70 and 90 strokes per minute. This should produce a palpable radial pulse with a blood pressure of 60 to 100 mm Hg. Rhythmic compression of the sternum, whilst giving good temporary artificial circulation, does not produce effective ventilation. This must be accomplished either by manual compression of the anaesthetic machine bag, or attachment of the endotracheal tube to a ventilator.

If the patient responds, the surgeon may instruct his assistant and the scrub nurse to complete any vital stage in the operation. Alternatively he will hand over cardiac massage to the assistant and complete the operation himself.

Immediately cardiac massage has been started, the circulating nurse or anaesthetic nurse fetches the cardiac resuscitation set which comprises various drugs, transfusion fluids and equipment, syringes and needles, electrical defibrillator (external or internal) and if possible an electrocardiograph monitor, which should be connected to the patient.

When ventricular asystole is responsible for the arrest of circulation, external massage may re-establish normal rhythm. If there is no response, intracardiac injections may be tried. The most generally used is adrenaline 1 in 10,000 dosage 3 to 5 ml intracardiac or if a very slow ventricular rate has been established, adrenaline 1 in 10,000, 1 ml per minute intravenously. This is for myocardial stimulation.

Calcium chloride, 10 per cent may be given intracardiac or intravenously in a dosage up to 10 ml, this increases tone in a flabby heart.

These measures may provoke ventricular fibrillation which can then be treated with a D.C. counter shock administered by the defibrillator. A D.C. counter shock may also be tried to provoke ventricular fibrillation (if massage is unsuccessful) which can be treated with a second shock. The shock should be given starting (manual control) at 300 J/2 to 4 millisecond.

If a defibrillator is unavailable, ventricular fibrillation can sometimes be treated by intravenous procaine amide (Pronestyl) 1 g or propranolol (Inderal) 5 mg given slowly.

With cardiac arrest of more than the briefest duration, acidosis, both metabolic and respiratory, is likely. If the period of arrest exceeds 2 minutes or if cardiac massage has been carried out for longer than 15 minutes, the patient should have 200/500 ml of 4·2 per cent sodium bicarbonate intravenously.

The blood pressure should be maintained if necessary by the addition of isoprenaline (Aleudrin) or metaraminol (Aramine) to the intravenous fluid.

If pulmonary oedema is suspected or if the volume of intravenous fluid given has exceeded 1500 ml, a diuretic may be given (e.g., frusemide (Lasix) 20 mg or more intravenously.

If normal consciousness does not return fairly quickly, there may be cerebral oedema (which invariably follows a period of anoxia) which may be treated by intravenous 50 per cent sucrose or Urevert.

Two indications for open thoracotomy and direct cardiac massage are (a) inability to restore a radial pulse and satisfactory blood pressure (e.g., in a stout patient when compression of the sternum is difficult or in chest injuries involving the rib cage) and (b) the absence of a D.C. defibrillator when only an A.C. defibrillator is available for direct application to a fibrillating heart.

General outline of procedure for cardiocirculatory arrest:
1. Arrested heart
2. External massage, controlled pulmonary ventilation
3. No beat; adrenaline given or attempt with D.C. shocks, this causes beat or
4. Fibrillation of the heart
5. D.C. defibrillator applied using large moistened, firmly attached electrodes with a surface area of at least 10 cm and supplying in adults 300 to 400 J D.C. over 2 to 4 milliseconds. All staff take hands off patient to avoid a personal electric shock.
6. Beat recommences
7. Intravenous transfusion of 200/500 ml of 4·2 per cent sodium bicarbonate, plus possibly noradrenaline to maintain blood pressure
8. Endotracheal tube passed at earliest opportunity, artificial ventilation continued until normal respirations recommence
9. If external massage unsuccessful, direct massage a thoracotomy may be considered. If the chest is opened, antibiotics should be given.

Cardiac-respiratory arrest trolley. It is prudent to assemble together the apparatus and drugs required for the treatment of cardiac-respiratory arrest. This may consist of a simple trolley for use within the operating suite or a more complex unit designed to transport the equipment to other parts of the hospital. In the latter case, in addition to laryngoscopes and endotracheal tubes with their connections, Ambu resuscitator, the

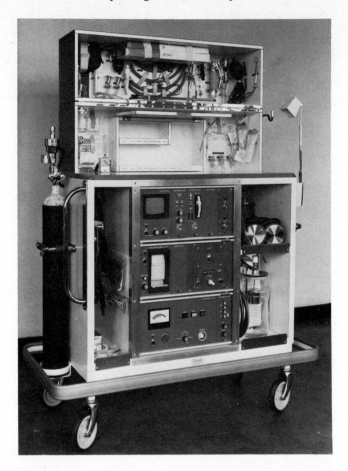

Figure 279   The Daniels Cardiac-arrest Trolley was designed in collaboration with the United Cardiff Hospitals. It embraces all the apparatus, instrumentation and drugs required within a minimum of space. The trolley measures 82 cm × 25 cm × 120 cm (33 in × 10 in × 48in) high and avoids the use of drawers and cupboards in which items can be so easily disarranged and therefore difficult to find at critical times. Each and every item is labelled and made readily accessible in its allotted position. All electrical apparatus is connected to the mains electricity supply via a Mains Control Unit with one mains cable fitted with a universal plug. The upper section contains drugs, endotracheal tubes, laryngoscopes, needles, syringes, etc., in two compartments one of which is hinged to allow closure of this section when not in use. The lower section contains equipment including, defibrillator, ECG, suction machine, Ambu resuscitator and oxygen cylinder. (A. C. Daniels & Co. Ltd.)

Contents of Cardiac Resuscitation Trolley

Top of Trolley:

Airways: Sizes 4–00.	Elastoplast 75 cm (3 in).
Laryngoscopes: Adult Blade.	I.V. Cut Down Set.
Child Blade.	I.V. Fluid (Sod. Bic. 8·4%, Glucose 5%,
Pen Torch.	Mannitol 20%).
Tongue Depressor.	Disposable Giving Set.
Mouth Gag.	Intracath.
Magill's Forceps.	2 I.V. Needles.
Tongue Forceps.	Stethoscope.
20 ml Syringe (Unsterile).	Receiver with suction catheters.

Middle Shelf:
Bronchoscopy Tray (Unsterile).
Tracheotomy Tray (with suture material) (Sterile).
Haemorrhage Arrest Tray (Sterile).

Bottom Shelf:
Defibrillator.
Electrode Jelly.
Suction Unit with Yankauers Sucker.
Rubber Gloves.
Battery Unit.
Cyclator Pump.

Left Side of Trolley:
Extension Lead.
Oxygen Cylinder.
Ambu Resuscitator.

Right Side of Trolley:
Drip Stand.
Oxygen Cylinder.
Cyclator Bracket.

Attached to Back of Trolley:
Cardiac Arrest Board.

Lid of Trolley (With Night Light):
Endotracheal Tubes (8).
Sizes from 9·5 to 5·5 (Sterile item) with connections.
Spencer Wells Artery Forceps.
Book for recording used items.
Sphygmomanometer.
3 Files.
Needles: 4 No. 15.
          4 No. 1.
Syringes: 2×1 cm^3.
           2×5 cm^3.
           2×2 cm^3.
Drug Box (with lid).

Connections (3)
  Ambu Bag to Endotracheal.
  Cyclator to Tracheotomy.
  Cyclator to Endotracheal.
Gauze and Lubricant.
Strapping: 12 mm (0·5 in).
Scissors: Small straight Mayo's.
2 Way Resuscitation Tubes (6)
  Sizes from: 00/000 to 3/4.
Labels.
Biro.
Emergency Drugs.
GORD H. Needle (Sterile).
Sterile Intracardiac Needle.

DRUGS ON TROLLEY

Calcium Chloride	10%	10 ml.
Atropine Sulphate		0·6 mgm
Suxamethonium (Scoline)		100 mgm.
Nikethamide		2 ml.
Aminophylline		250 mgm.
Digoxin		0·5 mgm.
Adrenaline		1/10·000.
Lorfan		1 mgm.
Prostigmine		2·5 mgm.
Methyl Amphetamine		30 mgm.
Methoxamine		20 mgm.
Hydrocortisone		100 mgm Sol.
Noradrenaline		100 mgm.
Procaine Amide		100 mgm. in 1 cm^3.
Procaine Hyd.	10%	20 ml.
Lignocaine	1%	10 ml.
Vandid	5% A.	
Propranolol		5 mgm in 5 ml.
Inj. Isoprenaline		5 mgm.
Inj. Aramine		2 mgm
Lasix		20 mgm in 2 ml.
Sodium Bicarbonate B.P.		8·4% or 4·2%.

trolley should contain, a portable suction device, bronchoscope, defibrillator, ECG monitor and equipment for setting up a transfusion.

The drugs most likely to be needed in the treatment of cardiac arrest are:

Cardiac arrest. Adrenaline (epinephrine) 1 in 10,000 10 ml
  Calcium chloride 10 per cent 10 ml
  Lignocaine (Xylocaine) 1 per cent 10 ml
  Sodium Bicarbonate 8·4 per cent i.v. (equivalent to 1 mEq/ml) dosage 100 ml initially after 30 seconds arrest or 4·2 per cent dosage 200 ml initially

Supportive cardiac therapy. Isoprenaline 1 mg diluted to 500 ml with a 5 per cent glucose solution i.v.
  Potassium chloride (1·5 g in 10 ml) diluted to 500 ml with a 5 per cent glucose solution i.v. (20 mEq potassium)

Myocardial failure. Digoxin 0·25 mg per ml i.v.
  Ouabain (Strophanthin G) 0·5 mg per ml i.v.
  Frusemide (Lasix) 20 mg in 2 ml i.v.

Vasopressors. Methoxamine (Vasoxine) 20 mg per ml (dose 4 mg i.v.)
   Methylamphetamine 30 mg in 1·5 ml (dose 5 mg i.v.)
   Cerebral dehydration and diuresis. Mannitol solution 20 per cent (dose 1 to 200 ml)
   Urevert or 50 per cent sucrose

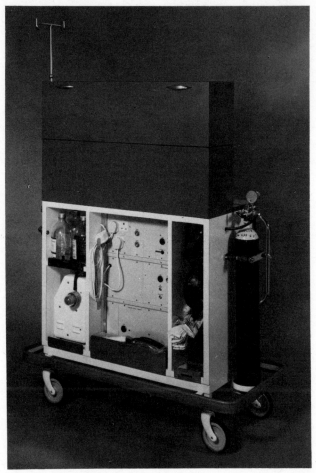

Figure 280   Rear view of the Cardiac Arrest trolley with the upper section closed. The top is covered with red Formica to distinguish it from other trolleys. (A. C. Daniels & Co. Ltd.)

Respiratory complications
   Adrenaline 30 ml per ml
   Aminophylline 250 mg per 10 ml i.v.
   Nikethamide 25 per cent 5 ml i.v.
   Nalorphine (Lethidrone) 10 mg per ml i.v.
   Levallorphan (Lorfan) 5 mg per 5 ml (dose 1 mg) i.v.
   Hydrocortisone 100 mg i.v.

When the operation is completed the anaesthetist will give instructions to the nurse accompanying the patient back to the ward. Under no circumstances must the patient leave the theatre suite until the anaesthetist is satisfied that he is fit to do so.

A good airway must be maintained in the manner described earlier but if there is any doubt regarding this or the possibility that the patient may vomit, he should be placed on his side with the underlying limb flexed, and the shoulders supported.

The patient is transferred carefully to the ward trolley with minimal movement, and covered with blankets before leaving the theatre suite. After returning him to his bed, if it is necessary to roll him to recover a stretcher, this must be done very gently, not only to avoid injury to the operation area, but a sudden rapid movement of the unconscious patient can cause cardiac arrest.

A tray containing mouth gag, tongue forceps, boxwood wedge, small towel, and vomit bowl or kidney dish should be carried with the patient during transit between the theatre and ward. These instruments must remain by the bed until the patient has recovered consciousness.

An airway or endotracheal tube left in position by the anaesthetist post-operatively should not be removed until the patient attempts to reject it. Attempts at rejection by the patient reveal that his swallowing reflex has returned and that unless there is any clinical contra-indication, the tube may be removed.

If oxygen has to be administered post-operatively to an unconscious patient, it should be given by means of a suitable catheter, mask or oxygen tent. If an endotracheal tube is *in situ*, oxygen may be given via a catheter passed into the lumen of the tube for a few inches. The oxygen flow in this latter case should not be above 3 litres per minute.

REFERENCES

SYKES, M. K. (1946) *British Medical Journal,* i, 561.

HAID, B. and HOSSLI, G. (1956) *Cardiac and Respiratory Arrest.* Roche Products Ltd.

JUDD, P. A., TOMLIN, P. J., WHITBY, J. L., INGLIS, T. C. M. & ROBINSON, J. S. (1968) *Lancet,* ii, 1019.

SELLICK, B. A. (1961) *Lancet,* ii, 494–406.

11
Glossary of Technical Terms and Words
Commonly Used in the Theatre

Some of the technical terms used in the theatre often appear very complicated, and may be rather difficult to understand at first. It is for this reason that the glossary has been placed before the chapters dealing with specific operations.

Definitions of some of the more common suffixes and roots may help the nurse to understand the descriptions of various operation instrument sets.

SUFFIXES

—desis: a fusion operation, e.g., arthrodesis or fusion of a joint.

—ectomy: describes the removal or excision of a structure, e.g., gastrectomy, or excision of the stomach.

—graphy: representing, recording or describing, e.g., ventriculography.

—otomy: refers to incising or dividing a structure, e.g., laparotomy, making an opening into the abdomen; or tenotomy, dividing a tendon.

—ostomy: making an artificial opening between one organ and another, or one organ and the surface of the body, e.g., gastroenterostomy, an opening between the stomach and small intestine; gastrostomy, an opening between the stomach and the surface of the abdomen, usually for the purpose of feeding.

—orrhaphy: a repair operation, e.g., herniorrhaphy, repair of a hernia; perineorrhaphy, repair of the perineum.

—oscopy: inspection of the interior of a duct, cavity or organ by means of an endoscopic instrument. These instruments usually incorporate their own illumination in the form of a minute electric lamp (or bundle of optic fibres which transmit light to the area being examined) and often having magnifying viewing attachments, e.g., the cystoscope, for examining the bladder; the sigmoidoscope, for examining the sigmoid flexure of the colon.

—pexy: suturing or fixing in place, e.g., nephropexy, suturing a 'wandering' kidney to the posterior abdominal wall.

—plasty: is used to describe a plastic operation for the repair of tissues or organs which have been damaged by injury or disease, e.g., rhinoplasty, the rotation of a skin flap from the forehead and scalp, to cover a defect of the nose; arthroplasty, an operation on a joint to increase mobility.

ROOTS

Adeno:	gland, e.g., Adenoma
Angio:	vessel, e.g., Angiography
Arthro:	joint, e.g., Arthroplasty
Broncho:	bronchus, e.g., Bronchoscopy

Cardio:	heart, e.g., Cardiotomy
Cholecyst:	gall bladder, e.g., Cholecystectomy
Col:	colon, e.g., Colectomy
Colpo:	vagina, e.g., Colporrhaphy
Cranio:	skull, e.g., Cranioplasty
Cysto:	sac containing fluid, e.g., Cystectomy
Gastro:	stomach, e.g., Gastrectomy
Herni:	abnormal aperture, e.g., Herniorrhaphy
Hyster:	uterus, e.g., Hysterectomy
Laryn:	larynx, e.g., Laryngoscopy
Mast:	breast, e.g., Mastectomy
Nephr:	kidney, e.g., Nephrectomy
Oöphor:	ovary, e.g., Oöphorectomy
Orchid:	testis, e.g., Orchidectomy
Osteo:	bone, e.g., Osteotomy
Pharyng:	throat, e.g., Pharyngotomy
Pneum:	lung, e.g., Pneumonectomy
Prostate:	prostate, e.g., Prostatectomy
Pyel:	kidney or pelvis, e.g., Pyelolithotomy
Rhino:	nose, e.g., Rhinoplasty
Thoraco:	chest, e.g., Thoracotomy
Ureter:	ureter, e.g., Ureterolithotomy
Vulv:	vulva, e.g., Vulvectomy

Adenoidectomy: Removal of adenoid tissue from the naso-pharynx.

Adrenalectomy: Excision of an adrenal gland for tumour, treatment of hypertension or relief of pain in malignant conditions e.g., carcinoma of breast.

Advancement: An operation to correct squint, also known as strabismus operation.

Albee's operation: *Hip* – arthrodesis effected by removing the upper surface of the femur and corresponding edge of acetabulum; *Spine* – arthodesis effected by splitting spinous processes and inserting a bone graft obtained from the tibia.

Anastomosis: The establishment of an intercommunication between two hollow organs, blood vessels or nerves.

Angiography: Serial X-ray examination of the cerebral vascular tree following injection of radio-opaque medium into a neck artery.

Antrostomy: Making an opening into the maxillary antrum to provide external drainage. The Caldwell Luc operation is an extensive form of antrostomy.

Appendicectomy: Removal of the appendix.

Arteriectomy: Excision of an artery or part of an artery.

Arteriorraphy: Suturing an artery.

Arteriotomy: Incision of an artery.

Arthrectomy: Excision of a joint.

Arthrodesis: An operation to permanently stiffen a joint and performed to prevent movement by obliterating the joint.

Arthrography: X-ray examination of a joint, often after the injection of a radio-opaque substance.

Arthroplasty: An operation to effect increased movement of a joint. The operation usually consists of replacing the joint surface or surfaces with a metallic or plastic prosthesis.

Arthroscopy: Examination of the interior of a joint by means of an arthroscope.

Arthrotomy: Incising a joint for the purpose of examination or subsequent drainage.

Bankhart's operation: For recurrent dislocation of the shoulder – repair of the glenoid rim defect supplemented by plication of the joint capsule and subscapularis muscle.

Bilroth's operation: A partial gastrectomy with either 1. anastomosis of the remaining section of the stomach to the duodenum or 2. closure of the lines of section followed by gastrojejunostomy.

Biopsy: Excision of small piece of tissue for examination.

Blalock's operation: Performed usually for Fallot's tetralogy – anastomosis of the pulmonary artery (distal to a pulmonary stenosis) to a branch of the aorta.

Bronchoscopy: Examination of the interior of the bronchial tree by means of a bronchoscope. Certain operative manipulations are possible through the instrument, including removal of a foreign body or section of a growth for pathological investigation.

Caesarean section: Removal of a foetus at or near term through an abdominal incision.

Capsulectomy: Excision of a capsule – generally a joint, lens or kidney.

Capsulotomy: Incision of a capsule e.g., that surrounding the lens of the eye.

Caudal block: see epidural.

Cervicectomy: Amputation of the uterine cervix.

Cholecystectomy: Excision of the gall-bladder.

Cholecytstenterostomy: Constructing an opening between the gall-bladder and the small intestine for the drainage of bile. This is performed when there is an obstruction of the common bile duct as may occur by pressure due to a growth. e.g., carcinoma of the head of pancreas.

Cholecystotomy: Making an opening into the gall-bladder, generally for the removal of gall-stones.

Choledochotomy: Making an opening into the common bile duct generally for the removal of stones.

Chordotomy: The division of nerve tracts within the spinal cord.

Circumcision: Excision of the prepuce or foreskin.

Coccygectomy: Excision of the coccyx.

Colpotomy: Incision of the vaginal wall, usually performed to drain an abscess in the pouch of Douglas through the vagina.

Colectomy: Excision of a portion of whole of the colon.

Colostomy and Caecostomy: These are terms used when making a fistula or an opening between the colon or caecum and the surface of the abdomen, to act as a temporary or permanent anus for the discharge of faeces. The most common sites for a colostomy are at the level of the transverse or pelvic colon.

Colporrhaphy: A repair operation of the vaginal wall in the treatment of pelvic prolapse. Prolapse of the uterus and stretching of the anterior vaginal wall may cause the bladder and urethra to bulge into the vaginal canal, creating the condition known as cystocele. Similarly, a posterior prolapse, with stretching of the posterior vaginal wall, allows prolapse of the rectum, forming a rectocele. A cystocele is treated by the operation of anterior colporrhaphy, and a rectocele by posterior colporrhaphy. Both these operations are often combined with perineorrhaphy.

Commissurotomy: Splitting a stenosed valve, e.g., mitral or aortic.

Corneoplasty: Excision of opaque corneal tissue and replacement with a healthy, transparent, human donor cornea (Keratoplasty).

Craniectomy denotes removal of bone from skull vault, e.g., osteoplastic flap.

Cranioplasty: A plastic operation on the skull.

Craniotomy: This is a term used when opening the cavity of the skull, e.g., in the treatment of cranial injuries such as depressed fractures; for the removal of an intracranial tumour; for the drainage of an abscess.

Cryosurgery: Using the effect of freezing on tissue in surgery.

Culdoscopy: Examining the uterus by passing a culdoscope through the posterior vaginal fornix behind the uterus to enter the peritoneal cavity.

Curettage: The removal of tissue by means of a curette, or spoon, using a scraping action. The most frequent curettage is that of the interior of the uterus and the removal of overgrown lymphatic tissue in the nasopharynx (adenoids).

Cyclotomy: An incision through the ciliary body as a drainage operation for the relief of glaucoma.

Cystectomy: Excision of the urinary bladder, most commonly for a malignant tumour.

Cystodiathermy: The application of a diathermy current to the walls of the urinary bladder via a cystoscope or by open operation.

Cystoscopy: Inspection of the interior of the bladder by means of an examining cystoscope. An operating cystoscope may be used for catheterising the ureters, cauterising papillomata, and obtaining a biopsy of bladder or tumour tissue. A resectoscope is used for resecting part of the prostate via the urethra.

Cystostomy: Temporary or permanent suprapubic drainage of the bladder.

Dacryocystectomy: Excision of part or all of the lacrymal sac.

Dacryocystorhinostomy: Performed for obstruction of the naso-lacrymal duct to establish drainage from the lacrymal sac to the nose.

Debridement: Thorough cleansing of a wound, removal of foreign matter, and damaged or infected tissue.

Decortication: Excision of the cortex or outer layer of an organ e.g., visceral pleura of the lung.

Diathermy: A high-frequency electric current in the form of electromagnetic waves. These waves are concentrated at the point of the surgeon's electrode, producing great heat which is utilised to coagulate the tissues (e.g., sealing blood-vessels). When the frequency of the current is increased, the diathermy electrode may be used like a knife to divide the tissues, giving minimal coagulation.

Disobliteration: Endarterectomy – removal of intimal plaques which are blocking an artery – rebore.

Dissect: To cut or separate tissues.

Ectopic Gestation: The implantation and development of a fertilised ovum outside the uterus, most frequently in a Fallopian tube. Rupture of the ectopic gestation causes severe bleeding and shock, requiring urgent surgical intervention.

Embolectomy: An operation for the removal of an embolus, usually a blood-clot, from an artery.

Encephalography: X-ray examination of the ventricular system and subarachnoid spaces surrounding the brain by fractional replacement of cerebrospinal fluid with filtered air. (See also ventriculography.)

Endarterterectomy: See disobliteration.

Endoscopy: Inspection of any body cavity by means of a scope.

Enterostomy: The establishment of an intestinal fistula.

Enucleation: Removal of the eye is described under this heading. The term means also the removal of a tumour as a whole, compared to its removal in sections (eviscerate or gut).

Epididymectomy: Excision of the epididymis, which is a series of tubules lying behind the testis, and continuous with the vas deferens.

Epidural block: Injection of local anaesthetic, usually into the lumbar or caudal region before surgery or for prolonged analgesia.

Episiotomy: Involves the incision of the perineum during labour, to prevent excessive laceration.

Excision: Cutting away or taking out.

Fasciotomy: Incision of fascia.

Fenestration: Establishment of a fenestra or window in the horizontal semicircular canal to re-establish sound conduction to the inner ear of a suitable patient suffering from otosclerosis.

Fothergills operation: Colpoperinorrhaphy including amputation of the cervix – i.e. repair of a cystocele and rectocele – see also Manchester repair.

Fulguration: Destruction of tissue by diathermy.

Gallie's operation: Radical repair of a hernia using fascia lata strips taken from the lateral aspect of the thigh.

Ganglionectomy: Excision of a ganglion.

Gastrectomy: Excision of the stomach. The most usual operation is partial gastrectomy in the surgical treatment of gastric or duodenal ulcers. Total gastrectomy although nowadays a relatively rare operation is generally reserved for malignant conditions.

Gastroenterostomy: Making an opening between the stomach and small intestine, usually the jejunum, for the purpose of short circuiting the stomach contents, which normally pass through the pylorus into the duodenum.

Gastroscopy: Inspection of the stomach cavity via the oesophagus, or via a gastrostomy, using a gastroscope.

Gastrostomy: Making an artificial opening between the stomach and the abdominal surface for the purpose of feeding. This is generally done for the patient having an oesophageal stricture which cannot be relieved by dilation with bougies.

Gastrotomy: Opening the stomach for the purpose of exploration, or the removal of a foreign body.

Gilliam's operation: Shortening of the round ligament to correct retroversion of the uterus. See also hysteropexy, ventrosuspension.

Girdlestones operation: The original procedure is described as removal of part of the acetabulum and the femoral head and neck with a muscle mass stitched between the bone ends. Nowadays removal of part of the femoral head and neck only is often called Girdlestones.

Glossectomy: Excision of the tongue.

Haemorrhoidectomy: The ligation and excision of internal piles.

Harris' operation: A transvesical, suprapubic prostatectomy.

Hemicolectomy: Excision of approximately half of the colon.

Hepatectomy: Excision of part of the liver.

Herniorrhaphy: The repair of an abnormal aperture in the walls of a cavity which has allowed the protrusion of a viscus. An example of this is the direct inguinal herniorrhaphy in which a sac containing viscera protruding from the abdomen through Hesselbach's triangle is obliterated.

Herniotomy: A simple operation for hernia, with return of hernia contents to their normal position and ligation of the sac.

Hymenectomy: Excision or trimming of an imperforate or rigid hymen.

Hypophysectomy: Excision of the pituitary gland.

Hysterectomy: Removal of the uterus via the abdomen or vagina. A subtotal hysterectomy means the removal of the body of the uterus, but leaving the cervix: total hysterectomy implies excision of the entire uterus: pan-hysterectomy generally means the excision of the uterus, Fallopian tubes and ovaries also: radical hysterectomy describes removal of the uterus, appendages, upper part of the vagina and adjacent connective tissue. This latter operation is known also as Wertheim's operation.

Hysteropexy: A plastic operation on the uterus performed in the treatment of a retroverted uterus. See also ventrosuspension.

Hysterotomy: Opening into the uterus usually for the removal of a foetus a good period before term.

Iridectomy: Removal of a section of the iris of the eye, thus forming an artificial pupil. This is performed as a preliminary to cataract extraction and in the relief of tension in glaucoma.

Ileocolostomy: A fistula or opening made between the ileum and colon to by-pass an obstruction or inflammation.

Ileocystoplasty: A plastic operation, utilising a section of isolated ileum to increase the urinary bladder.

Ileostomy: A fistula or opening made between the ileum and the surface of the abdomen.

Ileoureterostomy: Transplantation of the lower ends of the ureters into an artificial bladder formed from an isolated loop of ileum which is made to open on to the surface of the abdomen.

Jejunostomy: Making an opening into the jejunum.

Keller's operation: For hallux valgus or rigidus – excision of the proximal half of the proximal phalanx, also exostosis of the metatarsal head.

Keratectomy: Excision of a portion of the cornea.

Keratoplasty: see corneoplasty.

Laminectomy: Cutting through and removal of the spinal laminae as a preliminary of approach to the spinal cord or intervertebral discs.

Laparotomy: Opening the abdominal cavity for the purpose of inspection of or operation upon the organs within. An emergency laparotomy is performed for many conditions which come under the heading 'acute abdomen'. When an accurate diagnosis is uncertain this may reveal acute appendicitis, perforated ulcers of the stomach or bowel, intestinal obstruction, e.g., malignant growth, strangulated hernia, etc.

Laryngectomy: Excision of the larynx.

Laryngofissure: Splitting the thyroid cartilage of the larynx to expose the vocal cords.

Laryngoscopy: Inspection of the interior of the larynx, either by means of an illuminated laryngoscope (direct laryngoscopy) or by a mirror and reflected light (indirect laryngoscopy). The anaesthetist uses a laryngoscope to inspect the entrance to the larynx and to assist in the insertion of an endotracheal tube into the trachea by direct vision.

Laryngotomy: Opening the larynx to introduce a tube for the purpose of aiding respiration. This operation should more correctly be termed laryngostomy, meaning a temporary or permanent opening into the larynx. Like tracheostomy, this operation is often performed in cases of extreme urgency when the glottis is blocked.

Leucotomy: An operation in the frontal area of the brain for division of some white nerve fibres. Performed for relief of certain mental conditions associated with extreme anxiety or emotional stress.

Lithotomy: Incision for removal of a stone or calculus.

Lithotrity or **Litholapaxy:** The crushing and removal of a calculus or stone lying in the bladder by using a lithotrite passed per urethra.

Lobectomy: Excision of one lobe of the lung.

Lymphadenectomy: Excision of a lymph node or nodes.

Manchester repair: Colpoperinorrhapy including amputation and reconstruction of the cervix. See also Fothergill's operation.

Mastectomy: Removal of the breast. This operation is performed for carcinoma of the breast and is generally combined with some form of radiotherapy. A more extensive operation called radical mastectomy involves excision of the breast together with the underlying pectoral muscles and adjacent lymph glands.

Mastoidectomy: The removal of diseased mastoid air cells as a result of mastoiditis.

Meniscectomy: Removal of a torn semilunar cartilage usually from the knee joint.

Myomectomy: Removal of a fibroid from the uterus.

Myringotomy: Incision of the tympanic membrane of the ear to allow drainage of the middle ear.

Nephrectomy: Removal of a kidney.

Nephropexy: A plastic operation to secure a 'wandering kidney' to the posterior abdominal wall.

Nephrostomy: Making an opening between the pelvis of the kidney and the abdominal surface for the purpose of drainage. It is usual to employ a self-retaining catheter, such as the De Pezzer type, which may be connected to a suitable receptacle.

Nephrotomy: Incising the kidney, usually for the removal of a renal calculus. The operation is then called nephrolithotomy.

Neurectomy: Excision of a part of a nerve.

Neuroplasty: Surgical repair of nerves.

Neurorrhaphy: Anastomosis of the two ends of a divided nerve.

Neurotomy: Incision into a nerve.

Oesophagectomy: Excision of the oesophagus, generally for a malignant condition.

Oesophagoscopy: Inspection of the interior of the oesophagus by means of an illuminated oesophagoscope. Biopsy of a tumour or the removal of an impacted foreign body may also be carried out.

Oöphorectomy: Excision of one or both ovaries.

Oöphorosalpingectomy: Excision of an ovary and its associated Fallopian tube.

Orchidectomy: Removal of the testis.

Osteoplasty: Any plastic operation on a bone.

Osteotomy: Division of a bone. Normally an osteotome is used for this purpose and the instrument has two bevelled edges as opposed to a chisel which has only one bevelled edge, the other being straight. The operation is generally performed to correct bone deformity, or as a part of an arthroplastic procedure.

Pallidotomy: Division of nerve fibres from the cerebral cortex to the corpus striatum to relieve Parkinson tremor.

Pancreatectomy: or radical excision of the pancreatic head: Excision of the head of pancreas, duodenum, part of the jejunum, stomach, lower half of the common bile duct and part of the pancreatic duct.

Paul-Mikulicz operation: After excising a section of the colon, the two cut ends of the bowel are kept exposed outside the peritoneal cavity on the abdomenal surface. After a period these cut ends are anastomosed without the peritoneal cavity being opened.

Pericardectomy: Excision of a thickened pericardium of the heart.

Parathyroidectomy: Excision of one or more parathyroid glands.

Parotidectomy: Excision of the parotid salivary gland.

Patellectomy: Excision of the patella.

Perineorrhaphy: This is the repair carried out when the pelvic floor has become weakened, allowing the uterus to prolapse.

Pharyngolaryngectomy: Excision of the pharynx and larynx.

Pharyngotomy: Opening the pharynx as a preliminary to removing a malignant growth of the upper part of the oesophagus.

Phlebectomy: Excision of a vein or part of.

Phlebotomy: Incision into a vein.

Phrenic Avulsion: In order to produce paralysis of one dome of the diaphragm and collapse of the lower part of the lung on that side, the fibres of the phrenic nerve are torn from their attachment. Another operation is crushing of the phrenic nerve to produce a temporary effect.

Pneumonectomy: Excision of one lung in the treatment of malignant conditions and tuberculosis, etc.

Pneumothorax (Artificial): Air in the pleural space. The air is introduced into the pleura via a hollow needle and using the pneumothorax apparatus.

Proctoscopy: Examination of the rectum and anal canal, using a proctoscope.

Prostatectomy: Removal of the prostate gland either suprapubically, retropubically, transurethrally or by the perineal route.

Pyelography (Retrograde): The injection of a radio-opaque substance into the pelvis of the kidney via the ureteric catheter. Subsequent radiological examination reveals the outline of the renal pelvis on the X-ray plate.

Pyelolithotomy: Removal of a stone from the kidney pelvis.

Pyloro-myotomy: In the treatment of congenital pyloric stenosis in infants, the muscular coat of the pyloric section of the stomach is incised down to the level of the mucosa to provide relief. This is known as Ramstedt's operation.

Pyloroplasty: A plastic operation on the pylorus to widen the orifice.

Radium or Radiotherapy:

Atomic or Nuclear Reactor: A machine for producing radioactive isotopes, such as radioactive iodine and cobalt.

Cobalt: A radioactive isotope, which has a half-life of 5·3 years and decays eventually into nickel.

Disintegration or Decay: This is a spontaneous process in which the radioactive material emits an alpha, beta or gamma ray.

Half-Life: Radioactive material is made up of a large number of radioactive nuclei. As these disintegrate during the decay of the material and give off alpha, beta or gamma rays, the total number of nuclei in the material diminishes, and consequently the activity of the isotope gradually becomes weaker. The half-life is defined as 'the amount of time which is required for one half of a large number of identical nuclei (making up the isotope) to disintegrate'. For example, in the case of radium which has a half-life of roughly 1700 years; in 1700 years the radium contains half as many radioactive nuclei than when it was formed, and in 3400 years this figure will be approximately one quarter of the original number of nuclei.

Radiation: The diffusion of rays from a point (in this case gamma rays which cause biological damage to the tissues). Malignant tumours are often more susceptible to radiation than normal tissue but over-exposure to these rays may cause normal tissue to become damaged and produce diseases such as leukaemia (where the white cells of the body are over-produced).

Radium: A radioactive isotope, with a half-life of about 1700 years.

X-ray: A penetrating electromagnetic radiation which is generated by bombarding a metal target (in the X-ray tube) with energetic electrons. X-rays and gamma rays for practical purposes may really be regarded as the same thing.

Ramstedt's Operation: See pyloro-myotomy.

Rectosigmoidectomy: Excision of the rectum and sigmoid colon.

Rhinoplasty: A plastic operation on the nose for reformation due to injury or cosmetic reasons.

Salpingectomy: Excision of a Fallopian tube.

Salpingo – oöphorectomy: Excision of a Fallopian tube and ovary.

Shelf operation: Open reduction of congenital dislocation of hip.

Sigmoidoscopy: Inspection of the rectum or sigmoid flexure of the colon, using an illuminated endoscope passed per anum.

Skeletal Traction: The insertion of a pin or wire through a bone for the purpose of traction. A Steinmann pin and Kirschner wire are the two most commonly used, and these may be inserted into the fractured bone itself, or a bone below the fracture forming part of an appendage to it. The most usual sites are the tibial tubercle for fractures of the femoral shaft and the lower tibia for fractures of the tibial shaft.

Splenectomy: Removal of the spleen. The most common condition requiring its removal is traumatic rupture, although certain diseases involving enlargement of the organ may require surgery also.

Stapedectomy: Excision of stapes for otosclerosis and insertion of Teflon piston, vein graft or plug of fat.

Stereotactic Surgery: Deep ablative surgery of the white matter, basal ganglia or brain stem projection fibres by electro-coagulation or cryo-probe.

Sympathectomy: Partial excision of sympathetic nerve.

Synovectomy: Excision of a joint synovial membrane often in rheumatoid conditions.

Tarsorraphy: Suturing the eyelids together as a temporary measure in certain conditions, e.g., fifth cranial nerve damage.

Tenoplasty: A plastic operation on a tendon.

Tenorrhaphy: Anastomosis of the two ends of a cut tendon.

Tenotomy: Division of a tendon.

Thoracoplasty: Removal of several ribs on one side to produce collapse of the underlying lung.

Thoracotomy: Opening the chest cavity, e.g., as a preliminary to heart surgery.

Thoracoscopy: Inspection of the pleural space, using a thoracoscope passed through a small incision in the chest wall.

Thromboendarterectomy: Removal of a thrombus from an artery followed by reboring.

Thymectomy: Excision of the thymus.

Thyroidectomy: Removal of approximately seven-eights of each lobe of the thyroid gland leaving the parathyroid glands intact.

Tonsillectomy: Excision of the tonsils.

Trachelorrhaphy: Repair of a lacerated uterine cervix.

Tracheostomy: Often incorrectly termed tracheotomy, is an operation for the insertion of a tube into the trachea as an aid to respiration. Generally, the trachea is opened at the level of the thyroid isthmus, but in emergency the opening may be made through the upper rings of the trachea. This latter operation is called a 'high tracheostomy', and may be performed rapidly, as the tracheal rings are close to the skin.

Trendelenburg's Operation: Usually refers to ligation of internal saphenous vein in varicosed leg veins, also an operation describing pulmonary embolectomy.

Trephine Operation: This term is applied to the removal of a disc of tissue. Trephining of the skull, in the true sense of the word, involves the removal of a disc of bone, although today craniotomies are usually performed by drilling a hole with suitable perforators and burrs. The resultant pulverised bone may be returned to the hole after operation but this is not always considered necessary.

Removal of a small disc of the sclerotic coat of the eye in the treatment of chronic glaucoma is also called trephining.

Turbinectomy: Removal of the turbinate bones.

Ureterectomy: Excision of a ureter.

Ureterocolostomy: Transplantation of the ureters into the colon.

Ureteroileostomy: See ileoureterostomy.

Ureterolithotomy: This describes the operation for opening the ureter to remove a calculus.

Urethrotomy: A rather uncommon operation now for incising the urethra in the treatment of strictures. Internal urethrotomy is performed with a guarded knife passed into the urethra. External urethrotomy involves opening the urethra through an incision made in the perineum.

Vagotomy: Division of the vagus nerves often in conjunction with gastro-enterostomy in the treatment of peptic ulcer or pyloroplasty.

Valvotomy: Incision of a valve generally in the heart or major blood vessels.

Vasectomy: Excision of a section of the vas deferens.

Ventriculo-atrial or **ventriculo-peritoneal shunt**: The establishment of artificial CSF drainage to heart or peritoneal cavity in cases of primary or secondary hydrocephalus (Pudenz or Spitzholter valve).

Ventriculo-cysternostomy: The establishment of artificial drainage between the ventricles and cysterna magna. (Torkildsen operation.)

Ventriculography: This is radiography of the cerebral ventricles accomplished by removing cerebrospinal fluid and replacing it with a small quantity of air, using hollow ventricular needles. Trephine holes are made in the skull and the ventricular needles passed into the ventricles (see also encephalography).

Ventro-suspension: A plastic operation on the uterus for shortening the round ligaments which run forward to the inguinal canal, thereby suspending the uterus in the anteverted position. This operation is known also as hysteropexy.

Vulvectomy: Excision of the vulva.

Wertheim's hysterectomy: For carcinoma of the cervix – extensive excision involving the uterus, upper vagina, Fallopian tubes, ovaries and regional lymph glands.

Instruments for Particular Operations

There are two methods of instrument selection: (*a*) enough instruments are prepared for a particular operation; (*b*) basic instrument sets are used and specialised instruments are added to these as required.

In this book method (*a*) is used only for highly specialised or very minor procedures. Method (*b*) is used extensively, for it ensures that the instruments to which the surgeon is accustomed are always at hand and is a method which is suited to the pre-set tray system of sterilisation. Also, by arranging the instruments in groups, the teaching of nurses and technicians is simplified.

Except in minor procedures, the general set, or when only a few instruments are needed, the more common instruments are not illustrated. This is to allow greater prominence to the special instruments described.

12

General Instruments

The general set. Figure 281

The general set of instruments is arranged according to the kind of operation, and preference of the surgeon; but this set must include sufficient basic instruments for any of the operations performed in that particular theatre. However, the instruments listed, indeed any of the operation sets described in the following chapters, are intended to act only as a guide and must, of course, be adjusted to suit a surgeon's individual requirements.

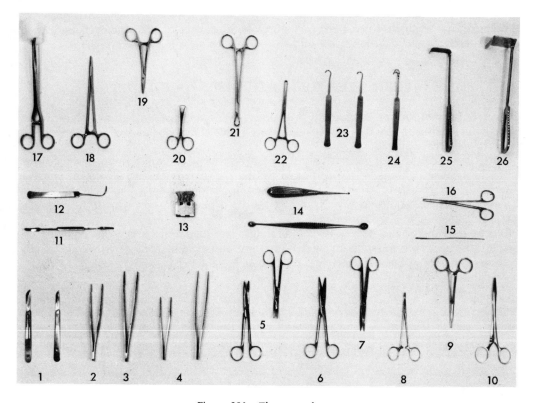

Figure 281   The general set.

1. Scalpel handles Nos. 3 and 4, with Nos. 10 and 20 blades (Bard Parker), 2.
2. Dissecting forceps, toothed, small (Lane), 2.
3. Dissecting forceps, toothed, large (Bonney), 2.
4. Dissecting forceps, non-toothed, small and large, 2.

5. Scissors, curved on flat, small and large (Mayo), 2.
6. Scissors, straight (Mayo).
7. Scissors, straight, stitch.
8. Artery forceps, curved on flat (Kelly Fraser), 10.
9. Artery forceps, straight (Moynihan), 10.
10. Artery forceps, straight 20 cm (8 in) (Spencer Wells), 5.
11. Dissector (MacDonald).
12. Aneurysm needle.
13. Photoclips for anchoring soiled dressing bag, diathermy leads or suction tubing etc., 3.
14. Curetting spoons, medium and large (Volkmann and Boyd Davies), 2.
15. Probe, malleable silver.
16. Sinus forceps.
17. Sponge-holding forceps (Rampley), 5.
18. Needle holder, large (Mayo), 2.
19. Needle holder, small (Kilner), 2.
20. Towel clips (Backaus), 5.
21. Tissue forceps (Lane), 5.
22. Tissue forceps (Allis), 5.
23. Retractors, single hook, sharp and blunt, 2.
24. Retractors, double hook, blunt, 2.
25. Retractors, medium (Langenbeck), 2.
26. Retractors, large (Morris), 2.

13
General Operations on the Abdomen

The laparotomy set. Figure 282

Combined with the general set, this is the basis for all major operations on the abdomen and is suitable for a midline, paramedian, transverse or elliptical incision. Bowel clamps and special instruments are added as required.

Types of central abdominal incisions

HIGH MIDLINE INCISIONS

These are used for operations on the stomach, liver, gall-bladder, spleen, etc. A vertical midline incision is made through the skin, extending from just below the xyphisternum to the umbilicus where it curves outwards to avoid this landmark. The incision is continued through the linea alba to expose the peritoneum, which is picked up with forceps and incised.

LOW MIDLINE INCISIONS

These are used for operations on the lower bowel, bladder, uterus and rectum, etc. A vertical midline incision is made through the skin, extending from the pubis to the umbilicus where it curves outwards. The anterior rectus sheath is split following the line of the linea alba, and the peritoneum is picked up with forceps and incised.

PARAMEDIAN INCISIONS

These are used primarily to gain access to one side of the abdomen and are placed accordingly. A vertical skin incision is made 2 cm from the midline. The extent of the incision depends upon the operative procedure; e.g., for caecal or lower colon operations the incision would extend from just above the level of the umbilicus to the pubis, for gastric or gall-bladder operations the incision would extend from just below the costal margin to the umbilicus. For extensive procedures the incision would be a combination of both types just given.

The anterior rectus sheath is incised 2 cm from the midline and the rectus muscle retracted laterally or split between its fibres. The posterior rectus sheath and peritoneum together are picked up with forceps and incised.

Transverse (Kocher's type) incisions are not often used as there is danger of damage to the nerves supplying the rectus muscle. An oblique skin incision is made below the costal margin. The rectus muscle, external oblique and underlying internal oblique and transversus muscles are divided across in line with the skin incision, and the peritoneum is opened in the usual manner.

PFANNENSTIEL TRANSVERSE ELLIPTICAL INCISION

This is favoured by the gynaecologists. The skin is incised elliptically just above the pubis. The anterior rectus sheath is incised transversely in line with the skin incision, and is retracted to expose the rectus muscles which are freed from the sheath. The rectus muscles are separated from the midline and the peritoneum is picked up with forceps and incised vertically.

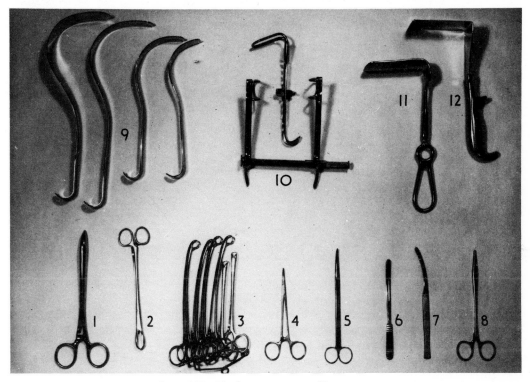

Figure 282   The laparotomy set of instruments

1. Gall-bladder forceps, curved on flat (Moynihan), 6.
2. Long tissue forceps (Lane), 6.
3. Tetra or skin forceps (Moynihan), 4 for sides of wound and 2 for ends of wound.
4. Artery forceps, curved on flat (Kelly Fraser), 25.
5. Long scissors, curved on flat (McIndoe).
6. Hernia director (Key).
7. Hernia bistoury, curved.
8. Artery forceps, straight 20 cm (8 in) (Spencer Wells), 25.
9. Deep retractors, curved narrow blade (Deaver), set of 4.
10. Retractor, self-retaining abdominal (Panting).
11. Deep retractor, right-angled narrow blade (Worrall).
12. Deep retractor, right-angled broad blade (Winsbury-White).

Not illustrated:

2·5 and 3 (2/0 and 0) Chromic catgut or Dexon for ligatures.*
2·5, 3, 4, and 5 (2/0, 0, 1 and 2) Silk or thread for ligatures.
4 or 5 (1 or 2) Chromic catgut, Dexon or silk on large half-circle, round-bodied needles for peritoneum, and large half-circle cutting needles for rectus or linea alba. (Proportionally smaller for children.)
5 (2) Nylon (strong) on curved cutting needles for tension sutures (optional).
2·5 (2/0) Nylon or silk on curved or straight cutting needles for skin.
Fine rubber tubing or buttons for tension sutures.
Michel or Kifa skin clips (optional).

Closure of central abdominal incisions

The peritoneum and posterior rectus sheath are sutured with a continuous chromic catgut or Dexon on a round-bodied needle. Non-absorbable tension sutures on curved cutting needles may be inserted in midline and paramedian incisions. These tension sutures pass from one side of the incision through the skin, figure-of-eight manner through the muscle, and out through the skin again on the opposite side of the incision. The sutures are tied over a button or thin rubber tubing after the muscles have been approximated. Alternatively, several interrupted sutures of silk, nylon or polyester material may be inserted to approximate the muscles before using chromic catgut.

For midline and paramedian incisions, the anterior rectus sheath or linea alba is sutured with interrupted or continuous chromic catgut, Dexon or monofilament nylon on a cutting or lance point needle.

Kocher's incision is closed by approximating the muscles with interrupted mattress sutures of chromic catgut or Dexon, which are left long and tied when all have been placed.

The skin is closed with interrupted or continuous silk or nylon on a curved or straight cutting needle, sometimes used in conjunction with Michel or Kifa skin clips (lower midline incisions especially).

Note: In all the following chapters, suture sizes are described as metric followed in parentheses by the original BPC sizing.

Appendicectomy

DEFINITION
    Removal of the appendix.
POSITION. Supine.

INSTRUMENTS
    General set (Fig. 281)
    Bowel-holding forceps (Hamilton Bailey)
    Long artery forceps, curved on flat (Moynihan gall-bladder or Gordon Craig artery
        forceps), 5
    Suction tubing, nozzles and tube anchoring forceps
    2·5 and 3 (2/0 and 0) Chromic catgut, Dexon or silk for ligatures
    2·5 (2/0) Chromic catgut or Dexon on a non-traumatic curved or straight intestinal
        needle for purse-string suture
    3 or 4 (0 or 1) Chromic catgut or Dexon on a small half-circle round-bodied needle for
        peritoneum and first muscle layer
    3 or 4 (0 or 1) Chromic catgut or Dexon on a small half-circle cutting needle for muscle
        aponeurosis
    2·5 (2/0) Silk or nylon on a medium-curved or straight-cutting needle for skin sutures
    (Michel or Kifa skin clips may be required)
    (Medium-sized tube drain or corrugated drain may be required).

OUTLINE OF PROCEDURE
    Incisions used for this operation include the McBurney 'grid iron', the Battle type and the right lower paramedian. (If a paramedian approach is used, the instruments for laparotomy are selected.)

The centre of a McBurney incision lies in the right iliac region, situated over a point which is at the junction of the outer with the inner two-thirds of an imaginary line joining the umbilicus with the anterior superior iliac spine. It is about five or seven cm in length, and is approximately parallel with the inguinal ligament. The aponeurosis of the external oblique is incised in line with the skin incision. The underlying fibres of the internal oblique and transversus muscles are separated at right angles to the external oblique to expose the peritoneum. The peritoneum is picked up with forceps and incised.

A Battle incision is made more towards the midline, and the rectus muscle is retracted medially to expose the peritoneum which is picked up with forceps and incised.

The caecum is identified and the appendix grasped with a pair of tissue forceps. The meso-appendix is ligated with chromic catgut, Dexon or silk, and the base of the appendix is crushed and ligated with chromic catgut or Dexon. A purse-string suture is placed around the appendix base, the appendix is removed and the stump invaginated before tying the purse-string suture. All instruments which have come in contact with the transected stump are discarded before the operation proceeds.

When the appendix is adherent in a retrocaecal position, the surgeon may divide it and invaginate the stump before ligating the meso-appendix.

The wound is closed by suturing the peritoneum with continuous chromic catgut or Dexon on a round-bodied needle, the internal oblique and transversus muscles with similar (but interrupted) sutures and the external oblique with a continuous chromic catgut or Dexon suture on a cutting needle. Finally the skin is closed with interrupted silk or nylon sutures on a cutting needle or by inserting skin clips.

If the appendix has perforated, the surgeon may insert a drainage tube through a separate stab incision before closing the wound.

Drainage of an intrapelvic abscess (1)

DEFINITION
The establishment of a temporary drainage tract for an intraperitoneal pelvic abscess.
POSITION. Supine.

INSTRUMENTS
General set (Fig. 281)
Artery forceps, straight, 20 cm (8 in) (Spencer Wells), 5
Deep retractors, narrow blade (Deaver), 2
Suction tubing, nozzles and tube anchoring forceps
Selection of drainage tubes
Ligatures and sutures as for appendicectomy (or laparotomy),

OUTLINE OF PROCEDURE
A rubber or plastic drainage tube is inserted into the pelvis through a McBurney or lower paramedian incision. A solution containing antibiotics may be instilled through the tube, which is sutured to the skin during wound closure, and transfixed with a safety-pin above the skin surface to prevent it being pushed farther into the wound. The wound is closed in the usual manner for that particular incision.

Drainage of an intrapelvic abscess (2)

DEFINITION. As above.

POSITION. Lithotomy.

INSTRUMENTS. As above, plus proctoscopes.

OUTLINE OF PROCEDURE

The proctoscope is inserted and the abscess drained through a small incision in the upper rectal wall when the abscess is pointing there. This operation is not generally performed to-day but may be of very great use if the patient's condition is too poor for an abdominal operation.

Drainage of subphrenic abscess

DEFINITION

The establishment of a temporary drainage tract for an abscess under the diaphragm.

POSITION

Lateral kidney, with bridge elevated.

INSTRUMENTS

As for kidney operations (Chapter 18, Fig. 317), plus drainage tubes.

OUTLINE OF PROCEDURE

An oblique incision is made, extending from the midpoint of the last rib towards the anterior superior iliac spine. The external oblique, internal oblique and transversus muscles are cut across to expose the peritoneum. It may be necessary to excise a rib in order to do this. A finger is inserted under the diaphragm to break through the inflamed peritoneum into the abscess. The peritoneum is picked up with forceps, opened, and the pus aspirated with a suction tube. A wide-bore drainage tube is inserted and the wound closed in layers. A firm gauze and wool dressing is then applied and secured with a many-tailed bandage. Sometimes the surgeon will insert a long drainage tube which is connected to a low vacuum suction apparatus. This reduced the amount of dressing required and keeps the cavity empty of fluid and pus.

OPERATIONS ON THE GALL-BLADDER AND COMMON BILE DUCT

Cholecystostomy

DEFINITION

An opening made into the gall bladder to establish drainage of bile.

POSITION

Supine, with liver bridge elevated (optional)

INSTRUMENTS

General set (Fig. 281)
Laparotomy set (Fig. 282)
Gall bladder set (Fig. 283)
10 ml syringe and exploration needle
Suction tubing, nozzles and tube anchoring forceps
Laparotomy ligatures and sutures
2·5 (2/0) Chromic catgut or Dexon on a small curved non-traumatic intestinal needle for purse-string suture.

OUTLINE OF PROCEDURE

Through a right paramedian or transverse incision, a purse-string suture is placed in the tip of the gall-bladder. A trocar and cannula is inserted at a point in the centre of this purse-string suture and the bile evacuated. Desjardin's forceps may be used through the stab opening to extract any gall-stones. A long drainage tube is inserted and secured by tying the purse-string suture.

The wound is closed in the usual manner and the drainage tube connected to a sealed bottle or disposable plastic bag.

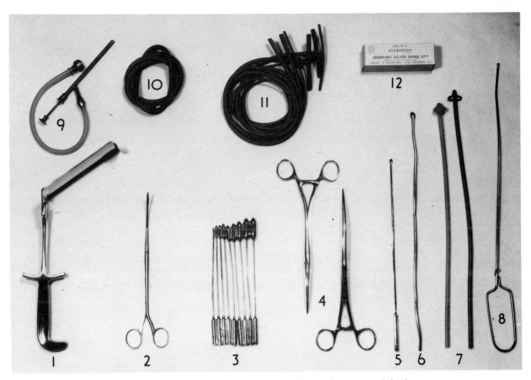

Figure 283   Operations on the gall-bladder and common bile duct.

1. Liver retractor (Nuttall).
2. Gall-stone forceps (Desjardin).
3. Common bile duct probes (Bake).
4. Intestinal occlusion clamp, curved (Doyen).
5. Gall-stone probe (Desjardin), 3 sizes.
6. Malleable scoop and probe (Moynihan).
7. Catheters, self-retaining (De Pezzer and Malecot, sizes 16 and 18 Charrière gauge).
8. Catheter introducer.
9. Gall-bladder trocar and cannula.
10. Long rubber drainage tube (alternatively plastic may be used).
11. 'T' drainage tubes (Kehr), assorted sizes.
12. Haemostatic agent (gelatine sponge).

Cholecystectomy

DEFINITION

Removal of the gall-bladder.

POSITION

Supine, with the liver bridge elevated (optional)

INSTRUMENTS. As above.

OUTLINE OF PROCEDURE

The incision is as above; the cystic duct and artery are identified, clamped, ligated with chromic catgut, Dexon or silk, clamped distally, and divided. The gall-bladder is freed from the liver and removed. The raw surface of the liver may either be sutured over with 2·5 (2/0) chromic catgut or Dexon on a small curved non-traumatic intestinal needle, or a haemostatic agent (e.g., gelatine sponge or Surgicel) applied.

A long drainage tube is inserted and the wound closed in the usual manner.

Choledochotomy

DEFINITION

An incision into the common bile duct, usually for the extraction of gall-stones.

POSITION

Supine, with the kidney bridge elevated (optional).

INSTRUMENTS

As above, plus malleable probes, bougies, irrigation syringe, catheter and warm saline.

OUTLINE OF PROCEDURE

The incision is as above; the common bile duct is identified and two long 'stay' sutures of 2·5 (2/0) chromic catgut or Dexon on a small (20 mm) non-traumatic intestinal needle are inserted. The duct is opened between these sutures, suctioned and explored with probes and Desjardin's forceps. The duct may be irrigated with saline before inserting a Kehr's T-tube which is secured by the two 'stay' sutures; and the incision in the duct is closed with further 2·5 (2/0) chromic catgut or Dexon sutures.

An additional long drainage tube is placed in the vicinity of the duct and the wound is closed in the usual manner.

Cholecystogastrostomy

DEFINITION

Anastomosis between the gall-bladder and the stomach.

POSITION. Supine.

INSTRUMENTS. As above.

OUTLINE OF PROCEDURE

The incision is as above; the gall-bladder is drained with a trocar and cannula and then approximated to the stomach. Curved occlusion clamps are applied and an anastomosis made with two layers of 2·5 (2/0) chromic catgut or Dexon sutures on a small or medium curved non-traumatic intestinal needle. A long drainage tube is inserted in the vicinity of the anastomosis and the wound closed in the usual manner.

Cholecystoenterostomy

DEFINITION

The procedure is as above but the anastomosis is made between the gall-bladder and the jejunum, often with jejuno-jejunostomy.

Choledochoduodenostomy

DEFINITION

Anastomosis between the common bile duct and the duodenum.

POSITION. Supine.

INSTRUMENTS

As above, plus 2 (3/0) chromic catgut or Dexon on a small curved non-traumatic intestinal needle.

OUTLINE OF PROCEDURE

The incision is as above; the common bile duct is mobilised and anastomosed to the duodenum with two layers of 2 (3/0) chromic catgut or Dexon. A long drainage tube is inserted in the vicinity of the anastomosis and the wound is closed in the usual manner.

Radical resection of the head of the pancreas

DEFINITION

The head of pancreas, duodenum, part of the jejunum and stomach are resected, together with the lower half of the common bile duct and part of the pancreatic duct.

POSITION. Supine.

INSTRUMENTS

General set (Fig. 281)
Laparotomy set (Fig. 282)
Gall-bladder set (Fig. 283)
Gastrectomy set (Fig. 286)
Suction tubing, nozzles and tube anchoring forceps
Diathermy leads, electrodes and lead anchoring forceps
Laparotomy ligatures and sutures
2, 2·5 and 3 (3/0, 2/0 and 0) Chromic catgut or Dexon on small and medium half-circle and curved non-traumatic intestinal needles for anastomoses
2·5 (2/0) Silk on small curved non-traumatic intestinal needles.

OUTLINE OF PROCEDURE

Through a midline incision a partial gastrectomy, duodenectomy, partial jejunectomy, pancreatectomy and choledochectomy is performed. The stump of the pancreas is joined to the remaining portion of the jejunum (pancreaticojejunostomy) as an end to end anastomosis. The end of the common bile duct is anastomosed to the jejunum (choledochojejunostomy), using interrupted silk sutures in both cases. The stomach is anastomosed to the jejunum (gastrojejunostomy) in the usual manner and the wound is closed.

Ramstedt's operation

DEFINITION

An operation performed for the relief of congenital pyloric stenosis and which consists of division of the circular muscle fibres of the pylorus.

POSITION

The patient is placed in the supine position or immobilised on a padded crucifix if local anaesthesia is being used.

INSTRUMENTS

Sponge-holding forceps (Rampley), 5
Towel clips, 5
Scalpel handles No. 3, with Nos. 10 and 15 blades (Bard Parker), 2
Fine dissecting forceps, toothed (Gillies), 2
Fine dissecting forceps, non-toothed (McIndoe), 2
Scissors, straight, 13 cm (5 in) (Mayo)
Scissors, curved on flat, 18 cm (7 in) (Mayo)
Long scissors, curved on flat (McIndoe)
Sinus forceps
Blunt dissector (Watson Cheyne)
Blunt dissector (MacDonald)
Fine artery forceps, curved on flat (mosquito), 5
Fire artery forceps, straight (mosquito), 5
Small retractors, double hook, 2
Medium retractors (Czerny), 2
Fine tissue forceps (McIndoe), 5
Skin or tetra towel forceps (Moynihan), 4 for the sides of the wound and 2 for the ends of the wound (Optional)
2 and 2·5 (3/0 and 2/0) Chromic catgut or Dexon for ligatures
2·5 and 3 (2/0 and 0) Chromic catgut or Dexon on small half-circle round-bodied needles for peritoneum and muscles
2 (3/0) Silk or nylon on a small curved or straight cutting needle for skin sutures.

OUTLINE OF PROCEDURE

Through a small midline or paramedian incision, the pylorus is delivered into the wound and an incision made through the tumour wall into the circular muscle fibres, care being taken to avoid incising the mucosa. These fibres are stretched with artery or sinus forceps until the mucosa herniates into the muscle incision. The wound is closed in the usual manner.

Gastroscopy

DEFINITION

The examination of the interior of the stomach, using an illuminated endoscope.

POSITION

Supine or left lateral, with the knees and thighs flexed. The eyes are covered with a towel.

INSTRUMENTS

Gastroscope (Fig. 284)
Oesophageal bougies, set
Oesophageal tubes, sizes 16 and 18 Charrière gauge
Mouth gag (Mason or Doyen)
Tongue forceps

Angled tongue depressor
Pharyngeal spray
Topical anaesthetic, e.g., 4 per cent lignocaine (Xylocaine)
Lubricant, e.g., lignocaine (Xylocaine) gel
Hot water in tall jar, for telescopes.

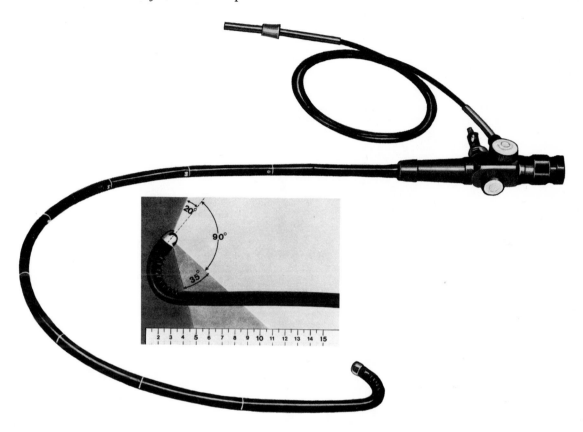

Figure 284   Flexible fibre gastroscope.
Visualisation of the entire stomach including proximal stomach, cardia and fundus is easily achieved by deflecting the distal tip up and down for 90°. Additionally, the head is rotatable along its axis for 40°. The deflecting portion of the tip is exceptionally short so as to permit this manoeuvre easily in most stomachs. The instrument accepts biopsy forceps utilising the insufflation channel thereby in no way diminishing its visualisation or photographic ability. The gastroscope has high intensity fibre optic illumination and is very suitable for cine-gastroscopy, still photography or teaching via closed circuit television. (Richard Wolf GmBH, Down Bros Ltd.)

OUTLINE OF PROCEDURE

Topical anaesthetic is applied and the patient's head placed in a position of extension so that the surgeon has a straight line to the stomach. This is accomplished, either by using a Negus or Haslinger head support, or by an assistant holding the head in extension after lowering the head of the table. The patient assists the surgeon by swallowing as the lubricated instrument is passed.

Gastrostomy

DEFINITION

The establishment of an opening between the stomach and the abdominal wall for the purpose of feeding. It is an operation which is not often carried out nowadays.

POSITION. Supine.

INSTRUMENTS

General set (Fig. 281)
Gastrostomy set (Fig. 285)

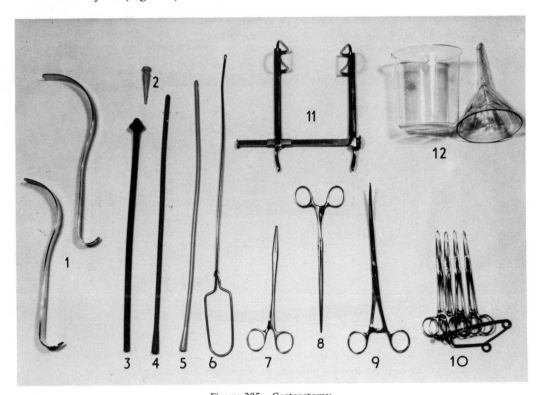

Figure 285   Gastrostomy

1. Deep retractors, narrow blade (Deaver, 25 mm (1 in) wide), 2.
2. Spigot.
3. Catheter, self-retaining (De Pezzer) size 20 Charrière gauge.
4 and 5. Catheters, rubber or plastic (Jaques), sizes 12 and 14 Charrière gauge.
6. Catheter introducer.
7. Artery forceps, straight, 20 cm (8 in) (Spencer Wells), 12.
8. Intestinal occlusion clamp, straight (Doyen).
9. Intestinal occlusion clamp, curved (Doyen).
10. Fine tissue forceps (McIndoe), 4.
11. Retractor, self-retaining abdominal (Gosset).
12. Beaker, funnel and sterile water to test efficiency of opening.

Suction tubing, nozzles and tube anchoring forceps
Local anaesthetic requisites
2·5 and 3 (2/0 and 0) Chromic catgut or Dexon for ligatures

3 (0) Chromic catgut or Dexon on a small curved non-traumatic needle for stomach suture

3 or 4 (0 or 1) Chromic catgut or Dexon on a small half-circle round-bodied needle for peritoneum and muscles

2·5 (2/0) Silk or nylon on medium curved or straight cutting needles for skin sutures.

OUTLINE OF PROCEDURE

As the patient is very often in a very emaciated condition and may be a poor general anaesthetic risk, local anaesthesia is usually employed. Another advantage of local anaesthesia is that the patient may be given gastric feeds if desired immediately after operation. Through a small paramedian or midline incision the stomach is grasped with Allis tissue forceps. A series of purse-string sutures are placed around the selected incision area through which the catheter is to be inserted. After incising the stomach, gastric contents (if any) are evacuated with a suction tube, the catheter inserted, and the purse-string sutures tightened to form an inverted valve of stomach wall around the catheter. The catheter is secured to the skin with sutures during wound closure.

Gastroenterostomy

DEFINITION

The establishment of an opening between the stomach and the jejunum.

POSITION. Supine.

INSTRUMENTS

General set (Fig. 281)
Laparotomy set (Fig. 282)
Intestinal occlusion clamps, straight (Doyen), 2
Intestinal occlusion clamps, curved (Doyen), 2
Twin occlusion clamps (Lane), optional
Fine tissue forceps (McIndoe), 5
Fine artery forceps, straight (mosquito), 5
Suction tubing, nozzles and tube anchoring forceps
Laparotomy ligatures and sutures
2·5 and 3 (2/0 and 0) Chromic catgut or Dexon on medium or small curved non-traumatic intestinal needles for anastomosis
2·5 (2/0) Silk on small curved non-traumatic intestinal needles for anastomosis.

OUTLINE OF PROCEDURE

Through a left paramedian or midline incision an opening is made in the avascular space of the transverse mesocolon. The posterior wall of the stomach is grasped with tissue forceps on the lesser and greater curvatures at each end of the proposed line of anastomosis. The jejunum is grasped with tissue forceps also, and occlusion clamps applied to the stomach and jejunum. A continuous 2·5 (2/0) chromic catgut or Dexon suture or interrupted silk sutures are used for the posterior seromuscular layer joining the stomach and bowel. The stomach and jejunum are then opened and gastric contents evacuated with the suction tube. The second posterior row of sutures consists of a continuous 2·5 or 3 (2/0 or 0) chromic catgut or Dexon through and through all layers of the stomach and bowel, and this is continued around the stoma to form the first anterior layer. If continuous chromic catgut has been used for the first posterior layer, this suture is continued to form the second seromuscular layer of the anastomosis; alternatively, interrupted silk sutures are used. The opening in the mesocolon is sutured to the stomach before wound closure. This operation is often combined with vagotomy.

Partial gastrectomy

DEFINITION

Resection of a portion of the stomach with anastomosis between the remaining portion of the stomach and the duodenum or jejunum.

POSITION. Supine.

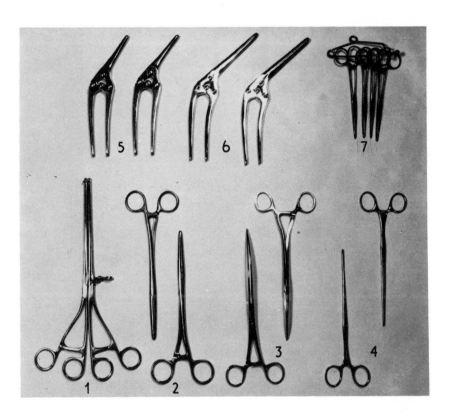

Figure 286   Gastrectomy and resection of bowel.

1. Twin occlusion clamp for stomach or intestine (Lane).
2. Intestinal crushing clamps (Joll), 2.
3. Intestinal occlusion clamps, curved (Doyen), 2.
4. Intestinal occlusion clamps, straight (Doyen), 2.
5 and 6. Intestinal crushing clamps, double action, small and large (Payr), 2 of each size.
7. Fine tissue forceps (McIndoe), 4.

INSTRUMENTS

General set (Fig. 281)
Laparotomy set (Fig. 282)

Gastrectomy set (Fig. 286)
Fine artery forceps, straight (McIndoe), 5
Suction tubing, nozzles and tube anchoring forceps
Laparotomy ligatures and sutures
2·5 and 3 (2/0 and 0) Chromic catgut or Dexon on small and medium curved and half-
    circle non-traumatic intestinal needles for anastomosis
2·5 (2/0) Silk on a small curved or half-circle non-traumatic needle for anastomosis.

OUTLINE OF PROCEDURE

There are several variations in the technique of gastric resection but basically the initial dissection is the same. The incision may be right paramedian or midline and possibly transverse.

The Billroth I or Schoemaker Operation. The omentum on the greater curvature of the stomach is dissected free down to the duodenum, clamping, dividing and ligating the blood vessels in the process. The right gastric vessels on the lesser curvature of the stomach are identified and divided between stout ligatures of chromic catgut or silk. A crushing clamp is placed across the duodenum at its junction with the stomach, and then alongside this but just distally an occlusion clamp is also applied. The duodenum is divided with a scalpel, which is then discarded. The left gastric or coronary vessels and the vessels in the omentum on the upper left side of the stomach are ligated with stout chromic catgut or silk and then divided. An occlusion clamp is applied across the stomach at the desired level and the organ resected.

The cut end of the stomach is funnelled with two layers of sutures towards the greater curvature and the anastomosis made to the duodenum. The first posterior and second anterior seromuscular layers of the anastomosis consist of continuous 2·5 (2/0) chromic catgut or Dexon suture or interrupted silk sutures. The second posterior and first anterior layers consist of a continuous 3 (0) chromic catgut or Dexon suture placed through and through all layers of the stomach and bowel. Instruments used for the anastomosis are discarded before wound closure.

Billroth II Operation. In all the following variations of this operation, the duodenum is divided between crushing clamps and closed with a continuous chromic catgut suture followed by a second layer of catgut or interrupted silk sutures. The stomach is resected and anastomosed to a loop of jejunum. With the original Billroth II operation, now rarely performed, the cut end of the stomach is closed and the jejunum joined to a fresh opening in the stomach. The Polya operation is perhaps the most common and consists of an end to side anastomosis between the entire cut end of the stomach and the jejunum, posterior to the transverse colon. An anterior Polya resection consists of an end to side anastomosis made in a similar manner but anterior to the transverse colon. The Hoffmeister resection consists of closing the cut end of the stomach, leaving a 51 mm (2 in) stoma on the greater curvature to which the jejunum is anastomosed. Alternatively, a central 51 mm (2 in) stoma may be formed by partially closing the cut end of the stomach from each side. The loop of jejunum is then anastomosed to the opening.

Total gastrectomy

This is occasionally performed for malignancy and the dissection approximates to that for partial gastrectomy but is more extensive. The procedure is generally performed via a thoraco-abdominal approach. A Billroth I type of anastomosis may be used, joining the oesophagus to the duodenum, but more commonly an oesophagojejunostomy is established.

Resection of small bowel

DEFINITION
Resection of a portion of the small intestine.

POSITION. Supine.

INSTRUMENTS
As for gastrectomy.

OUTLINE OF PROCEDURE
The incision may be paramedian or midline (an exception being when treating a strangulated hernia and in this case the bowel may be delivered via the hernial orifice).

The mesenteric vessels supplying the loop of bowel are identified and ligated with chromic catgut or silk. Crushing and occlusion clamps are applied at each side of the affected section of bowel which is then resected. The occlusion clamps are retained until an end to end anastomosis has been made, using two layers of continuous chromic catgut or Dexon. Anastomosis instruments are discarded before wound closure in the usual manner.

Intussusception

DEFINITION
Obstruction from invaginated bowel.

POSITION
Supine with Trendelenburg for colonic invagination.

INSTRUMENTS
As for gastrectomy (resection of bowel may be necessary).

OUTLINE OF PROCEDURE
Through a paramedian or midline incision, the deformity is reduced by gentle pressure exerted on the head of the invaginated portion of the bowel. Warm packs are applied and if the bowel is non-viable, it is resected in the usual manner and the wound closed.

Right hemicolectomy

DEFINITION
Resection of the right half of the colon.

POSITION. Supine.

INSTRUMENTS
As for gastrectomy.

OUTLINE OF PROCEDURE
Through a right paramedian or midline incision, the ascending colon and distal part of the ileum are mobilised from the lateral peritoneal fold. The ureter and duodenum are identified, the mesentery incised, and the mesenteric vessels ligated with chromic

catgut or silk before division. If the anastomosis is to be made side to side, crushing clamps are applied across the transverse colon and the ileum. The bowel is then resected and the stumps closed with a layer of continuous 3 (0) chromic catgut or Dexon through and through sutures and a seromuscular layer of interrupted silk sutures. Curved occlusion clamps are applied and a side to side anastomosis made in the usual manner. If the anastomosis is to be end to end, crushing and occlusion clamps are applied transversely across the colon and obliquely across the ileum. The bowel is resected and the occlusion clamps retained until the anastomosis is completed in the usual manner. The instruments used for the anastomosis are discarded, the defect in the posterior peritoneum and mesentery sutured and the would closed.

Total colectomy

DEFINITION
    Resection of the ascending, transverse and descending colon.

POSITION
    Supine with some degree of Trendelenburg.

INSTRUMENTS
    As for gastrectomy
    Intestinal occlusion clamps, right-angled (Finch), 2.

OUTLINE OF PROCEDURE
    The incision may be midline or paramedian. The colon is mobilised from the distal end of the ileum to the sigmoid flexure, ligating and dividing the mesenteric and superior haemorrhoidal vessels with stout chromic catgut, Dexon or silk. Resection of the colon between two sets of crushing and occlusion clamps is performed and anastomosis made between the ileum and the rectum (ileorectostomy) in the usual manner, or the rectum is closed with interrupted silk sutures and an ileostomy performed. If the resection is low, the rectal anastomosis may be made with a series of interrupted mattress sutures of 3 (0) chromic catgut, Dexon or silk which are left long and not tied until all have been placed in position.

Abdominoperineal resection of the rectum and part of the colon

DEFINITION
    Mobilisation of the diseased portion of the colon which is pushed into the hollow of the pelvis for removal via the perineal route, and the establishment of a terminal colostomy.

POSITION
    Lithotomy and Trendelenburg with a sandbag or similar support under the buttocks.

INSTRUMENTS
    Anterior Part of the Operation
        General set (Fig. 281)
        Laparotomy set (Fig. 282)
        Long scalpel handle No. 4L with No. 20 blade (Bard Parker)
        Long dissecting forceps, toothed, 25 cm (10 in)
        Long dissecting forceps, non-toothed, 25 cm (10 in)

Long scissors, curved on flat, 23 cm (9 in) (Nelson)
Scissors, straight, 20 cm (8 in) (Mayo)
Intestinal occlusion clamps, straight (Doyen), 2
Intestinal occlusion clamps, curved (Doyen), 2
Intestinal crushing clamps (Payr or Joll), 2
Intestinal crushing clamps (de Martel or Zachary Cope), set of 3
Suprapubic retractor (Doyen)
Suction tubing, nozzles and tube anchoring forceps
Diathermy leads, electrodes and lead anchoring forceps
Ligatures and sutures as for laparotomy.
Long tissue forceps, 20 cm (8 in) (Lane's or Fagge's), 5

Posterior Part of Operation
General set (Fig. 281)
Extra towel clips, 5
Long scalpel handle No. 4L with No. 20 blade (Bard Parker)
Long tissue forceps, 20 cm (8 in) (Lane's or Fagge's), 5
Deep retractors, narrow blade (Paton), 2
Rugines curved and straight (Faraboeuf)
Bone nibbling or gouge forceps (single action)
Bone nibbling or gouge forceps (compound action)
Bone cutting forceps, curved (Liston)
Long scissors, straight, 20 cm (8 in) (Mayo)
Long scissors, curved on flat, 20 cm (8 in) (Mayo)
Urethral catheter, 18 to 20 Charrière gauge (Jaques, Nélaton, or Foley self-retaining)
(If Foley catheter is used, a syringe containing 5 to 30 ml of sterile water to inflate the
    catheter cuff, and a ligature for the pilot tube will be required, unless this is
    self-sealing.)
Spigot
Large rubber or plastic drainage tube
3 and 4 (0 and 1) Chromic catgut or Dexon for ligatures
4 or 5 (1 or 2) Chromic catgut or Dexon on a large half-circle cutting needle for deep
    sutures
5 (2) Silk on a large half-circle cutting needle for anal purse-string sutures
2·5 (2/0) Silk or nylon in large curved cutting needles for skin sutures.

OUTLINE OF PROCEDURE

Generally this operation is performed as a synchronous-combined procedure by two operation teams. In this case the instrument sets must be available on two trolleys for simultaneous use and it is very important that the swab count of each team is kept separate. To assist this, the instrument nurse assisting the surgeon performing the anterior part of the operation will ensure that only 'taped' swabs or packs are used in the vicinity of the pelvis and that instruments are not interchanged between the teams.

The Anterior Part of the Operation. Through a lower midline incision the bowel is mobilised from the point of transection to the coccyx, ligating and dividing the inferior mesenteric vessels. Slender crushing clamps such as the de Martel's are applied across the colon, above the diseased portion. The bowel is divided and the proximal end brought out through an incision at the selected site for the permanent colostomy. A rubber glove is secured over the distal clamp to prevent soiling of the peritoneum, and the diseased portion of the bowel and rectum is pushed into the hollow of the pelvis for removal by the surgeon performing the perineal part of the operation. The pelvic peritoneum is sutured with a continuous 2·5 (2/0) or 3 (0) chromic catgut or Dexon before general wound closure.

The Posterior Part of the Operation. A urethral catheter is inserted and the bladder emptied. The rectum is sealed by placing two purse-string sutures around the anus, and an elliptical incision made round the rectum exposing the levator ani muscles, which are divided. The urethra is identified and in co-operation with the surgeon performing the anterior part of the operation, the rectum is freed with scissors. The diseased bowel and rectum is removed through the posterior incision and the muscles approximated with chromic catgut. A long drainage tube (which will be attached to a suitable sterile bottle) is used to drain the pelvic space before skin closure with silk or nylon.

Anterior resection of the rectum and part of the colon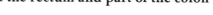

DEFINITION

A sphincter-saving resection of the rectum and part of the colon with re-establishment of continuity by anastomosis.

POSITION

As for abdominoperineal resection.

INSTRUMENTS

As for abdominoperineal resection
Minus de Martel clamps
Plus Intestinal occlusion clamps, right-angled (Finch), 2
Plus Proctoscope (Fig. 288).

OUTLINE OF PROCEDURE

Through a lower midline incision, the colon is mobilised from the point of transection to the ano-rectal junction, ligating and dividing the inferior mesenteric vessels. It is then divided between clamps, one a right-angled clamp (Finch) placed proximally to the two.

The mesorectum is separated from the back of the rectum at the level selected for division below the growth (not less than 6 cm from its inferior edge). The mesorectum is then clamped with two large artery forceps, divided and ligated leaving the rectum bared all round over a segment about 4 cm long.

The bowel is then clamped at the upper end of this bared segment with right-angled clamps and the rectum irrigated from below with an antibacterial solution, via a proctoscope. The rectum is then transected and the colon clamp brought into proximity to the open stump of the rectum. A row of seromuscular mattress Lembert sutures are inserted both laterally and medially and left untied. A further row of through and through mattress sutures are inserted and when all are placed the sutures are tied. This slides the colon down to the cut edge of the rectum, invaginates the suture line and completes the anastomosis. Finally the clamp is removed and the pelvic peritoneum sutured over the anastomosis to extraperitonealise the suture line.

A drainage tube is inserted and the wound closed in layers in the normal manner.

Colostomy

DEFINITION

The establishment of a temporary or permanent opening in the colon.

POSITION. Supine.

INSTRUMENTS

 General set (Fig. 281)
 Laparotomy set (Fig. 282)
 Colostomy set (Fig. 287)
 Ligatures and sutures as for laparotomy.

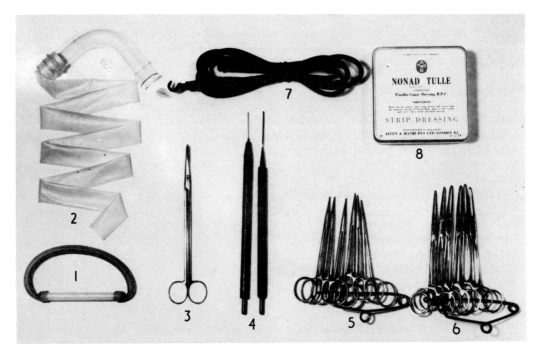

Figure 287 Colostomy

1. Glass or plastic colostomy rod and tubing.
2. Glass drainage tube and rubber or plastic tubing (Paul), optional, for use if colostomy is opened immediately.
3. Long scissors, curved on flat (McIndoe).
4. Diathermy electrodes (optional, as No. 2).
5. Fine artery forceps, straight (mosquito), 6.
6. Fine tissue forceps (McIndoe), 6.
7. Diathermy cable or lead (optional, as No. 2).
8. Paraffin gauze dressing.

OUTLINE OF PROCEDURE

 The incision can be paramedian, midline or in the iliac region as described for appendicectomy. The colon is mobilised and a loop brought either through the original incision or through a separate stab wound (inguinal colostomy). An opening is made in the mesentery of this loop of bowel, and a glass or nylon rod (attached at one end to a short piece of tubing) is passed between the skin and bowel. The tubing is then attached to the other end of the rod, forming a D-shaped loop which retains it in position. The wound is closed and petroleum jelly gauze placed around the exteriorised bowel. The colostomy is usually opened in the ward with a cautery or diathermy knife, but the apparatus should be available in case the surgeon decides to open the bowel in theatre. If the colostomy is opened immediately after operation, a Paul's drainage tube will be found very useful, especially if the faecal matter is semi-liquid.

Ileostomy

DEFINITION

The establishment of an opening into the ileum (generally permanent).

POSITION. Supine.

INSTRUMENTS

As for colostomy
Intestinal occlusion clamps, straight (Doyen), 2
2·5 (2/0) Chromic catgut or Dexon on a small curved non-traumatic intestinal needle for
    ileum closure. Ileostomy bag.

OUTLINE OF PROCEDURE

This operation is usually done for ulcerative colitis. Through a low paramedian or
midline incision, the ileum is mobilised and two occlusion clamps applied at the selected
point for ileostomy. The ileum is transected and the proximal end brought out through a
small circular wound made in the right side of the abdomen. The distal end of the ileum
is closed with 2·5 (2/0) chromic catgut or Dexon and the wound is closed. The base of the
exteriorised ileum is sutured to the abdominal wall and the mucosa is then everted. The
cut edge of the mucosa is sutured to the skin with 2·5 (2/0) chromic catgut or Dexon. An
ileostomy bag is usually applied immediately at the end of the operation.

Closure of colostomy

DEFINITION

Re-establishment of intestinal continuity.

POSITION. Supine.

INSTRUMENTS

General set (Fig. 281)
Deep retractors, narrow blade (Paton), 2
Intestinal occlusion clamps, straight (Doyen), 2
Fine tissue forceps (McIndoe), 5
Fine artery forceps, curved on flat (mosquito), 10
2·5 (2/0) Chromic catgut, Dexon or silk for ligatures
2·5 (2/0) Chromic catgut or Dexon and silk on a small curved non-traumatic intestinal
    needle for closure of bowel
3 or 4 (0 or 1) Chromic catgut or Dexon on a medium half-circle round-bodied or Mayo
    needle for peritoneum and muscle
2·5 (2/0) Silk or nylon on a large curved or straight cutting needle for skin sutures.

OUTLINE OF PROCEDURE

An extraperitoneal or intraperitoneal closure may be performed. If an extraperitoneal
closure is contemplated, the spur between the upper and lower portion of the colostomy
will have been crushed previously by an enterotribe.

For extraperitoneal closure an elliptical incision is made around the colostomy and the
skin and bowel freed down to the peritoneum. The segment of skin attached to the
colostomy is excised and the opening in the colon closed with one layer of continuous

chromic catgut or Dexon and one layer of interrupted silk sutures. The peritoneum and muscle are plicated over the sutured colon and the wound is closed.

For intraperitoneal closure the dissection is the same except that the peritoneum is opened at each side of the exteriorised colon. The bowel is sutured in the manner already described or is divided at each side of the colostomy, and an end to end anastomosis made. The wound is closed.

Splenectomy

DEFINITION
Removal of the spleen.

POSITION. Supine.

INSTRUMENTS
As for laparotomy, including ligatures and sutures.

OUTLINE OF PROCEDURE
A midline, left paramedian or transverse incision is made. The spleen is palpated, and if there are any adhesions these are clamped with forceps before dividing. The gastrosplenic ligament is first divided and then the lateral peritoneal fold of the lienorenal ligament is incised, allowing the spleen to be brought forward into the wound. The major splenic vessels are either clamped with sets of two strong artery forceps and divided, or are individually ligatured with double strong silk or thread and cut after the ligatures have been tied. The spleen is then free and may be removed. The wound is closed in layers.

Diaphragmatic hernia (abdominal approach)

(See also chapter on thoracic surgery.)

DEFINITION
The repair of an abnormal opening in the diaphragm (usually at the oesophageal hiatus) which allows protrusion of abdominal organs into the chest.

POSITION. Supine.

INSTRUMENTS
General set (Fig. 281)
Laparotomy set (Fig. 282)
Long tissue forceps (Littlewood or Vulsellum), 5
Long dissecting forceps, 25 cm (10 in) toothed
Long dissecting forceps, 25 cm (10 in) non-toothed
Long scissors, curved on flat, 23 cm (9 in) (Nelson)
Long needle holders (Halstead), 3
Ligatures and sutures as for laparotomy
2·5 (2/0) Silk or 30 S.W.G. stainless steel wire on small half-circle round-bodied needle for diaphragm repair.

OUTLINE OF PROCEDURE
A midline, left paramedian or transverse incision is made. The edges of the hernial

orifice are grasped with tissue forceps and the abdominal organs returned to the abdomen. The herniorrhaphy is performed with interrupted silk or wire sutures, which are usually left long until all have been placed, and then tied. The wound is closed.

Inguinal or scrotal herniorrhaphy

DEFINITION

The obliteration of a sac containing viscera, which have protruded from the abdomen, either as a direct hernia through Hesselbach's triangle, or as an indirect hernia through the internal ring.

POSITION. Supine.

INSTRUMENTS

    General set (Fig. 281)

    2·5 and 3 (2/0 and 0) Chromic catgut or Dexon for ligatures

    3 or 4 (0 or 1) Chromic catgut or Dexon on a small or medium half-circle round-bodied needle for the hernial sac, and on a half-circle cutting needle for the muscle tendon

    Repair material of choice, e.g., monofilament, braided nylon; braided silk; polyethylene; polyester; linen thread; stainless steel wire; and mesh made from nylon, braided silk or wire (Chapter 7); small or medium stout half-circle needles, such as Mayo needles, or special types such as fish-hook shape may be used to facilitate the suturing with the chosen material

    2·5 (2/0) Silk or nylon on medium or large curved or straight cutting needles for skin sutures

    (Alternatively, Michel or Kifa clips may be used.)

    Gallie's Repair, Extra Instruments

    Fascia forceps, right and left, 2

    Fasciatome or fascia stripper

    Gallie's living suture needles – small, medium and large

    2·5 and 3 (2/0 and 0) Silk on small half-circle round-bodied needles for securing graft.

OUTLINE OF PROCEDURE

Through an incision overlying the inguinal canal, the spermatic cord is mobilised and retracted with a piece of ribbon gauze or tubing. By separating the coverings of the cord, the hernial sac is found and isolated. It is opened to make quite sure that it is empty, transfixed, ligated with 3 or 4 (0 or 1) chromic catgut or Dexon at the internal ring, and is cut off. This is all that is necessary in infants who require no repair of the muscles at this stage.

There are many repair procedures, including *the Bassini operation* which consists of interrupted silk sutures from the border of the internal oblique and transversus abdominus muscles to the inguinal ligament deep to the spermatic cord. *In Gallie's repair* a strip of fascia lata is removed from the lateral aspect of the thigh either with a fasciatome or via a long incision extending from just above the knee to the greater trochanter. This fascia is then sutured 'zigzag' fashion across the posterior inguinal wall to strengthen it. *A nylon darn* consists of a continuous monfilament or braided nylon suture, introduced forwards and backwards across the posterior inguinal wall, extending from the internal oblique and transversus abdominus muscles to the inguinal ligament without actually drawing them into approximation.

Stainless steel wire or braided nylon/silk mesh may be used to strengthen the posterior wall. A piece of suitable shape and size is sutured around its periphery to the muscles described above.

The hernia repair may be further strengthened by overlapping the external oblique, suturing the upper margin to the inguinal ligament and using the part below the incision for an overlap. This means that the anterior wall of the inguinal canal has a double instead of a single layer of external oblique. The wound is closed.

Femoral herniorrhaphy

DEFINITION

This is similar to an inguinal hernia but the sac protrudes through the femoral ring into the femoral canal.

POSITION

As for inguinal hernia.

INSTRUMENTS

As for inguinal hernia.

OUTLINE OF PROCEDURE

The hernial sac is exposed below the inguinal ligament, freed, ligated and excised as previously described. The femoral canal is then usually closed from above by opening the inguinal canal and suturing the conjoined tendon to the pectineal ligament with interrupted silk or thread sutures. The operation then proceeds as for inguinal hernia.

Umbilical hernia

DEFINITION

A protrusion of intestine through the umbilicus or muscles surrounding the umbilicus. (In congenital form, the loop of intestine can easily be seen through a thin transparent membrane and is not strictly speaking a true hernia, for the bowel has never been inside the abdomen. The acquired hernia in children is due to the scar of the umbilicus giving way because of some strain (e.g., coughing). In adults, usually the obese patient, the hernia occurs above or below the umbilical scar itself.)

POSITION. Supine.

INSTRUMENTS

As for inguinal hernia.

OUTLINE OF PROCEDURE

A transverse elliptical incision is made above or below the umbilicus. The sac is isolated, opened, and the omentum contained either dissected free or clamped and resected. The redundant sac is excised, and the peritoneal opening closed with 4 or 5 (1 or 2) chromic catgut or Dexon. Repair is accomplished by overlapping the aponeurosis transversely with interrupted silk or thread mattress sutures (Mayo procedure). The skin wound is closed.

Ventral hernia

DEFINITION

A protrusion of abdominal viscera through an opening in the linea semilunaris, linea alba or through the scar of an abdominal incision.

POSITION. Supine.

INSTRUMENTS

As for inguinal hernia.

OUTLINE OF PROCEDURE

Through the selected incision the sac is identified and obliterated. The abdominal wall is repaired either with a fascial strip or a non-absorbable suture material (see inguinal hernia) and the wound is then closed.

Strangulated hernia

DEFINITION

Gangrene of an intestinal loop contained within a hernial sac, due to compression of its mesentery and blood-vessels.

POSITION. Supine.

INSTRUMENTS

As for inguinal hernia
Fine tissue forceps (McIndoe), 5
Fine artery forceps, straight (mosquito), 5
Intestinal occlusion clamps, straight (Doyen), 2
Intestinal occlusion clamps, curved (Doyen), 2
Intestinal crushing clamps (Payr, Joll or Schoemaker), 2
Artery forceps, straight, 20 cm (8 in) (Spencer Wells), 10
Long artery forceps, curved on flat (Moynihan gall-bladder), 5
Hernia director and bistoury
2·5 and 3 (2/0 and 0) Chromic catgut or Dexon on small or medium non-traumatic intestinal needles for resection anastomosis
Ligatures and sutures as for inguinal hernia.

OUTLINE OF PROCEDURE

The approach and dissection follows that for inguinal hernia or umbilical hernia, etc. The sac is opened and the gangrenous contents prevented from slipping into the abdomen whilst the constricting area is divided, perhaps with a director and bistoury under direct vision. Warm, moist packs are applied to the bowel and if it does not appear viable after five minutes, a resection of the affected part is carried out in the usual manner. Repair is carried out in the usual manner.

Proctoscopy and sigmoidoscopy

DEFINITION

An examination of the rectum or sigmoid flexure of the colon, using an illuminated endoscope passed per anum.

POSITION

Left lateral, lithotomy or kneeling.

INSTRUMENTS. As Figure 288.

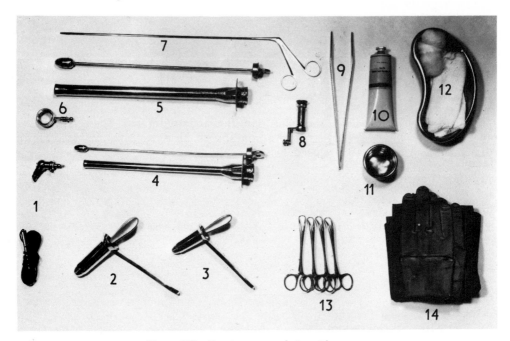

Figure 288   Proctoscopy and sigmoidoscopy.

1. Sigmoidoscope light lead and light attachment.
2 and 3. Large and small proctoscope (Kelly).
4 and 5. Large and small sigmoidoscopes (Norton Morgan).
6. Eyepiece for sigmoidoscope.
7. Biopsy forceps, cutting jaws (e.g., Brunings cup, Yeaman, etc.).
8. Telescope attachment.

9. Dissecting forceps, non-toothed.
10. Soft paraffin lubricant.
11. Gallipot containing Savlon 1 per cent.
12. Wool and gauze swabs.
13. Towel clips.
14. Rubber gloves and dressing towels.

Not Illustrated:
Double inflation bellows, and battery or transformer.

OUTLINE OF PROCEDURE

The lubricated endoscope is passed via the anus. When the surgeon uses a sigmoidoscope, the walls of the colon are kept separate by inflating with air. Small pledglets of cotton-wool are held with the long forceps to swab the area in view, and the biopsy forceps may be used to obtain a specimen of tissue for histology. Sometimes a rectal or colonic polyp may be diathermised and in this case the indifferent electrode is applied to the patient's leg, observing the precautions listed in Chapter 2. The active electrode is inserted through a special attachment at the proximal end of the endoscope.

Haemorrhoidectomy

DEFINITION

The excision of internal piles.

POSITION
Lithotomy or jack-knife.

INSTRUMENTS
Sponge-holding forceps (Rampley), 5
Towel clips, 5
Rectal speculum (Kelley, Gabrial, etc.)
Scalpel handle No. 3 with No. 10 blade (Bard Parker)
Dissecting forceps, toothed, 2
Scissors, straight, 15 cm (6 in) (Mayo)
Scissors, curved on flat, 15 cm (6 in) (Mayo)
Artery forceps, straight (Moynihan), 10
Dissectors (MacDonald and Durham), 2
Pile clamps (Kocher, curved), 6
Aneurysm needle
2·5 (2/0) Chromic catgut or Dexon for fine ligatures
6 (3) Chromic catgut, Dexon or silk on a medium curved round-bodied needle for pile
    transfixion and ligation
Stout rubber or plastic drainage tube and safety-pin
(Three small packs made from petroleum jelly gauze, or ribbon gauze soaked in anti-
    septic, may be required to pack around the tube to control oozing from pile areas
    after operation.)

OUTLINE OF PROCEDURE
The three piles are each clamped with forceps and individually dissected upwards off
the muscular coat of the anal canal until a pedicle is formed. This pedicle is transfixed at
the base, ligated and two-thirds of the pile cut off together with the tag of skin corresponding to the pile. A drainage tube may be inserted.

Anal fissure

DEFINITION
A small vertical ulcer at the anal margin.

POSITION
Lithotomy or jack-knife.

INSTRUMENTS
As for haemorrhoidectomy
Malleable probe
Small retractors, double hook, 2
Sinus forceps
Curetting spoon, double end (Volkmann)
Petroleum jelly gauze roll.

OUTLINE OF PROCEDURE
The anal margins are retracted and a knife directed against the floor of the ulcer
dividing the internal sphincter fibres. There is usually a small tag of skin (the so-called
'sentinel pile') in the region of the fissure, and this is cut away to provide free drainage.
The wound is plugged with petroleum jelly gauze.

Fistula in ano

DEFINITION

A sinus or sinuses between the anal canal and the skin in the region of the anus.

POSITION

Lithotomy or jack-knife.

INSTRUMENTS

As for anal fissure.

OUTLINE OF PROCEDURE

The sinuses are opened to provide free drainage, care being taken to divide only the subcutaneous sphincter muscle, otherwise incontinence may result. The surgeon may require a sterile dye to assist identification of the sinuses and indigo carmine or methylene blue together with a syringe and cannula should be available.

14
Operations on the Breast

Incision of breast abscess

DEFINITION
The incision and drainage of an abscess due to acute mastitis.

POSITION. Supine.

INSTRUMENTS
  Sponge-holding forceps (Rampley), 2
  Towel clips, 5
  Scalpel handle No. 3 with No. 10 blade (Bard Parker)
  Dissecting forceps, toothed, 2
  Dissecting forceps, non-toothed, 2
  Scissors, curved on flat, 13 cm (5in) (Mayo)
  Sinus forceps, 18 cm (7 in)
  Probe, malleable silver
  Artery forceps, straight (Moynihan), 5
  20 ml syringe with wide-bore exploration needles
  Sterile culture tube
  2·5 (2/0) plastic drainage tubing and safety-pin
  Latex rubber or plastic drainage tubing and safety-pin
  2·5 (2/0) Silk or nylon on a large curved cutting needle for securing drainage tubing.

OUTLINE OF PROCEDURE
An incision or incisions are made radiating from the nipple. If the abscess is loculated, care is taken to drain each compartment. A split drainage tube is inserted and secured to the skin with a suture. A firm dressing is applied.

Excision of simple adenoma or amputation of the breast. (Simple mastectomy)

DEFINITION
The removal or a simple adenoma; or amputation of the mammary gland, most commonly for chronic mastitis.

POSITION
Supine, with arms extended on narrow arm boards (Fig. 66).

INSTRUMENTS
  General set (Fig. 281)

Local infiltration set (Fig. 271) with adrenaline 1 : 400,000, optional
Artery forceps, curved on flat (Kelly Fraser, Dunhill, etc.), 25
Large tissue forceps (Lane or Fagge), 5
Diathermy leads, electrodes and lead anchoring forceps
Short rubber or plastic drainage tube and safety-pin for adenoma; or long drainage
    tube and Redi-vac for mastectomy
2·5 and 3 (2/0 and 0) Chromic catgut or Dexon for ligatures
2·5 (2/0) Silk or nylon on a large curved or straight cutting needle for skin sutures.

OUTLINE OF PROCEDURE

A simple adenoma is removed through an incision placed over the swelling, but
extending radially from the nipple to conserve the secreting ducts. The wound is closed
with or without drainage.

For simple mastectomy, the skin and subcutaneous tissues over the incision line may
be infiltrated with 100 to 300 ml of a 1 : 400,000 adrenaline solution to minimise bleeding.
An elliptical, vertical incision is then made extending from the axilla to the sternum,
enclosing the nipple in the centre of the ellipse. The skin is dissected from the breast
until the surgeon has reached the limits of the gland in all directions. The breast is peeled
off the deep fascia (without cutting into it) towards the axilla, using light strokes of the
knife, until the axillary tail of the gland is reached. The blood vessels at this point are
ligated before freeing the breast, which is then removed. A drain is placed in the lower
end of the wound which is closed in the usual manner. A negative pressure may be
applied to this drainage tube in the manner described below.

Radical mastectomy

DEFINITION

Removal of the mammary gland, together with the pectoralic minor and major muscles,
and the axillary glands. The operation is performed for malignant tumours of the breast.

POSITION

Supine with arms extended on narrow arm boards, or only one secured and the other
(operation side) held by a seated assistant. The arm is more easily supported in a flexed
position, holding the elbow in one hand and the wrist in the other. The elbow must not be
allowed to drop below the plane of the operation table or abducted more than a right
angle to the body, for the nerves may be stretched over the humeral head and cause
paralysis.

INSTRUMENTS

General set (Fig. 281)
Local infiltration set (Fig. 271) with adrenaline 1 : 400,000, optional
Artery forceps, curved on flat (Kelly Fraser, two-thirds serrated jaws), 25
Artery forceps, curved on flat (Dunhill, fully serrated jaws), 25
Large tissue forceps (Lane or Fagge), 6
Diathermy leads, electrodes and lead anchoring forceps
Long plastic drainage tube and Redi-vac
2·5 and 3 (2/0 and 0) Chromic catgut or Dexon and silk or thread for ligatures
3 (0) Chromic catgut or Dexon on a medium half-circle round-bodied needle for
    axillary sutures
2·5 (2/0) Silk or nylon on a large curved or straight cutting needle for skin sutures
(Skin graft instruments may be required (Fig. 359).)

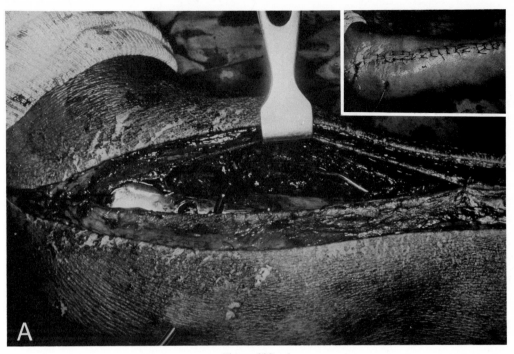

Figure 289   A
Perforated suction catheter in position prior to wound closure (inset shows catheter protruding from separate stab incision). Operation depicted is that on a limb although a similar
technique is used for draining a mastectomy wound. (Zimmer Orthopaedic Ltd.)

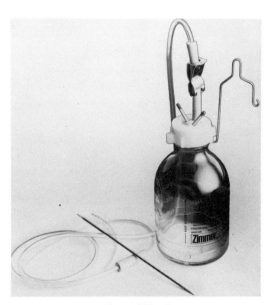

Figure 289   B
The Redi-vac suction device showing vacuum bottle, suction catheter and insertion trocar.
(Zimmer Orthopaedic Ltd.)

OUTLINE OF PROCEDURE

The skin and subcutaneous tissues over the incision line may be infiltrated with 100 to 300 ml of 1 : 400,000 adrenaline solution to minimise bleeding. An elliptical, vertical incision is then made, keeping at least 51 mm (2 in) from the growth all round, which is in the centre of the ellipse. The skin flaps over the axilla are reflected to expose the pectoralis major and minor muscles which are severed from their insertions. The fat and glands contained in the axilla are cleared by dissection, carefully avoiding damage to the major blood vessels, subscapularis nerve and the nerve of Bell. The skin flaps overlying the breast are reflected and the breast removed together with the pectoralis muscles underneath, extending from the sternum medially to the border of the latissimus dorsi muscle. A long drainage tube is inserted into the axilla through a separate stab incision, the skin flaps are approximated with tissue forceps and the wound is closed.

The long drainage tube is either coupled to an under-water collection bottle (Chapter 25), or preferably a slight negative pressure is applied by connecting a Redi-vac bottle* to the open end of the tube.

* Zimmer Orthopaedic Ltd.

15
Dental Operations

Dental extraction

DEFINITION
The removal of a tooth or root either under local or general anaesthesia.

POSITION
Supine, or sitting with the head and neck extended slightly.

INSTRUMENTS
Mouth gag (Mason or Doyen)
Dental props, set
Tongue forceps
Angled tongue depressor
Dental conveying forceps, stout and fine, 2
Dental extraction forceps, set
Dental elevators and probes, set
Mouth mirror
Local anaesthetic, e.g., 2 per cent lignocaine (Xylocaine) and dental syringe may be
    required
Mouth wash.

OUTLINE OF PROCEDURE
If general anaesthesia is to be administered, mouth props are inserted to prevent the patient from closing his jaw. Following the administration of a local anaesthetic, five minutes are allowed to elapse before the operation is commenced. The teeth are extracted and the patient is allowed a gentle mouth wash before leaving the dental chair.

Removal of impacted wisdom tooth

DEFINITION
The removal of the third molar tooth, the eruption of which is partially or completely prevented by its contact against the second molar tooth.

POSITION
Supine, with some reverse Trendelenburg.

INSTRUMENTS. As Figure 290.

OUTLINE OF PROCEDURE

An incision is made in the gum overlying the impacted tooth. The cortex of the bone which covers the tooth is drilled or gouged away. The tooth is removed and the incision closed either with 2 (3/0) chromic catgut, Dexon or silk.

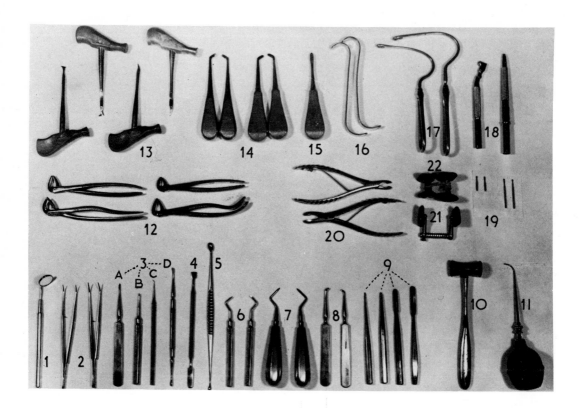

Figure 290   Removal of impacted wisdom tooth

1. Dental mirror.
2. Dental conveying forceps, fine and stout, 2.
3. A. Root elevator straight.
   B. Probe.
   C. Probe and scaler.
   D. Specula and spoon.
4. Spatula.
5. Curette (Volkmann).
6. Apical elevators, left and right, 2.
7. Apical elevators, left and right, 2.
9. Small gouges (Jenkins), 3 mm, 4 mm, 6 mm, and 8 mm, 4.
10. Small mallet (Rowland).
11. Dental cavity syringe.
12. Dental extraction forceps, appropriate shape.
13. Root elevators (Winter), 4.
14. Root elevators (Hospital), right and left, 4.
15. Root elevator (Read).
16. Retractors, cheek, 2.
17. Retractors, cheek, 2.
18. Dental drill handpieces, straight and angled, 2.
19. Dental burrs, fissure and rose-end type.
20. Bone-nibbling or gouge forceps, 2 sizes.
21. Gag (Brunton).
22. Mouth prop (Hewitt).

Not Illustrated:
Suction tubing, fine nozzles and tube anchoring forceps.

Treatment of a fractured mandible

DEFINITION

Reduction of a fractured mandible, followed by immobilisation, in this case by wiring the upper and lower teeth together.

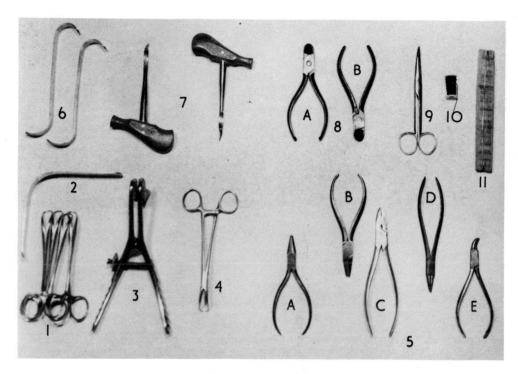

Figure 291   Wiring of mandible, utilising teeth.

1. Towel clips, 4.
2. Right-angled tongue depressor.
3. Mouth gag (Mason).
4. Tongue forceps (Mayo).
5. A. Collar pliers.
    B. Collar pliers.
    C. Collar pliers.
    D. Snipe nose pliers.
    E. Contouring pliers.
6. Cheek retractors, 2.
7. Root elevators (Winter), right and left, 2.
8. A. Wire-cutting forceps, straight.
    B. Wire-cutting forceps, angled on flat.
9. Scissors, curved on flat, 13 cm (5 in) (Mayo).
10. Silk or thread, stout.
11. Stainless-steel wire.

POSITION

Supine, with some reverse Trendelenburg.

INSTRUMENTS. As Figure 291.

OUTLINE OF PROCEDURE

With a pharyngeal pack in position, wires with loops are wound around the necks of tw adjacent teeth on one side of the lower jaw. The wires are twisted together so that the loops or eyelets protrude at gum level from the space between the two teeth.

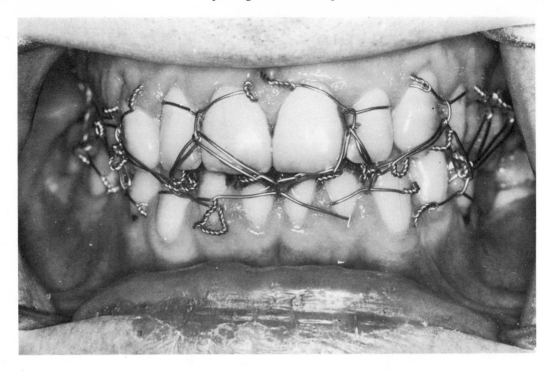

Figure 292 Interdental eyelet wiring. (Photo, courtesy Mr N. L. Rowe, F.D.S.R.C.S., M.R.C.S., L.R.C.P. Consultant in Oral Surgery, Queen Mary's Hospital, Roehampton.)

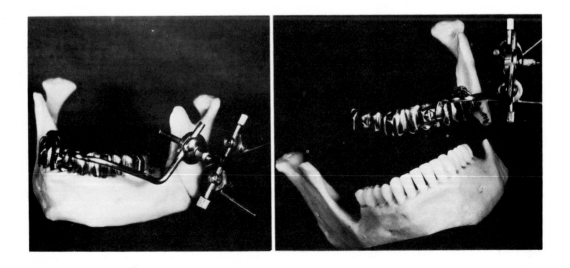

Figures 293 A. and B.
Mandibular splints for extra-oral fixation of mandible fractures.

   This procedure is repeated on the other side of the lower jaw and at correspondingly opposite positions around the teeth in the upper jaw. This results in protruding eyelets spaced evenly around the jaw.

   The wires are now passed through eyelets on opposing jaws. The pharyngeal pack is removed, the tie wires tightened and the lower teeth secured in normal occlusion with the upper teeth; this immobilises the fracture.

   An alternative method of jaw immobilisation is shown in Figures 293A and B.

16
Ear, Nose and Throat Operations

OPERATIONS ON THE EAR

Myringotomy

DEFINITION
Incision of the tympanic membrane in otitis media.

POSITION
Supine, with the head inclined away from the affected ear.

INSTRUMENTS. As Figure 294.

OUTLINE OF PROCEDURE
The surgeon wears a head lamp, uses a frontal mirror and reflected light or uses an operating microscope. A speculum is placed into the outer ear and a myringotome used to make an incision in the tympanic membrane. The discharge which wells forth is gently mopped or sucked away.

In secretory otitis media (blue drum, or 'glue' ear) it is sometimes advisable to put a Shepard's teflon grommet drain tube in the ear drum to ventilate the middle ear and to leave it in for some months (Fig. 295).

Mastoidectomy

DEFINITION
The removal of diseased mastoid air cells as a result of mastoiditis.

POSITION
Supine, with some reversed Trendelenburg and the head inclined away from the affected side.

INSTRUMENTS
Mastoidectomy set (Fig. 296)
Sponge-holding forceps (Rampley), 5
Towel clips, 5
Scalpel handles No. 3 with No. 10 and No. 15 blades (Bard Parker), 2
Fine dissecting forceps, toothed (Lane and Gillies), 2
Fine dissecting forceps, non-toothed (McIndoe), 2
Scissors, curved on flat, 13 cm (5 in) (Mayo)
Fine scissors, curved, 10 cm (4 in) (Kilner)

Stitch scissors, 13 cm (5 in)
Artery forceps, curved on flat (Kilner), 10
Needle holder (Kilner multiple joint or Gillies)
Suction tubing, fine nozzles and tube anchoring forceps
B.I.P.P. paste
5 ml syringe

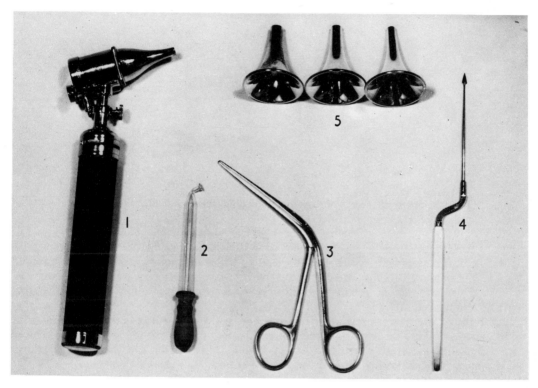

Figure 294   Myringotomy.

1. Auriscope.
2. Pipette.
3. Dressing forceps, angled (Tilley).
4. Myringotome.
5. Aura speculae (Pritchard), 3.

Fine exploring needles, sizes 18 and 14
(Alternatively, cartridge syringe and needles for 2 ml adrenaline cartridges)
2 (3/0) Plain catgut or Dexon for ligatures
2 (3/0) Plain catgut or Dexon on a small half-circle cutting needle for subcutaneous
   sutures
2 (3/0) Silk or nylon on a small curved cutting needle for skin sutures.

OUTLINE OF PROCEDURE

If the operation is for *acute mastoiditis*, a conservative mastoidectomy is performed.

The skin over the incision line is infiltrated with a 1 in 250,000 adrenaline solution to minimise bleeding. A curved incision is made behind the junction of the auricle with the scalp, and a periosteal elevator used to reflect this skin flap and ear to expose the underlying bone above and behind the external auditory meatus.

The bone over the mastoid antrum is gouged or drilled away and the diseased cells removed, but the middle ear is not opened. Either the mastoid cavity is packed with ribbon gauze impregnated with B.I.P.P., etc., and a portion of the gauze left protruding from the wound, or a post-auricular drain consisting of rubber or plastic drainage tubing is inserted. The wound is closed with catgut or Dexon, and silk or nylon skin sutures. The surgeon may also pack the external auditory canal with suitably impregnated ribbon gauze.

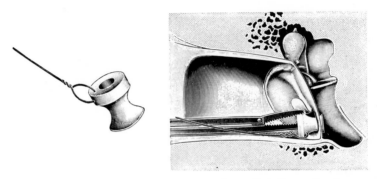

Figure 295   Shepard Grommet Drain tube, Teflon. (Down Bros.)

Radical mastoidectomy

In a radical mastoidectomy the middle ear and mastoid are turned into one cavity, drained permanently to the outside through an enlarged external auditory meatus. It is now customary to complete the operation with the creation of a new ear drum with a graft of temporal fascia.

The bone of the posterior wall of the external auditory meatus is removed and any middle ear pathology dealt with. Care is taken to avoid damage to the facial nerve which runs along the inner wall of the middle ear. The mastoid cavity and the middle ear are packed as previously described and the wound closed.

Mastoidectomy may also be performed through an endaural incision. This is known as Lempert's approach.

Microtia and atresia of the external auditory canal

DEFINITION

Correction of an abnormally small pinna and placing it farther back (as in this deformity it usually lies too far forward), and creation of an external auditory canal and meatus, and reconstruction of the ossicles when they are abnormal.

POSITION

As for mastoidectomy.

INSTRUMENTS

As for mastoidectomy
Dental drill and burrs (as for fenestration)
Operating microscope
General set (Fig. 281)
Skin grafting set (Fig. 359)

OUTLINE OF PROCEDURE

This abnormality may be due to maternal rubella, or the taking of thalidomide during pregnancy. The new pinna may have to be reconstructed in stages with a skin tube pedicle (Chapter 24). Cartilage taken from the patient's rib, from the mother or from another person is sometimes employed. A new ear drum is constructed with fascia lata and the newly constructed external auditory canal is skin grafted.

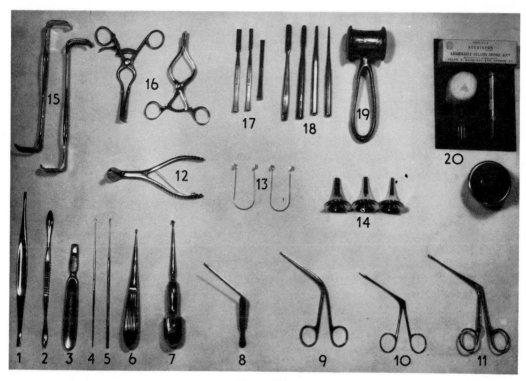

Figure 296

1. Raspatory (Howarth).
2. Raspatory (Durham).
3. Rugine (Faraboeuf).
4. Aural probe (Jobson Horne).
5. Aural hook (Hartmann).
6. Mastoid scoop (Lempert).
7. Mastoid burr (Heath).
8. Dressing forceps (Wilde or Keen).
9. Dressing forceps, angled (Tilley).
10. Aural forceps (Mathieu).
11. Aural forceps (Heath).
12. Aural speculum (Kramer).
13. Nasal specula (Thudichum), 2.
14. Aural specula (Pritchard), set of 3.
15. Medium retractors (Czerny), 2.
16. Retractors, self-retaining (Mayo angled, and West straight), 2.
17. Small chisels, 6 mm, 8 mm and 10 mm, 3.
18. Small gouges (Jenkins), 4 mm, 6 mm, 8 mm and 10 mm, 4.
19. Mallet (Heath).
20. Gelatine sponge, ribbon gauze, adrenaline, bone wax, B.I.P.P. paste in gallipot.

Otoplasty (See Chapter 24.)

Osteoma of the external auditory canal

DEFINITION

Removal of a bony tumour of the external auditory canal that blocks it and which may lead to serious complications.

POSITION

As for mastoidectomy.

INSTRUMENTS

As for mastoidectomy. (Drill and burrs may be needed.)

OUTLINE OF PROCEDURE

The exposure is similar to that for mastoidectomy. This skin is elevated off the tumour which is gouged out. Diamond paste burrs may be used to break through the bony wall of the tumour.

Operations to Improve Aural Function

Mobilisation of stapes

DEFINITION

The mobilisation of an otosclerotic fixed stapes, in order to re-establish sound conduction to the inner ear.

POSITION

As for mastoidectomy, but with a Zeiss operating microscope draped with sterile covers and placed so that it can be rotated over the operation field without disturbing the operation drapes. Sterile caps are fitted over the microscope knobs enabling the surgeon to adjust focus without contaminating his gloves. Saline irrigation apparatus is placed in a convenient position, together with the dental engine. Unless it has been sterilised the flexible drive of this engine must be covered with sterile cotton sleeving extending from the drill hand piece to the pulley wheels or connection on the supporting column.

INSTRUMENTS

As for mastoidectomy
Fenestration set, etc. (Fig. 297)
Local anaesthetic requisites may be required (Fig. 271).

OUTLINE OF PROCEDURE

This is sometimes performed under local anaesthesia so that an audiogram may be taken during operation to see if any gain of hearing has occurred.

The incision area is infiltrated with a 1 in 250,000 solution of adrenaline to provide local haemostasis. If a local anaesthetic is to be employed, this is combined with the adrenaline solution. An incision is made inside the ear canal and the middle ear exposed by elevating the tympanic membrane forward. In order to obtain exposure of the stapes and footplate area, some of the posterior bony canal at the annulus is drilled or chiselled away.

Using the operating microscope, the otosclerotic foci on the footplate are broken down with small chisels and picks. When the surgeon considers the stapes is sufficiently mobile, the tympanic membrane is rolled back into position and the external ear packed with an antibiotic impregnated ribbon gauze or gelatine sponge.

Stapedectomy

Mobilisation of the stapes seldom gives permanent results as the stapes usually becomes fixed again. The favoured procedure is to remove the stapes, to seal off the oval window into the labyrinth with a piece of temporal fascia, vein, or gelatin sponge and to replace the stapes with a prosthesis such as a specially shaped polyethylene tube of suitable length, or a teflon piston, or a piece of stainless steel hooked over the incus.

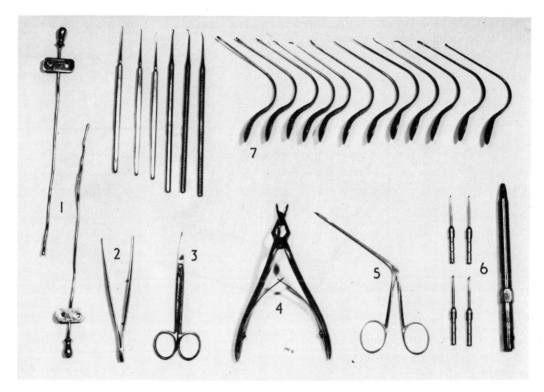

Figure 297   Fenestration, mobilisation of stapes, tympanoplasty.* See also appendix, page 589.

1. Irrigation cannulae.
2. Fine dissecting forceps, toothed.
3. Fine scissors, curved on flat, sharp points.
4. Gouge forceps (Jansen).
5. Malleus nipper.
6. Fine polishing burrs and dental hand-piece.
7. Fenestration picks and mobilisation instruments.

Fenestration

DEFINITION

The establishment of a fenestra or window in the horizontal semi-circular canal to re-establish sound conduction to the inner ear of a suitable patient suffering from otosclerosis.

POSITION

As for mobilisation of stapes.

INSTRUMENTS

As for mobilisation of stapes.

OUTLINE OF PROCEDURE

The initial stages of the operation are as for mastoidectomy through an endaural incision. The tympanic membrane and posterior wall of the membranous canal are fashioned into a flap which is turned back.

Utilising the operating microscope, a window is made with small polishing burrs in the horizontal semi-circular canal. The skin and tympanic membrane flap are positioned over the fenestra to transmit sound waves.

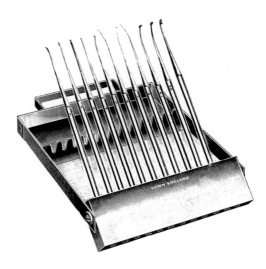

Figure 298   Instruments for Platinectomy and vein grafting. (Down Bros.)

The mastoid cavity is either packed with antibiotic impregnated ribbon gauze and skin grafted two weeks later, or a primary skin graft is performed as described for tympanoplasty.

Fenestration of the labyrinth is now only performed when stapedectomy is impossible for anatomical or pathological reasons. Continuous suction irrigation with a special sucrose-saline is advisable through special tubes attached to the mastoid retractor.

Tympanoplasty

DEFINITION

Repair of the ear drum by myringoplasty (a graft of temporal fascia, vein, fibrous fat or skin) and reconstruction of the ossicular chain with polyethylene, teflon, or stainless steel, or grafts of cartilage taken from the nasal septum, or bone chips, or sterile preserved ossicles taken from cadavers or other patients and preserved in the deep freeze.

POSITION

As for mobilisation of stapes.

INSTRUMENTS

As for mobilisation of stapes.
Skin graft knife or stout razor blade.

OUTLINE OF PROCEDURE

The incision area is infiltrated in the usual manner with 1 in 250,000 adrenaline solution and a modified endaural incision made.

The skin of the posterior canal wall and mastoid periosteum are elevated and a U-shaped flap reflected up from the anterior canal wall. The overhanging bone of the canal wall is removed with burrs or curettes, and the squamous epithelium scraped off the tympanic membrane and adjacent canal wall.

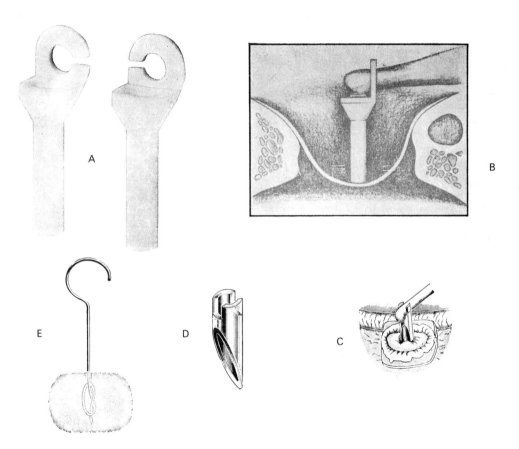

Figure 299 A & B.   Shea Teflon piston attached to tip of the incus with the lenticular process seated in a cup at the prosthesis head. By fitting on to the tip of the incus where the stapes was formerly attached, the prosthesis closely approximates the original angle to the oval window and provides a more normal reconstruction.

C. & D.   Shea slotted prosthesis.

E.   Prefabricated wire loop with gelatine sponge. (Down Bros. Ltd.)

An area of skin behind the ear is infiltrated with sterile saline, and a split-skin graft the size of the defect removed. The graft is trimmed to the approximate size and manoeuvred into position on the drum. The U-shaped flap is rotated back and the graft secured with gelatine sponge or small strips of antibiotic impregnated ribbon gauze over it.

The endaural incisions are closed and the external auditory canal packed in the usual manner so that an even pressure is applied to the graft.

Other Operations on the Middle and Inner Ear

Ménière's disease

DEFINITION

Surgical relief of Ménière's disease (attacks of rotational vertigo, tinnitus and deafness) after failure of conservative treatment. The best operation is division of the vestibular nerves without injuring the facial nerve or the cochlear nerve. This requires mastoidectomy instruments, operating microscope, diamond paste drills and a self-retaining dural retractor, such as de Martel's. This is a very difficult operation.

A much simpler and frequently successful procedure is to treat the vestibular labyrinth with ultra-sound. A mastoidectomy is done and a semi-circular canal of the labyrinth is drilled under continuous suction saline irrigation until the membranous labyrinth is almost exposed. Ultra-sound is then applied, 1 watt for 15 minutes; larger dosage or longer time may damage the facial nerve. An ultrasonic generator and transducer are required, and preferably also an electric thermometer to make sure that excessive heat does not damage the facial nerve.

Labyrinthectomy

The membranous labyrinth is removed either after drilling a semi-circular canal, or by suction through the oval window in a procedure similar to stapedectomy. This operation abolishes further attacks of vertigo, but produces total deafness in the operated ear. It is, therefore, used only when the ear is already very deaf. Other operations recommended for Ménière's disease are less successful.

Acoustic neuroma

DEFINITION

Removal of tumour of eighth cranial (acoustic and vestibular) nerve through the mastoid and labyrinth.

INSTRUMENTS

As for mastoidectomy and also stapedectomy type microscopic instruments; microscope; dental drill with diamond paste burrs, general surgery set to take fat from abdomen or thigh to seal cerebrospinal fluid leak.

OPERATIONS ON THE NOSE AND ACCESSORY SINUSES

Pre-operative nasal packing

DEFINITION

Packing of the nasal cavity before operation either to effect local anaesthesia (e.g., lignocaine (Xylocaine) 4 per cent) or to provide local vasoconstriction and haemostasis for the surgeon (e.g., 5 to 10 per cent cocaine solution with a very little adrenaline added. Too much adrenaline may cause ventricular fibrillation if halothane or trilene general anaesthesia is used).

POSITION. Supine.

INSTRUMENTS

Nasal specula (Thudichum), set
Nasal dressing forceps (Tilley or Wilde)
Roll of 25 mm (1 in) ribbon gauze
Lignocaine 4 per cent
Adrenaline 1 in 1000
Graduated measure, 15 ml ($\frac{1}{2}$ oz)
Head light, or head mirror and lamp
Towel or swab to protect the patient's lips.

OUTLINE OF PROCEDURE

The ribbon gauze is impregnated with solution, and one or both nasal cavities are packed, using a nasal speculum and dressing forceps. The ribbon gauze is first passed into the most posterior part of the cavity and successive layers are applied until it is filled. The pack is left in place for at least 15 minutes before operation, and is removed gently to avoid trauma of the nasal mucosa. Spraying the nose with 5 per cent cocaine first makes packing with ribbon gauze less unpleasant if the patient is conscious.

Reduction of a nasal fracture

DEFINITION

Anatomical re-alignment of a fractured nasal bone.

POSITION. Supine.

INSTRUMENTS

Nasal specula (Thudichum), set
Nasal dressing forceps (Tilley)
Nasal re-dressing or re-fracture forceps (Walsham)
Small mallet (Rowland), optional
25 mm (1 in) ribbon gauze which may be impregnated with petroleum jelly
Scissors, dressing
Stent material, and hot water in a small bowl
Adhesive strapping and a few small swabs.

OUTLINE OF PROCEDURE

If the injury is old the nasal bone may be re-fractured with the small mallet, utilising a swab to protect the skin.

One jaw of the Walsham's forceps is introduced into the nose and pressed against the nasal bone on the selected side. The other jaw provides counter-pressure against a swab placed on the outside of the nose.

The fragments of the nasal bone are manipulated into anatomical position and the nose is packed with ribbon gauze. A surface splint is fashioned from Stent by softening the material in hot water and moulding it into shape. This splint is retained in position on the outside of the nose with adhesive plaster.

Nasal polypectomy

DEFINITION

Removal of nasal polypi, either under general or local anaesthesia.

POSITION. Supine.

INSTRUMENTS

    Nasal specula (Thudichum), set
    Nasal specula (St Clair Thompson), set
    Nasal dressing forceps (Tilley or Wilde)
    Nasal snare, wire
    Punch forceps, small and large (Weil), 2
    25 mm (1 in) ribbon gauze impregnated with petroleum jelly
    Suction tubing and fine nozzles.

OUTLINE OF PROCEDURE

Using a nasal speculum, either the wire loop of the snare is manoeuvred around each polyp in turn and withdrawn, bringing the excised polyp with it; or the Weil's forceps are used to grasp and remove each polyp with a twisting action. Packing the nasal cavity or cavities completes the operation.

Turbinotomy or turbinectomy

DEFINITION

The removal of part of all of a hypertrophied nasal turbinate bone.

POSITION. Supine.

INSTRUMENTS

    Nasal specula (Thudichum), set
    Nasal specula (St Clair Thompson), set
    Nasal dressing forceps (Tilley or Wilde)
    Nasal snare, wire
    Punch forceps, small and medium (Weil or Luc), 2
    Nasal scissors, angled (Heymann)
    25 mm (1 in) ribbon gauze impregnated with petroleum jelly
    Suction tubing, fine nozzles and Robin tube anchoring forceps.

OUTLINE OF PROCEDURE

Using a nasal speculum, the surgeon inserts the angled scissors and divides the turbinate bone along its base for a short distance. The wire snare is inserted and the loop passed over the turbinal with the barrel of the snare lying along the cut made. The snare is withdrawn and the enlarged portion of the turbinal removed with forceps.

    The nasal cavity or cavities are packed with ribbon gauze in the usual manner.

Submucous resection of the nasal septum

DEFINITION

The removal of a deflected nasal septum to rectify an obstructed airway.

POSITION. Supine.

INSTRUMENTS

    S.M.R. set (Fig. 300)
    Sponge-holding forceps (Rampley), 5

Scalpel handles No. 3 with No. 10 and No. 15 blades (Bard Parker), 2
Towel clips, 5
Probe, malleable silver
Small retractors, single hook, 2
Mallet (Heath)
Tongue forceps (Mayo)

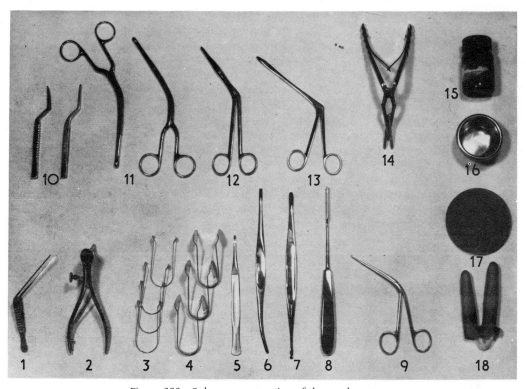

Figure 300   Submucous resection of the nasal septum.

1. Dressing forceps, angled (Wilde).
2. Nasal speculum, self-retaining (Killian).
3. Small nasal specula (Thudichum), set of 4.
4. Long nasal specula (St Clair Thompson), set of 3.
5. Nasal knife (Dundas Grant).
6. Nasal raspatory (Hill).
7. Nasal raspatory (Howarth).
8. Swivel knife (Ballenger).
9. Dressing forceps, angled (Tilley).
10. Nasal gouges, angled (Tilley and Killian).
11. Punch forceps (Luc), medium and small.
12. Nasal scissors, angled (Heymann).
13. Punch forceps (Weil).
14. Nasal septum forceps (Jansen Middleton).
15. B.I.P.P. (optional).
16. Lubricant in gallipot, e.g., liquid paraffin.
17. Stent impression material for nasal splint.
18. Rubber glove fingers for nasal pack (distended with ribbon gauze).

Mouth gag (Mason)
Angled tongue depressor
Suction tubing, fine nozzles and tube anchoring forceps
Needle holder (Kilner multiple joint)
Fine dissecting forceps, toothed (Gillies)
2 (3/0) Chromic catgut or Dexon on a small half-circle cutting needle for mucosa sutures.

OUTLINE OF PROCEDURE

A small incision is made at the junction of the skin and mucous membrane on one side of the nasal septum. A Thudichum's nasal speculum is inserted, and using a long raspatory through this incision, the mucoperichondrium is dissected free from the septum along one side.

An incision is then made through the cartilage along the line of the original incision and the raspatory introduced to strip off the mucoperichondrium on the other side of the septum. Care is taken not to puncture the mucosa on this side. The small nasal speculum is changed for a longer one (St Clair Thompson's), which is inserted so that the blades pass between the nasal septum and mucosa on each side. This separates the mucosa away from the septum and the cut edge of the septal cartilage lies in the centre of the speculum.

As much as possible of the cartilage is removed with a Ballenger's swivel knife, which is first passed backwards and then downwards, and finally forwards. Pieces of the vomer and vertical plate of the ethmoid are removed with punch forceps and the irregular spur which is usually present along the lower edge of the septum is removed with an angled gouge. The long speculum is removed and the tubinates are examined, using a Thudichum's speculum. If these are hypertrophied, a turbinotomy or turbinectomy may be performed.

Some surgeons suture the mucosal incision before inserting two rubber glove fingers (one in each nostril) which have been packed with petroleum jelly gauze.

Antrostomy (intranasal operation)

DEFINITION

An intranasal opening into the maxillary antrum performed for chronic suppuration.

POSITION. Supine.

INSTRUMENTS

Sponge-holding forceps (Rampley), 5
Scalpel handle No. 3 with No. 15 blade (Bard Parker)
Towel clips, 5
Nasal specula (Thudichum), set
Nasal specula (St Clair Thompson), set
Nasal dressing forceps (Tilley or Wilde)
Nasal snare, wire
Punch forceps, small and medium (Luc)
Punch forceps, small and medium (Weil)
Antrum trocar and cannula
Antrum harpoon (Tilley)
Antrum burr (Tilley)
Dissector (Hill)
Angled nasal scissors (Heymann)
Antrum punch forceps (Citelli)
Curetting spoon (Volkmann)
Probe
Small gouges, 4 mm, 6 mm, 8 mm (Jenkins)
Mallet (Heath)
Irrigation syringe and warm saline

Suction tubing, nozzles and tube anchoring forceps
(Two rubber glove fingers distended with petroleum jelly ribbon gauze may be
    required.)

OUTLINE OF PROCEDURE

The simplest operation consists of inserting an antrum trocar and cannula through
the lateral nasal wall and into the antrum. The antrum is then irrigated and the cannula
removed (antrum wash-out or lavage). Care should be taken to ensure there is no air in
the Higginson syringe which could cause air embolism.

A more extensive operation consists of performing a turbinectomy or turbinotomy
(removing the anterior end of the inferior turbinate), followed by the insertion of an
antrum harpoon, or using small gouges to make an opening through the lateral nasal
wall into the antrum. This opening is then enlarged with a burr and punch forceps,
followed finally by irrigation of the antrum with warm saline. The nasal cavity may be
packed, using two rubber glove fingers as previously described.

Radical antrostomy or Caldwell Luc operation

DEFINITION

An opening into the antrum through the mouth and superior maxilla, and the nose.

POSITION

Supine, with the head thrown back.

INSTRUMENTS

Caldwell Luc set (Fig. 301)
Sponge-holding forceps (Rampley), 5
Scalpel handle No. 3 with Nos. 10 and 15 blades (Bard Parker)
Towel clips, 5
Scissors, curved on flat, 13 cm (5 in) (Mayo)
Scissors, stitch, 13 cm (5 in)
Medium retractors, malleable copper, 2
Angled tongue depressor
Mouth gag (Mason)
Tongue forceps (Mayo)
Needle holder (Kilner multiple joint)
Dissecting forceps, toothed (Lane), 2
Dissecting forceps, non-toothed, 13 cm (5 in), 2
Curetting spoon (Volkmann)
Irrigation syringe and warm saline
Antrum trocar and cannula
Suction tubing, nozzles and tube anchoring forceps
3 or 2·5 (0 or 2/0) Chromic catgut, Dexon or silk on a small half-circle round-bodied
    needle for mucosa suture.

OUTLINE OF PROCEDURE

The anterior end of the inferior turbinate is removed as previously described above,
and the nasal cavity is packed with ribbon gauze impregnated with adrenaline 1 in 1000
or less.

The upper lip on the affected side is retracted upwards and an incision made in the mucosa lying over the superior maxilla. The mucous membrane is reflected from the surface of the bone, and the anterior wall of the antrum is removed, using the harpoon followed by a small gouge or punch forceps.

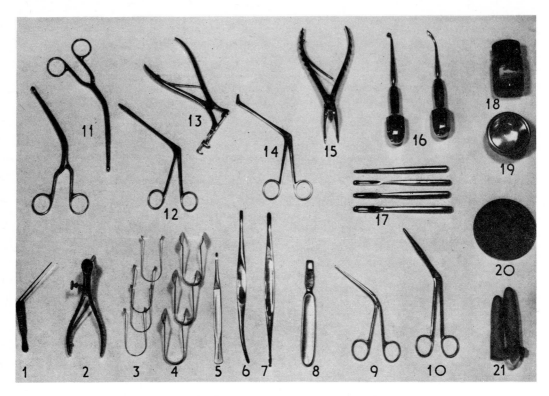

Figure 301   Caldwell Luc or radical antrostomy.

1. Dressing forceps, angled (Wilde).
2. Nasal speculum, self-retaining (Killian).
3. Small nasal specula (Thudichum), set of 4.
4. Long nasal specula (St Clair Thompson), set of 3.
5. Nasal knife (Dundas Grant).
6. Nasal raspatory (Hill).
7. Nasal raspatory (Howarth).
8. Rugine (Faraboeuf).
9. Dressing forceps, angled (Tilley).
10. Nasal scissors, angled (Heymann).
11. Punch forceps (Luc), large and medium.
12. Punch forceps (Weil).
13. Gouge or punch forceps (Citelli).
14. Nasal punch forceps (Grunwald).
15. Gouge forceps (Jansen).
16. Antrum harpoon and burr (Tilley).
17. Small gouges (Jenkins), 4 mm, 6 mm, 8 mm and 10 mm, 4.
18. B.I.P.P. (optional).
19. Lubricant in gallipot, e.g., liquid paraffin.
20. Stent impression material (optional).
21. Rubber glove fingers for nasal pack (distended with ribbon gauze).

Any polypoid inflammatory material in the antrum is scraped away, and the cavity is irrigated with warm saline. The cavity may then be packed with B.I.P.P. ribbon gauze, and the opening in the gum closed with catgut sutures.

The surgeon then proceeds to perform an intranasal antrostomy as previously described, to provide an opening for drainage and irrigation when the oral opening is finally closed. Some surgeons perform this procedure from within the antrum, after the superior maxilla has been opened.

OPERATIONS ON THE FRONTAL SINUS

Ethmoidectomy (intranasal operation)

DEFINITION
Removal of the anterior wall of the ethmoidal labyrinth and ethmoidal cells for chronic inflammatory conditions and to prevent recurrence of polypi.

POSITION. Supine.

INSTRUMENTS
As for submucous resection
Frontal sinus probe
Frontal sinus curette.

OUTLINE OF PROCEDURE
A submucous resection of the nasal septum may be performed to provide better access to the ethmoidal labyrinth.

Basically, the operation consists of removing the ethmoid cells which lie around the passage leading from the nasal cavity to the frontal sinus. The operation is performed almost entirely with a long nasal speculum, frontal sinus probe, punch forceps, such as Luc's and the frontal sinus curette.

Sphenoidectomy (intranasal operation)

DEFINITION
Removal of the lining from the sphenoidal sinuses for chronic inflammatory conditions.

POSITION
As ethmoidectomy.

INSTRUMENTS
As ethmoidectomy.

OUTLINE OF PROCEDURE
This is a similar operation to that described under intranasal ethmoidectomy, but in this case the clearance is carried out to a higher and more posterior limit to clear-out the diseased sphenoidal sinuses.

Fronto-Ethmoidectomy (Killian's operation)

DEFINITION
An opening made into the frontal sinus through an incision above the orbit, and removal of diseased ethmoid cells.

POSITION. Supine.

INSTRUMENTS
Sponge-holding forceps (Rampley), 5
Towel clips, 5

Scalpel handles No. 3 with Nos. 10 and 15 blades (Bard Parker), 2
Dissecting forceps, toothed (Gillies and Lane), 2
Dissecting forceps, non-toothed, 13 cm (5 in), 2
Small retractors, double hook, 2
Retractors, self-retaining (Mayo hinged and West straight), 2
Fine artery forceps, curved on flat, mosquito, 10
Fine tissue forceps (McIndoe), 5
Skin hooks (Gillies), 2
Scissors, curved on flat, 13 cm (5 in) (Mayo)
Fine scissors, curved, 10 cm (4 in) (Kilner)
Scissors, stitch, 13 cm (5 in)
Small rugines, curved and straight (Faraboeuf), 2
Bone-nibbling forceps, curved on flat
Frontal sinus punch forceps (Citelli)
Punch forceps, small and medium (Luc)
Frontal sinus rasps (Watson-Jones), set of 3
Frontal sinus curette
Nasal specula (St Clair Thompson), set
Nasal dressing forceps (Tilley)
Small gouges, 4 mm, 6 mm, 8 mm and 10 mm (Jenkins), 4
Mallet (Heath)
Needle holder (Kilner multiple joint, or Gillies)
Suction tubing, fine nozzles and tube anchoring forceps
2 (3/0) Plain catgut or Dexon for ligatures
2 and 2·5 (3/0 and 2/0) Chromic catgut or Dexon on small half-circle round-bodied
    needles for subcutaneous sutures
1·5 (4/0) Silk or nylon on a small curved cutting needle for skin sutures.

OUTLINE OF PROCEDURE

An incision is made over the supra-orbital margin in line with the eyebrow, and it
extends slightly down towards the nose. The skin flap is reflected together with the
periosteum overlying the frontal sinus.

An opening is made into the sinuses with gouges, and this is enlarged with punch
forceps. Care is taken to leave the supra-orbital margin by gouging above and below
this ridge, which if removed would result in deformity or spread of infection to cancellous bone. The lining is removed from the ethmoid and frontal sinuses and sometimes
also from the sphenoid sinus and it may be removed also from the maxillary antrum by
extending the incision downwards a little alongside the nose (Patterson's approach).

A plastic or rubber tube may be inserted between the cavity and the nose, being left
to protrude at one end from the nostril, where it is secured with a suture. Haemostasis
is secured and the subcutaneous tissues approximated before closing the skin with fine
silk or nylon sutures.

OPERATIONS ON THE THROAT AND MOUTH

Direct laryngoscopy

DEFINITION

Direct examination of the larynx with an endoscope which places the mouth, pharynx
and larynx in a straight line (the Boyce position).

POSITION. Supine.

INSTRUMENTS

Laryngoscope with appropriate size of blade (Mackintosh, Magill or Chevalier Jackson, etc.)
Tongue forceps (Mayo)
Angled tongue depressor
Laryngeal swab holders and small mops
Laryngeal biopsy forceps
Adrenaline 1 in 1000
Graduated measure
Suction tubing, nozzles and tube anchoring forceps
Diathermy leads, electrodes and lead anchoring forceps.

OUTLINE OF PROCEDURE

The patient is anaesthetised and, with his neck in a position of extension with the head well thrown back, the laryngoscope is inserted. A biopsy may be taken with the biopsy forceps and the area swabbed with small mops soaked in adrenaline solution, or diathermised.

For bronchoscopy and oesophagoscopy, see chapter on Thoracic Operations.

Peritonsillar abscess or quinsy

DEFINITION

An abscess between the anterior pillar of the fauces and the tonsil (in the peritonsillar space).

POSITION

Sitting, facing the surgeon, or lateral position with the table in slight Trendelenburg.

INSTRUMENTS

Scalpel handle No. 3 with No. 15 blade (Bard Parker) wrapped with adhesive plaster, tip only exposed
Sponge-holding forceps (Rampley) and small sponges or swabs, 5
Mouth gag (Mason or Doyen)
Tongue forceps (Mayo)
Angled tongue depressor
Scissors, straight with sharp outer edges
Pharyngeal spray and 4 per cent lignocaine
Sterile throat swab
Mouth washes (used with great caution and with patient bending forwards).

OUTLINE OF PROCEDURE

A little topical local anaesthesia is generally employed. An incision is made with the guarded knife through the maximum bulge in the soft palate, parallel with the posterior margin and extending approximately about 2 cm inwards from the anterior pillar of the fauces. Scissors with a sharp outer edge are introduced quickly into the incision and separated.

Tonsillectomy and adenoidectomy

DEFINITION
Enucleation of the tonsils either by dissection or guillotine, and curetting of the adenoids.

POSITION
Dissection. Supine, with the head and neck in extension. A 'jack' may be used to support the mouth gag during operation. One of the best gag supporters is two Draffin poles, one on each side, resting on the operating table, thus leaving the patient's chest unobstructed. Adenoidectomy as below. *Guillotine:* First supine with the head to one side, and then lateral for the adenoidectomy.

INSTRUMENTS
As for tonsillectomy (Fig. 302)

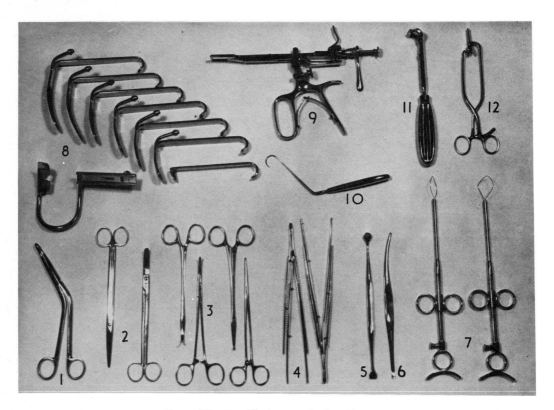

Figure 302   Tonsillectomy and adenoidectomy.

1. Tonsil-holding forceps (Denis Browne).
2. Tonsil scissors, curved and straight.
3. Tonsil artery forceps, curved and straight.
4. Long, fine dissecting forceps, toothed and non-toothed (Waugh).
5. Tonsil dissector and pillar retractor (Beavis).
6. Dissector (Hill).
7. Tonsil snare (Eve).
8. Mouth gag and blades (Boyle-Davis).
9. Haemostatic tonsil guillotine.
10. Tonsil ligature needle.
11. Adenoid curette (St Clair Thompson).
12. Tonsil-compressing forceps (Courtenay Yorke).

Sponge-holding forceps (Rampley), 5
Towel clips, 5
Mouth gag (Mason)
Tongue forceps (Mayo)
Angled tongue depressor
Suction tubing, nozzles and tube anchoring forceps
2 (3/0) Silk, linen thread, catgut, or Dexon for ligatures
Adrenaline 1 in 1000 (optional)
Graduated measure
Iced water.

OUTLINE OF PROCEDURE

Dissecting Operation. A Boyle-Davis mouth gag is inserted and if an endotracheal tube has not been placed in position, the anaesthetic gases are conveyed to the back of the pharynx through a tube attached to the side of the tongue blade.

The tonsil is grasped with holding forceps and drawn inwards, exposing the anterior pillar of the fauces. Using curved scissors, or a dissector, an incision is made through the mucous membrane at the junction between the tonsil and the anterior pillar. The tonsil is freed by blunt dissection, first at the upper part and then the lower, clamping any vessels which may be seen bleeding as the dissection proceeds. After the tonsil has been removed, other bleeding vessels are clamped and tied, or under-run and tied with silk or linen thread. The other tonsil is removed in a similar manner and both tonsil beds are inspected for complete haemostasis before the gag is removed.

If the adenoids are to be removed the patient is turned on his side.

Guillotine Operation. A mouth gag is inserted and the tongue grasped with tongue forceps. The guillotine is passed into the mouth and the right tonsil positioned in the ring. With the haemostatic type instrument (tonsil enucleator), the clamp mechanism is closed to crush the tonsil 'pedicle' for about 20 seconds before depressing the knife blade to separate the tonsil from its bed. With the simple type instrument, when the tonsil has been pressed well into the ring, the knife blade is depressed and the tonsil removed by a slight twist of the guillotine. The second tonsil is removed, and compression clamps are applied to a taped swab in each tonsil fossa. The child is immediately turned on its side for removal of the adenoids. The guillotine operation is now less common than dissection.

Adenoidectomy. The adenoids are removed with a curette which is passed behind the soft palate, pressed hard against the posterior pharyngeal wall, and moved in a downwards sweeping action. Care is taken to avoid damage to the mucosa of the posterior pharyngeal space.

The patient's face and neck are bathed with ice-cold water, and if haemorrhage persists a Boyle-Davis gag may be inserted for further inspection of the tonsil fossae.

Tracheostomy

DEFINITION

The establishment of an opening into the trachea below the larynx, and the insertion of a tube for the purpose of supplying an airway.

POSITION

Supine, with a sandbag between the shoulder blades, neck extended, with the head thrown well back and the chin in the midline (Fig. 67).

INSTRUMENTS

As for tracheostomy (Fig. 303)
Sponge-holding forceps (Rampley), 5
Towel clips, 5
Needle holder (Kilner)
Suction tubing, nozzles and tube anchoring forceps
2·5 and 3 (2/0 and 0) Chromic catgut or Dexon for ligatures
3 (0) Chromic catgut or Dexon on a small half-circle round-bodied needle for muscle sutures

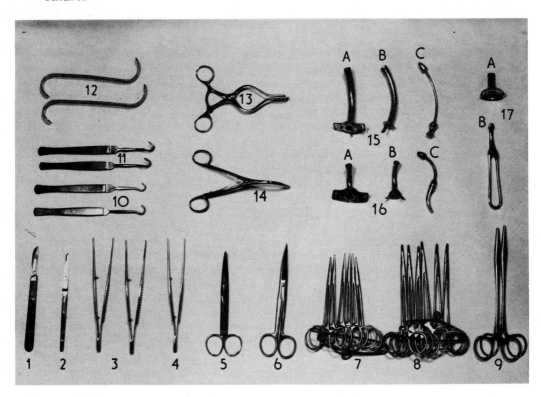

Figure 303   Tracheostomy or laryngostomy.

1. Scalpel handle No. 3 with No. 10 blade (Bard Parker).
2. Scalpel handle No. 9 with No. 15 blade (Bard Parker).
3. Fine dissecting forceps, toothed (Gillies), 2.
4. Fine dissecting forceps, non-toothed (McIndoe), 1.
5. Scissors, curved on flat, 13 cm (5 in) (Mayo).
6. Scissors, stitch.
7. Fine artery forceps, straight, mosquito, 6.
8. Fine artery forceps, curved on flat, mosquito, 6.
9. Artery forceps, straight, 18 cm (7 in) (Spencer Wells), 2.
10. Small retractors, sharp and blunt, single hook, 2.
11. Small retractors, double hook, 2.
12. Medium retractors, malleable copper.
13. Retractor, self-retaining (West).
14. Tracheal dilating forceps (Bowlby or Trouseau).
15. Long tracheostomy tubes (Chevalier Jackson), assorted sizes. A, outer tube; B, inner tube; C, pilot or introducer.
16. Medium tracheostomy tubes (Parker), assorted sizes. A, outer tube; B, inner tube; C, pilot or introducer.
17. Laryngotomy tube (Butlin), 3 sizes. A, tube; B, pilot or introducer.

2 (3/0) Silk or nylon on a small curved cutting needle for skin sutures
(Local anaesthetic requisites (Fig. 271) may be required.)

OUTLINE OF PROCEDURE

This operation is often performed with extreme urgency. The patient may have a
general or local anaesthetic, and sometimes none whatsoever, especially if he is unconscious. Although the operation may be performed for obstruction due to foreign
bodies or laryngeal stridor (and could then be termed *tracheotomy*), many surgeons
like to use it as a routine for the unconscious patient suffering from a serious head injury
and some jaw injuries.

A tracheostomy set of tubes and instruments arranged in the correct order of use
should be kept sterile and ready in all operating theatres. It is important that the tapes
are ready attached to the outer tubes, as many valuable minutes may be lost placing
these in position during operation.

It is important that the head and neck are maintained perfectly in the midline during
the whole of the operation. A vertical midline incision is made over the upper part of
the trachea just below the cricoid cartilage. The incision is extended through the deep
fascia, and the sternothyroid and hyoid muscles retracted laterally.

The isthmus of the thyroid gland is either clamped across, divided and ligated, or
displaced. Another layer of fascia is incised, the cricoid cartilage steadied with a single
sharp hook, and the trachea is opened through a vertical stab wound which divides
about two rings of cartilage. The tracheal dilators are inserted into this incision, separated,
and a tracheal tube inserted. Some surgeons cut a small flap of cartilage when making
their incision in order to accommodate the circumference of the tube better, especially
the cuffed, rubber variety (which may be used as an alternative to those illustrated).
This cartilage flap is sutured to the skin to prevent it slipping back accidentally into the
trachea should the tube become displaced.

A few sutures of catgut may be required to approximate the muscles around the
tube, and the skin is closed in the usual manner. The tapes are secured round the neck
and a dressing of tulle gras applied under the tube flange.

Laryngofissure

DEFINITION

An opening through the thyroid cartilage into the larynx to remove a tumour or
tumours.

POSITION

As for tracheostomy.

INSTRUMENTS

General set (Fig. 281)
Laryngofissure and laryngectomy set (Fig. 304)
Tongue forceps (Mayo)
Angled tongue depressor
Mouth gag (Mason)
Suction tubing, nozzles and tube anchoring forceps
Diathermy leads, electrodes and lead anchoring forceps
Connection and tubing for anaesthetic machine
Corrugated rubber or plastic drainage tubing

2·5, 3 and 4 (2/0, 0 and 1) Chromic catgut or Dexon for ligatures

2·5 and 4 (2/0 and 1) Chromic catgut or Dexon (or stainless-steel wire) on medium half-circle cutting and round-bodied needles for larynx and muscle sutures

2·5 or 2 (2/0 or 3/0) Silk or nylon on a medium curved cutting needle for.skin sutures.

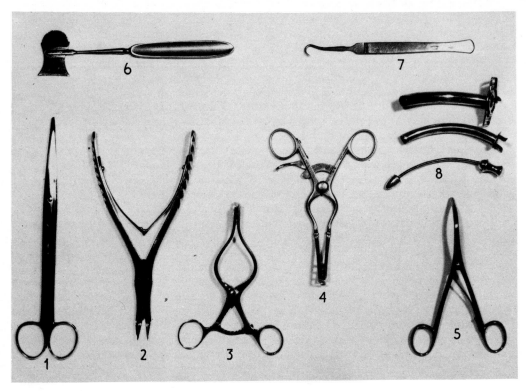

Figure 304   Laryngofissure or laryngectomy.

1. Scissors, straight 20 cm (8 in) (Mayo).
2. McIndoe bone cutting forceps.
3. Retractor, self-retaining (West).
4. Retractor, self-retaining (Mayo, angled).
5. Tracheal dilators (Bowlby or Trouseau).
6. Cartilage saw.
7. Small retractor, sharp single hook.
8. Long tracheostomy tube (Chevalier Jackson, large size).

OUTLINE OF PROCEDURE

A preliminary tracheostomy may have been performed. A midline incision is made from the hyoid bone to the cricoid cartilage. Soft tissues are retracted and the thyroid cartilage divided with shears or a cartilage saw, care being taken to divide the mucous membrane of the larynx in the midline. (This is to avoid damage to the vocal cords.) The cut edges of the cartilage are retracted to expose the interior of the larynx. The tumour is excised, haemostasis secured with diathermy, and the wound closed in layers, with drainage. Stainless-steel wire or chromic catgut is used to close the larynx.

Laryngectomy

DEFINITION

Removal of the entire larynx, and establishment of a permanent tracheostomy.

POSITION
As for laryngofissure.

INSTRUMENTS
As for laryngofissure
Silk may be used in preference to catgut sutures for the deep closure.

OUTLINE OF PROCEDURE
A midline incision is made from the hyoid bone to the cricoid cartilage. The body of the hyoid bone may be divided in the midline and the ends retracted.

The muscle attachments at the sides of the larynx are freed and the trachea is severed. The endotracheal tube is withdrawn, and a wide tracheostomy tube (wrapped with tulle gras) is inserted and connected to the anaesthetic machine.

The larynx is elevated and freed, clamping the vessels as dissection proceeds. The pharynx is then opened and the larynx removed. When haemostasis is complete, the pharnyx is closed with interrupted chromic catgut, Dexon or silk sutures.

The incision is closed, with drainage, and the skin margins in the lower part of the wound are sutured around the tracheal opening.

There are a variety of post-laryngectomy tracheostomy tubes (e.g., Lombard's, which is metallic), but a very satisfactory tube can be fashioned from the lower 6 cm (2·5 in) or so of a size 10 Magill endotracheal tube with a safety pin put across it. If the rubber produces skin irritation, a plastic tube can be used. In laryngectomy and pharyngo-laryngectomy a nasogastric feeding tube is passed either beforehand in the ward, or towards the end of the operation in the theatre.

Partial amputation of the tongue

DEFINITION
Removal of varying amounts of the tongue for carcinoma, but usually not less than half when the growth is limited to one side. Radical dissection of the cervical glands (Chapter 20) will also be performed, either before, during, or after this operation.

POSITION. Supine.

INSTRUMENTS
As for tracheostomy
General set (Fig. 281)
Mouth gag (Doyen or Mason)
Tongue forceps (Mayo)
Angled tongue depressor
Fine artery forceps, curved on flat, mosquito, 10
Fine artery forceps, straight, mosquito, 10
Fine tissue forceps (McIndoe), 5
Suction tubing, nozzles and tube anchoring forceps
Diathermy leads, electrodes and lead anchoring forceps
2 and 2·5 (3/0 and 2/9) Chromic catgut or Dexon for ligatures
2·5 and 3 (2/0 and 0) Chromic catgut or Dexon on small half-circle round-bodied needles for sutures
3 (0) Silk on a medium half-circle round-bodied needle for stay sutures.

OUTLINE OF PROCEDURE

A preliminary tracheostomy is performed and the pharynx packed with ribbon gauze. Three stay sutures are inserted into the tongue and left long. One of the sutures is placed behind the growth and the other two at each side of the tip of the tongue.

The mucous membrane on the floor of the mouth is freed and the tongue split longitudinally down the centre. The tongue is freed from the hyoid bone and the posterior postion divided across well behind the growth. Any blood-vessels seen during dissection are picked up with artery forceps and ligated or under-run, if possible before they are divided. Haemostasis may be achieved also with diathermy.

The cut edge of the tongue is sutured and the mucous membrane approximated also if possible.

Partial excision of the jaw

DEFINITION

Partial removal of the mandible for malignancy. This operation is usually combined with radical dissection of the cervical glands (Chapter 20).

POSITION

Supine, with sandbag between the shoulder blades, neck extended, and head thrown well back, with the chin central and in the midline.

INSTRUMENTS

As for partial amputation of the tongue
Wire saw and handles (Gigli or Olivecrona)
Saw guide (de Martel)
Jaw saw (Wood)
Bone awls, set
Bone-nibbling forceps, small and medium, 2
Bone-cutting forceps (Liston)
Bone-cutting forceps (Horsley compound action)
Small rugines, curved and straight (Faraboeuf), 2
Bone-holding forceps (St Thomas)
Ligatures as for partial amputation of the tongue, plus 2/0 and 0 Silk.

OUTLINE OF PROCEDURE

An L-shaped or T-shaped incision is made over the neck and lower mandible. Radical dissection of the cervical glands is carried out and the muscles attached to the mandible are freed. The tongue and the parotid gland are retracted and the portion of the jaw to be removed is divided with a saw. The bone is disarticulated from the joint and resected.

The wound is closed in layers with drainage in the usual manner. If the mucosa cannot be approximated, the wound will be partially packed and an intra-oral or buccal skin graft will be performed at a later date by the plastic surgeon. In order to restore the facial contours after such an extensive excision, the dental surgeon may co-operate with the otolaryngologist and plastic surgeon to provide a prosthesis, which will also help to maintain the graft in position during healing.

Operations on the Face

Excision of superficial ulcer of the face

DEFINITION

The removal of a superficial dermal ulcer.

POSITION. Supine.

INSTRUMENTS

Sponge-holding forceps (Rampley), 2
Towel clips, 4
Scalpel handles Nos. 3 and 9 with Nos. 10 and 15 blades (Bard Parker)
Fine dissecting forceps, toothed (Gillies), 2
Fine dissecting forceps, non-toothed (McIndoe), 2
Scissors, curved 10 cm (4 in) (Kilner or strabismus)
Fine pointed scissors, curved (Iris)
Fine double-hook retractors, 2
Skin hooks (Gillies or Kilner), 2
Fine tissue forceps (McIndoe), 4
Artery forceps, straight, mosquito, 5 to 10.
Artery forceps, curved on flat, mosquito, 5 to 10
Fine needle holder (Gillies, Kilner, etc.)
2 and 1·5 (3/0 and 4/0) Plain catgut or Dexon for ligatures
2 (3/0) Plain catgut or Dexon on a small curved round-bodied needle for fat sutures
1·5 or 1 (4/0 or 5/0) Silk or nylon on a small curved non-traumatic cutting needle for skin sutures
(Skin graft instruments may be required (Fig. 359).)

OUTLINE OF PROCEDURE

An elliptical incision is made following the facial lines and with the ulcer in the centre of the ellipse. The ulcerated skin is dissected free and the surrounding skin flaps undermined. If the skin can be approximated, it is closed with fine interrupted sutures; if it cannot, a skin flap is rotated or a split-skin graft performed, using a soft textured graft such as that which can be obtained from the inner aspect of the upper arm.

Removal of sebaceous or dermoid cysts, naevi, etc.

This is similar to the operation above but with the addition of the following instruments:
Dissector (MacDonald or Durham)
Double-end curetting spoon (Volkmann)
Medium retractors, double hook, 2.

Catheter sizes compared (Figs. 305, 306)

Catheters, bougies and sounds are made in three sizes, English, Charrière and Béniqué. The English gauge varies 0·5 mm between each size, and the Charrière gauge 0·33 mm in

Catheter sizes compared. (J. G. Franklin & Sons Ltd.)

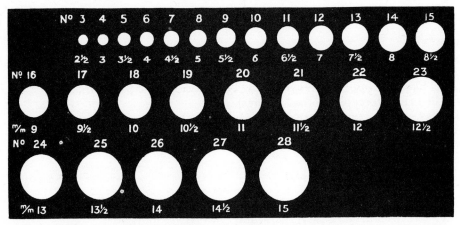

Figure 305   English catheter gauge.

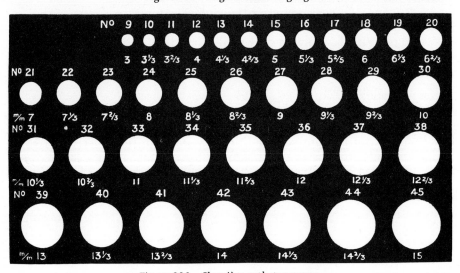

Figure 306   Charrière catheter gauge.

diameter between each size – e.g., English gauge No. 8 is equivalent to 5 mm, No. 9 equals 5·5 mm, and No. 10 equals 6 mm; Charrière gauge No. 15 is equivalent to 5 mm, No. 16 equals 5·5 mm, No. 17 equals 5·66 mm and No. 18 equals 6 mm.

It is worth remembering that Béniqué gauge is double Charrière gauge numbers throughout, and Béniqué gauge is treble the English gauge numbers plus 6 throughout – e.g., No. 12 English gauge equals $12 \times 3 + 6 = 42$ Béniqué gauge = 21 Charrière gauge.

Bougies, catheters and sounds (Fig. 307)

These are available in a number of materials – rubber, plastic, metal (silver or stainless steel). Some catheters have one lumen whereas other have several for the purpose of irrigation.

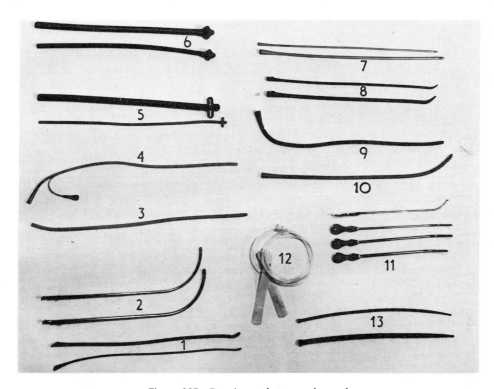

Figure 307   Bougies, catheters and sounds.

1. Catheters, coudée and bi-coudée, gum elastic.
2. Catheters, metal, silver.
3. Catheter (Jaques or Nélaton), rubber.
4. Catheter, self-retaining (Foley, inflatable balloon), rubber.
5. Catheters, self-retaining (Malecot), rubber.
6. Catheters, self-retaining (De Pezzer), rubber.
7. Catheters (Nélaton), plastic.
8. Catheter (Tiemann or Marshall), rubber.
9. Catheter (Harris, two eyes), rubber.
10. Catheter (whistle tip, oblique terminal opening and two eyes), rubber.
11. Bladder sounds or bougies (Clutton), stainless-steel.
12. Catheter (Gibbon), and retaining strap, plastic.
13. Bladder sounds or bougies, plastic.

Catheters may be obtained with inflatable cuffs or balloons at their distal tip which prevent accidental withdrawal. Full details of care and sterilisation of catheters is given in Chapter 6.

Circumcision

DEFINITION
Partial excision of the penile foreskin.

POSITION. Supine.

INSTRUMENTS
Scalpel handle No. 3 with No. 10 blade (Bard Parker)
Fine dissecting forceps, toothed (Gillies)
Fine dissecting forceps, non-toothed (McIndoe)
Probe, malleable silver
Artery forceps, straight, 18 cm (7 in) (Spencer Wells) *or*
Bone cutters or sinus forceps
Scissors, straight, blunt points (Mayo 13 or 15 cm (5 or 6 in))
Fine scissors, curved on flat, dissection points (Kilner)
Fine artery forceps, straight, mosquito, 5
2 (3/0) Chromic catgut or Dexon for ligatures
2 (3/0) Chromic catgut or Dexon on a small curved cutting needle, preferably non-traumatic, for prepuce sutures
Dressing of gauze impregnated with petroleum jelly Tinct. Benz. Co., or Whiteheads varnish.

OUTLINE OF PROCEDURE
Two artery forceps are clipped to each side of the prepuce opening, and a probe inserted to separate the glans from the prepuce. More traction is applied to the foreskin and a pair of artery forceps or bone cutters is placed obliquely across the prepuce, but distal to the underlying glans. The excess foreskin is excised with a knife and the cut edge allowed to retract. The inner layer of the prepuce has to be slit up the dorsum of the penis to the glans and the redundant piece of skin excised. Any bleeding vessels are picked up and ligated before the cut edge of the skin is sutured to the inner layer of the prepuce.

Radical amputation of the penis

DEFINITION
Complete removal of the penis, and the lymphatic glands in the groin for malignancy.

POSITION
Supine, with the legs separated, and then lithotomy.

INSTRUMENTS
General set (Fig. 281)
Bladder sounds (Lister, Clutton, etc.) set
Urethral catheter, self-retaining (Foley size 18 to 20 Charrière gauge)
20 ml syringe and sterile water for inflating cuff of catheter
Catheter lubricant
Diathermy leads, electrodes and lead anchoring forceps
2·5 and 3 (2/0 and 0) Chromic catgut, Dexon or silk for ligatures
2 (3/0) Chromic catgut or Dexon on a small curved non-traumatic round-bodied needle for urethral suture

3 or 4 (0 or 1) Chromic catgut or Dexon on a medium half-circle round-bodied needle
    for muscle sutures
2·5 (2/0) Silk or nylon on a medium curved cutting needle for skin sutures
(Corrugated drain may be required.)

OUTLINE OF PROCEDURE

An incision, slightly convex downwards, is made just below the inguinal ligament on
both sides. The skin flaps are reflected to expose Scarpa's triangle, and the superficial fat,
fascia and glands are dissected out right down to the femoral vessels. The mass is reflected towards the pubis and left attached by a thin pedicle for subsequent removal with
the penis. A corrugated drain may be inserted and the wounds partially sutured.

The legs are separated or the patient is placed into lithotomy position, and a bladder
sound is inserted. The urethra, exposed through an incision in the perineum, is dissected
free from the corpora cavernosa, and divided at a point about one and a half inches
from where it emerges from the perineum. The two corpora cavernosa are severed from
the rami of the pubis, and the arteries to the penis ligated. The skin incision is continued forwards across the scrotum to the root of the penis which it encircles. The
scrotum and testicles are dissected away from the penis, and the skin incision around its
base is continued up to join the two groin incisions. The skin flaps are reflected and the
penis removed together with the mass of glands from each groin.

The skin incisions are closed, with the urethra split and sutured to the posterior end
of the wound. A self-retaining catheter is inserted as a temporary measure.

Excision of hydrocele or encysted hydrocele of the cord

DEFINITION

Removal of a hydrocele sac (formed by the tunica vaginalis surrounding the testicle) or
removal of an encysted hydrocele of the cord (formed by the prolongation of the tunica
vaginalis from the testicle along the spermatic cord).

POSITION. Supine.

INSTRUMENTS

General set (Fig. 281)
Hydrocele trocar and cannula
Diathermy leads, electrodes and lead anchoring forceps
Corrugated drain
2 and 2·5 (3/0 and 2/0) Chromic catgut or Dexon for ligatures
2·5 and 3 (2/0 and 0) Chromic catgut or Dexon on a small half-circle round-bodied
    needle for deep sutures
2 (3/0) Silk or nylon on a small or medium curved cutting needle for skin sutures.

OUTLINE OF PROCEDURE

Hydrocele. The testicle is exposed through an incision made over the external inguinal
ring, extending downwards and inwards towards the pubis. Unless the testicle is very
large the incision stops just short of the scrotal skin. The spermatic cord is dissected free
and traction applied under the hydrocele sac appears in the lower part of the wound.
A trocar and cannula may then be inserted to drain the fluid, and the collapsed tunica
vaginalis is cut away with scissors or a diathermy needle, and the innumerable vessels
which have been divided during dissection are ligated or diathermised. When haemostasis

is complete, a corrugated drain is inserted through a stab wound in the bottom of the scrotum, and the testicle is returned to its normal position.

The wound is closed in layers. Some surgeons remove a hydrocele through an upper scrotal incision, and instead of excising the sac it may be slit up the front, turned back and sutured behind the testicle.

An Encysted Hydrocele of the Cord. The incision, which generally is made over the swelling, usually lies over the inguinal canal, which is incised. The distended sac is freed from other structures of the cord, and ligated above and below before excision. The surgeon will search towards the internal ring in case there is an extension to the sac, which may form a hernia at a later date. Any sac so found is treated as a hernial sac (Chapter 13). The wound is closed in layers.

Orchidectomy

DEFINITION
Removal of the testicle.

POSITION. Supine.

INSTRUMENTS
General set (Fig. 281)
Corrugated drain
2·5 and 3 (2/0 and 0) Chromic catgut, Dexon or silk for ligatures
3 or 4 (0 or 1) Chromic catgut or Dexon on a small half-circle round-bodied needle for muscle (inguinal incision)
2·5 (2/0) Silk or nylon on a small or medium curved cutting needle for skin sutures.

OUTLINE OF PROCEDURE
The testicle is exposed through an inguinal (or scrotal) incision. The spermatic cord is dissected up and the vessels and vas deferens ligated individually, and the testicle is removed. A corrugated drain is inserted into the scrotum through a stab incision and the wound is closed. A pressure dressing is applied.

Vasectomy

DEFINITION
Excision of part of the vas deferens.

POSITION. Supine.

INSTRUMENTS
Sponge-holding forceps (Rampley), 2
Towel clips, 4
Scalpel handle with No. 10 blade *or*
Diathermy scalpel with ball attachment
Fine dissecting forceps, toothed (Gillies), 2
Fine dissecting forceps, non-toothed (McIndoe), 2
Fine scissors, curved on flat (McIndoe or Lahey), 1
Scissors, curved on flat, 13 cm (5 in) (Mayo), 1
Fine artery forceps, curved on flat (Mosquito), 5

Artery forceps, curved on flat (Criles), 2
Tissue forceps, 15 cm (6 in) (Allis), 2
Special vasectomy mobilisation clamp (Tinkler), 1 (Optional)
Diathermy leads and electrodes
Local anaesthetic requisites (Fig. 271)
2·5 and 3 (2/0 and 0) Chromic catgut or Dexon for ligatures
2 or 2·5 (3/0 or 2/0) silk or nylon on straight or curved non-traumatic cutting needle
    for skin sutures.

OUTLINE OF PROCEDURE

The skin and underlying tissues are infiltrated with local anaesthetic. The vas is palpated and either mobilised between the fingers or with a special vasectomy clamp. The skin overlying the vas is incised longitudinally for a few centimetres and the vas is picked up out of the incision with tissue forceps. It is usual to infiltrate the covering sheath of the vas with a few millilitres of local anaesthetic before proceding further.

The spermatic cord coverings are incised to display the vas deferens proper, a white avascular structure similar in appearance to a strand of spaghetti. The vas is gently lifted and the sheath teased away to free about 5 or 6 cm of vas. The vas is clamped at each end with an artery forceps and the segment between excised and sent for histological examination. The severed ends are ligated with catgut, Dexon (or silk) and a careful inspection made for haemostasis.

The skin is closed with mattress sutures of silk or nylon (some surgeons use catgut or Dexon to avoid having to remove the sutures) and the wound dressed with plastic spray solution such as Nobecutane.

Excision of varicocele

DEFINITION

The ligation and excision of varicose veins in the spermatic cord.

POSITION. Supine.

INSTRUMENTS

General set (Fig. 281)
2·5 and 3 (2/0 and 0) Chromic catgut or Dexon for ligatures
3 or 4 (0 or 1) Chromic catgut or Dexon on a small half-circle cutting needle for muscle
    tendon suture
2·5 (2/0) Silk or nylon on a small or medium curved or straight cutting needle for skin
    sutures.

OUTLINE OF PROCEDURE

An incision is made over the external inguinal ring and the spermatic cord dissected out. Some of the varicose veins are isolated from the rest of the spermatic vessels and are separated from the cord for about 8 cm (3 in) of their length. These vessels are ligated above and below the varicocele which is then excised. Some surgeons leave these ligatures long and tie them together, so pulling the testicle a little away from the scrotum. The wound is closed.

Orchidopexy

DEFINITION

Placing an undescended testicle into the scrotum (in a child).

POSITION. Supine.

INSTRUMENTS
    General set (Fig. 281)
    Fire artery forceps, curved on flat, mosquito, 10
    Fine tissue forceps (McIndoe), 5
    Fine-toothed dissecting forceps (Gillies), 2
    Fine scissors, curved on flat, 10 cm (4 in) (Kilner or strabismus)
    2 and 2·5 (3/0 and 2/0) Chromic catgut or Dexon for ligatures
    2·5 (2/0) Chromic catgut or Dexon on a small half-circle or curved non-traumatic
        round-bodied needle for testicle fixation and hernial sac transfixion
    2·5 or 3 (2/0 or 0) Chromic catgut or Dexon on a small half-circle round-bodied needle
        for muscle sutures
    2 (3/0) Silk or nylon on a small or medium curved cutting needle for skin sutures.

OUTLINE OF PROCEDURE
    Through a groin incision, the testicle is mobilised and the hernial sac is excised and the
neck transfixed. By dissecting the structures of the cord from the extraperitoneal tissues,
the testicle is eventually brought down into the scrotum. It is retained there either by
transposing the organ into the opposite side of the scrotum, or by constructing a tunnel
between the scrotum and the thigh and sewing the testicle to the fascia lata. In the
latter case, a second operation must be performed three months later to separate the
scrotum and thigh.

Cystoscopy

DEFINITION
    Examination of the urinary bladder with an endoscope for diagnosis.

POSITION. Lithotomy.

INSTRUMENTS
    As Figure 308
    (A supply of sterile water, normal saline or antiseptic colution (see Chapter 6, chemical
        disinfection) at a temperature of 34·5° to 35·5°C (104° to 106°F) should be available
        to fill the bladder and provide irrigation. This fluid should be dispensed from closed
        inverted flasks, 1 or 2 litre, via a suitable flask connector, tubing and the cystoscope
        irrigation connection. If large quantities of fluid are required several flasks can be
        interlinked with one another (Fig. 309). The flasks should be renewed for each
        operation.

OUTLINE OF PROCEDURE
    If the urethra is constricted, bladder sounds of a progressively larger diameter are
passed until the passage is dilated sufficiently to accept the cystoscope. A lubricated
cystoscope is passed into the bladder and a specimen of urine taken for bacteriological
examination. The light cable is attached, the bladder filled with solution and the telescope inserted to examine the bladder. (When a biopsy is required the surgeon changes
his instrument for an operating cystoscope and would then need Riches or similar
biopsy forceps. If bleeding is persistent after biopsy the surgeon may complete the
procedure by leaving an indwelling catheter.) For the due excretion test, 10 ml of intra-

venous 0·4 per cent indigo carmine is used, and a tray should be prepared for intravenous injection.

The bladder is emptied, the light cable detached and the instrument removed.

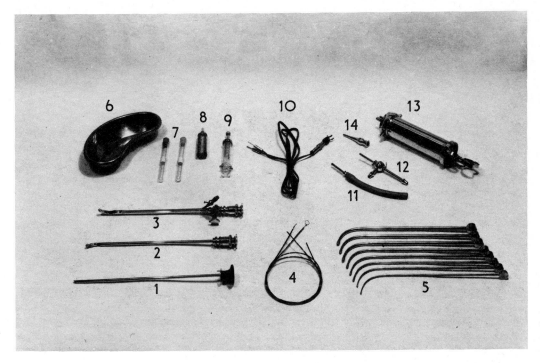

Figure 308   Cystoscopy and retrograde pyelography.

1. Telescope.
2. Cystoscope (Ringleb), for examination and irrigation.
3. Cystoscope, double catheterising (Ringleb).
4. Ureteric catheters, assorted sizes.
5. Bladder sounds or bougies (Lister), set of various sizes.
6. Kidney dish.
7. Sterile specimen tubes marked right and left kidney.
8. Radio-opaque medium, e.g., hypaque 45 per cent.
9. 10-ml syringe with connection for ureteric catheters.
10. Electric cable for connection to lamp circuit on cystoscope.
11. Irrigation nozzle, one-way.
12. Irrigation nozzle, two-way.
13. Bladder syringe.
14. Nozzle for bladder syringe.
(*Note*. Alternatively, a closed flask of irrigation solution may be used instead of the bladder syringe.)

Not Illustrated:
Transformer or battery.
Irrigation solution.

Urethroscopy

DEFINITION

Examination of the interior of the urethra.

POSITION

Supine with legs separated slightly, or lithotomy.

INSTRUMENTS

    Bladder sounds or bougies (Lister, Clutton, etc.), set

    Urethroscope or appropriate cystoscope (e.g., Canny Ryall, Brown Beurger, Braasch direct vision, Geiringer, etc.)

    Supply of sterile irrigation solution

    Connecting tubing and nozzles for urethroscopes

    Electric cable and batteries.

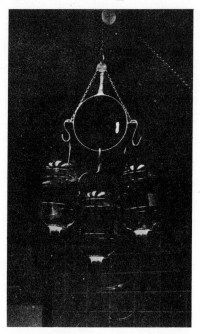

Figure 309   Macbic closed irrigation system. (A.O.R.N. Journal, U.S.A.)

OUTLINE OF PROCEDURE

All instruments used for urethroscopy have an attachment for continuous irrigation, as compared with simple cystoscopy when continuous irrigation is not generally necessary. For anterior urethroscopy an instrument similar to the Ringleb's cystoscope shown in Figure 308 and having a concave tip is used. Alternatively, an instrument incorporating a straight closed-end sheath, or a straight open-end sheath may be used, e.g., the Canny Ryall or Geiringer respectively. For posterior urethroscopy, the end of the sheath is convex in shape although the straight open-end instrument can be used for this also.

The lubricated instrument is inserted and if urethral constrictions are present, these are dilated first in the usual manner with sounds. The telescope is inserted, the light cable attached and the irrigation commenced.

Three types of telescopes are available, the fore-oblique, the right wide-angled field, and the direct vision. The fore-oblique telescope is similar to the one used for simple cystoscopy when the surgeon generally wishes to examine a field of view which lies in front of and a little to one side of the distal tip of the instrument. This type of instrument can be used for urethroscopy, but it is preferable to use a wide-angle lens telescope which gives a field of view at right angles to the aperture in the tip of the instrument. The direct vision telescope can only be used if the instrument has an open-end sheath.

The Braasch cystoscope does not incorporate a telescope, and the surgeon views the interior of the urethra through a glass window in the proximal part of the instrument.

After the urethra has been examined, the instrument may be passed into the bladder for a general examination unless this was performed at the beginning of the procedure. Alternatively, the instrument is removed and replaced with an ordinary cystoscope.

Any fluid left in the bladder is evacuated, the light cable detached and the instrument removed.

Fibre optics are now replacing conventional optic and light systems in endoscopic instruments. It is a term applied to a system for transmitting light and images through thin fibres of optical glass by the phenomenon of total internal reflection.

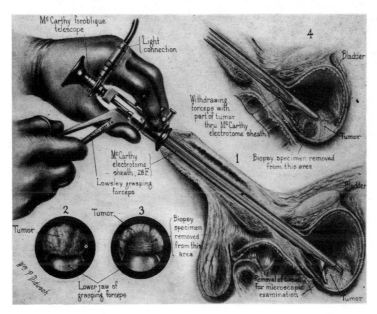

Figure 310   Lowsley grasping forceps being used with a fibre optic for oblique telescope.
(A.C.M.I.)

The system consists of three basic parts:
1. The light source or generator unit
2. The cable or optical bundle
3. The instrument or endoscope.

1. The light is supplied by a high intensity bulb having an inbuilt Parabolic reflector. This reflector, which although focusing the short light rays into the optical bundle, allows the long (or hot) infra-red rays to pass through. This ensures only cold light is allowed to pass to the instrument.

2. The optical bundle which is connected at one end to the light source and at the other to the instrument contains approximately 200,000 flexible optical fibres, which are coherent (capable of carrying an image). This means that they transmit a pre-focused light of a very high intensity and even density to the instrument.

The bundles are covered in PVC and are very flexible.

3. The telescope or instrument sheath contains a layer of optical fibres placed in an annular fashion between two tubes to form a sheath. In the former case the inner tube contains the optical viewing system and in the latter case a channel for insertion of a

telescope. These fibres are grouped together at the distal end of the instrument to form a rod or bar. At the proximal end of the instrument the fibres are grouped together to form a connection for the light cable. The maximum intensity of light output at the distal end of optical bundle depends on the working distance in cm (inches) from the object.

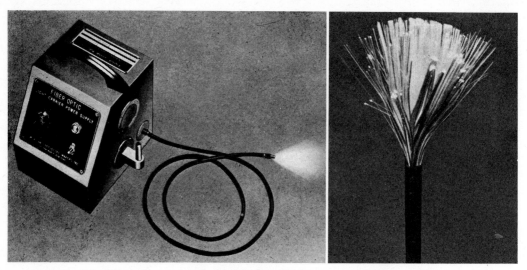

Figure 311   Fibre light source and optical bundle which is connected to the endoscope in use. (A.C.M.I.)

Figure 312   Section of the optical bundle showing light transmitted to the distal end of the fibres.   (A.C.M.I.)

This may be as high as 5000 ft candles at 25 mm (1 in) distance but averages 1600 to 2800 ft candles intensity. The degree of intensity can be adjusted.

Fibre optics can also be used for image transmission but this is more applicable to the flexible endoscope such as the gastroscope illustrated on p. 291 (Chapter 13). Fibre optic instruments cannot be autoclaved but should be disinfected by cold chemicals (e.g., ethylene oxide) or sub-atmospheric steam (Chapter 6).

Producing a cold intense light, fibre optic instruments are very suitable for photography of cavities.

Ureteric catheterisation and retrograde pyelography

DEFINITION

The insertion of a ureteric catheter into the ureter and the kidney pelvis to obtain a specimen of urine from that kidney, or for the retrograde injection of a radio-opaque fluid for X-ray examination of the kidney.

POSITION. Lithotomy.

INSTRUMENTS

As Figure 308.

OUTLINE OF PROCEDURE

A lubricated catheterising cystoscope is inserted, the obturator removed and the telescope inserted to visualise the ureteric orifices. A ureteric catheter of appropriate size is passed into each orifice in turn by using the movable platform at the distal end of the instrument. The stilette is left in the catheters until it has been advanced a few centimetres into the ureter, and it is then removed before the catheter is advanced any further. The bladder is emptied, the light cable detached and the cystoscope carefully removed, leaving the catheters in position.

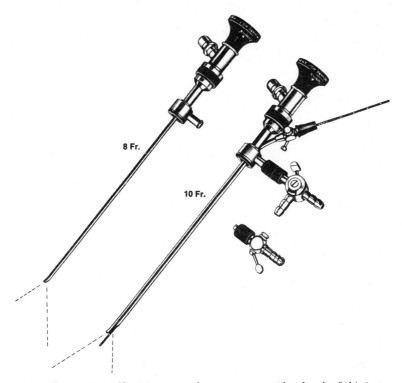

8 Fr.

10 Fr.

Figure 313   Fibre optic Wolf miniature urethro-cystoscope. The sheath of this instrument is of 8 or 10 Charrière gauge and contains a layer of optical fibres placed in an annular fashion between two tubes. The distal end is fenestrated and the fibres are formed into a rectangular bar adjacent to the objective. The telescope has an angle of view of 170° and has built-in fibre optic bundles. (Richard Wolf GmBH, Down Bros Ltd.)

The instrument nurse must ensure that the ureteric catheter marked with a red band at its proximal end is used for the right kidney. Similarly, the left ureter is catheterised with a catheter marked blue or green at its proximal end. Two test tubes marked Right and Left are strapped to each thigh (right and left respectively) to collect urine specimens from the kidneys. The catheters are each passed, either through the holes of a rubber teat which fits over the test tube, or through a cotton-wool plug in the neck of each tube. In the X-ray department, a radio-opaque medium such as 35 per cent Pyelosil or Hypaque will be injected into each catheter before making a radiographic examination of the kidneys.

Transurethral prostatectomy

DEFINITION
Transurethral removal of the prostate gland.

POSITION. Lithotomy.

INSTRUMENTS

    Bladder sounds or bougies (Lister, Clutton, etc.), set
    Supply of sterile water, etc., for irrigation (see cystoscopy)
    Connecting tubing and nozzles for resectoscope
    Electric resectoscope (Fig. 314) or 'cold punch' instrument
    Electric cable and batteries

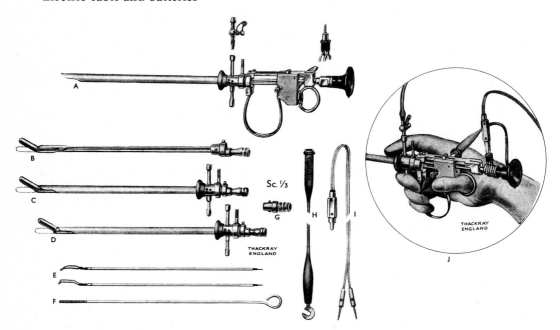

Figure 314   Raper resectoscope.   (Chas. F. Thackray Ltd.)

A, Resectoscope assembled in insulated sheath, 30 Charrière gauge. *Note.* Double-prong connector for light lead: small irrigating nozzle with tap.

B, Obturator for above.

C and D, Insulated sheaths, 28 and 26 Charrière gauge, with obturators.

E, Cutting loops (active diathermy electrode slides inside sheath).

F, Probe for cleaning.

G, Large irrigation nozzle.

H, Diathermy lead.

I, Light lead.

J, Resectoscope ready for use. *Note.* Irrigation tube attached to side nozzle; light lead coupled to double-prong connector.

    Diathermy leads, lead anchoring forceps and diathermy apparatus
    Urethral catheter, self-retaining (Foley size 18, 20 or 22 Charrière gauge)
    20 ml syringe and sterile water for inflating cuff of catheter.

OUTLINE OF PROCEDURE

    The indifferent diathermy electrode is applied to the patient's thigh with the usual precautions. (Alternatively the resectoscope sheath incorporates the indifferent diathermy electrode.) Progressively larger sizes of sounds are passed into the urethra followed by the resectoscope. The obturator is removed and the telescope/resecting loops inserted. Irrigation and diathermy connections are made and the interior of the bladder examined together with the prostatic area.

The prostate is resected by advancing and withdrawing the diathermy loop with the current switched on. It may be necessary to change the diathermy loops several times during operation as they become charred.

A special electrode is used to coagulate bleeding vessels. A self-retaining catheter is inserted and the bladder irrigated until the water returns clear.

Alternatively, the 'cold punch' instrument is used for prostatic resection via the urethra. In this case the instrument is introduced in a similar manner to the electric resectoscope, but the hypertrophied prostate gland is excised with a punch mechanism at the distal end of the instrument.

Fulguration of bladder tumours

DEFINITION
Removal of bladder tumours or lesions by diathermy.

POSITION. Lithotomy.

INSTRUMENTS
As for cystoscopy (Fig. 308)
    Operating cystoscope, preferably an irrigating instrument, having channels through which flexible diathermy electrodes can be introduced and manipulated: *or* an operating cystoscope which incorporates its own electrode at the distal end.
Diathermy electrodes, set of flexible variety leads and anchoring forceps
    (Self-retaining urethral catheter occasionally required (e.g., Foley 18, 20 or 22 Charrière gauge).)

OUTLINE OF PROCEDURE
The indifferent diathermy electrode is applied to the patient's thigh with the usual precautions. The lubricated cystoscope is inserted, the obturator removed, the irrigation tubing and diathermy connections are made and the telescope inserted to visualise the lesion.

The electrode is applied to the tumour and diathermy used until fulguration is complete. The bladder is emptied, the cystoscope removed and if necessary the catheter is inserted.

Lithotrity or litholapaxy

DEFINITION
Crushing and removal of bladder stones via the urethra.

POSITION
Lithotomy, with the head of the table slightly lowered.

INSTRUMENTS
As Figures 308 and 315.

OUTLINE OF PROCEDURE
A cystoscopy is performed. When the stones have been visualised, the cystoscope is removed and progressively larger sizes of sounds are inserted followed by the lithotrite. The stone or stones are crushed, the lithotrite removed and an evacuation catheter

inserted. The Bigelow's evacuator is used to irrigate the bladder and extract the fragments of stone by suction. It may be necessary to repeat this procedure several times
before all the stone or stones have been completely crushed and removed.

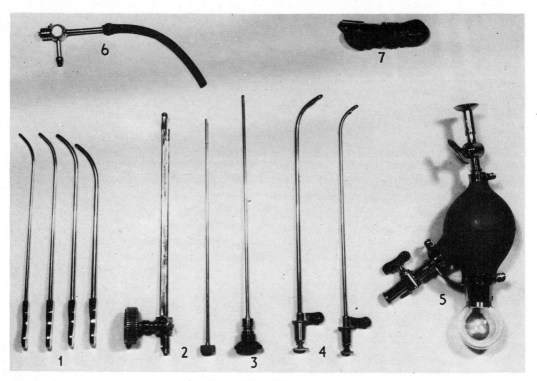

Figure 315 Lithrotrity.
1. Bladder sounds or bougies (Clutton), set   5. Evacuator (Bigelow).
   of various sizes.   6. Irrigation nozzle, two-way.
2. Lithrotrite and obturator.   7. Electric lead for connection to lamp
3. Telescope.   circuit on lithrotrite.
4. Evacuation catheters, metal.

Suprapubic cystostomy

DEFINITION
    Temporary or permanent suprapubic drainage of the bladder.

POSITION
    Supine, with some Trendelenburg.

INSTRUMENTS
    General set (Fig. 281)
    Suprapubic trocar
    Catheter introducer
    Catheter, self-retaining (De Pezzer, 30 to 34 Charrière gauge)
    Spigot
    Urethral catheter (Jaques or Nélaton size 18 Charrière gauge). To distend bladder if
        required.

Catheter lubricant
Bladder syringe and warm irrigation solution
Corrugated drain and safety-pin
Suction tubing, nozzles and tube anchoring forceps
2·5 and 3 (2/0 and 0) Chromic catgut or Dexon for ligatures
3 or 4 (0 or 1) Chromic catgut or Dexon on a medium half-circle cutting needle for
    bladder and muscle sutures
2·5 (2/0) Silk or nylon on a medium or large curved or straight cutting needle for skin
    sutures.

OUTLINE OF PROCEDURE

If the bladder is not distended, it is first filled with irrigation solution. A 7–10 cm
(3–4 in) midline incision is made just above the pubis. The incision is deepened and the
rectus sheath opened in the midline, followed by a transverse opening in the transversalis fascia. The fascia and peritoneum are pushed upwards, and two stay sutures are
inserted into the bladder wall and left long. Any veins in the vicinity of the proposed
opening into the bladder are under-run and tied off. A stab incision is made, the bladder
fluid suctioned away and a De Pezzer catheter inserted. The stay sutures are used to
secure the catheter in position and these are reinforced if necessary with further interrupted sutures of chromic catgut or Dexon.

Some surgeons make a smaller incision in the abdomen and use a large trocar and
cannula to insert the catheter. The wound is closed in layers with a corrugated drain in
the lower part. The catheter is secured to the skin with a suture which is tied round the
catheter near to the point where it emerges from the wound.

Transvesical prostatectomy

DEFINITION

Removal of the prostate gland via a suprapubic incision into the bladder.

POSITION. Trendelenburg.

INSTRUMENTS

General set (Fig. 281)
Skin or tetra-towel forceps (Moynihan), 4 for sides of wound and 2 for ends of wound
Artery forceps, 20 cm (8 in) (Spencer Wells), 10
Long scissors, curved on flat (Nelson's)
Long dissecting forceps, toothed, 25 cm (10 in)
Long dissecting forceps, non-toothed
Deep retractors, narrow blade (Deaver or Paton), 2
Illuminated bladder retractor, self-retaining (Morson)
Vulsellum forceps (Teale), 2
Boomerang needles (Harris or Millin) for reconstruction of prostatic bed, 3 sizes
Ligature-carrying forceps (Harris or Millin), 2
Bladder syringe and irrigation solution at 43·3° to 46°C (110° to 115°F)
Urethral catheter (Harris or Jaques size 18 Charrière gauge)
Large drainage tube or self-retaining catheter (De Pezzer size 36 Charrière gauge)
Catheter lubricant
Corrugated drain
Suction tubing, nozzles and tube anchoring forceps
Diathermy leads, electrodes and lead anchoring forceps

2·5 and 3 (2/0 and 0) Chromic catgut or Dexon for ligatures, and on ligature-carrying forceps for prostatic bed sutures

3 (0) Chromic catgut or Dexon on a small half-circle round-bodied needle for bladder sutures

3 or 4 (0 or 1) Chromic catgut or Dexon on a medium half-circle cutting needle for muscle

2·5 (2/0) Silk or nylon on a large curved or straight cutting needle for skin sutures

2·5 (2/0) Nylon on a large Colts needle for catheter suture.

OUTLINE OF PROCEDURE

There are several prostatectomy operations via this route and the following is a description of the Harris procedure:

If the bladder is not distended, it is first filled with sterile irrigation solution. A 13 cm (5 in) or longer midline incision is made just above the pubis. The incision is deepened and the rectus sheath opened in the midline, followed by a transverse opening in the transversalis fascia. The fascia and peritoneum are pushed upwards and two stay sutures are inserted into the bladder wall and left long. Any veins in the vicinity of the proposed opening into the bladder are under-run and tied off. A stab incision is made, the bladder fluid suctioned away, the incision extended and a self-retaining bladder retractor inserted.

The mucous membrane over the prostate is incised under direct vision with a pair of scissors. The retractor is removed and the gland shelled out with two fingers. The retractor is reinserted and any bleeding points picked up with forceps and diathermised. Using the boomerang needle, the torn mucous membrane is sutured well down into the prostatic cavity so that its posterior wall is covered.* A urethral catheter is inserted into the bladder and a figure-of-eight suture introduced in front of the catheter so that when it is tied, the side walls of the prostatic cavity are brought together. This manoeuvre largely obliterates the cavity and acts as a haemostatic suture also.

A long nylon suture is inserted through the abdominal wall at one side of the incision and passes into the bladder, through the tip of the catheter, and out again through the abdominal wall at the opposite side of the incision. When the incision has been closed, these ends are tied together over a gauze pad or are threaded through a short length of rubber tubing in the manner described for tension sutures (Chapter 13). This suture serves to suspend the catheter in the bladder until it is withdrawn about the tenth day post-operatively.

When all bleeding has stopped, the bladder drainage tube is inserted and the wound closed in layers around this tube. A corrugated drain extending down to the bladder is left at the lower end of the wound. The suprapubic drain and corrugated drain are usually removed on the fourth or fifth day post-operatively.

It is worth mentioning here that this type of operation was performed in two stages as the Freyer's procedure. In this operation a preliminary suprapubic cystostomy is performed and when the patient's general and bladder condition are considered suitable, the prostate is enucleated between two fingers of one hand in the bladder, and two fingers of the other hand in the rectum. Haemostasis is secured with hot packs and the operation

---

* The Harris or Millin boomerang needle (Fig. 316) consists of a spring-loaded holder to which the needle is attached. The needle has an open eye at its distal point and can be rotated through about 60 degrees by depressing the handle. In operation the surgeon approximates the needle to the tissues being sutured, and advances it through them by depressing the handle. The assistant positions a loop of suture material (usually catgut) in the open eye of the needle by means of ligature-carrying forceps and the surgeon releases the tension on the spring-loaded handle. The needle rotates back through track created by it, withdraws the catgut and thereby completes the suture. The boomerang needle may be used for single or continuous sutures.

concludes with the insertion of a wide-bore drainage tube into the bladder. The operation has largely been superseded by the Harris and similar procedures or by a retropubic or Millin's prostatectomy.

Millin's retropubic prostatectomy

DEFINITION
Removal of the prostate gland through a suprapubic incision but without opening the bladder.

POSITION. Trendelenburg.

INSTRUMENTS
General set (Fig. 281)
Millin's prostatectomy set (Fig. 316)

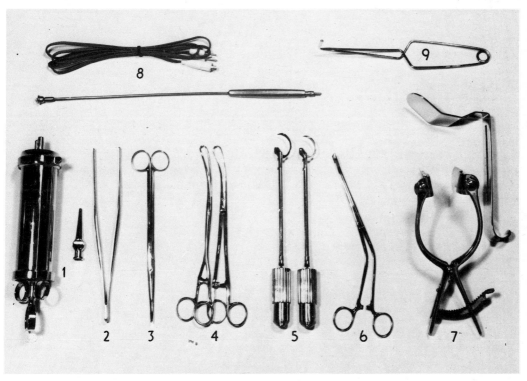

Figure 316   Millin's retropubic prostatectomy.

1. Bladder syringe.
2. Long dissecting forceps, toothed (Millin).
3. Long scissors, curved, 23 cm (9 in) (Nelson).
4. Vulsellum forceps, 2.
5. Boomerang needles (Millin or Harris), 2.
6. Ligature-carrying forceps (Young).
7. Retractor, self-retaining (Millin).
8. Malleable light with electric lead.
9. Bladder-neck spreader (Millin).

Skin or tetra-towel forceps (Moynihan), 4 for sides of wound and 2 for ends of wound
Artery forceps, 20 cm (8 in) (Spencer Wells), 10
Long artery forceps, curved on flat (Gordon Craig), 5

Deep retractors, narrow blade (Paton or Deaver 25 mm (1 in))
Irrigation solution at 43·3° to 46°C (110° to 115°F)
Urethral catheter (whistle tip or similar, size 20 Charrière gauge)
Catheter lubricant
Spigot
Suction tubing, nozzles and tube anchoring forceps
Diathermy leads, electrodes and lead anchoring forceps.

OUTLINE OF PROCEDURE
A transverse suprapubic incision is made and the prostate exposed behind the pubis.
Blood-vessels running across the anterior aspect of the gland are ligated before opening
the capsule in the front. The gland is enucleated, haemostasis secured with diathermy and
sutures and a urethral catheter inserted into the bladder. The prostatic capsule is sutured
and the wound closed in the usual manner with a corrugated drain down to the prostate
capsule in the lower end of the wound.

With any form of prostatectomy the vas deferens may be ligated on both sides to
prevent any possibility of infection reaching the testicles by this route.

Total cystectomy and ureterosigmoidostomy

DEFINITION
Removal of the urinary bladder and transplantation of the ureters into the sigmoid
colon.

POSITION. Trendelenburg.

INSTRUMENTS
General set (Fig. 281)
Laparotomy set (Fig. 282)
Fine tissue forceps (McIndoe), 5
Fine dissecting forceps, non-toothed (McIndoe), 2
Fine dissecting forceps, toothed (Gillies), 2
Scalpel handle No. 9 with No. 15 blade (Bard Parker)
Fine artery forceps, straight, mosquito, 10
Fine artery forceps, curved on flat, mosquito, 10
Intestinal occlusion clamps, curved (Doyen), 2
Suction tubing, nozzles and tube anchoring forceps
Diathermy leads, electrodes and lead anchoring forceps
Laparotomy ligatures and sutures
2 (3/0) Chromic catgut or Dexon on a small curved non-traumatic intestinal needle size
    20 mm for ureteric anastomosis.

OUTLINE OF PROCEDURE
Sometimes the ureters are transplanted as a first procedure and the cystectomy follows
at a later date.

Ureterosigmoidostomy. Through a lower midline incision, the sigmoid colon is mobilised. The posterior peritoneum is incised and the ureters are mobilised for a considerable
length. A ligature is placed at the junction of each ureter with the bladder and they are
divided proximal to this ligature.

Curved occlusion clamps are applied longitudinally to the colon at the point selected for the anastomosis. A small longitudinal incision is made in the bowel wall through the serosa, muscle and mucosa. The ureters are united to the colon mucosa by direct mucosa to mucosa sutures, using fine non-traumatic chromic catgut or Dexon sutures (Leadbetter's operation). The ureters may be immobilised further by suturing the serosa over them for a short distance from the anastomosis, and the sigmoid colon is immobilised to the wing of the pelvis. The wound is closed and a rectal tube inserted.

Cystectomy. If this is done as a second stage, the approach is as before. The peritoneum is stripped off the bladder, which is then dissected free from the surrounding tissue. The urethra is ligated and severed and the blood-vessels divided between forceps to complete mobilisation so that the bladder can be removed. The blood-vessels are diathermised or ligated, and when haemostasis is complete, the peritoneum is sutured to reconstruct the pelvic floor. The wound is closed in layers.

It may be mentioned here that the ureters can be transplanted into a loop of ileum (uretero-ileostomy) instead of the sigmoid colon. In this case 15 cm (6 in) or so of ileum are transected with the mesentery left intact, and the remaining proximal and distal bowel are anastomosed to re-establish intestinal continuity. The short section of ileum is closed at one end and the ureters transplanted in the manner previously described for uretero-sigmoidostomy. The open end of the ileum is brought through the abdominal wall as for ileostomy (Chapter 13) and the urine drains into this, so forming an artificial bladder. It is usual to leave a small Paul's tube in the ileostomy, or apply an ileostomy bag immediately after operation.

Partial cystectomy

DEFINITION
Removal of part of the urinary bladder, and if necessary transplantation of one or both ureters to another part of the bladder.

POSITION. Trendelenburg.

INSTRUMENTS
As for cystectomy
Urethral catheter (Jaques or Nélaton size 18 Charrière gauge)
Bladder syringe and irrigation solution
3 or 4 (0 or 1) Chromic catgut or Dexon on a small half-circle round-bodied needle for bladder sutures.

OUTLINE OF PROCEDURE
The bladder is distended with irrigation solution and an approach made through a lower midline incision.

Two stay sutures are inserted into the bladder wall and left long. Any vessels which are overlying the area for incision are under-run with chromic catgut or Dexon and tied. The bladder is opened and the fluid evacuated with the suction tube. The segment of bladder for removal is excised by the clamp and cut method whereby artery forceps are applied across the tissue before excision. If the ureter or ureters are involved in this area, they are divided and immobilised for sufficient of their length to enable transplantation into another part of the bladder by the direct mucosa to mucosa anastomosis. The bladder is closed with two layers of chromic catgut or Dexon sutures and a urethral catheter inserted. The wound is closed as before with drainage.

Adrenalectomy

DEFINITION
Removal of whole or part of one or both adrenal glands.

POSITION
Supine (the operation may also be performed through a posterolateral incision, and in this case the position is that for kidney operations).

INSTRUMENTS
Abdominal Approach
  General set (Fig. 281)
  Laparotomy set (Fig. 282)
  Long scissors, curved on flat, 23 cm (9 in) (Nelson)
  Long dissecting forceps, non-toothed, 25 cm (10 in)
  Long dissecting forceps, toothed, 25 cm (10 in)
  Silver ligature clips and insertion forceps (McKenzie)
  Suction tubing, nozzles and tube anchoring forceps
  Diathermy leads, electrodes and lead anchoring forceps
  Laparotomy ligatures and sutures.

OUTLINE OF PROCEDURE
A midline or paramedian approach is made and the upper pole of the kidney visualised by incising the posterior peritoneum and mobilising and retracting the overlying organs. The gland is palpated and grasped with tissue or sponge-holding forceps. It is carefully dissected free from the vena cava if it is on the right side. The adrenal vessels are clamped with long artery forceps or silver ligature clips and divided with the long scissors. The gland is removed and haemostasis secured either by ligatures, silver clips, chromic catgut or Dexon sutures or diathermy. The posterior peritoneum is reconstructed with chromic catgut or Dexon sutures and the wound closed in the usual manner.

INSTRUMENTS
Posterolateral Approach
  As nephrectomy, minus stone forceps, ureteric bougies and catheters.

OUTLINE OF PROCEDURE
A posterolateral incision is made and the kidney exposed through the bed of the twelfth rib. Removal of the gland follows that described above except that the peritoneum is not opened. The wound is closed as for nephrectomy.

Kidney and Ureteric Operations

Nephrectomy

DEFINITION
Removal of the kidney.

POSITION
Lateral, with kidney bridge elevated, Figure 41.

INSTRUMENTS
General set (Fig. 281)
Nephrectomy set (Figure 317)
Artery forceps, 20 cm (8 in) (Spencer Wells), 10

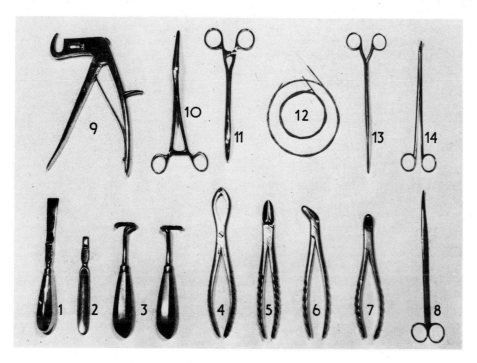

Figure 317   Nephrectomy and other kidney operations.

1. Rugine (Mitchell).
2. Rugine (Faraboeuf).
3. Rib raspatories (Doyen), left and right side.
4. Bone-holding forceps (Fergusson).
5. Bone-cutting forceps (Liston).
6. Bone-nibbling forceps, angled on side.
7. Bone-nibbling forceps, angled on flat.
8. Long scissors, curved on flat, 23 cm (9 in) (Nelson).
9. Rib shears (Exner).
10. Kidney pedicle clamp.
11. Long artery forceps, curved on flat (Moynihan gall-bladder), 8.
12. Ureteric catheters.
13. Renal calculi forceps (Desjardin).
14. Renal calculi forceps (Thompson Walker).

Long artery forceps, curved on flat (Moynihan gall-bladder), 5
Long artery forceps, curved on flat (Gordon Craig), 5
Long dissecting forceps, non-toothed, 25 cm (10 in)
Long dissecting forceps, toothed, 25 cm (10 in)
Deep retractors, narrow blade (Deaver), set of 4
Deep retractors, broad blade (Winsbury-White and Worrall), 2
Long, medium-diameter drainage tube and safety-pin
2·5, 3, 4 and 5 2/0, 0, 1 and 2) Chromic catgut or Dexon and silk or thread for ligatures
4 or 5 (1 or 2) Chromic catgut or Dexon on a large half-circle cutting needle for muscle sutures
2·5 (2/0) Silk or nylon on a large curved cutting needle for skin sutures.

OUTLINE OF PROCEDURE

An oblique incision is made commencing just below the mid-point of the last rib and continuing downwards and forwards towards the anterior superior iliac spine. The external oblique, transversus and internal oblique muscles are divided in line with the incision and the twelfth rib may or may not be excised.

The kidney is separated from its surrounding fat by blunt dissection and is delivered into the wound. The ureter and renal vessels are either clamped separately and divided distal to each forcep; or double ligatures are passed round each vessel and the ureter, which are divided between these ligatures. The kidney is removed and if artery forceps have been applied, the vessels and ureter are ligated. A drainage tube is inserted, the kidney bridge lowered and the wound closed in layers.

Nephrostomy

DEFINITION

The establishment of a temporary drainage of the kidney.

POSITION

Lateral with kidney bridge elevated.

INSTRUMENTS

As nephrectomy
Catheter, self-retaining (De Pezzer, size 26 or 28 Charrière gauge)
3 (0) Chromic catgut or Dexon on a small curved non-traumatic intestinal needle.

OUTLINE OF PROCEDURE

The kidney is exposed as previously described and an incision made through the capsule and substance of the organ. A self-retaining catheter is inserted and two or three stout chromic catgut or Dexon sutures are inserted at each side of the catheter through the substance of the kidney. These are tied to secure the catheter, and the capsule is closed with a non-traumatic suture of 3 (0) chromic catgut or Dexon.

The kidney bridge is lowered and the wound closed in layers following the insertion of a long drainage tube down to the kidney incision.

Nephropexy

DEFINITION

Fixation of an unduly mobile kidney.

POSITION

Lateral, with kidney bridge elevated.

INSTRUMENTS

As for nephrectomy.

OUTLINE OF PROCEDURE

The kidney is exposed as previously described and carefully mobilised, freeing any kinks which may be present in the ureter. The kidney is secured to the posterior abdominal wall with sutures of chromic catgut or collagen tape which are placed through the substance of the organ or attached to strips of capsule which have been raised from the kidney. The kidney bridge is lowered and the wound closed in layers, with or without drainage.

Nephrolithotomy or pyelolithotomy

DEFINITION
Removal of a stone from the kidney or pelvis of the ureter.

POSITION
Lateral, with kidney bridge elevated or break back position (Fig. 64).

INSTRUMENTS
As for nephrectomy
20 ml syringe, fine catheter and irrigation solution
2 (3/0) Chromic catgut or Dexon on a small curved non-traumatic intestinal needle.

OUTLINE OF PROCEDURE
The kidney is exposed in the usual manner and freed from surrounding fat. For *nephrolithotomy*, the calculus is palpated by holding the kidney between the finger and thumb. The calculus is steadied carefully through the kidney substance and an incision made over it starting on the convex border of the organ. When the knife reaches the calculus it is removed and an examination made for others. The incision is closed with two or three stout chromic catgut or Dexon sutures placed through the kidney substance, followed by several fine sutures to approximate the capsule. A drainage tube is inserted down to the kidney, the bridge is lowered and the wound closed in layers.

For *pyelolithotomy* exposure and mobilisation are the same as above, but care is taken to free the pelvis of the ureter by rotating the kidney forwards, as all the vessels pass in front of the ureter in their normal course. The calculus is palpated, steadied between the forefinger and thumb, and an incision made into the pelvis. The stone is extracted and the kidney probed for other stones, finally irrigating with sterile irrigation solution (e.g., saline). The incision is closed with fine non-traumatic sutures of chromic catgut or Dexon which may be reinforced with a piece of fat. A drainage tube is inserted down to the kidney, the operation table levelled and the wound closed in layers. (Sometimes the operation may be completed with a nephrostomy, especially if the stone removed is large.)

The operation of nephrolithotomy may be replaced by partial nephrectomy in suitable cases. In this procedure, the approach, dissection and closure follow that for nephrolithotomy. The stone is located and the overlying capsule incised and carefully peeled off the area of excision. As bleeding is usually profuse, a special occlusion clamp is applied across the renal pedicle for a limited time. A segment of kidney is removed together with the stone contained and the kidney pelvis may be irrigated. The stump of the calyx is closed with fine catgut and the substance of the kidney with several mattress sutures of strong chromic catgut which are so placed that when they are tied, the cut edges of the kidney tend to invaginate slightly. When haemostasis is complete, the capsule is sutured over the kidney with fine chromic catgut on a non-traumatic needle.

Ureterolithotomy

DEFINITION
Removal of a stone from the ureter.

POSITION
   Supine, or lateral as for nephrectomy.

INSTRUMENTS
   As for nephrectomy
   20 ml syringe, fine catheter and irrigation solution
   Fine rubber or plastic tubing, or nylon tape
   2 (3/0) Chromic catgut or Dexon (or plain catgut at the surgeon's discretion) on a small
      curved rounded-bodied non-traumatic needle.

OUTLINE OF PROCEDURE
   The ureter is approached either through an extension of the kidney incision, or
through a paramedian incision. In the former case, the kidney incision is continued
forwards to the centre of Poupart's ligament, deepened through the muscles to the
peritoneum which is not opened but reflected inwards from the posterior abdominal
wall.
   The ureter lies on the psoas muscle and may be adherent to the peritoneum from which
it is dissected free.
   In the latter case, a lower midline incision is made and the peritoneum not opened but
peeled inwards from the anterior and lateral abdominal wall. The ureter is then mobilised
as before and the stone palpated.
   A piece of tubing or nylon tape is passed around the ureter just above and below the
stone, which is manoeuvred a little beyond the point of impaction. An incision is made
into the ureter, the stone removed and the incision closed with fine non-traumatic catgut
or Dexon sutures which pass through the muscular coats only. A drain is inserted down
to the ureteric incision and the wound closed in layers. Some surgeons irrigate the ureter
and probe with fine ureteric bougies to search for other stones.

19

Gynaecological and Obstetric Operations

Excision of Bartholinian cyst

DEFINITION
  The removal of a cyst due to blockage of the duct of the Bartholin gland which is in the labium majora on either side.

POSITION
  Lithotomy, Figure 65.

INSTRUMENTS
  Sponge-holding forceps (Rampley), 5
  Towel clips, 5
  Scalpel handle No. 3 with No. 10 blade (Bard Parker)
  Dissecting forceps, toothed (Lane), 2
  Dissecting forceps, non-toothed, 15 cm (6 in)
  Scissors, curved on flat, 13 cm (5 in) (Mayo)
  Tissue forceps (Allis), 5
  Dissector (MacDonald or Durham)
  Fine artery forceps, straight, mosquito, 10
  Needle holder (Mayo)
  2·5 (2/0) Chromic catgut or Dexon for ligatures
  3 (0) Chromic catgut or Dexon on a small half-circle round-bodied needle for deep sutures.

OUTLINE OF PROCEDURE
  An incision is made over the swelling in the long axis of the labium majora, and deepened down to the cyst wall. The cyst is removed by blunt dissection and any blood-vessels encountered are picked up and ligated. The incision is closed with chromic catgut, drawing the walls of the cyst cavity together.

Excision of the vulva

DEFINITION
  Removal of the vulva.

POSITION. Lithotomy.

INSTRUMENTS
  General set (Fig. 281)

Urethral catheter, self-retaining (Foley size 18 Charrière gauge)
20 ml syringe and sterile water for inflating cuff of catheter
Proflavine emulsion or similar gauze pack
2·5 and 3 (2/0 and 0) Chromic catgut or Dexon for ligatures
4 or 5 (1 or 2) Chromic catgut or Dexon on a medium half-circle Mayo's needle with a
    trocar point for sutures.

OUTLINE OF PROCEDURE

An outer, oval incision is made, surrounding both labia majora if necessary. An inner, oval incision is also made and this lies just within the mucocutaneous junction, to include the urethral orifice, passing around the vaginal orifice. The incisions are extended down to the urethra. Just above the urethra the cut edges are united together, but the cut edge of the vagina below is approximated to the cut edge of the skin all around. A self-retaining catheter is inserted and the vagina packed with a length of gauze to control bleeding.

Perineorrhaphy

DEFINITION

Repair of a complete or incomplete rupture of the perineum.

POSITION. Lithotomy.

INSTRUMENTS

As vulvectomy
Ligatures and sutures as vulvectomy
3 (0) Chromic catgut or Dexon on a small half-circle round-bodied needle for plication
    of rectum
3 (0) Chromic catgut or Dexon on a curved non-traumatic intestinal needle for rectal
    closure (complete rupture only).

OUTLINE OF PROCEDURE

Incomplete Rupture, where a Segment of Perineum Remains. Tissue forceps are applied to the estimated edge of the original vaginal opening. Traction on these forceps stretches the torn edge of the perineum which is cut away between the forceps to expose an edge of mucosa and skin. The edge of the mucosa is dissected up and the posterior vaginal wall freed from the rectum. A triangular-shaped piece of vaginal wall (with its base at the perineum) is excised, and the levator ani muscles identified and drawn together with mattress sutures of chromic catgut or Dexon. The triangular gap is approximated longitudinally with a continuous chromic catgut or Dexon suture, and the vagina is packed in the usual manner. The procedure is completed by inserting a self-retaining catheter into the bladder.

Complete Rupture. This operation is similar to that just described, but in addition it is necessary to reconstruct the rectum and the anal sphincter.

The septum separating the rectum and vagina is cut away, so exposing the mucous membrane of both. The rectum is freed and the torn ends of the sphincter identified. The rectum is sutured and the sphincter brought together with strong chromic catgut or Dexon. The operation then resembles incomplete rupture with repair of the levator ani muscles and closing the triangular gap formed by partial excision of the posterior vaginal wall. Finally, a catheter and vaginal pack are inserted.

Anterior colporrhaphy, amputation of cervix and posterior colpoperineorrhaphy (Manchester repair)

DEFINITION

Repair of a cystocele (prolapse of the bladder into the vagina) and repair of a rectocele (prolapse of the rectum into the vagina).

POSITION. Lithotomy.

INSTRUMENTS

General set (Fig. 281)
Dilation and curettage set (Fig. 318)
Artery forceps, straight (Moynihan), 24
Urethral catheter, self-retaining (Foley size 18 Charrière gauge)
20 ml syringe and sterile water for inflating the cuff of the catheter
2·5 and 3 (2/0 and 0) Chromic catgut or Dexon for ligatures
3 (0) Chromic catgut or Dexon on a small half-circle round-bodied needle for plication of the bladder
4 or 5 (1 or 2) Chromic catgut or Dexon on a small half-circle Mayo needle with a trocar point for sutures
Proflavine emulsion or similar gauze pack for the vagina.

OUTLINE OF PROCEDURE

Anterior Colporrhaphy. An Auvard's speculum is inserted and the cervix grasped with Vulsellum forceps. The surgeon may then perform a dilation and curettage of the uterus if the patient is over the menopause and has cervical bleeding.

Traction is placed on the Vulsellum forceps, pulling the cervix down and thereby stretching the anterior vaginal wall. An incision is made just above the junction of the cervix with the vaginal wall and blunt pointed scissors are inserted to separate the bladder from the vagina. A bladder sound is inserted, and the dissection continued up to a point just below the urethra, and the vaginal wall is then slit up the midline along the extent of the separated portion. These skin flaps are retracted laterally and the bladder mobilised from the cervix and up and away from view. The cystocele is repaired by plicating the pubocervical fascia with 3 (0) chromic catgut or Dexon, thereby making a buttress between the bladder and vagina.

Amputation of the Cervix. If there is a vault prolapse, then a partial amputation of the cervix is performed. This is done after dissecting up two flaps of mucous membrane from the cervix, one in front and one behind. The partial amputation of the cervix is performed and the two flaps of mucous membrane sutured so that the mucosa is invaginated towards the lining of the cervix to form a reconstructed cervical os.

The anterior incision is closed with several mattress sutures which are placed lateral to the cut edge of the vaginal wall on each side. These sutures are tied and the redundant vaginal wall excised, so narrowing the vagina. The procedure is completed with a row of interrupted chromic catgut or Dexon sutures.

Posterior Colpoperineorrhaphy. The Auvard's speculum is removed and an elliptical transverse section of skin excised with scissors. The rectum is freed with dissecting scissors and the posterior vaginal wall is slit up the midline. The rectocele is repaired by approximating the levator ani muscles with mattress sutures of chronic catgut or Dexon. The redundant vaginal mucosa is excised and the edges brought together with continuous chromic catgut sutures.

The transverse incision in the posterior vaginal wall is sutured longitudinally, which again tightens the vagina. The operation is completed by inserting a self-retaining catheter into the bladder and packing the vagina with a proflavine emulsion gauze or similar pack.

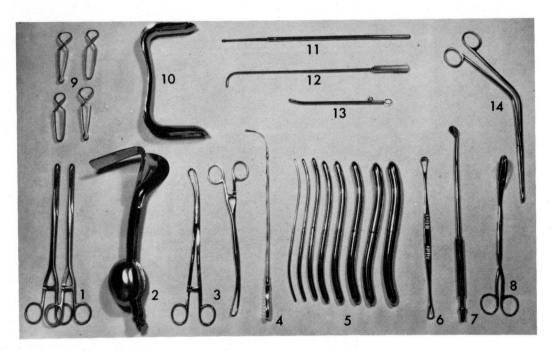

Figure 318　　Dilatation of the cervix and uterine curettage.

1. Sponge-holding forceps (Rampley), 2.
2. Vaginal speculum (Auvard).
3. Vulsellum forceps (Teale), 2.
4. Uterine sound (Horrock).
5. Uterine dilators (Hegar), set of various sizes.
6. Uterine curette (Sim), double end.
7. Flushing curette (Rheinstadter).
8. Ovum forceps (Greenhalgh).
9. Towel clips, 4.
10. Vaginal speculum (Sim).
11. Spiked-end probe (Playfair).
12. Bladder sound.
13. Female catheter, metal.
14. Uterine dressing forceps (Jessop Hospital pattern).

Dilation of the cervix and curettage of the uterus

DEFINITION

Dilation of the cervix and scraping away the uterine mucosa.

POSITION. Lithotomy.

INSTRUMENTS

As Figure 318.

OUTLINE OF PROCEDURE

An Auvard's speculum is inserted and the cervix drawn down and steadied with one or two vulsellum forceps. The position and length of the uterus are gauged with a uterine sound and progressively larger sizes of uterine dilators are inserted until the os is large enough to introduce the curette. The surgeon always holds each dilator between his thumb and forefinger, with the other fingers extended at the side, so that should the dilator slip, these extended fingers will come into contact with the buttocks and prevent the dilator penetrating too deeply. A uterine curette is inserted and the mucosa scraped gently and systematically. The curetted mucosa is sent for histological examination.

If the procedure is being carried out for retained products of conception, the initial stages follow that described above, but in this case the retained products are removed preferably with ovum or sponge-holding forceps instead of a curette, and the uterine sound is not used. A gauze pack may then be inserted into the vagina.

Fallopian insufflation and salpingography

DEFINITION

Insufflation of the Fallopian tubes with CO_2 to test their patency; and injection of a radio-opaque medium for X-ray examination of the interior of the uterus and Fallopian tubes.

POSITION. Lithotomy.

INSTRUMENTS
   Salpingography (Fig. 319).

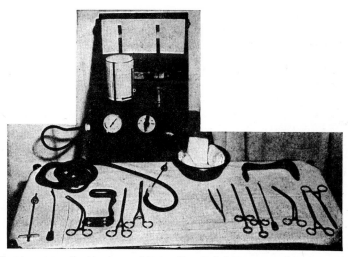

Figure 319   Apparatus for Testing and Recording Tubal Patency and Functional Activity.
(From *A Textbook of Midwifery* by Margaret Myles, by kind permission.)

Instruments for endometrial biopsy:	Instruments for tubal insufflation:
2 sponge-holding forceps.	2 cannulae.
1 Sim's speculum.	1 uterine sound.
1 teneculum forceps.	1 teneculum forceps.
1 uterine sound.	1 Sim's speculum.
2 endometrial biopsy curettes.	2 sponge-holding forceps.
1 dissecting forceps.	

OUTLINE OF PROCEDURE
   A bi-valve speculum is inserted and the cervix drawn down and steadied with one or

two pairs of vulsellum forceps. The position and length of the uterus are gauged with a uterine sound and progressively larger sizes of uterine dilators are inserted up to the outside diameter of the insufflation nozzle. The insufflation nozzle is inserted into the cervical canal and CO_2 under pressure is injected into the uterus up to 180 mm Hg. Patency of the Fallopian tubes is determined either by applying a stethoscope to the abdominal wall and listening to the gas escaping into the peritoneal cavity from each tube as the pressure is applied, or observing a direct reading Kymograph which records pressure variations as the CO_2 is injected. (The dilation may then be continued followed by endrometrial biopsy.)

For salpingography, a Sim's speculum is inserted and the radio-opaque medium (Urografin 76 per cent) injected into the uterine cavity with a special syringe. An X-ray is taken immediately.

Cervical and uterine polypus, biopsy and cauterisation of the cervix

DEFINITION

Removal of a polypus from the cervix or interior of the uterus; biopsy of the cervix for histological examination; cauterisation for cervical erosion and chronic cervicitis.

POSITION. Lithotomy.

INSTRUMENTS
  Dilation and curettage (Fig. 318)
  Scalpel handle No. 3 with No. 10 blade (Bard Parker)
  Dissecting forceps, toothed (Lane), 2
  Dissecting forceps, non-toothed, 18 cm (7 in), 2
  Scissors, curved on flat, 18 cm (7 in) (Mayo)
  Needle holder (Mayo)
  Diathermy or cautery apparatus, leads and electrodes for cervical cauterisation
  3 or 4 (0 or 1) Chromic catgut or Dexon on a small half-circle Mayo needle with a
     trocar point for sutures.

OUTLINE OF PROCEDURE

Cervical Polypus. A Sim's speculum is inserted and the polyp grasped with ring forceps or artery forceps. The polypus is twisted until it comes away, and the cervical canal is gently scraped with a small curette.

Uterine Polypus. A Sim's speculum is inserted and the cervical os dilated until the opening is large enough to grasp the polyp with forceps and twisted as described above. If bleeding is persistent and cannot be stopped with hot irrigations, the surgeon will pack the uterine cavity with a length of gauze.

Cervical Biopsy. This operation is generally performed in conjunction with dilatation and curettage of the uterus, sometimes following a Papanicolaou cervical smear in which suspicious cells have been found. A small wedge or cone of cervix is excised and sent for histological examination, and the incision is approximated with chromic catgut or Dexon. The vagina may be packed with a proflavine emulsion or similar gauze pack.

Cervical Cauterisation. A bi-valve or Sim's speculum is inserted and heat applied to the ulcerated area by means of a cautery or diathermy electrode. If diathermy is being used, the indifferent electrode is applied to the patient's thigh with the usual precautions (Chapter 2). The vagina will be packed with a proflavine emulsion or similar gauze pack.

Spiritous antiseptics must not be used for skin preparation due to the danger of explosion with diathermy or cautery.

Laparoscopy (peritoneoscopy)

DEFINITION
Inspection of the peritoneal cavity by means of a laparoscope introduced through the abdominal wall.

POSITION
Either supine or slight Trendelenburg with legs in lithotomy.

INSTRUMENTS
Laparoscopy
Sponge-holding forceps (Rampley), 2
Towel clips, 5
Scalpel handle No. 3 with No. 10 blade (Bard Parker)
Dissecting forceps, toothed (Lane), 2
Dissecting forceps, non-toothed, 15 cm (6 in)
Scissors, curved on flat, 13 cm (5 in) (Mayo), 1.
Needle holder (Mayo), 1
Laparoscope, such as the Frangeheim (as Fig. 320)
Palmer biopsy drill forceps (Fig. 321)

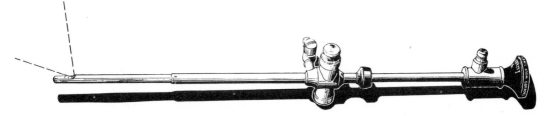

Figure 320   Frangenheim laparoscope.

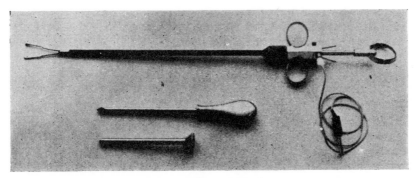

Figure 321   Palmer Biopsy forceps.

Verres trocar and cannula
Diathermy leads and electrodes
Fibre light projector

2·5 or 3 (2/0 or 0) chromic catgut or Dexon for ligatures and on small half-circle
   cutting needle for subcutaneous sutures if required
2·5 (2/0) silk or nylon on straight or curved cutting needle for skin sutures.
Vaginal examination
Instruments as for D and C may be required
Gentian violet solution and 10 ml syringe with cannula.

OUTLINE OF PROCEDURE

The Verres needle is inserted through a small 2 cm skin incision made transversely just
below the umbilicus. The same incision is used later for inserting the laparoscope trocar
and cannula. (The point of the Verres needle is first covered with K-Y or similar jelly.)

The needle is manipulated until the point is felt to pass through the outer layer of the
rectus sheath then impinging upon the posterior layer and with a little more pressure
enter the abdominal cavity. The sudden dropping of the inner core into the needle (Fig.
322) is a further indication that the point has entered the abdominal cavity.

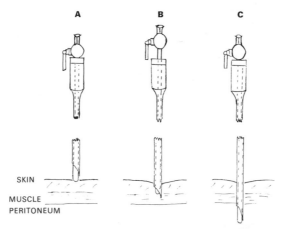

Figure 322   A. Needle at skin surface, inner core fully extended.
B. Needle in abdominal wall, inner core fully retracted at point, air intake raised above
shoulder.
C. Needle point through abdominal wall, inner core descends rounded end now prevents
point of outer sheath from damaging bowel, etc. Air intake sits down on shoulder as point
enters peritoneal cavity.

The needle is then connected to a carbon dioxide supply controlled through an
apparatus such as the Semm's automatic insufflator and some three litres of gas are allowed
to pass into the abdominal cavity. This takes three to four minutes and care is taken not
to raise the intra-abdominal pressure by more than 20 mm Hg as this could seriously
interfere with the return of blood to the heart by stopping the flow in the inferior vena
cava which could lead to acute hypotension.

The lubricated laparoscope trocar and cannula are now inserted slightly diagonally
(alongside the Verres needle) through the rectus sheath and into the abdominal cavity.
The trocar is removed and the telescope with its accompaning light carrier is passed
through the cannula into the abdominal cavity.

PROCEDURES CARRIED OUT WITH THE LAPAROSCOPE (FISHER, 1970)

1. *Infertility.* Tubal patency can be demonstrated by dye installation through a
cervical canula by a second operator. A solution of gentian violet, is instilled into the

uterus; with the laparoscope the surgeon by visualising dye transit can confirm tubal patency. Similarly the restriction of dye dispersal by fine adhesions is easily demonstrated. At the same time ovarian biopsy can be taken to establish the presence of primordial follicles or functioning corpora lutea or graffian follicles.

2. *Ectopic Pregnancy.* When there are doubts in cases of early tubal abortion laparoscopy can reveal the presence of the tubal gestation and the surgeon can then proceed to laparotomy and definitive surgery. Conversely, a ruptured retention cyst which is settling can be left alone and thus laparotomy avoided.

3. *Acute Infection.* In the presence of abdominal pain where the differential diagnosis includes acute salpingitis, ectopic pregnancy and ruptured retention cysts, laparoscopy has been used to identify the engorged and distended Fallopian tubes in cases of acute salpingitis, thus permitting conservative treatment and avoiding laparotomy.

4. *Amenorrhoea.* The investigation of amenorrhoea today will include a laparoscopy, visualising the ovaries and enabling a biopsy to be taken. This step can be most useful in establishing the likelihood of the ovaries responding to treatment. In the absence of primordial follicles there is little evidence that stimulation by gonadotrophins will be of value. Similarly, the presence of multiple micro-cysts in the ovary indicate the need for extreme caution in the management of gonadotrophin stimulation therapy.

5. *Sterilisation.* It is possible by introducing suitably insulated forceps through a second small incision to divide the Fallopian tubes by diathermy coagulation in one or more places and thus effect sterilisation by interrupting tubal continuity.

6. *Unexplained Abdominal Pain.* Much of the gynaecologist's practice concerns pain in the pelvis. In these instances laparoscopy provides a means of obtaining a correct diagnosis in cases of unsuspected endometriosis and other causes of pelvic inflammatory response. Thus definitive treatment is possible and the patient's pain relieved.

At the close of the operation the carbon dioxide is first expelled from the abdominal cavity via the cannula which is then removed. The skin incision is closed with silk or nylon, alternatively subcutaneous sutures of catgut or Dexon may be used.

Abdominal hysterectomy

DEFINITION
Partial or entire removal of the uterus through an abdominal incision.

POSITION
Trendelenburg, Figure 45.

INSTRUMENTS
General set (Fig. 281)
Laparotomy set (Fig. 282)
Hysterectomy set (Fig. 323)
2·5 and 3 (2/0 and 0) Chromic catgut or Dexon for ligatures, fine and medium
5 (2) Chromic catgut or Dexon on large half-circle Mayo needles with trocar points for transfixion sutures and uterine, vaginal vault, peritoneum and muscle sutures
3 (0) Chromic catgut or Dexon on a medium half-circle round-bodied needle for reconstruction of pelvic floor
2·5 (2/0) Silk or nylon on a large straight or curved cutting needle for skin sutures
(Kifa and Michel clips may be required.)

OUTLINE OF PROCEDURE
The vagina is swabbed with antiseptic solution and plugged with a length of anti-

septic gauze, which is left protruding for subsequent removal during operation. Removal and safety ensuring removal will be easier if a pair of sponge-holding forceps is attached to this pack and left lying between the patient's legs.

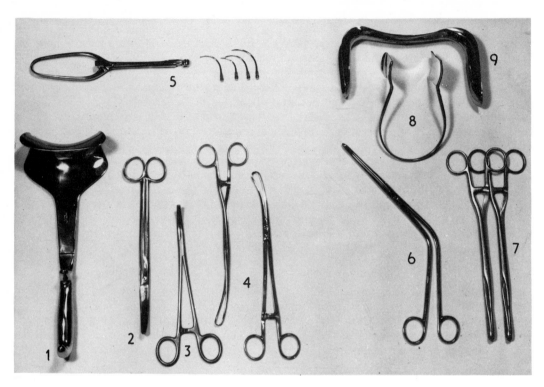

Figure 323　　Abdominal hysterectomy, etc.

1. Suprapublic retractor (Doyen).
2. Long, heavy scissors, curved on flat 25 cm (10 in).
3. Artery forceps, curved on flat (Mayo-Oschner), 6.
4. Vulsellum forceps (Teale), 2.
5. Needle holder and needles (Bonney-Reverdin), 3 sharp point and 1 blunt point.
6. Uterine dressing forceps (Jessop Hospital pattern).
7. Sponge-holding forceps (Rampley), 2.
8. Vaginal retractor (Collins).
9. Vaginal speculum (Sim).

The abdomen is opened through a subumbilical midline incision which passes through the skin, linea alba and peritoneum. The bowel which may protrude is displaced towards the diaphragm with two or three large gauze packs. The uterus is drawn out of the pelvis and two pairs of Kocher's or Mayo-Oschner forceps are applied across the broad ligament either inside or outside the ovaries, depending on whether they are to be removed or not. It is usual to try to leave at least one ovary for endocrine function. The broad ligament is opened on each side between these forceps and a flap of peritoneum is cut from the front of the uterus. The bladder is separated from the front of the cervix by blunt dissection and is pushed well below the point of transection. Pairs of clamps are placed across the cardinal ligaments and uterine arteries on each side, carefully avoiding the ureters, and the vessels are divided between the clamps.

For subtotal hysterectomy, the uterus is removed by cutting across the cervix; for pan or total hysterectomy the pack is removed from the vagina, the fornix of the vagina is cut into, the cervix seized with a pair of vulsellum forceps and drawn upwards, and the uterus is removed by dividing the vagina from the cervix all round.

Transfixion sutures are placed and tied around the clamped stumps of the ovarian vessels, round ligament and uterine arteries. For subtotal hysterectomy, the stump of the cervix is closed over with a few interrupted chromic catgut or Dexon sutures, and for total hysterectomy the cut edge of the vagina is closed with interrupted or continuous chromic catgut or Dexon sutures. The flap of peritoneum is sutured over the cut edge of the posterior peritoneum, covering the cervical or vaginal stump and the transfixed round ligaments. The surgeon may suture the round ligaments to the vault of the vagina before reconstructing the pelvic floor with No. 0 chromic catgut or Dexon sutures. The abdominal wound is closed in layers.

Wertheim's hysterectomy

DEFINITION

Total hysterectomy, bilateral salpingo-oöphorectomy, with removal of the upper part of the vagina and lymphatic glands which drain the pelvis.

POSITION

Trendelenburg, Figure 61.

INSTRUMENTS

As for abdominal hysterectomy
Hysterectomy clamps, right-angled (Wertheim), 2
Diathermy leads, electrodes and lead anchoring forceps
Urethral catheter, self-retaining (Foley size 18 Charrière gauge)
20 ml syringe, and sterile water to inflate cuff of catheter
Ligatures and sutures as for hysterectomy.

OUTLINE OF PROCEDURE

This follows the procedure of total hysterectomy but with the following additions.

The rectum is freed from the vagina which is divided across well beyond the cervix after applying strong right-angled clamps (Wertheim's). In this way, when the uterus is removed, the growth on the cervix is covered by a section of the vagina clamped over it, thereby preventing soiling of the peritoneal cavity. After the vagina has been closed and the vessels ligatured, the connective tissue on the side walls of the pelvis and around the vessels is carefully dissected free, together with the iliac and obturator glands.

The pelvic floor is reconstructed as before and the wound closed in layers. As the bladder has been extensively separated, it is usual to leave a catheter *in situ* for a few days post-operatively.

Vaginal hysterectomy

DEFINITION

Removal of the uterus through the vagina.

POSITION. Lithotomy.

INSTRUMENTS

General set (Fig. 281)
Artery forceps, straight, 20 cm (8 in) (Spencer Wells), 10

Deep retractors, narrow blade (Deaver or Paton), 2
Artery forceps, heavy curved on flat (Mayo-Oschner or Kocher), 6
Vulsellum forceps (Teale), 2
Scissors, heavy curved on flat, 20 cm (8 in) (Mayo)
Vaginal speculum (Auvard)
Urethral catheter, self-retaining (Foley size 18 Charrière gauge)
20 ml syringe, and sterile water to inflate cuff of catheter
4 and 5 (1 and 2) Chromic catgut or Dexon for all ligatures, transfixion sutures and
   closure sutures on large half-circle Mayo needles with trocar points
Proflavine emulsion or similar gauze pack may be required for vagina.

OUTLINE OF PROCEDURE

An Auvard's speculum is inserted, and the cervix grasped with vulsellum forceps,
pulled down and steadied. An incision is made below the urinary orifice and round the
cervix. The bladder is freed from the uterus in front, and the rectum from the uterus
posteriorly. The anterior and posterior peritoneum is opened and traction applied to the
cervix so that clamps can be applied to the cardinal ligament and uterine arteries. The
fundus of the uterus is delivered from the abdomen and clamps applied to each round
ligament. The round ligament is severed between the clamps and the uterus is removed.
The vessels and ligaments are transfixed and ligated with chromic catgut or Dexon. The
anterior and posterior peritoneum are sutured together, exteriorising the round ligaments and uterine vessels which are sutured over by closing the vaginal wall.

A catheter is inserted and the vagina plugged with a proflavine emulsion gauze or
similar pack.

Oöphorectomy, salpingectomy, myomectomy

DEFINITION

Removal of an ovary; Fallopian tube; or one or more uterine fibroids.

POSITION

Trendelenburg. (Supine for ectopic gestation.)

INSTRUMENTS

As for abdominal hysterectomy.
Suction tubing, nozzles and tube anchoring forceps for ectopic gestation.

OUTLINE OF PROCEDURE

The uterus is exposed through a subumbilical midline incision. The *oöphorectomy* and
removal of ovarian cyst, the pedicle of the ovary or tumour is transfixed with strong
chromic catgut or Dexon, clamping with Mayo-Oschner forceps before division. The
tumour is removed and the raw edges of the tied pedicle are covered with peritoneum
secured with fine chromic catgut sutures.

In *salpingectomy*, the inflamed tubes are usually adherent behind the uterus. They are
carefully freed by blunt dissection and clamped across with double clamps before dividing. A catgut or Dexon transfixion ligature is now passed around the cut tube and vessels
at each side of the division. This operation is performed also for ruptured ectopic gestation and in this case suction is used to remove blood from the peritoneal cavity.

In *myomectomy*, the uterus is incised and the fibroids shelled out. The uterine incision
is closed with two layers of chromic catgut or Dexon and the abdominal incision closed
in the usual manner. The common complications are haemorrhage and sepsis.

Hysteropexy

DEFINITION

A plastic operation on the uterus, performed for retroversion.

POSITION. Trendelenburg.

INSTRUMENTS

As for laparotomy (Figs. 281 and 282)
Artery forceps, curved (Mayo-Oschner or Kocher), 2.

OUTLINE OF PROCEDURE

There are several operations for this condition, but only one, that of ventrosuspension or shortening of the round ligaments, will be described here.

A transverse, curved incision is made just above the pubis. This incision is carried down to the rectus sheath only, which is then incised in a vertical direction and the peritoneum is opened. The uterus is raised and a transfixion ligature placed on each round ligament about 1 cm (half and inch) from where it joins the uterus. The two ends of this ligature are left about 25 cm (10 in) long.

The skin is separated from the anterior rectus sheath for a small area on each side of the incision. Using scissors, the anterior rectus sheath is separated from the rectus muscle in a downward and outward direction towards the internal abdominal ring. Curved artery forceps are manoeuvred along this so-formed track on each side of the incision to the internal ring. They pass through the internal abdominal ring and are manoeuvred along the round ligament to the point of ligature, where they are pushed through a stab incision in the peritoneum. The ligature is grasped and the forceps withdrawn, pulling the round ligament through the internal abdominal ring to appear between the anterior rectus sheath and muscle. The round ligaments are secured to the anterior rectus sheath with sutures of strong silk and the ligatures are used as an additional sutures to make fixation doubly sure.

This procedure shortens the round ligaments by doubling them over and the suspension of the uterus is tightened, thereby correcting retroversion. The wound is closed in layers.

Caesarean section

DEFINITION

Removal of the foetus through an incision in the abdominal wall and the uterus.

POSITION

Supine, followed by Trendelenburg. 10°–20°.

INSTRUMENTS

As for hysterectomy
Uterine forceps (Green-Armytage), 5
Obstetric forceps
Suction tubing, nozzles and tube anchoring forceps
2 ml syringe and needles with ergometrine 0·5 mg
Mucus extractors and general apparatus for resuscitation of the child (cord clamps, scissors, etc.).

OUTLINE OF PROCEDURE

The patient comes to theatre with a catheter *in situ* which is released but not removed during the operation. A midline incision is made extending from the umbilicus to the pubis. The bowel is displaced towards the diaphragm with packs and a 10 cm (4 in) incision made in the uterus. For lower segment operations (the majority of procedures), the incision is made horizontally in the uterus (after separating the bladder from the uterus) just where the peritoneum is reflected off the bladder, and for upper segment operations, the incision is in the midline vertically. This requires a clean scalpel. The incision is completed with scissors and by manual stretching. The foetus is delivered and the umbilical cord clamped with forceps and divided. Whilst the midwife or paediatrician resuscitates the child, the placenta is delivered and the cut edges of the uterus grasped with Green-Armytage forceps. Suction is used to remove amniotic fluid.

Ergometrine is injected intravenously to cause contraction of the uterine muscles and thereby arrest haemorrhage. The incision in the uterus is closed with two layers of chromic catgut or Dexon sutures, the first layer passing through the muscle coat but not the mucosa, and the second layer is inserted to inverted the first layer. The uterovesical peritoneum is sutured and the wound closed in the usual manner.

Clots are expressed from the vagina by pressure on the abdomen and a pad applied to the vulva.

REFERENCES

FISHER, A. M. (1970) *Natnews*, Autumn, p. 21.

20

Operations on the Neck

Radical cervical node dissection

DEFINITION
Removal of the submental, submaxillary and deep cervical glands, together with the sternomastoid muscle.

POSITION
Supine, with a sandbag under the shoulder blades, and the neck in extension (Fig. 67).

INSTRUMENTS
General set (Fig. 281)
Long scissors, curved on flat (McIndoe)
Large aneurysm needle
Artery forceps, curved on flat (Kelly Fraser), 10
Artery forceps, curved on flat (Dunhill), 25
Retractors, self-retaining (Travers and West), 2
Corrugated drainage tube and safety-pin or long plastic drainage tubing and Redivac
    suction bottle
Suction tubing, nozzles and tube anchoring forceps.
Diathermy leads, electrodes and lead anchoring forceps
2, 2·5 and 3 (3/0, 2/0 and 0) Chromic catgut, Dexon or silk for ligatures
3 (0) Chromic catgut or Dexon on a medium half-circle round-bodied needle for muscle
    sutures
2·5 (2/0) Silk or nylon on a small or medium curved cutting needle for skin sutures
(Michel or Kifa clips may be used.)

OUTLINE OF PROCEDURE
An oblique incision is made from the mastoid process to the sternum. This incision is extended Y-fashion to the chin just beyond the midline. The skin flaps are reflected and the platysma incised at the lower end of the sternomastoid muscle which is then divided across. This muscle is dissected up and the lower part of the internal jugular vein clamped and ligated. Dissection is continued, turning up the sternomastoid muscle and jugular vein and removing all tissue which lies behind as far as the trapezius muscle. When the dissection reaches the bifurcation of the common carotid artery, the tissues below the chin, including the submaxillary gland, are then dealt with and reflected towards the carotid bifurcation also. The insertion of the sternomastoid muscle into the skull is severed and the mass of tissue removed, together with the lower pole of the parotid gland. During this dissection the facial artery and vein and the upper part of the jugular

vein will be ligated, but the carotid vessels and the vagus and other essential nerves are carefully preserved. The wound is closed with drainage after haemostasis is complete.

Excision of parotid tumour

DEFINITION
    Removal of a tumour in the parotid gland.

POSITION
    As radical cervical dissection.

INSTRUMENTS
    As radical cervical dissection, except
    2 (3/0) Silk or nylon on a small curved cutting needle for skin sutures.

OUTLINE OF PROCEDURE
    An incision is made commencing near the lobe of the ear and extending along the crease of the neck. The parotid gland is exposed and the tumour freed by dissection. Haemostasis is secured, a drain inserted and the wound is closed.

Excision of thyroglossal duct or cyst

DEFINITION
    Removal of a congenital duct between the thyroid gland and the pharynx, which may be cystic, and have an external opening in the neck.

POSITION
    As radical cervical dissection.

INSTRUMENTS
    As radical cervical dissection
    Small bone cutting forceps.

OUTLINE OF PROCEDURE
    Sistrunk's operation consists of a transverse curved incision which is made over the site of the cyst, or an elliptical incision around the sinus opening. The cyst and sinus tract are grasped with tissue forceps and dissected down to the hyoid bone, the centre of which is removed, thereby dividing the bone. Dissection is continued down to the base of the tongue and the extent of this dissection confirmed by palpating through the mouth. The sinus and cyst are removed and the tissues of the tongue are closed with chromic catgut or Dexon sutures. The hyoid bone is approximated with chromic catgut or Dexon, a drain inserted and the wound closed.

Partial thyroidectomy or excision of adenoma of thyroid

DEFINITION
    Removal of part of the thyroid gland or removal of thyroid adenoma.

POSITION
    As radical cervical dissection.

INSTRUMENTS
   General set (Fig. 281)
   Thyroidectomy set (Fig. 324)
   Long scissors, curved on flat (McIndoe)

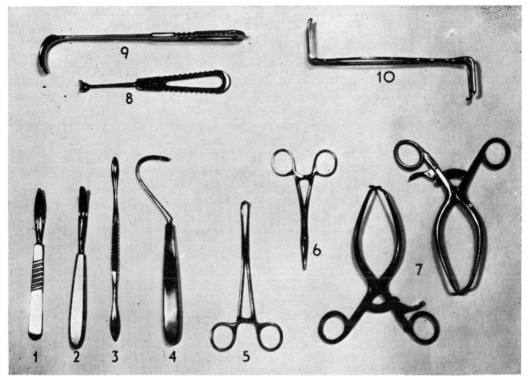

Figure 324   Partial thyroidectomy, etc.

1. Thyroid dissector with eye at point (Kocher).
2. Thyroid dissector (Kocher).
3. Dissector (Durham).
4. Large aneurysm needle.
5. Thyroid-holding forceps (Laney), 2.
6. Artery forceps, curved on flat (Dunhill), 36.
7. Retractors, self-retaining, thyroid, 2 (Jackson Burrow, or alternatively one Joll type).
8. Small short blade retractors, thyroid (Kocher), 2.
9. Small, long blade retractors, thyroid (Kocher), 2.
10. Medium retractors (Czerny), 2.

Corrugated drainage tube and safety-pin
Suction tubing, nozzles and tube anchoring forceps
Diathermy leads, electrodes and lead anchoring forceps
Local infiltration requisites and adrenaline 1 in 400,000 in saline (Optional)
2·5 and 3 (2/0 and 0) Chromic catgut or Dexon and silk for ligatures
2 and 3 (3/0 and 0) Chromic catgut or Dexon on small half-circle round-bodied needles
   for muscle and subcutaneous sutures
2 (3/0) Silk on a medium curved cutting needle for skin sutures *or* Michel or Kifa clips.

OUTLINE OF PROCEDURE
   Some surgeons infiltrate the skin of the incision area and the platysma with a solution of

1 in 400,000 adrenaline in saline which acts as a vasoconstricting agent, lessens bleeding and provides a plane of cleavage between the platysma and the deeper structures.

A low transverse incision is made in the neck, in line with the skin creases. The skin flaps and platysma are reflected widely and a self-retaining retractor or retractors inserted. The deep cervical fascia is incised in the midline and the infra-hyoid muscles retracted laterally or divided. The gland is carefully freed one lobe at a time by first clamping and dividing the middle thyroid vein, and then elevating the upper pole with a gland enucleator and ligating the superior thyroid artery. The lower lobe of the gland is then dislocated forwards and the inferior thyroid artery is ligatured in continuity.

This process may then be repeated on the other lobe before any glandular tissue is excised. A small portion of the posterior part of one or both lobes which contains the parathyroid glands is left and the remainder excised, first clamping with forceps as the excision proceeds. These divided vessels and tissue are ligated to secure haemostasis, a drain is inserted through a stab incision in the deep fascia on each side, and the muscles and fascia are sutured. The skin is closed with sutures or skin clips.

For excision of adenoma, the gland is exposed in the usual manner, and artery forceps are placed along the line where the tumour has caused the gland tissue to thin out. An incision is made just in front of these into the adenoma capsule. The tumour is then shelled out and the resultant cavity sutured over. The wound is closed as above.

21
Neurosurgical Operations

Angiography

DEFINITION

Serial X-ray examination of the cerebral vascular tree following the injection of a radio-opaque medium into a main artery in the neck, the needle being introduced percutaneously.

POSITION

Supine, with the head extended, preferably on a Lysholm skull table.

INSTRUMENTS

Sponge-holding forceps (Rampley), 5
Towel clips, 5
Scalpel handle (Bard Parker) with No. 11 blade
20 ml syringes, 3
Sterile normal saline, pyrogen free, 60 ml
Arterial puncture needles, i.e., Lindgren arterial needles; carotid or vertebral type
   needles, adult and child size
Adaptors and silicone tubing, 15 cm in length
Local anaesthetic requisites (Fig. 271)
Contrast medium, e.g., Hypaque 35 per cent or Conray 420.

OUTLINE OF PROCEDURE

A skin bleb of local anaesthetic is raised anterior to the sternomastoid and then the carotid sheath or region of the vertebral artery is infiltrated. The needle is mounted on a syringe filled with saline and is inserted into the appropriate artery through a nick in the skin. After ensuring that there is a good backflow of blood from the selected vessel the assembly is kept patent by slow injection of saline.

After positioning the patient for radiography, the saline-filled syringe is exchanged for a syringe containing contrast medium which is then rapidly injected intra-arterially whilst X-rays are taken. Normally these consist of three views, antero-posterior, lateral and oblique taken serially. Each time 8 to 10 ml of contrast medium is injected.

Air encephalography

DEFINITION

X-ray examination of the ventricular system and subarachnoid spaces surrounding the brain by fractional replacement of cerebrospinal fluid with filtered air.

POSITION
Sitting, with head flexed 20°, usually in an encephalography chair.

INSTRUMENTS
Spinal set (Fig. 272).

OUTLINE OF PROCEDURE
Local anaesthesia and lumbar puncture is performed, omitting manometry. Using 5 ml quantities, 30 to 40 ml of c.s.f. is gradually replaced with air (filtered through a swab whilst being sucked into the syringe), an X-ray being taken after 10 ml replacement to check that air is entering the brain ventricles. After adequate air replacement the lumbar puncture needle is removed, the patient placed supine and further X-rays are taken. A sample of the aspirated c.s.f. is sent for analysis.

Myelography

DEFINITION
X-ray examination of the spinal canal after the injection of an oily radio-opaque medium into the subdural space.

POSITION
Lateral with knees and neck moderately flexed, or sitting.

INSTRUMENTS
Spinal set (Fig. 272)
Myodil contrast medium.

OUTLINE OF PROCEDURE
Local anaesthesia and lumbar puncture is performed in the third or fourth lumbar interspace. Pressure readings without, and then with jugular compression are taken and 5 to 6 ml of c.s.f. withdrawn for analysis. The patient is then X-rayed supine and prone on a tilting table. The Myodil is left *in situ*.

Cysternal puncture

DEFINITION
The subarachnoid injection of Myodil for myelography in cases of 'failed lumbar puncture' due to 'dry tap' secondary to total spinal block. The contrast medium is injected into the cysterna magna.

POSITION
Sitting with the neck flexed.

INSTRUMENTS
Spinal set (Fig. 272)
Cysternal puncture (short bevel) needle
Needle guard
Steel rule, 15 cm (6 in).

OUTLINE OF PROCEDURE

A skin bleb of local anaesthetic is raised in the mid-line of the neck, halfway between the external occipital protuberance and the sixth cervical spinous process. After infiltration of the neck musculature, the cysternal puncture needle (with the guard set at 55 mm) is then slowly inserted in the mid-line to traverse the posterior atlanto-occipital membrane and enter the cysterna magna at the base of the brain. After withdrawing 5 to 6 ml of c.s.f. for analysis, Myodil is injected, the needle withdrawn and X-rays taken as in myelography.

Ventriculography

DEFINITION

An X-ray examination of the ventricular system of the brain after partial replacement of the ventricular c.s.f. with air, or occasionally Myodil.

POSITION

Supine or sitting in the neurosurgical chair.

INSTRUMENTS

Burr hole set (Fig. 325)
Sponge-holding forceps (Rampley), 5
Scalpel handle No. 4 with No. 22 blade (Bard Parker)
Fine dissecting forceps, non-toothed (McIndoe)
Fine dissecting forceps, toothed (Gillies)
Medium dissecting forceps, non-toothed
Medium dissecting forceps, toothed (Lane's)
Artery forceps, straight (Moynihan), 5
Scissors, stitch
Fine needle holder (West)
Diathermy leads, electrodes, scabbard and lead anchoring forceps
Spinal manometer
Pint measure with warm saline
Local anaesthetic requisites (Fig. 271)
Suction tubing, fine nozzles and tube anchoring forceps
Fine Nélaton catheters, polyvinyl or latex rubber with spigots, 5
250 ml conical flask fitted with a two-holed rubber stopper, glass air-vent and 100 cm of silicone tubing and fine metal concentric connector
Horsley's bone wax
2 or 1·5 (3/0 or 4/0) Silk on small curved round-bodied needles for dura
2 (3/0) Silk on small curved cutting or straight cutting needles for skin.

OUTLINE OF PROCEDURE

Local anaesthetic is infiltrated into the areas selected for ventricular puncture. A 5 cm straight incision is made 3·5 cm from the midline either on the frontal or parietal eminences. Two artery forceps are clipped on to the deepest galeal layer as retractors and after clearing back the periosteum, the artery forceps are replaced with a self-retaining retractor which by virtue of pressure from the blades creates haemostasis.

The hole is drilled first by using the perforator and then the appropriate matching burr. The dura is elevated with a dural hook, incised in a cruciate fashion and the lifted edges diathermised. The underlying brain is diathermised and incised at the entry point for insertion of the cannula. The lateral ventricles are cannulated on either side and c.s.f. pressure measured if required. Samples of c.s.f. are taken separately fom each side for analysis.

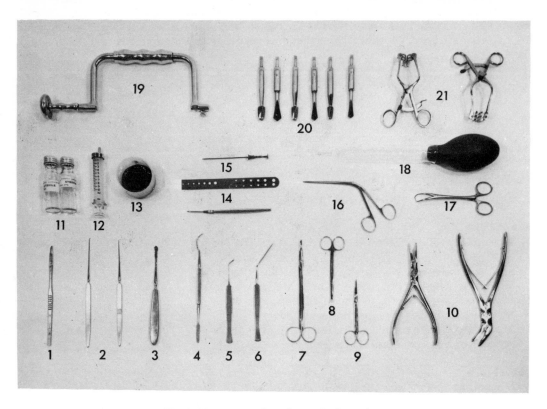

Figure 325   Burr Hole and ventriculography.

1. Scalpel handle No. 5 with No. 15 or 11 blade (Bard Parker).
2. Dura hooks, sharp and blunt.
3. Periosteal elevator (Adson).
4. Dissector (McDonald).
5. Trephine seeker/small aneurysm needle.
6. Dura separator (Sergeant's).
7. Scissors curved (Metzenbaum).
8. Scissors curved (strabismus).
9. Scissors straight (Iris).
10. Bone nibblers, curved on flat and angled on side.
11. CSF specimen bottles.
12. 10 ml syringe.
13. Bonney's Blue.
14. Steel rule and skin pen.
15. Ventricular cannula.
16. Nasal dressing forceps.
17. Towel clips (5).
18. Irrigation syringe.
19. Skull brace (Hudson).
20. Skull perforators and burrs (Hodson).
21. Retractors, self-retaining (Shnitkers).

Not Illustrated:
Sponge-holding forceps (Rampley), 4.
Scalpel handle No. 3 with No. 10 blade (Bard Barker).
Artery forceps, straight (Moynihan), 4.
Local anaesthetic requisites. Diathemy requisites.
2·5 (2/0) silk or braided nylon on straight or curved cutting needles.

The cannulae may be exchanged for fine catheters through which c.s.f. is fractionally replaced with filtered air in 5 to 10 ml increments to give a total replacement of 30 to 40 ml with normal size ventricles. If Myodil is used only 5 to 6 ml is injected.

The catheters are spigoted and the scalp closed in two layers after haemostasis has been secured. Following radiography, the catheters (which project through the suture line) are either removed, or in cases of chronic raised intracranial pressure, one is left coupled to the drainage flask for 24 to 48 hours to minimise the risk of brain compression or 'coning'.

Burr hole and biopsy abscess drainage

DEFINITION

Diagnostic needle biopsy of pathological intracerebra tissue or cyst drainage via a burr hole.

POSITION

Supine, lateral or prone depending on selected site for biopsy.

INSTRUMENTS

As for ventriculography

Glass microscope slides, 7·6 cm × 2·5 cm (3 in × 1 in)

In cases of brain abscess a selection of short rubber tubing of medium bore, 5 cm long will be required. Also either Micropaque or Steripaque radio-opaque emulsion.

OUTLINE OF PROCEDURE

Up to an including the dural incision the procedure approximates that for ventriculography. The burr hole is sited so that on 'needling' the brain a relatively 'silent' area is traversed.

The brain substance is explored with a fine brain needle passed in radiate fashion, to discover pathological tissue or cysts. When a possibly pathological area of brain is entered, a gentle aspiration biopsy is taken through the needle and pressure-smeared between two microscope slides which are placed in formol saline and sent for pathological examination.

Cysts and abscess cavities are drained through medium-bore tube drains. Abscess cavities are irrigated and Micropaque or Steripaque instilled. This emulsion adheres to the cavity wall and serial radiographs will chart alterations in cavity size. The scalp is closed in two layers.

Craniotomy and craniectomy

DEFINITION

Craniotomy is incision through the scalp and underlying muscle with fashioning of a muscle-hinged osteoplastic flap of the skull in order to gain access to the brain. *Craniectomy* denotes removal of bone from the skull vault either by enlargement of burr holes or removal of osteoplastic bone flap, again to afford access to the brain. Included under this heading is reduction of a depressed fracture of the skull vault.

POSITION

Supine for frontal, temporal or parietal exposures; prone for occipital and posterior fossa exposures; sitting for posterior fossa exposures or lateral for temporo-parietal flaps.

INSTRUMENTS

General set (Fig. 281), except large retractors

Burr hole set (Fig. 325)

Craniotomy set (Fig. 326)
Mallet (Heath's)
Small gouges, 3 mm, 4 mm, 6 mm, 8 mm, 10 mm (Hahn or Jenkins), 5
Retractors, self-retaining (West, Mayo hinged, etc.), 2

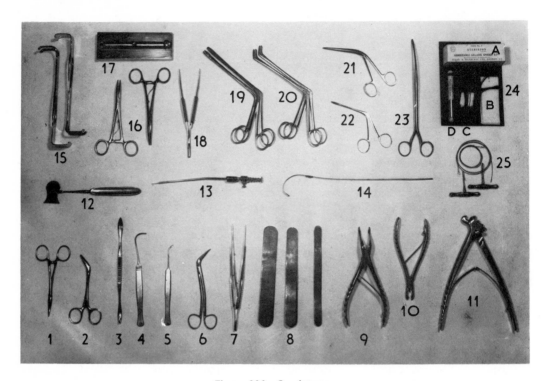

Figure 326 Craniotomy.

1. Artery forceps, curved on flat (Cairn, Kelly, Fraser, etc.), 36
2. Artery forceps, curved on side, 24.
3. Dissector, double end (Durham).
4. Medium aneurysm needle.
5. Small aneurysm needle.
6. Dura mater scissors (Schmieden).
7. Fine dissecting forceps, toothed and non-toothed (Gillies and McIndoe).
8. Brain retractors, malleable copper, 3 sizes, $\frac{1}{2}$ in, $\frac{3}{4}$ in and 1 in (13 mm, 19 mm and 25 mm).
9. Gouge forceps (Jansen).
10. Gouge forceps, angled on flat.
11. Punch forceps (de Vilbiss skull-cutting forceps).
12. Cranial saw (Hey).
13. Brain suction nozzle (Sloan Robertson).
14. Saw guide (de Martel).
15. Medium retractors (Czerny), 2.
16. Silver-clip insertion forceps (McKenzie), 2.
17. Silver-clip galley (McKenzie).
18. Fine diathermy forceps (Brigden).
19. Pituitary forceps, straight (Cairn Cushing), small, medium and large.
20. Pituitary forceps, angled on side (Cairn Cushing), small and medium.
21. Dressing forceps, angled (Tilley).
22. Aural forceps, angled, crocodile jaws (Mathieu).
23. Foreign body forceps (Desjardin).
24. A. Gelatine sponge. B. and C. Patties, D. Bone wax.
25. Olivecrona's wire saw and handles.

Fine needle holders (West or Kilner), 2
20 ml syringe
Elastic rubber bands for securing forceps in groups
Plastic or rubber drainage tubing either corrugated or tubular

Suction tubing, fine nozzles and tube anchoring forceps

Diathermy leads, electrodes, scabbard and lead anchoring forceps

(Bone awl or micro hand drill with twist drills and drill guard may be needed, plus
    stainless steel wire)

2 or 1·5 (3/0 or 4/0) Silk on small curved round-bodied needles for dura

2 (3/0) Silk on small curved cutting or straight cutting needles for skin.

OUTLINE OF PROCEDURE

Depending on the site and extent of brain exposure required, either a solitary burr
hole will be made which is enlarged as necessary to form a limited craniectomy (e.g., for
access to the Gasserian ganglion, certain temporal haematoma, subtemporal decompres-
sions or emergency intracranial vascular surgery); or alternatively several burr holes are
made in rhombic form and linked with a wire saw to form a bony 'trapdoor' hinged on the
temporal muscle. This is the classical osteoplastic flap.

Elevation of a depressed fracture of the skull vault. To gain access to the fracture margins,
a skin incision is made which possibly will include existing scalp wounds if the fracture
be compound. The galeal bleeding is arrested with artery forceps which are grouped
conveniently with rubber bands and clipped to the drapes.

The periosteum is reflected from the fracture lines for 5 to 10 mm each side and a burr
hole made on sound bone to one side of the depression in order to afford access to the
extradural space. Alternatively small comminuted fragments of bone often found
impacting the fracture in the depressed position are nibbled away, any extradural haematoma being removed by suction. The dura is freed from the skull and an Adson elevator
or bone spike inserted into the burr hole or bony defect. Using intact bone as the fulcrum,
the depressed fragments are gently elevated into anatomical position and haemostasis is
secured.

If the dura is penetrated resulting in a c.s.f. leak, the rent must be exposed and explored. Minimal pulped brain is gently irrigated, removed with suction and finally
haemostasis secured with diathermy or Cushing clips. The dural rent is closed with fine
silk interrupted sutures or a fascial patch, the donor site being conveniently temporal
fascia or even fascia lata.

The scalp is closed (after inserting a drain) as for ventriculography.

Evacuation of extradural haematoma. (This may only require instruments as for
ventriculography providing the additional cranial instrument set is kept sterile for
immediate use.)

A limited temporal craniectomy is made as previously described. The bleeding point is
exposed – usually where the middle meningeal vessels emerge from the bony tunnel in
the temporal bone to cross to the dura. Bleeding is arrested by coagulation or by under-
running the vessel with a fine suture or applying a Cushing clip. The dura is then secured
with dural 'hitch' stitches to the pericranium thereby occluding dead space and preventing extradural ooze under the bone edges, which can predispose towards extradural clot
reaccumulation. After haemostasis is secured and a drain inserted the scalp is closed
routinely with two layers of silk sutures to both muscles and scalp.

Subdural haematoma. (This may only require instruments as for ventriculography as
above.) These are removed normally by making two burr holes at suitable sites and then
after dural incision the fluid or clot is aspirated by suction. Any remaining clot is flushed
out by gentle irrigation utilising a fine catheter, the saline being introduced at one burr
hole and the clot expelled via the other. If the clot be solid and too firm to evacuate, an
osteoplastic flap must be turned and the clot removed under direct vision.

In chronic subdural haematoma the brain shrinks and there is often some difficulty in
expanding it to refill the space left by the evacuated haematoma. In this case saline is

injected either via a lumbar puncture, or the lateral ventricle is cannulated and filled directly with saline via a Cushing brain needle.

Raising an osteoplastic flap. This is a preliminary procedure for all extensive intra-cranial procedures. The initial stages follow those previously described but a larger planned scalp incision is made. After scalp reflexion to the base of the planned incision, bleeding points are diathermised and the scalp flap covered with a saline soaked pack.

Two radial diathermy incisions are made down to bone in the temporal muscle, so that a fan-shaped section over the site of the osteoplastic bone flap will remain attached to temple and also to the reflected bone. This soft-tissue bridge is responsible for revas-cularisation of the bone flap after replacement when the operation is completed.

Five or six trephine holes are made at intervals on the circumference of the proposed bone flap. After deflecting the underlying dura from beneath the margins of the burr holes, first the bone base of the flap beneath the temporalis muscle is divided or narrowed enough to fracture through when the flap is reflected. The remaining burr holes are then linked one after the other with a de Martel saw guide and wire saw, chamfering the bone edges to prevent the replaced bone flap from sinking inward.

The bone is then rapidly prised up and reflected, followed by removal of any bone spikes at the base. It is then wrapped with a saline soaked pack, which is secured to the drapes with rubber bands and towel clips. Occasionally the bone flap may be totally removed at this stage when a large decompression is needed rapidly. Bone haemostasis is secured with diathermy or bone wax and the edges are then covered with moist lintine strips followed by a fresh towel to cover all instruments *in situ* to that moment.

The dura is always reflected toward the vertex of the skull. A point near to the bone margins toward the base of the skull and free from blood vessels is selected and picked up with a sharp hook. It is then nicked with a scalpel and the nick enlarged with a director and scalpel sufficiently to introduce a small patty. The brain being protected by the patty, the dura is opened with dural scissors. Vessels to be traversed are coagulated, under-run or occluded with clips. The dural flap is reflected and covered with a moist patty or gutta-percha strip. The dura is kept moist throughout the operation.

Tumours are gently separated out with brain retractors, scissors, diathermy and suc-tion tube, or removed 'piecemeal' with a diathermy loop as in the case of large meningio-mata. The cavity left by infiltrative tumours is gently irrigated until haemostasis is complete. Oozing is controlled with gelatin sponge, Oxycel or Surgicel covered with a moist cotton-wool pack which is sucked dry. This pack is later removed with the aid of irrigation.

For closure the dura is first 'hitch stitched' to the pericranium as described previously, then closed with interrupted silk sutures. The bone flap is replaced *in situ* and sutured in place with periosteal silk sutures. In some cases the flap is fixed with twisted loops of stainless steel wire inserted in holes drilled in the flap and surrounding intact vault bones. Whilst drilling, the brain is guarded to avoid accidental deep penetration. The scalp may be drained using a subgaleal suction drain.

Posterior fossa exploration. A midline, 'crossbow' or lateral linear incision is made through previously infiltrated neck musculature. Artery forceps on each side of the incision are grouped together with rubber bands. The neck musculature is incised with diathermy down to bone and the occipital bone bared widely, stripping the muscles back with a periosteal elevator and large self-retaining retractors.

Two burr holes are made one on either side of the midline over the cerebellum. Using nibblers, a large craniectomy is made bilaterally and the crest of midline bone between these removed. The posterior aspect of the foramen magnum rim is removed, as is usually the posterior arch of the atlas and even the axis together with the axis' spinous process.

The dura is opened widely in stellate fashion and held back with 'hitch stitches'. The brain is explored by 'needling' and retraction, pathological tissue being dealt with as previously described. The dura is left open and the muscles closed in layers to effect a watertight closure. Skin is then closed in two layers.

Cranioplasty

DEFINITION
Repair of skull defects with bone, acrylic resin or Vitalium prostheses.

POSITION
As for the appropriate craniotomy. If iliac bone or rib is to be used for a bony cranio-plasty, the patient is placed in the lateral or half-lateral position.

INSTRUMENTS
As for craniotomy
Bone graft set (Fig. 346)
Pistol grip hand drill, twist drills and drill guard
Stainless steel wire
Prosthesis; acrylic polymer and monomer, acrylic plate or Vitallium plate.

OUTLINE OF PROCEDURE
The cranial defect is exposed by reflexion of the scalp flap and careful sharp dissection to leave freshened bone margins and intact dura underlying the defect. The bone edges are 'stepped or chamfered' until the prepared prosthesis sits snugly in position. Holes are drilled in the surrounding bone at suitable intervals and the prosthesis is firmly wired into place with stainless steel wire. After twisting the wire ends these are cut and buried in the drill holes. The scalp is closed in two layers often with a suction drain in place for 24 hours post-operatively.

If an autogenous bone graft is used to repair the defect the bone is removed from the appropriate donor site. A plate of cortical and cancellous bone can be removed *en bloc* from the inner aspect of the ileum, alternatively two or three sections of rib of sufficient length to bridge the skull defect may be used. A rib is split lengthwise and wired *in situ* in parallel strips to roof over the defect. Any cancellous chippings are lightly packed in the interspaces and the scalp closed routinely.

Prefrontal leucotomy

DEFINITION
Severing of the fronto-thalamic association fibres in both frontal lobes of the brain.

POSITION
Sitting or supine, with head flexed forward.

INSTRUMENTS
As for ventriculography (page 389)
Narrow brain retractors, 4
Leucotome.

OUTLINE OF PROCEDURE
There are many individual variations of the operation, the usual procedure is a modified

Freeman and Watts operation. The coronal suture is localised by skin markings 13 cm along the midline from the nasion toward the vertex. A small vertical incision is made bilaterally along the coronal suture centred 3 cm behind the zygomatico-frontal suture and 6 cm above the superior margin of the zygoma. A burr hole is made and enlarged to 2 by 3 cm. The dura is incised in cruciate fashion, haemostasis being secured with diathermy.

A brain needle is inserted horizontally just in front of the anterior horn of the lateral ventricle and the depth to the falx determined which is usually 55 mm or thereabouts. If the ventricle is opened section is made anterior to the needle track to avoid the former.

A leucotome is inserted with the blade held horizontally and a cut made parallel to the zygoma, 10 mm less in depth to that of the falx in order to avoid the pial vessels on the medial orbital gyrus. The section is carried forward as far as possible using a sweeping action, with the brain surface as the axis. The leucotome is then withdrawn and a vertical section made of similar depth in the coronal plane. After finally withdrawing the leucotome the wound is irrigated until bleeding stops and then closed routinely.

Stereotactic surgery

DEFINITION

Deep ablative surgery of the white matter, basal ganglia or brain stem projection fibres by means of a special probe utilising electro-coagulation or extreme cold (cryoprobe) as the destructive agent. Accuracy of siting is accomplished by means of a stereotactic frame applied to the skull coupled with contrast radiography demonstrating fixed intracerebral landmarks as points of reference.

POSITION

Sitting (Leksell and cryoprobe); or prone (Guiot) depending on which stereotactic frame is used.

INSTRUMENTS

As for ventriculography (page 389)
Micro hand drill, twist drills and drill guard
Lead shot
Cryoprobe or electro-coagulation unit
Stereotactic frame (Leksell, Cooper, Guiot Gillingham, etc.).

OUTLINE OF PROCEDURE

One stage procedure. The ventricles are outlined by contrast radiography and the stereotactic frame applied to the skull. By reference to a standard stereotactic atlas, the probe is inserted and localised into the required position and a lesion performed in increments until the desired effect is obtained in the conscious patient.

Two stage procedure. The preliminary stage is performed followed two days later by the main operation. An example is stereotactic thalamopallidotomy, designed to relieve the tremor and rigidity of Parkinsonism.

Stage one consists of inserting lead shot landmarks on the surface of the skull. Using the stereotactic frame bar as a guide, three incisions are made through the scalp one traverse frontally as low as possible towards the nasion; another longitudinally over the coronal suture and a third longitudinal or transverse incision low on the occipital bone towards the external occipital protuberance. All the incisions are placed in the midline. Using a guarded drill, several holes are drilled in the outer table of the skull so that five or six lead shot can be inserted and secured with bone wax, arranged in a W fashion to give a 'spread' of shot across the skull midline at the three sites.

The scalp is closed routinely and an air encephalogram taken with several radiographic views to include the lines of shot and the septum pellucidum as well as the third ventricle. By computation by consideration of the position of lead shot and various other intra-cranial landmarks, accurate co-ordinates of the globus pallidus and ventro-lateral nucleus of the thalamus are worked out. From this, the position of the parietal burr hole required in a direct line behind these targets is also worked out.

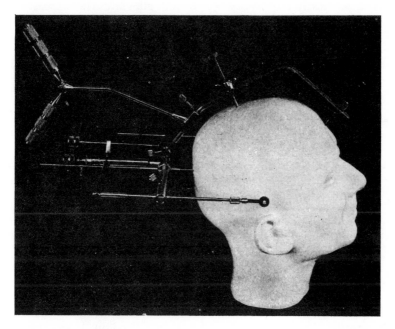

Figure 327   Guiot Gillingham stereotactic frame.   (Eschmann Bros and Walsh Ltd.)

Stage two, the patient is conscious, placed in the prone position, with the head resting in a neurosurgical horseshoe and the limbs exposed. The original incisions are re-opened and the lines of lead shot exposed. The shot selected for siting an anchor point for the Guiot frame is removed and after enlarging the socket left behind, a special screw is driven home into the outer skull table. The procedure is repeated at the other incisions and after removing all surplus lead shot markers, the bar of the Guiot frame is secured to the anchor points and the wounds closed around the screws.

Two burr holes are then made and the dura incised to expose brain. The first is sited over the frontal horn of the lateral ventricle which is then catheterised. The second burr hole is made over the parietal eminence on the side for the lesion, a pre-determined site, usually about 3 to 3·5 cm above the external occipital protuberance and centred 16 mm from the midline.

The Guiot frame is secured to the central bar with the depth electrode touching the brain surface. Myodil 3 ml is instilled into the ventricle and by manipulating the head is manoeuvred into the third ventricle to outline the anterior and posterior commissure. The sights of the Guiot frame are then aligned on the globus pallidus by using these points of reference and an image intensifier.

The Myodil is aspirated and the frontal burr hole closed. The electrode is slowly inserted into the brain 16 mm from the midline until the ventro-lateral nucleus of the thalamus is entered, this usually results in a dramatic cessation or diminuation of tremor. A radiofrequency current of known strength and duration is then passed through the electrode to make a small spherical lesion in the thalamus. Alternatively the cryoprobe tip is cooled to -30 to $-100°C$. and after a predetermined time, warmed up again (Chapter 22).

After an acceptable result is achieved, the electrode is pushed further anteriorly, traversing the internal capsule to enter the globus pallidus. A second lesion is then made, which usually dramatically improves dexterity and alleviates the increased rigidity. The apparatus is then removed and the incisions closed.

By similar techniques, electrodes and probes can produce lesions in the frontal association to cause a controlled, more exact leucotomy; suprafellar cysts can be approached and ascending pain fibres in cases of intractable pain can be destroyed in the brain stem, with minimal interference to brain function.

Torkildsen operation (Ventriculo-cysternostomy)

DEFINITION
The establishment of artificial drainage between the lateral ventricles and cysterna magna.

POSITION
Prone with the neck flexed.

INSTRUMENTS
As for craniotomy
Silicone tubing 8 to 10 Charrière gauge.

OUTLINE OF PROCEDURE
A vertical midline incision is made in the occipital region, haemostasis secured and self-retaining retractors placed to retract the muscles. Two parietal burr holes are made followed by a limited posterior fossa craniectomy, the dura not being opened initially. Silicone drainage tubes are introduced into both lateral ventricles via supratentorial dural incisions. These tubes are laid in channels cut in the outer skull table between the burr holes and the craniectomy.

The cerebellar dura is opened for 1 cm, and the silicone tubes, after trimming for length, are inserted through the arachnoid into the cysterna magna. The dura is then closed around the tubes and the scalp sutured in layers.

Insertion of ventriculo-atrial or ventriculo-petritoneal shunt

DEFINITION
The establishment of artificial c.s.f. drainage to heart or peritoneal cavity in cases of primary or secondary hydrocephalus.

POSITION
Supine, with head rotated to the left, sandbag under the shoulders and an X-ray film cassette beneath the patient's chest.

INSTRUMENTS

As for ventriculography (page 389)
Fine arterial bulldog clamps, 3
Small gauges, 3 mm, 4 mm, 6 mm, (Hahn or Jenkins), 3
Suitable valve (Pudenz or Spitz-Holter)
Fine bore silicone tubing assorted sizes
Eynard connectors, 2.

OUTLINE OF PROCEDURE

Ventriculo-atrial shunt, (Pudenz valve insertion). A preliminary chest radiograph confirms the level of the right atrium. A right sub-mandibular incision is made and the posterior branch of the common facial vein or the right internal jugular vein is exposed and freed from surrounding tissues.

A supramastoid occipital scalp incision 5 cm (2 in) long is made well above the line of the lateral sinus, and using a small gouge a hole is drilled in the attenuated skull. The dura is incised and the enlarged occipital horn of the lateral ventricle is catheterised with the top-half of the Pudenz catheter. This is then occluded with the bulldog clip to prevent leakage of c.s.f.

(It is not normally necessary to insert the patent flushing disc in the shunt circuit. If this is required, the gouge-hole must be enlarged to fit the rim of the disc snugly and bone haemostatis secured with bone wax. A 5 cm length of top catheter is then cut off and tied to the centre of the outlet of the flushing disc with fine silk. The disc is then inserted and sutured to the periosteun margins of the bone defect. This step is omitted if no flusher is required.)

Two silk ligatures are passed around the right internal jugular vein, or the posterior branch of the common facial vein if the latter is of sufficiently large calibre to admit the Pudenz tube valve. The top ligature is tied to occlude the vessel. The Pudenz atrial catheter is checked for correct functioning of the four slit valves at the atrial end. The vessel is nicked and the catheter inserted toward the superior vena cava until it is estimated to be within the right atrium.

A few millilitres of Hypaque 35 per cent is injected via an Eynard connector whilst a radiograph of the chest is taken to verify correct positioning of the valve. After any necessary adjustment, so that the valve tip is well within the right atrium, the Pudenz tube is secured in the neck with the lower ligature. The tubing of the lower end of the valve is then tracked from the neck incision to the scalp incision, using large artery forceps forced along the subcutaneous tissues. After trimming to a suitable length, the top and bottom tubes are linked over a fine connector supplied with the valve (or to the flushing disc) with silk ties. After checking fontanelle tension and the flusher if fitted, for correct function, both wounds are closed in two layers.

Ventriculo-peritoneal shunt. Ventricular catheterisation is performed as above with a single length of fine silicone tubing with several side holes cut near the top end. The tubing is then tunnelled subcutaneously, if necessary with supplementary small incisions down the neck and across the right anterior chest wall to a secondary incision sited just below the right costal margin.

The peritoneal cavity is opened at this site and after trimming to length and cutting several side holes in the silicone tubing, the latter is inserted into the suprahepatic space and sutured to peritoneum with watertight closure. The wounds are closed in layers.

Repair of spina bifida and meningocoele

DEFINITION

The repair of a congenital defect in the vertebral column which allows herniation of the malformed meninges and the spinal cord or caudu equina.

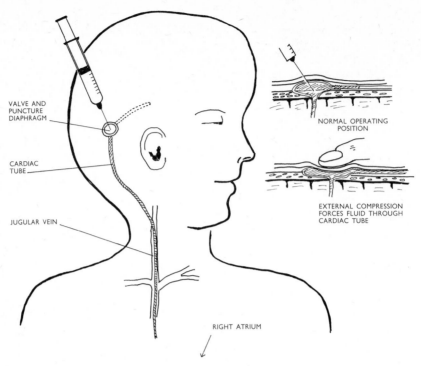

Figure 328   Pudenz valve for ventriculo-atrial shunt.

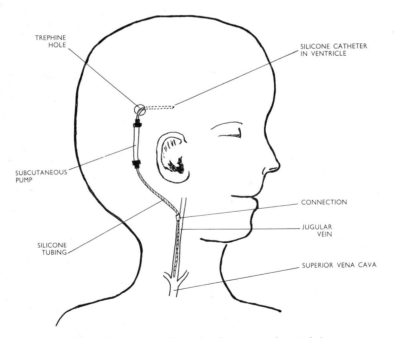

Figure 329   Spitz-Holter valve for ventriculo-atrial shunt.

POSITION. Prone.

INSTRUMENTS

General set (Fig. 281)
Fine artery forceps, curved on flat, mosquito, 25
Fine dissecting forceps, toothed (Gillies), 2
Fine dissecting forceps, non-toothed (McIndoe), 2
Fine tissue forceps (McIndoe), 12
Fine scissors, curved on flat, iris, 2
Long scissors, curved on flat (McIndoe)
Suction tubing, fine nozzles and tube anchoring forceps
Diathermy leads, electrodes, scabbard and lead anchoring forceps
2 (3/0) Plain catgut or Dexon on small curved round-bodied needles
2 (3/0) Silk on small curved cutting needles.

OUTLINE OF PROCEDURE

The margins of the herniated sac or exposed neural disc are freed from the overlying skin which is then retracted gently. The underlying neural tissue is gradually freed from the surrounding fascia on the margins of the lamina defect with preservation of all possible neural tissue. Haemostasis must be meticulous. The edges of the neural disc are then sunk beneath a flap of reflected fascia tailored from the paravertebral tissues. This layer is closed with fine silk, plain catgut or Dexon to secure a watertight closure.

In the case of meningocoele when no neural disc is exposed, after freeing adherent nerve roots from the sac of the meningocoele, the sac is excised, the roots returned to the spinal canal and the sac edges resutured together.

The skin is closed, if necessary with the formation of rotation flaps and extensive undermining, in two layers to give a tensionless three layer closure in all.

Excision of spinal cord tumour

DEFINITION

The removal of a spinal cord tumour following cervical, dorsal or lumbar laminectomy.

POSITION

Prone neurosurgical position (Fig. 69) with some flexion of the spine; lateral flexed position or laminectomy position (Fig. 71).

INSTRUMENTS

As for laminectomy (Chapter 23, Fig. 353)
Silver clips and galley (Cushing's)
Insertion forceps for silver clips
Dura scissors (Schmeiden)
Gall-stone scoop and probe, malleable
Wound irrigation catheter, size 6 and 8 Charrière gauge
Spinal puncture needle, size 18
Ligatures and sutures as for laminectomy.

OUTLINE OF PROCEDURE

Three or four laminae overlying the tumour site are removed as described for laminectomy (Chapter 23). The dura is incised over the tumour with a fine knife and Schmeiden scissors. Stay sutures are placed in the edges of the cut dura to act as retractors and these lie over moist lintine strips arranged along each side of the wound.

The tumour is freed by sharp and blunt dissection together with adherent meninges, and haemostasis is secured with diathermy, gelatine sponge, Oxycel or Surgicel. The dura is closed with interrupted silk sutures, and if excision of the tumour has left a defect this is covered with gelatine sponge or film. The wound is closed as for laminectomy, with or without drainage.

Lumbar sympathectomy

DEFINITION

Removal of the lower three lumbar sympathetic ganglia and intervening trunk for vasospastic disturbances.

POSITION. Supine.

INSTRUMENTS

As for laparotomy (Chapter 13, Figs. 281 and 282)
Illuminated retractor (Coldlight)
Long dissecting forceps, non-toothed, 25 cm (10 in) 2
Long dissecting forceps, toothed, 25 cm (10 in)
Long scissors, curved on flat, 23 cm (9 in) (Nelson)
Silver clips and galley (McKenzie)
Insertion forceps for silver clips
Ligatures and sutures as for laparotomy (page 283).

OUTLINE OF PROCEDURE

The chain of ganglia may be approached by either of two incisions. If the sympathectomy is unilateral, an incision, rather like a kidney incision is made, but rather further forward. This incision extends from the margin of the twelfth rib towards the umbilicus, splitting the external oblique and transversus muscles in line with their fibres in the manner described for appendicectomy in Chapter 13. The ganglia are approached by retracting the peritoneum which is not opened.

If the sympathectomy is bilateral, the approach *may* be midline or paramedian, opening the peritoneum anteriorly, retracting the viscera and opening the posterior peritoneum to expose the ganglia situated on each side of the abdominal aorta.

The second, third and fourth lumbar ganglia and the intervening trunk are dissected free and removed after ligating the proximal and distal points with silver clips. The wound is closed in the usual manner for laparotomy.

Division of the sensory root of the trigeminal nerve (Dandy's operation)

DEFINITION

Intracranial fractional division of the sensory root of the trigeminal nerve for the relief of intractable trigeminal neuralgia.

POSITION

Sitting with the head in a frontal horse-shoe to afford access to the temporal region and face on affected side.

INSTRUMENTS
As for ventriculography (page 389)
Trigeminal retractor, large self-retaining (Dandy's)
Brain retractors, malleable
Headlight
Blunt meningeal hooks, 2
Silver clips and galley (Cushing's)
Insertion forceps for silver clips
Bone-cutting forceps (de Vilbiss)
Dural scissors (Dott).
Ligatures and sutures as for ventriculography (page 389)

OUTLINE OF PROCEDURE
A moderate sized temporal craniectomy is made extending well downward to the floor of the middle cranial fossa. The middle meningeal vessels are clipped or diathermised and divided. An extradural subtemporal dissection is made toward the midline until the dural fold overlying the trigeminal ganglion is exposed.

The dura is incised and by blunt dissection with meningeal hooks the sensory root of the trigeminal nerve is isolated and the motor root identified. The appropriate sensory division of the trigeminal nerve is then divided and the temporalis muscle is sutured in two layers after haemostasis has been secured. The scalp is sutured routinely in two layers without drainage.

Peripheral nerve anastomosis

DEFINITION
Repair of an injured peripheral nerve by anastomosis.

POSITION
Musculospiral (radial), ulnar or median nerves; supine, with the arm extended on an arm table. Sciatic or popliteal; prone.

INSTRUMENTS
General set (Fig. 281)
Peripheral nerve set (Fig. 330)
Fine dissecting forceps, toothed (Gillies), 2
Fine dissecting forceps, non-toothed (McIndoe), 2
Plaster of Paris back slab, or similar splint.

Ligatures and Sutures for an Arm Operation
2 and 2·5 (3/0 and 2/0) Plain catgut or Dexon for ligatures
3 (0) Chromic catgut or Dexon on a medium half-circle cutting needle for muscle sutures
2·5 (2/0) Silk or nylon on a medium curved cutting needle for skin sutures.
Ligatures and Sutures for a Leg Operation
2·5 and 3 (2/0 and 0) Plain catgut or Dexon for ligatures
4 or 5 (1 or 2) Chromic catgut or Dexon on a medium or large half-circle cutting needle for muscle sutures
2·5 or 0 (2/0 or 0) Silk or nylon on a large or medium curved cutting needle for skin sutures.

Nerve Sutures for both Operation Areas
   1 or 0·75 (5/0 or 6/0) Silk or Dacron on a small curved round-bodied non-traumatic
      needle.
   (The suture material should be silicone coated.)

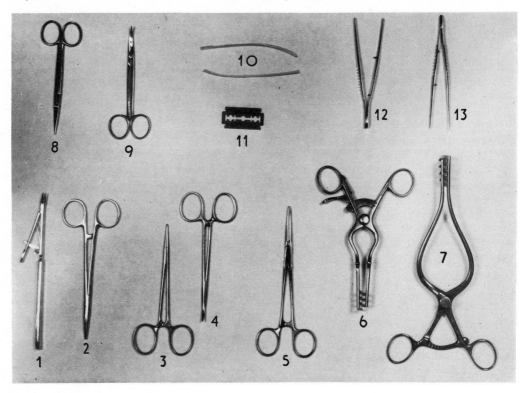

Figure 330   Peripheral nerve suture.

1. Fine needle holder (Silcock).
2. Fine needle holder (Fulcrum lever type).
3. Fine artery forceps, straight, mosquito, 6.
4. Fine artery forceps, curved on flat, mosquito, 12.
5. Fine tissue forceps (McIndoe), 6.
6. Retractor, self-retaining (Mayo, angled).
7. Retractor, self-retaining (Travers).
8. Iris scissors, straight, sharp points.
9. Iris scissors, curved on flat, sharp points.
10. Plastic or rubber tubing for nerve retractors.
11. Razor blade.
12. Fine dissecting forceps, toothed, fixation, 2.
13. Fine dissecting forceps, non-toothed, fixation, 2.
(See also microinstruments in Appendix, p. 663).

OUTLINE OF PROCEDURE

The incision is made and the muscles split or retracted to expose the nerve. The proximal and distal portions of the divided nerve are mobilised so that they can be brought together without tension. This usually means that the skin incision must be extended and the nerve mobilised for a considerable distance proximal to the division.

The bulbous fibrous neuroma is excised with the razor blade, and 'stay' sutures are placed in the nerve sheath. These 'stay' sutures are used as temporary retractors and to approximate the nerve ends, which are anastomosed with interrupted silk sutures placed through the nerve sheath only. Care is taken to complete the anastomosis without rotation of the nerve ends. A piece of Millipore or Dacron silastic material may be wrapped around the anastomosis to form a protective tunnel.

The muscle is sutured over the nerve and the skin is closed. The limb is immobilised with a splint and bandages in a position which affords the least tension on the nerve suture line.

Transposition of ulnar nerve

DEFINITION

Anterior translocation of the ulnar nerve from its normal position behind the medial epicondyle to a soft tissue channel made medially in the flexor carpi ulnaris, thereby alleviating recurrence of symptoms due to stretching of the nerve.

POSITION

Supine, with the arm extended on an arm table and small sandbag.

INSTRUMENTS

As for peripheral nerve suture.

OUTLINE OF PROCEDURE

A curved incision is made, extending above and below the elbow, with its centre lying over the medial epicondyle. The skin flaps are reflected and the nerve dissected free from behind the epicondyle. Loops of rubber tubing or tape are placed around the nerve which is retracted medially. The flexor carpi ulnaris is partially detached from the epicondyle, and reflected to form a channel into which the nerve is laid.

The muscle can be sutured over the nerve with interrupted chromic catgut, Dexon or left unsutured and the skin closed with interrupted silk or nylon.

A very large proportion of ophthalmic operations are performed under local anaesthesia if the patient is co-operative. In small children and restless adults general anaesthesia is usually administered.

Local anaesthesia consists of instillation of cocaine 4 per cent at intervals before operation. In addition, for operations on the eyelids a 1 or 2 per cent lignocaine (Xylocaine) is injected subcutaneously. For operations on the eyeball itself and ocular muscles, a subconjunctival and retrobulbar injection of lignocaine (Xylocaine) is made. The lignocaine (Xylocaine) solution is often combined with 1 in 10,000 adrenaline which acts as a haemostatic agent. Local anaesthesia is often used in conjunction with sedatives such as pethidine and Largactil.

Excision of chalazion

DEFINITION
The removal of a cystic degenerated Meibomian gland in the eyelid.

POSITION. Supine.

INSTRUMENTS. As Figure 331.

OUTLINE OF PROCEDURE
The cyst is usually removed via the conjunctiva but occasionally through the skin. In either case, the skin overlying the lesion is infiltrated with local anaesthetic, and if the cyst is to be removed through the conjunctiva, this may be ballooned out with local anaesthetic injected into the inferior or superior cul-de-sac.

A chalazion clamp is applied with the cyst projecting into the ring of the forceps. Approach to the cyst through the conjunctiva is made through an incision vertical to the lid margin, for this type of wound closes readily without sutures. The cyst is curetted unless it is large, or has recurred in which case it is dissected out with sharp scissors or a scalpel.

If the cyst is approached through the skin, the incision is made parallel with the lid margin and is closed afterwards with a few interrupted silk sutures.

Ectropion correction

DEFINITION
The correction of an eylid deformity (usually the lower lid), where relaxation of the skin and muscles of the eyelid cause permanent exposure of the conjunctiva.

POSITION. Supine.

INSTRUMENTS. As Figure 331.

OUTLINE OF PROCEDURE

There are several operations for this condition, including skin grafting procedures. Basically the operation consists of tightening the lower lid to correct the abnormal position.

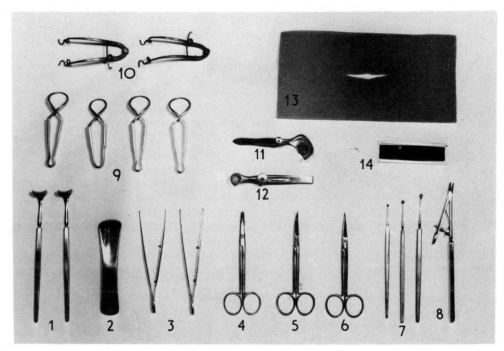

Figure 331   Lid operations.

1. Eyelid retractors (Desmarre), 2.
2. Lid spatula (MacCallan).
3. Fine dissecting forceps, toothed and non-toothed, fixation.
4. Fine scissors, curved, blunt points.
5. Iris scissors, curved on flat, sharp points.
6. Iris scissors, straight, sharp points.
7. Meibomian cyst curettes, 3 sizes.
8. Fine needle holder (Silcock).
9. Towel clips, 4.
10. Eyelid specula, left and right (Clark).
11. Entropian forceps (Desmarre), 2, left and right.
12. Tarsal cyst forceps (Greene).
13. Foam plastic towel for isolating operation area. (Alternatively a self adhesive polyvinyl sheet with a central aperture may be used, e.g., Steridrape, ViDrape or OpSite.)
14. Black silk (1·5 to 2·5 (4/0 to 2/0)) may be needed and small curved cutting needle.

An incision is made along the entire eyelid margin, and a triangular section of conjunctiva and tarsus is excised at the mid-point of the lid. The base of the triangle lies along the lid margin and is made so that when the two edges of the defect are approximated, the conjunctiva tends to turn in towards the eyeball. A triangular section of skin is then excised at the outer canthus, and the skin of the lower lid is undermined. The conjunctival triangular defect is sutured together and the lower lid sutured laterally to close the other skin defect at the outer canthus. A final suture is placed at the junction of the tarsal resection. This is a double-needle suture which passes through the conjunctiva and skin at each side of the resection. The loop of the suture bridges the tarsal suture line on the conjunctival aspect and is tied over fine rubber tubing outside the lid.

Entropion correction

DEFINITION

The correction of an eyelid deformity where inward rotation or inversion of the eyelid may cause trauma by the rubbing of the lashes on the cornea.

POSITION. Supine.

INSTRUMENTS. As Figure 331.

OUTLINE OF PROCEDURE

The operation consists basically of everting the eyelid by shortening the skin.

An incision is made 2 or 3 mm from the lid margin for the entire length. A second elliptical incision is made, joining the lower incision at each end, and a crescentic piece of skin a few millimetres wide is excised. The skin is undermined on each side of the incision and a section of orbicularis muscle fibres may be picked up with forceps and excised for the entire length of the eyelid. Some surgeons then remove thin slices from the underlying tarsus.

The wound is closed with silk sutures, usually four in number, each of which passes through the upper skin edges of the incision, then the upper edge of the tarsus and orbicularis muscle, across the wound and out through the lower lip of the skin incision. When tied, these sutures approximate the skin and defect in the eyelid muscle, causing eversion of the lid to its normal position.

Dacryocystorhinostomy

DEFINITION

The establishment of a permanent opening between the lacrimal sac and the nasal cavity.

POSITION. Supine.

INSTRUMENTS

Scalpel handles No. 3 with Nos. 10 and 15 blades (Bard Parker), 2
Fine dissecting forceps, toothed, fixation, 2
Fine dissecting forceps, toothed (Gillies), 2
Fine dissecting forceps, non-toothed (McIndoe), 2
Fine scissors, curved dissecting points (Kilner)
Scissors, angled (Heymann)
Fine artery forceps, curved on flat, mosquito, 10
Fine tissue forceps (McIndoe), 5
Small rugines, curved (Faraboeuf and Traquair), 2
Retractor (Muller)
Retractor (Rollet)
Dissectors (Howarth and Hill), 2
Punch forceps (Citellis or Duggan)

Punch forceps (Weil or Luc)
Small gouges, 4 mm, 6 mm, 8 mm, 10 mm
Small chisels or osteotomes, 4 mm, 6 mm, 8 mm, 10 mm
Small mallet (Rowland)
Nasal speculum (St Clair Thompson)
Canaliculus dilator (Nettleship)
Lacrimal probes, set
Fine needle holder (Kilner multiple joint)
Eye needle holder (Silcock)
Suction tubing, fine nozzles and tube anchoring forceps.
2 (3/0) Plain catgut for ligatures
2 (3/0) Chromic catgut or Dexon on a small half-circle round-bodied non-traumatic
   needle for the anastomosis
2 or 2·5 (3/0 or 2/0) Chromic catgut or Dexon on a small half-circle round-bodied
   needle for subtanceous sutures
1·5 (4/0) silk or nylon on a small curved cutting needle for skin sutures
Ribbon gauze impregnated with 1 in 1000 adrenaline.

OUTLINE OF PROCEDURE

This operation is usually performed under general anaesthesia. The tip of the middle
turbinate bone on the affected side may be resected, and the nasal cavity packed with
ribbon gauze impregnated with adrenaline. A vertical or slightly curved incision is made
over the lacrimal sac about 6 millimetres from the inner canthus of the eye, extending
from a level with the upper eyelid to just below the bony orbit.

The lacrimal sac is exposed and freed from its bed. The bone of the lacrimal fossa and
the lacrimal crest is chiselled or punched away until a hole has been made equal to the
size of the sac. The inner wall of the lacrimal sac is incised, or excised, and an opening is
made through the nasal mucosa. An anastomosis is made between these openings with a
non-traumatic catgut or Dexon suture, and the wound is closed with catgut or Dexon
sutures for the subcutaneous tissues, and silk or nylon for the skin.

Strabismus operations

DEFINITION

Advancement or recession of the ocular muscles in the treatment of squint.

POSITION. Supine.

INSTRUMENTS. As Figure 332.

OUTLINE OF PROCEDURE

These operations are usually performed under general anaesthesia, but for adults local
anaesthesia may be employed.

An eye speculum is inserted and a crescentic incision made in the conjunctiva, parallel
with the limbus of the eye. The conjunctiva is freed from the underlying fascia and insertion of the ocular muscle on the sclera, to a point well beyond that selected for the
introduction of the muscle hook. A slit is made in the capsule of the muscle on one side
and a strabismus hook inserted under the muscle. The capsule on the other side of the
muscle, where the hook presents its point, is incised and a second hook introduced from
this side.

The two hooks are separated and a muscle forcep clamped across the muscle at a point near to its insertion in the sclera. The muscle is divided across and sutured to a new scleral insertion usually in the same meridian as the original insertion. This lies behind the original insertion for recession and in front for advancement. In addition, during advancement procedures, a portion of the muscle may be resected before suturing. If silk sutures are used they pass through the muscle tendon, sclera, and out of the conjunctiva for subsequent removal. Catgut or Dexon sutures, if used, are tied under the conjunctival flap. The conjunctiva is closed with interrupted silk sutures.

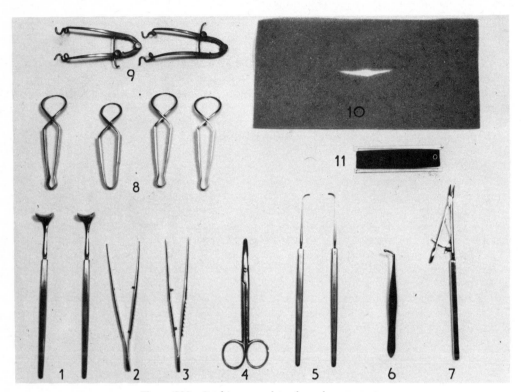

Figure 332   Strabismus and tendon advancement.

1. Eyelid retractors (Desmarre), 2.
2. Fine dissecting forceps, toothed, fixation.
3. Fine dissecting forceps, non-toothed, fixation.
4. Strabismus scissors, curved, blunt points.
5. Strabismus hooks (Graefe), 2.
6. Strabismus forceps (Prince), left or right.
7. Fine needle holder (Silcock).
8. Towel clips, 4.
9. Eyelid specula, left and right (Clark).
10. Foam plastic towel for isolating operation area. (Alternatively a self adhesive polyvinyl sheet with a central aperture may be used, e.g. Steridrape, ViDrape or OpSite.)
11. 2·5 (2/0) black silk on small curved cutting needle.

Corneal transplants

DEFINITION

Transplantation of a corneal graft from an enucleated eye of another human being in the treatment of suitable corneal opacities, or irregularities such as keratoconus and keratectasis.

POSITION. Supine.

INSTRUMENTS

(These are the essential instruments required, as there are many individual instruments which may only be of use to a particular surgeon.)
Eye speculum
Fine dissecting forceps, toothed, fixation, 2
Fine dissecting forceps, non-toothed, fixation, 2
Graft manipulators
Support for donor eye
Scissors, angled, sharp points
Fine keratomes
Double-bladed knife or corneal trephines of various sizes
Fine needle holder (Silcock)
1·5 (4/0) Silk on a small curved non-traumatic cutting needle for graft fixation, and traction sutures for opaque corneal excision area.

OUTLINE OF PROCEDURE

There are many corneal transplant operations, but basically each consists of grafting a circular piece of healthy corneal tissue on to a prepared central area of the recipient's cornea.

In Castroviejo's operation, the opaque corneal area to be removed is outlined with a double-bladed knife. A continuous corneal suture is placed 'criss cross' fashion from outside the outlined area, and the loops are left loose and arranged on each side. A suture is passed through the segment to be excised and traction is applied. The segment is removed by passing a keratone through the upper edge of the outlined area and then dividing the other three sides with angled scissors.

A graft of equal size and shape to the excised segment is removed from the donor cornea and held in position over the prepared recipient area by pulling the continuous corneal suture tight.

In other types of operations, the graft may be cut and the recipient area prepared with a circular trephine. Instead of utilising the loops of a continuous suture to hold the graft in place, it may be secured by interrupted sutures which will be placed according to the surgeon's individual technique.

Iridectomy

DEFINITION

Excision of a segment of iris. This is performed for many conditions, including cysts or tumours of the iris, anti-glaucoma operations, iris prolapse, as part of cataract extraction, etc.

POSITION. Supine.

INSTRUMENTS

(Here again, essential instruments only are listed as there are many kinds of forceps, etc., which are personal and only of interest to a particular surgeon.)
Eye speculum
Von Graefe knife
Fine dissecting forceps, toothed, fixation
Iris forceps of appropriate shape to suit a particular surgeon

Eye scissors (De Wecker)
Iris scissors, sharp points, curved and straight
Iris hook
Iris spatula
Fine needle holder (Silcock)
Irrigation cannula and undine with warm saline or similar solution
1·5 (4/0) Silk on a small curved cutting or Stallard needle for conjunctival suture.

OUTLINE OF PROCEDURE

An eyelid speculum is inserted and the eyeball fixed with toothed forceps at a point close to the limbus and opposite the site for the limbal incision. A knife is inserted about one millimetre from the corneoscleral junction and is depressed as it enters the anterior chamber. The blade is then withdrawn, and the assistant rotates the eye downwards with the fixation forceps. If visibility is obscured by haemorrhage, the anterior chamber is gently irrigated by holding the irrigation nozzle against the posterior lip of the incision and depressing it slightly. The closed tip of an iris forceps is introduced into the anterior chamber just beneath the cornea. When the iris sphincter is reached, the forceps are opened and a tiny fold of iris grasped as close to the sphincter as possible. This fold of iris is withdrawn and cut off with De Wecker's scissors held at the lips of the wound. Either a complete iridectomy or peripheral iridectomy is performed. Reposition of the iris pillars is done by gentle irrigation or an iris spatula.

The corneoscleral incision may or may not be sutured with interrupted silk sutures.

Cataract extraction

DEFINITION

The removal of an 'opaque' crystalline lens.

POSITION. Supine.

INSTRUMENTS. As Figure 333.

OUTLINE OF PROCEDURE

This operation is performed under local anaesthesia, consisting of 4 per cent cocaine conjunctival instillation, retrobulbar injection of 2 per cent lignocaine (Xylocaine) and facial nerve injection of 2 per cent lignocaine to prevent the patient from closing his eyelids. In children and the mentally disturbed a general anaesthetic is preferable.

An eye speculum is inserted and a silk stitch may be placed under the superior rectus muscle to enable a little traction to be applied and thereby prevent the patient from rolling his eye upwards.

The eye is steadied by grasping the conjunctiva with fixation forceps at a point immediately below the cornea. A Von Graefe knife traverses the anterior chamber, and by cutting upwards a corneal section is made, extending from two fifths to a half of the periphery of the cornea.

The lens is extracted either extracapsularly or intracapsularly. With the former procedure, the lens capsule is incised with a cystotome and the lens expressed with a little pressure exerted on the lower part of the eye with a lens spoon. With the latter procedure, the capsule is grasped with forceps and withdrawn by traction.

An iridectomy may be performed and the chamber gently irrigated with saline. The conjunctival flap is closed with interrupted silk sutures.

Cryosurgery

A lens may be removed by cryoextraction. Basically the instrument consists of a probe or stilette which can be cooled to a temperature of between $-35°C$ and $-150°C$. Bringing this fine pointed instrument in contact with the lens causes it to adhere to the tip. The lens can then be removed without the use of forceps.

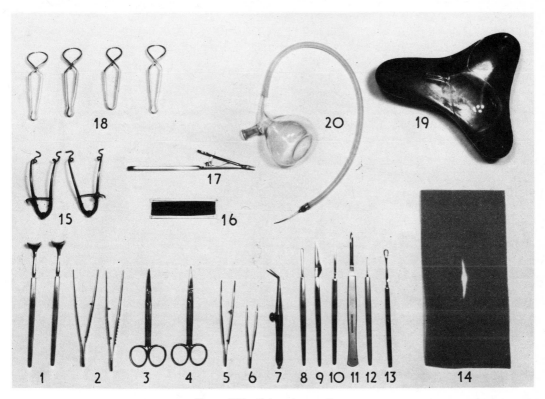

Figure 333   Cataract operations.

1. Eyelid retractors (Desmarre), 2.
2. Fine dissecting forceps, toothed and non-toothed, fixation.
3. Iris scissors, curved on flat, sharp points.
4. Iris scissors, straight, sharp points.
5. Capsule forceps (Arruga).
6. Iris forceps (Barraquer).
7. Eye scissors (De Wecker).
8. Iris repositor (Nettleship).
9. Cataract knife (Beer), *or*
10. Cataract knife (Smith), *or*
11. Cataract knife (Graefe).
12. Iris hook (Tyrrell).
13. Vectis (Snellen).
14. Foam plastic towel for isolating operation area. Alternatively a self-adhesive polyvinyl sheet with a central aperture may be used, e.g. Steridrape, ViDrape or OpSite.
15. Eye specula, left and right (Clark).
16. 2·5 or 2 (2/0 or 3/0) black silk on small curved cutting needle.
17. Fine needle holder (Silcock).
18. Towel clips, 4.
19. Undine in triangular tray for first irrigation.
20. Undine with plastic tubing and fine nozzle for second irrigation.

One type of instrument consists of a hollow probe attached to a small insulated handle which can be filled with a quantity of liquid nitrogen. The nitrogen cools the tip of the probe to approximately $-35°C$ (Cryostylet, U.S.A.).

Another instrument called the Rubinstein cryoprobe is cooled by liquid nitrogen being pumped from a storage machine to the probe tip. It differs from the Cryostylet in that the probe also incorporates a heating element. In use the probe is brought into contact with the lens, the liquid nitrogen is then introduced which cools the extreme tip of the probe down to $-150°$C. After extracting the lens, it is released from the probe tip by sending a small surge of electricity through the heating element which warms the instrument. Various temperatures can be selected for the probe tip ranging between $-35°$C to $-150°$C.

Great care is necessary with this technique for if the probe is left in contact with lens for too long a period the intense cold will damage other parts of the eye.

Corneoscleral trephining

DEFINITION

Trephining a hole at the corneoscleral junction into the anterior chamber to effect drainage of aqueous fluid in the treatment of glaucoma.

POSITION. Supine.

INSTRUMENTS
    Eye speculum
    Fine dissecting forceps, toothed, fixation
    Fine dissecting forceps, non-toothed, fixation
    Scleral fixation clamp, toothed
    Iris spatula
    Iris hook
    Iris scissors, curved and straight, 2
    Eye scissors (De Wecker)
    Iris forceps, toothed
    Von Graefe knife
    Took's corneal splitter
    Scleral trephines, 1·5 mm and 2 mm
    Fine needle holder (Silcock)
    1·5 (4/0) Silk on a small curved cutting or Stallard needle for conjunctival suture.

OUTLINE OF PROCEDURE

This operation is generally performed under local anaesthesia. The patient rotates his eye strongly away from the operation site.

The conjunctiva is grasped with non-toothed forceps as far away from the limbus as possible. A crescentic incision is made and a flap of conjunctiva is reflected up with its base at the corneoscleral junction. The eyeball is then fixed with scleral fixation clamps and the conjunctival flap folded over the cornea. Using a knife, the cornea is split for 1 mm in the centre of the flap base and a trephine hole is made which lies centrally over the corneoscleral junction. An iridectomy is then performed.

The wound may be irrigated gently, and the flap of conjunctiva returned to its normal position and sutured with a continuous silk to make a watertight closure.

Simple enucleation

DEFINITION

Removal of the entire eyeball for disease or injury.

POSITION. Supine.

INSTRUMENTS
   Eye speculum
   Fine dissecting forceps, toothed, fixation
   Fine dissecting forceps, non-toothed, fixation
   Scleral fixation clamps, toothed
   Iris scissors, sharp points, curved and straight, 2
   Scissors, curved on flat, 13 cm (5 in) (Mayo)
   Muscle hook
   Tonsil snare (optional)
   Fine artery forceps, curved on flat, mosquito, 5
   Fine artery forceps, straight, mosquito, 5
   Fine artery forceps, straight, mosquito, 5
   Fine needle holder (Silcock, Kilner multiple joint)
   2·5 (2/0) Plain catgut or Dexon may be required for ligatures
   1·5 (4/0) Silk on a small curved cutting needle for conjunctival suture.

OUTLINE OF PROCEDURE
   General anaesthesia is usually administered for this operation.
   The conjunctiva is incised close to the limbus and is undermined into the internal and external commissures and into the superior and inferior fornices. The internal rectus, superior rectus, inferior rectus and external rectus muscles are divided in that order, utilising a muscle hook and sharp-pointed scissors. The external rectus is usually cut, leaving a small tab of muscle adherent to the sclera so that a scleral clamp or mosquito artery forceps can be applied to control the eyeball for subsequent enucleation.
   The eyeball is prolapsed from the orbit utilising this clamp, and the enucleation completed either by threading a tonsil snare over the eyeball and optic nerve, or dividing the nerve with Mayo's scissors. A snare is never used if the eyeball is perforated.
   Haemorrhage is controlled by pressure or catgut or Dexon ligatures and the conjunctiva is closed with a running suture of silk, which is not tied.

23
Orthopaedic Operations

Tourniquets

Many orthopaedic operations are performed under tourniquet in a bloodless field. A correctly applied tourniquet will compress the vessels just sufficiently to stop blood flow, and no more. Excessive pressure is not only unnecessary but carries with it the danger of irreversible ischaemia in the muscles and damage to nerve fibres.

A tourniquet on the lower limb should be applied to mid-thigh, well clear of the knee joint; and for the upper limb, it should be placed at mid-biceps level well above the elbow joint. If a tourniquet is applied near a joint or over a bony prominence, there is little padding effect of muscle and fat, therefore the pressure exerted may damage vessels or nerves by compressing them directly against the bone.

Although Esmarch's rubber bandages or Samway's anchor tourniquets may be used, there should be some means of measuring the pressure exerted by a tourniquet and for this reason the pneumatic type is regarded as the most satisfactory. The Conn pneumatic tourniquet enables the pressure to be measured with an aneroid gauge, which is marked in millimetres of pressure of mercury up to 550 mm. Also, with a pneumatic tourniquet, this pressure is applied evenly around the limb, and the chance of 'pinching' the skin or causing areas of irregular pressure is almost eliminated.

The limb is exsanguinated with a rubber bandage applied over a towel, from extremity to the level of the tourniquet. The Conn tourniquet, which should be in direct contact with the skin and **not** applied over a towel (Fig. 334), may then be inflated with a hand pump, or by oxygen under pressure, and the Esmarch's bandage is removed. The pressure applied to an arm should not exceed 275 mmHg (5 lb p.s.i.); and to a leg, 550 mmHg (10 lb p.s.i.). Whilst this is in excess of the usual blood-pressure, it is still within safe limits and is necessary to compensate for the padding effect of muscle and fat overlying the vessel wall.

After inflating the cuff with a hand pump, the non-return valve remains closed until release of the tourniquet is required. If the pressure should drop, e.g., due to leaks, it must be raised again with the pump which remains connected to the apparatus. In order to do this the non-return valve is opened slightly, and closed again after the correct pressure has been reached. However, this tourniquet does not compensate for variations of pressure in the cuff due to movement of the limb and drapes, or accidental pressure by an assistant directly on the outside of the cuff.

The Kidde tourniquet is an apparatus which permits the rapid inflation of a tourniquet cuff to a pre-set pressure which is automatically maintained until change is desired. Variation in pressure (between a range of 0–1000 mmHg) can be achieved easily during lengthy operative procedures.

The apparatus utilises a non-toxic gas in liquid form, which is delivered from a replaceable pressurised can. The level of gas is indicated in a visible gas reservoir.

The Kidde tourniquet may be used with any pneumatic cuff although a special neoprene tourniquet secured with velcro tape is available.

Generally, surgeons do not leave a tourniquet in position for too long a time. If the limb has been exsanguinated, 1 hour is within safe limits, but for operations lasting much longer than this, the surgeon may release and re-inflate the tourniquet at hourly intervals.

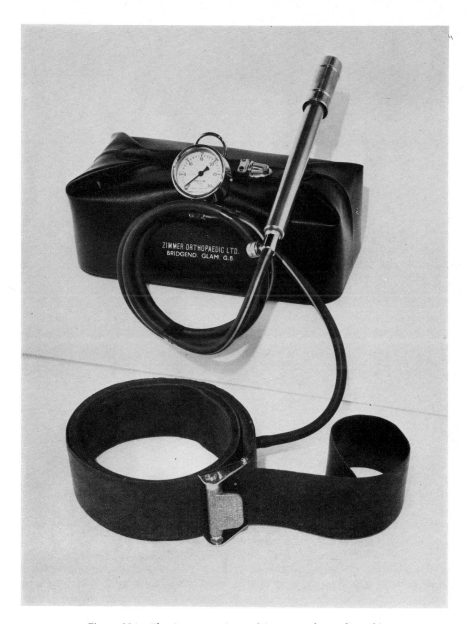

Figure 334   The Conn tourniquet. (Zimmer Orthopaedic Ltd.)

An efficient system of recording the application and removal of tourniquets must be in operation. A tourniquet forgotten and left in position when the patient returns to the ward can be disastrous and result in the loss of a limb.

Skeletal traction (long bones)

DEFINITION
The insertion of pins or wires through a bone in order to apply traction as an alternative to skin traction.

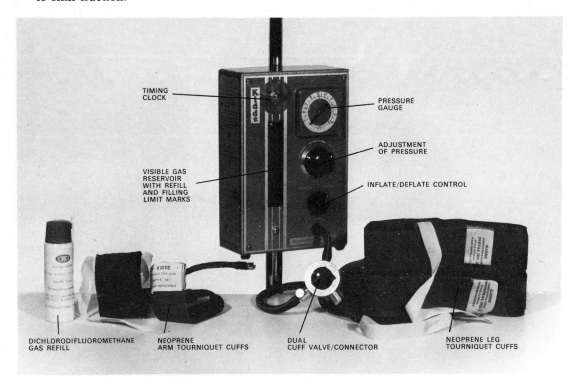

TIMING
CLOCK

PRESSURE
GAUGE

ADJUSTMENT
OF PRESSURE

VISIBLE GAS
RESERVOIR
WITH REFILL
AND FILLING
LIMIT MARKS

INFLATE/DEFLATE CONTROL

DICHLORODIFLUOROMETHANE
GAS REFILL

NEOPRENE
ARM TOURNIQUET CUFFS

DUAL
CUFF VALVE/CONNECTOR

NEOPRENE LEG
TOURNIQUET CUFFS

Figure 335   The Kidde automatically compensated tourniquet. (Howmedica U.K. Ltd.)

POSITION
Usually supine, but varies with the site for insertion.

INSTRUMENTS
As Figure 336
Splints, weights, pulleys, traction frame, etc.

OUTLINE OF PROCEDURE
Skeletal traction may be used as a temporary procedure for the manipulation of a fracture during operation, or as a permanent means of maintaining this reduction after operation until the fracture heals. It is used either as fixed traction, or as sliding traction with weights and pulleys, etc., in combination with a splint.

For average adults with a traction of up to 9 kg (20 lb) a Steinmann pin size 4 mm$\frac{5}{32}$ in) diameter is usually adequate, although for larger patients and a greater degree of traction it may be necessary to increase this diameter to 4·8 mm $\left(\frac{3}{16}\right.$ in). If the pin is to be inserted with a hand or power drill, it should have a diamond-shaped point; but if a hand chuck and mallet are used, the point needs to be of a trocar shape.

When inserting a Steinmann pin, a small skin incision is first made at the entrance and then the exit of the pin. Each end is then attached to a Bohler's stirrup and the limb is immobilised on a splint in the usual manner.

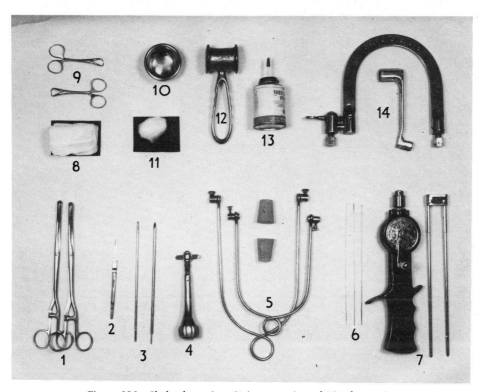

Figure 336   Skeletal traction, Steinmann pin and Kirschner wire

1. Sponge-holding forceps (Rampley), 2.
2. Scalpel handle No. 9 with No. 15 blade (Bard Parker).
3. Traction pins (Steinmann) of appropriate diameter; diamond and trocar points illustrated.
4. Hand chuck for Steinmann pins.
5. Traction pin stirrups (Bohler), and corks for points of pins.
6. Traction wires (Kirschner), 3 sizes.
7. Drill with telescopic guide for insertion
   of Kirschner wires. (Chuck keys may be required.)
8. Swabs.
9. Towel clips, 2.
10. Gallipot containing skin antiseptic.
11. Cotton-wool for sealing around the protruding pins.
12. Mallet (Heath).
13. Nobecutane for sealing puncture wounds.
14. Traction wire stirrup (Kirschner) and key.

Kirschner wires are very thin in comparison with Steinmann pins. However, when these wires are maintained under tension in a special stirrup (in a manner similar to a piano wire) the degree of traction obtainable is quite considerable and as a very small hole is made, bone damage is minimal. There are three sizes of wires, 0·9 mm (0·035 in), 1·15 mm (0·045 in), 1·6 mm (0·062 in) in diameter, the middle size being the most popular. Kirschner wires are inserted with a special hand or power drill, having a telescopic attachment which is extended to support the wire. This attachment collapses as the wire is inserted, the wire is stretched taut in the special Kirschner stirrup and splints applied as before. In both cases the point at which the pin or wire enters and leaves the skin is sealed with a piece of cotton-wool and plastic skin or collodion.

For fractures of the femoral shaft, a pin or wire is passed through the upper part of the tibia; and for fractures of the tibial shaft, the pin or wire is passed through the lower end of the tibia or os calcis.

Skeletal traction (skull)

DEFINITION

Traction applied to the skull in the treatment of cervical lesions, e.g., cervical dislocations, by means of a caliper.

POSITION

Supine, with no pillow.

INSTRUMENTS

Batchelor's Zygoma Hooks
    Sponge-holding forceps (Rampley), 2
    Scalpel handle No. 3 with No. 15 blade (Bard Parker)
    Zygoma hooks (2) and frame (Fig. 337)
    Local anaesthetic requisites (Fig. 271)
    Traction cord, weights and pulleys, etc.

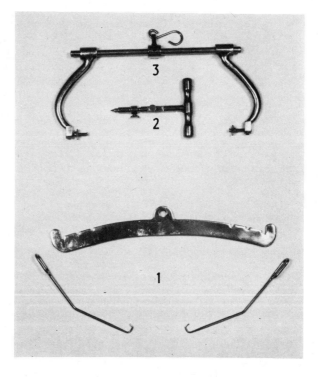

Figure 337   Skeletal traction, skull calipers
1. Zygoma hooks and traction bar (Batchelor).
2. T-handle trephine (Blackburn).
3. Skull traction apparatus (Blackburn).

Blackburn's Skull Calipers
  Sponge-holding forceps (Rampley), 2
  Scalpel handles No. 3 with Nos. 10 and 15 blades (Bard Parker)
  Dissecting forceps, toothed (Lane), 2
  Scissors, curved on flat, 13 cm (5 in) (Mayo)
  Small retractors, double hook, 2
  Artery forceps, curved on flat (Kilner, etc.), 5
  Rugine, curved (Faraboeuf)
  Skull trephine (Blackburn) (Fig. 337)
  Skull caliper (Blackburn) (Fig. 337)
  Allen key for caliper
  Small needle holder (Kilner)
  Local anaesthetic requisites (Fig. 271)
  2·5 (2/0) Silk or nylon on a small curved cutting needle for skin sutures
  Traction cord, weights and pulleys, etc.

OUTLINE OF PROCEDURE
  The Batchelor's zygoma hooks are the simplest to insert and many surgeons regard them as more satisfactory, for they have little tendency to slip out after insertion.
  The zygoma area is infiltrated with local anaesthetic, and a small stab incision is made sufficient for insertion of the hook. A hook is inserted under the zygoma on each side and connected to the frame to which traction is applied by weights and pulleys attached to the patient's bed.
  For insertion of the Blackburn caliper, under local anaesthesia, an incison about 1·3 cm ($\frac{1}{2}$ in) long is made in the parietal region on each side of the skull. The trephine is set to the depth required by adjusting the guard, and a small disc of bone is removed. The caliper is inserted, the retaining screw adjusted down to the wound, and if necessary one or two skin sutures are inserted to close the ends of the wound round the caliper. Traction is applied as previously described.

The bone and fracture set of instruments

  The basic set illustrated in Figure 338 consists of suitable instruments for the average bone operation. The very small or large bone instruments are added as required, and do not form part of the basic set unless they are in constant use.
  Bone levers, hooks and holding forceps are generally used in pairs, especially for the manipulation of fractures. Bone-cutting and nibbling or gouge forceps may have single joints; or multiple joints (compound action), which allows considerable force to be applied with the minimum of effort, and are of great value when the bone is very hard.

Open reduction of a fracture

DEFINITION
  Reduction of a fracture by open operation.

POSITION
  Dependent upon the location of the fracture.

INSTRUMENTS
  General set (Fig. 281)
  Bone and fracture set (Fig. 338)

(If internal fixation is contemplated, instruments for this are added. See appropriate section, e.g., plating and screwing.)

2·5 or 3 (2/0 or 0) Plain catgut or Dexon for ligatures

3, 4 or 5 (0, 1 or 2) Plain or chromic catgut or Dexon sutures on appropriate needle for that area of the body

2·5 or 3 (2/0 or 0) Silk or nylon on a curved or straight cutting needle for skin sutures.

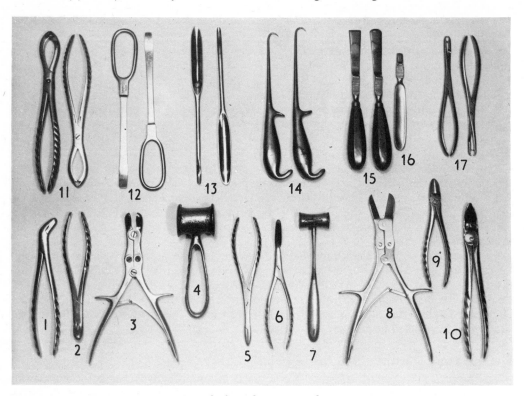

Figure 338   The bone fracture set of instruments

1. Gouge or nibbling forceps, angled on side.
2. Gouge or nibbling forceps, angled on flat.
3. Gouge or nibbling forceps, compound action.
4. Mallet (Heath).
5. Necrosis or sequestrum forceps, straight.
6. Necrosis or sequestrum forceps, angled on flat.
7. Mallet (Rowland).
8. Bone-cutting forceps, compound action (Horsley).
9. Bone-cutting forceps, straight (Liston).
10. Bone-cutting forceps, angled on flat (Liston).
11. Bone-holding forceps (Fergusson lion), 2.
12. Bone elevators or levers (Bristow), 2.
13. Bone elevators or levers (Lane), minimum of 2.
14. Bone hooks (Lane).
15. Large periosteal elevators or rugines (Mitchell), straight and round end.
16. Small periosteal elevator or rugine (Faraboeuf).
17. Bone-holding forceps (St Thomas's Hospital).

OUTLINE OF PROCEDURE

The open reduction of a fracture is performed when adequate reduction by closed methods has been unsuccessful or is impossible; when displacement, angulation or deformity are likely following closed reduction, e.g., fractures of the patella; to promote union and reduce stay in hospital, e.g., internal fixation of fractures of the middle and upper femoral shaft; to reduce mortality, e.g., internal fixation of femoral neck fractures and intertrochanteric fractures.

The fracture is exposed through a skin incision which is sufficiently long to provide adequate exposure with minimal retraction of soft tissues. This incision is generally not placed directly over bony prominences, and the fracture is approached through intermuscular planes rather than through muscle bellies.

The bone is exposed by minimal periosteal stripping and reduction is accomplished with bone levers, hooks or bone-holding forceps. If internal fixation is contemplated, the reduction may be maintained with ordinary bone-holding forceps or the self-retaining kind.

If the fracture has not been fixed internally some type of external splintage will be needed (Chapter 29). Occasionally internal fixation may be combined with external splintage as a temporary measure.

Drills, plates and screws (Fig. 339)

Internal fixation for bone surgery can take the form of a plate screwed into position on the surface of a bone; a screw passing through the bone to transfix the fracture; or an intramedullary nail or pin inside the bone.

There are very few metals which can be left inside the body without causing at least a severe reaction, if not complete corrosion. The 'noble' metals including gold and silver may be used, but are very expensive and often mechanically weak. It must be mentioned that tantalum is another metal which has been used for implants, but it has been shown that this metal can cause severe tissue reaction (not corrosion) and its use is now rather limited.

There are three metals which have been found suitable for surgical implants, although none of these is regarded as perfect. The three implant metals are: special stainless-steel of the SMo or EN58J type; Vitallium or Vinertia; and Titanium.

The SMo or EN58J is called an austenitic stainless-steel containing about 18 per cent of chromium, 8 per cent nickel and 2 to 4 per cent molybdenum, in addition to iron residue and traces of other elements. It has excellent corrosion resistant properties, great toughness and can be worked by machine.

Austenitic stainless-steel is non-magnetic, but may become slightly magnetic as a result of cold working such as the drawing process used to manufacture Kirschner wires, Kuntscher nails and Steinmann pins. It cannot be hardened much more than a Rockwell C35 (a degree of hardness determined with a special testing machine) and is therefore not suitable for osteotomes which require a lasting sharp edge.

The resistance of austenitic stainless-steel to corrosion lies in its 2 to 4 per cent addition of molybdenum, but equally important are the highly polished surface finish, careful cleansing process, the creation of an oxide surface layer and removal of debris left in the implant during the polishing operations by 'passivating' the implant in a chemical bath and adequate inspection after manufacture of detect flaws. It is interesting to note that the most satisfactory method of polishing implants is by reverse plating. In this method, which is the exact opposite of electrolytic plating (e.g., chromium plating), debris is 'thrown' off the implant even from the most inaccessible areas such as the threads of screws and cannulations of pins.

Under normal circumstances the protective oxide layer is self-sealing if the surface of an implant becomes slightly scratched. In spite of this, care must be taken to avoid scratching any implant during handling, as a point of corrosion may be set up which could cause severe reaction in the tissues.

It is appropriate here to mention the martensitic stainless-steels which are used in the manufacture of most surgical instruments. These stainless-steels are magnetic and can be hardened to a Rockwell C56 to C60 which is adequate for osteotomes and chisels, etc. Ordinary plated carbon steel can be hardened to a Rockwell C55 to C65 and for this reason some surgeons contend that carbon steel osteotomes retain a better edge than stainless-steel osteotomes. However, with improved manufacturing techniques, stainless-steel is fast approaching carbon steel in quality from this point of view.

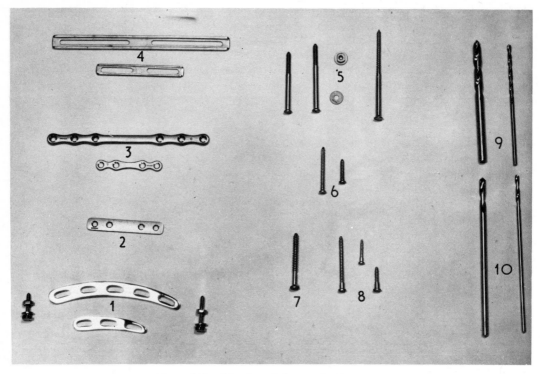

Figure 339   Selection of plates and screws, etc.

1. Spinal plates and bolts (Wilson).
2. Bone plate (Venable).
3. Bone plates, sizes 7 and 0 (Sherman).
4. Bone plates with slots for screws, sizes 7·5 cm and 15 cm (3 in and 6 in) (Egger).
5. Barr bolts, tibial, with nut and washer.
6. Bone screws, 3·6 mm ($\frac{9}{64}$ in) diameter (Sherman).
7. Bone screw, transfixion, size 4 mm ($\frac{5}{32}$ in) diameter.
8. Bone screws, wood type thread, sizes 3·6 mm ($\frac{9}{64}$ in) and 2·8 mm ($\frac{7}{64}$ in) diameter.
9. Bone drills, Vitallium, conventional flutes, sizes 6·14 mm (0·25 in) and 3·2 mm (0·13 in) diameter.
10. Bone drills, stainless-steel, short flutes to prevent enlarging the hole in the proximal cortex during drilling of the distal cortex, sizes 4 mm ($\frac{5}{32}$ in) and 2·8 mm ($\frac{7}{64}$ in) diameter.

Martensitic stainless-steel is rust resistant but it corrodes if left in the tissues and is therefore entirely unsuitable for internal use. A surgeon will take steps to remove a fragment of martensitic stainless-steel which has 'flaked off' from a surgical instrument and become embedded in the tissues.

Vitallium (American), Vinertia (British) are non-ferrous alloys (they do not rust) containing 65 per cent cobalt, 30 per cent chromium and 3 per cent molybdenum with traces of other elements. The metal is virtually inert in the body tissues and is very strong but very difficult to work by machine. Most implants, even screws, are cast from molten metal because of this difficulty. The tensile strength is in the order of 63 to 66 kgf per mm^2 (40 to 42 tons per in^2).

Non-ferrous alloys do not rely upon a high surface polish for part of their corrosion resistance, and slight damage to the surface is not quite so important as with the stainless-steels. But this does not mean that any less care should be taken during handling, for a highly polished smooth surface of an implant may be essential, e.g., for arthroplasty of joints.

Titanium used for surgical implants is commercially prepared by Imperial Chemical Industries to within 99 per cent of purity. The minute trace elements remaining to a maximum of 1 per cent are oxygen, iron, carbon, nitrogen and hydrogen, and these are completely dissolved throughout the metal. These trace materials in wrought Titanium are less significant amounts than in the case of SMo stainless steel and cobalt, chromium, molybdenum alloys.

Unlike austenitic stainless-steels such as SMo, Titanium cannot be 'work hardened' by machining or cold drawing, so that the high tensile strength achieved in cold drawn stainless-steel wire as used for staples, Kirschner wires, Steinmann pins, Rush type pins cannot be reproduced in Titanium. However those implants usually made from the annealed material of stainless-steel, have less tensile strength and yield point (or ductility) as compared with Titanium before permanent deformation of the implant occurs under stress.

Implants suitable for manufacture in Titanium include, hip prostheses, hip nails, bone plates and screws. For its strength the metal is exceptionally light being about half the weight of the equivalent size in stainless-steel. It is extremely inert and resistant to corrosion by body tissue and fluids. Its ultimate tensile strength can be as high as 95 kgf per mm^2 (60 tons per in^2) but on average is in the region of 70 kgf to 79 kgf per mm^2 (44 to 50 tons per in^2). Titanium has been used clinically since 1957 and as a result of many papers on its successful use it is for some purposes replacing the other metallic implant materials.

To use different metals in contact with one another in the body is very undesirable. Although all three metals described are relatively inert when used alone, severe reactions can occur if, for instance, a stainless-steel screw is used in contact with a Vitallium plate. This reaction is said to be partially an electrolytic and partially a chemical process. Whatever the cause, the end result is corrosion of the implant, and often non-union of the fracture or a discharging wound. *The scrub nurse must ensure that she does not give the surgeon implants made from different metals and which are to be used in contact with one another in the tissues.*

It is possible for small fragments of metal to 'flake off' from instruments used for the insertion of implants. For this reason, it is desirable that all instruments used for handling implants are made from or tipped with the same metal as the implant; otherwise small fragments of metal may be transferred from the insertion instruments and set up local points of corrosion in the tissues. This is especially so with screwdrivers, which may slip off the screw during insertion.

Drills

Bone drills are made from three materials, martensitic stainless-steel, Vitallium and plated carbon steel. The first two types of drills are sterilised by steam, but the carbon steel drills must be dry-heat sterilised or submerged in chemicals.

Drill points must be kept sharp and at slightly less than the 45 degrees angle point of the conventional industrial drills. If the drill shaft is not straight, or has been incorrectly aligned in the drill chuck, the result will be an oval hole in the bone. Correct alignment is checked by looking along the drill shaft as the chuck is rotated. A drill end (up to 6·4 mm ($\frac{1}{4}$ in) in diameter) should appear as a point about the size of a full stop on this page. A blunt drill appears as a larger point, and a wobbling drill as an oval-shaped point. In this case the drill must be re-aligned in the chuck, or discarded for straightening and re-sharpening before further use.

Vitallium drills appear to have several advantages over the other two types. They are rustless, have lasting sharpness and the ability to bend 90 degrees without breaking.

Screws

Bone screws have fine or coarse threads which either extend for the full length of the screw or for only three-quarters of the length.

The screw slot varies in shape within three varieties: the plain slot, the Phillip's recessed head/Duodrive and the cruciform or cross slot (see Appendix of Instruments). A standard shape of screwdriver is used for the first variety but a special 'cross point' screwdriver must be used for the other two.

Screws used for holding bone plates in position are of two main diameters, 3·6 mm ($\frac{9}{64}$ in) and 4 mm ($\frac{5}{32}$ in). Sherman, Phillips and cruciform are 3·6 mm ($\frac{9}{64}$ in) and 4 mm ($\frac{5}{32}$ in) diameter.

As the screw always passes through both cortices in the fixation of bone plates, this type of screw is fully threaded in order that the threads may gain the greatest purchase in both sides of the bone.

Screws used alone for the fixation of bone fragments are partially threaded and termed 'wood or transfixion' screws. In this case the screw is usually inserted through the fragment and into the area of cancellous bone adjacent, e.g., fracture of the medial malleolus. The partially threaded portion of the screw near the head allows the surgeon to 'draw up' the loose fragment against the larger one without causing the bone to split. This type of screw can be used also for fixing together two fragments, e.g., a spiral fracture of the tibia.

The holding power of a screw is almost at its maximum in bone when the size of the hole drilled is approximately equivalent to half the distance between the outside diameter and root diameter of the screw threads. Therefore, the hole drilled in cortical bone should approximate 85 per cent of the outside diameter of the screw. This obviates both the weak holding power of larger holes and the tendency of the screws to split the bone with smaller holes. However, when the bone is of a soft composition, i.e., cancellous bone, the hole drilled should be only slightly larger than the root diameter of the threads.

For a 2·8 mm ($\frac{7}{64}$ in) diameter screw, size No. 9, 2·4 mm ($\frac{3}{32}$ in) diameter drill is used; 3·6 mm ($\frac{9}{64}$ in) diameter screws require a size No. 31 approx. 2·8 mm ($\frac{7}{64}$ in) diameter drill; 4 mm ($\frac{5}{32}$ in) diameter screws require a 3·6 mm ($\frac{9}{64}$ in) or 3·2 mm ($\frac{1}{8}$ in) diameter drill; and 4·5 mm approx. ($\frac{11}{64}$ in) diameter screws require a 4 mm ($\frac{5}{32}$ in) or 3·6 mm ($\frac{9}{64}$ in) diameter drill. A more complete list of drill to screw diameters is shown in the Appendix.

After drilling a hole the surgeon measures its depth with a screw measure. This measure has a hooked end with which he feels the outer edge of the hole in the opposite cortex. The handle of the instrument is then slid down to touch the proximal cortex and the depth read off against a scale engraved on the handle.

If the surgeon does not wish to drill right through the bone, the depth of the hole is determined by probing the bottom with his measure and reading off the scale as before.

A self-retaining or automatic screwdriver is used to insert the screw up to 6·4 mm ($\frac{1}{4}$ in) from the head. The Williams or Burns are probably the ones most popular for standard single-slot screws. Alternatively there are a number of power operated screwdrivers including the Stryker bit which fits into the Stryker power tool and the Howmedica Universal Air Drill.

The Williams screwdriver is adjustable for various sizes of screw heads by means of the large screw connected to the retaining lever on the handle (illustrated in Fig. 340 and Appendix of Instruments). When loading screws, care must be taken to avoid force as the lever is closed. The adjusting screw must be altered until the lever closes easily with the screw in position. Failure to do this will result in breakage of the sleeve which supports the screw head. Both the Williams and the Burns screwdrivers must be dismantled, cleaned, lubricated regularly and sent for repair when the tip becomes worn and does not fit snugly into the screw head.

The screw is finally tightened home with a plain-end screwdriver, such as Lane's, which must fit tightly into the screw slot. Nothing is more irritating than a screwdriver which keeps slipping out of the slot as the screw is driven home, and in addition, there is a grave danger of scratching the screw, with risk of corrosion.

Plates

Bone plates are designed to provide maximum strength with minimal dimensions, although no plate will take full weight bearing until the fracture has almost healed. Plates may be contoured slightly to accommodate the curvature of a bone, but if great angles are needed, the manufacturer will incorporate these when the implant is cast or machined. Once a plate has been contoured, it must not be re-bent in the reverse direction, otherwise metal fatigue may occur.

Plates such as Sherman's, Venable's and Lane's have holes for screw fixation, but there are other types including the Egger's contact plates which have slots instead. Slotted bone plates are designed to permit the fractured ends of the bone to move together slightly under the plates after they have been inserted. This allows constant contact of the bone ends (due to muscular pressure) while slight necrosis, absorption, and osteogenesis at the traumatised ends occurs. The other advantage is that the surgeon is able to insert his screws at any selected position along the slot.

The Hicks plates have lateral lugs in which the screw holes are positioned and which prevent rotation of the fragments after insertion of the plate (see Appendix page 642).

In order to minimise bacterial contamination of implants such as screws and plates, etc., these should always be handled with sterile forceps and not the gloved hands.

Plating and screwing

DEFINITION
Internal fixation of a fracture by means of plates and screws.

POSITION
Generally supine, but dependent upon the location of the fracture.

INSTRUMENTS
General set (Fig. 281)
Bone and fracture set (Fig. 338)
Plating and screwing set (Fig. 340)
2·5 or 3 (2/0 or 0) Plain catgut or Dexon for ligatures
3, 4 or 5 (0, 1 or 2) Plain or chromic catgut or Dexon sutures on appropriate needle for that area of the body
2·5 or 3 (2/0 or 0) Silk or nylon on a small, medium or large cutting needle for skin sutures
Plaster of Paris or splints may be required.

OUTLINE OF PROCEDURE

The fracture is exposed and reduced. If plating is to be performed, the plate is adjusted to the correct contour and applied to the bone subperiosteally, and screwed in position.

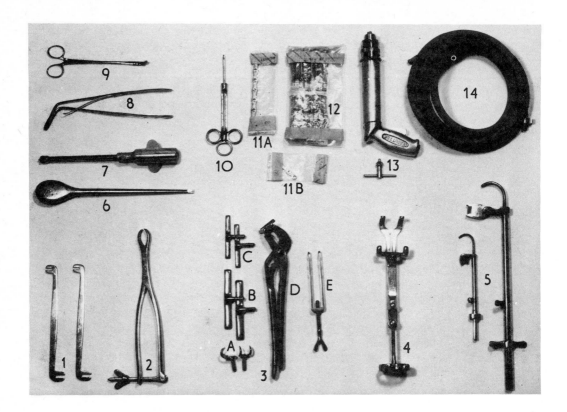

Figure 340   Instruments for screwing and plating.

1. Plate benders, 2.
2. Bone clamp, self-retaining (Hey Grove), 2.
3. Bone clamp, adjustable and self-retaining (Charnley).
   A. Hook jaws suitable for fractured patella, olecranon, etc., 2.
   B. Large jaws suitable for femur, 2.
   C. Medium jaws suitable for tibia, etc., 2.
   D. Adjustable handle with two small jaws.
   E. Self-retaining screw clamp for handle.
4. Bone clamp, self-retaining (Lowman).
5. Bone clamps, self-retaining (Sinclair), large and small.
6. Ordinary screwdriver (Lane).
7. Automatic screwdriver (Williams).
8. Plate-holding forceps.
9. Screw-holding forceps.
10. Screw measuring device (Crawford Adams).
11. Bone plate, sterile in nylon packet, appropriate size.
    A. Shows a large size, and B. a small size of plate.
12. Set of screws and drills in nylon packet.
13. Power drill and chuck key (Desoutter compressed air drill).
14. Rubber air hose for power drill.

If screw fixation only is required, one or more screws are introduced obliquely across the fracture line.

The wound is closed in the usual manner and temporary splints applied if required.

Wiring

DEFINITION

Internal fixation of a fracture by means of cerclage wire loops.

POSITION

Generally supine, but dependent upon the location of the fracture.

INSTRUMENTS

General set (Fig. 281)
Bone and fracture set (Fig. 338)
Wiring set (Fig. 341)

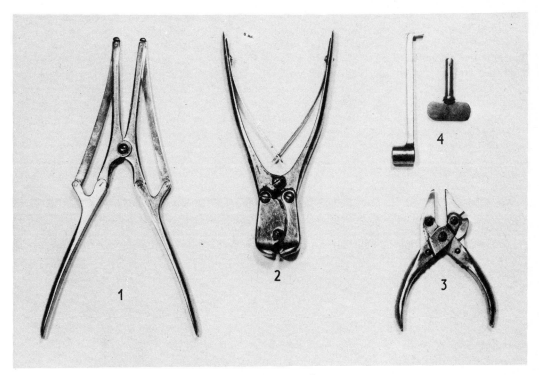

Figure 341   Instruments for wiring
1. Wire knot-tying forceps (Harris).
2. Wire-cutting forceps, compound action.
3. Pliers and wire-cutting forceps combined.
4. Wire-twisting apparatus (Hey Grove).

Bone clamps illustrated in Figure 340 may be required
Bone awl or drill
2·5 or 3 (2/0 or 0) Plain catgut or Dexon for ligatures
3, 4 or 5 (0, 1 or 2) Plain or chromic catgut or Dexon sutures on appropriate needles for that area of the body
2·5 or 3 (2/0 or 0) Silk or nylon on a small, medium or large cutting needle for skin sutures
Plaster of Paris or splints may be required.

OUTLINE OF PROCEDURE

The fracture is exposed and reduced. Austenitic stainless-steel wire within the range of 29 SWG and 18 SWG (Chapter 7) is generally used, although sizes 20, 24 and 28 SWG are the most useful.

The fracture may be immobilised by a circumferential wire loop, e.g. a butterfly fracture of a bone shaft; or a loop is passed through holes drilled in each fragment, e.g., fracture of the patella.

The surgeon will require a bone awl or drill if holes are needed in the bone fragment. If the wire is sufficiently stiff it is passed directly round the bone or through the holes made. If a smaller gauge of wire is used, it is first threaded on to a large suture needle and is twisted back upon itself for about one inch. Alternatively, an aneurysm needle or wire passer (e.g., Sharps) may be used and the wire is threaded through the eye but not twisted back upon itself. Sometimes the surgeon may find it easier to pass the aneurysm needle round the bone first and then thread the wire through the terminal hole.

When the wire is in position, a final check is made on correct alignment of the fragments and the wire is twisted or tied in a knot. If the wire is to be twisted, this is accomplished either with special twisting forceps or two pairs of pliers. If a knot is being tied and unless the wire is very fine, a special forceps for tying wire knots is needed. Fine wire is then cut with heavy scissors reserved for the purpose and heavy wire with wire-cutting forceps.

It is essential the scrub nurse ensures that wire is free from kinks before she hands it to the surgeon. A kink is a weak point and is very liable to break, either during insertion or after operation.

The wound is closed in the usual manner and splints or plaster of Paris may be applied.

Internal fixation by nail or pin. Femoral neck fractures, Smith Petersen nail

DEFINITION

The internal fixation of a subcapital or transcervical fracture of the femoral neck with a trifin pin. This procedure may be used also to immobilise a slipped upper femoral epiphysis in adolescents.

POSITION

Immobilised on a fracture table (Fig. 73).

INSTRUMENTS

General set (Fig. 281)
Bone and fracture set (Fig. 338)
Set of trifin nails (Smith Petersen) (Fig. 342), or four flange nails (illustrated in Appendix)
Steel rule, 15 cm (6 in)
Plate benders, 2
3 (0) Plain catgut or Dexon for ligatures
3 or 4 (0 or 1) Plain catgut or Dexon on a medium half-circle cutting or Mayo needle with a trocar point for muscle sutures
2·5 or 3 (2/0 or 0) Silk or nylon on a medium curved cutting needle for skin sutures.

OUTLINE OF PROCEDURE

The patient is immobilised on a fracture table and if necessary the fracture is manipulated and reduced. This fracture table may be a Plaistow which is illustrated in Fig. 73,

Bell, Albee or Hawley table, Shropshire horse, or a special attachment on a general operation table. The position of the patient's legs is adjusted to maintain reduction of the fracture during operation, and this usually means in abduction and extension with some degree of internal rotation of the affected limb.

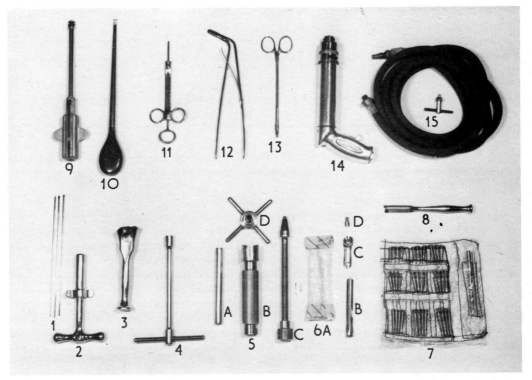

Figure 342   Femoral neck fracture, Smith Petersen nail

1. Three guide wires of exactly the same diameter and length 2·3 cm × 25 cm ($\frac{3}{32}$ in × 10 in).
2. Guide wire hand chuck (Watson-Jones).
3. Fracture impactor (Smith Petersen).
4. Box spanner for bolt (Smith Petersen).
5. Driver/extractor for trifin nail (Smith Petersen).
   A. Tommy bar for additional leverage on capstan during extraction of nail.
   B. Extractor barrel.
   C. Driver/extractor, threaded bar.
   D. Extraction capstan.
6. A. Trifin nail of appropriate size (Smith Petersen), sterile in packet.
   B. Showing Smith Petersen trifin nail.
   C. Small retaining plate (Coventry).
   D. Bolt and spring washer for attaching plate to nail (Coventry).
7. Set of screws and drills in nylon wallet.
8. Trifin nail starter (Smith Petersen).
9. Automatic screwdriver (Williams).
10. Ordinary screwdriver (Lane).
11. Screw measuring device (Crawford Adams).
12. Plate-holding forceps.
13. Screw-holding forceps.
14. Power drill (Desoutter compressed air drill).
15. Rubber air hose for power drill, and chuck key.

X-ray apparatus is positioned to give anterior and lateral position films during the course of operation.

An incision is made about 25 mm (1 in) below the tip of the trochanter, and is carried 5 cm to 8 cm (2 to 3 in) down the lateral aspect of the thigh parallel with the femoral shaft. Dissection is made down to the fascia lata which is incised and split with scissors in line with the skin incision. The fascia lata is retracted to expose the vastus lateralis which is incised and retracted away from the femur with bone levers. Further blunt dissection with a periosteal elevator exposes the region of the trochanter.

A Smith Petersen nail, like many implants used for the fixation of fractures in the femoral neck region, has a central cannulation to accommodate a guide wire. It is important that a guide wire is checked for correct size by passing it through the cannulation of the nail. If the wire it too tight, or does not run smoothly through it (perhaps due to a bent wire or some manufacturing error), either the wire or the nail must be replaced. There is grave danger of a tight wire being carried through into the pelvis as the nail is driven home.

After drilling a 4·8 mm ($\frac{3}{16}$ in) to 6·4 mm ($\frac{1}{4}$ in) hole in the bone about 25 mm (1 in) below the trochanter along the shaft, the guide wire is inserted into the femoral neck and an X-ray taken to confirm its position. The guide wire may require several adjustments before the correct position is achieved.

The length of the nail required is determined by placing another identical guide wire alongside the portion of the wire which projects from the bone, and the amount projecting is deducted by measurement from the total length of the guide wire. This measurement is the same as that in the femoral neck.

If a small plate is to be used to retain the nail in position, it is usual to add a 6·4 mm ($\frac{1}{4}$ in) to the required measurement of nail.

A three or four flange nail of appropriate length is hammered home over the guide wire within 13 mm ($\frac{1}{2}$ in) of the cortex. The guide wire is then removed, and the fracture impacted with a blow on a Smith Peterson impactor positioned over the head of the protruding nail. The nail is then driven home either flush with the femoral cortex (no retaining plate) or with approx 6 mm ($\frac{1}{4}$ in) left projecting (small, one hole retaining plate).

If required, the small retaining plate may then be secured to the nail with a threaded bolt and screwed to the femoral shaft.

The wound is closed in layers and the patient may require a plaster boot which incorporates a short splint across the heel and at right angles to the leg to prevent rotation of the foot after operation.

There are many other types of intra-medullary appliances for immobilising femoral neck fractures, these include sliding nails (Pugh) and compression screws (Charnley, Garden). Some of these are illustrated in the Appendix.

Internal fixation by nail or pin. Femoral trochanteric fractures, McLaughlin and McKee

DEFINITION

The internal fixation of a basal, pertrochanteric or subtrochanteric fracture of the upper femur.

POSITION

As for Smith Petersen nail (Fig. 73).

INSTRUMENTS

McLaughlin Appliance
   General set (Fig. 281)
   Bone and fracture set (Fig. 338)
   Set of trifin nails (Smith Petersen) (Fig. 342)

Intertrochanteric plate, five or seven hole, with bolt and locking washer (McLaughlin). Illustrated in Appendix.
Ligatures and sutures as for Smith Petersen nail

McKee Nail and Plate
General set (Fig. 281)
Bone and fracture set (Fig. 338)
Femoral neck fracture set (Fig. 342 minus items 4, 5 and 6)
Driver/extractor (McKee)
Box spanner (McKee)
Trifin nail of appropriate size (McKee), sterile in packet. Illustrated in Appendix
Intertrochanteric plate (McKee), sterile in packet. Illustrated in Appendix
Plate benders, 2
Ligatures and sutures as for Smith Petersen nail.

OUTLINE OF PROCEDURE
The initial stages of the immobilisation of the patient, fracture reduction and incision are similar to that for Smith Petersen nail. In the case of the McLaughlin appliance and McKee plate, however, the incision extends several centimetres further down the femoral shaft in order to provide adequate exposure to insert the longer plate.

A McLaughlin Plate is bolted to a Smith Petersen nail which is inserted as described previously, with 6 mm ($\frac{1}{4}$ in) of the nail head left protruding from the bone. The plate is secured to the femoral shaft with five or seven screws, depending upon the length of the plate. The design of this plate (see Instrument Appendix), which has a curved shoulder, allows adjustment of the angle between the nail and plate without having to actually bend the plate itself.

A McKee Plate is bolted to a McKee nail which is inserted in a manner similar to a Smith Petersen nail. The difference between the two nails is that whereas the Smith Petersen nail has a threaded hole in the head portion, the McKee nail has a threaded projection. The plate is fitted over this threaded projection and secured with a hexagonal nut. However, this type of plate may first require adjustment of its angle with the plate benders in order that the plate lies flush along the shaft when bolted to the nail. The plate is then secured to the shaft by four or six screws, depending upon the length of plate selected.

The wound is closed in layers in the usual manner.

Slipped upper femoral epiphysis

It has been mentioned that the Smith Petersen trifin nail can be used to immobilise a slipped upper femoral epiphysis. Alternatively, Austin Moore pins, Knowle's pins or fine Steinmann pins may be used for this procedure.

These pins resemble guide wires but are made from austenitic stainless steel or Vitallium. The procedure is as for Smith Petersen nail up to the insertion of the guide wire, but in this case an Austin Moore pin, Knowle pin or Steinmann pin is drilled into the femoral neck and across the epiphyseal line.

The position and length of the pin are checked radiologically and when satisfactory, several other pins, up to four, may be inserted alongside the first pin within the neck but generally at slightly different angles. Any excess pin projecting from the bone is cut off and the wound is closed in the usual manner.

One of the advantages of this technique is said to be that these pins occupy less space within the femoral neck than the conventional trifin nail, and there is consequently less interference with bone formation (it is also less traumatic).

Intramedullary fixation of the femoral shaft fracture, Kuntscher nail

DEFINITION
Intramedullary fixation of fractures of the middle and upper shaft of the femur.

POSITION
Either supine, with a sandbag under the affected buttock, or full lateral.

INSTRUMENTS
General set (Fig. 281)
Bone and fracture set (Fig. 338)
Kuntscher nail set (Fig. 343)

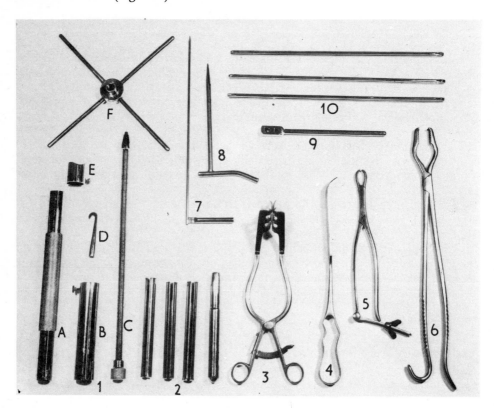

Figure 343   Femoral shaft fracture, Kuntscher nail

1. Extractor for Kuntscher nails (Brigden).
    A. Extractor barrel.
    B. Extension tube for extractor barrel (long nails).
    C. Threaded extractor bar.
    D. Extractor hook.
    E. Sleeve designed for contact with trochanter or end of fractured bone.
    F. Extractor capstan.
2. Drivers and set for Kuntscher nails, one driver for each diameter of nail in use.
3. Retractor, self-retaining (Adson).
4. Large bone-levers (Lane), 2.
5. Bone clamp, self-retaining (Hey Grove), 2.
6. Large bone-holding forceps (Lane), 2.
7. Guide for Kuntscher nails.
8. Reamer for Kuntscher nails.
9. Nail bender.
10. Femoral shaft nail (Kuntscher). Those illustrated show 8·5 mm, 9 mm and 9·5 mm diameter.

Diathermy leads, electrodes and lead anchoring forceps

Power Drill.

Intramedullary reamers, appropriate size

3 and 4 (0 and 1) plain catgut or Dexon for ligatures

4 or 5 (1 or 2) Chromic catgut, Dexon or silk, etc., on a large half-circle cutting or
   Mayo's needle with a trocar point for muscle sutures

3 (0) Silk or nylon on a large curved or straight cutting needle for skin sutures

OUTLINE OF PROCEDURE

There are several surgical approaches to the femur but the one most used for Kuntscher nailing is the lateral approach.

The leg is angulated at the fracture site, and a short incision made over the fracture on a
line which extends between the greater trochanter and the external condyle of the femur.
The superficial and deep fascia are incised and the vastus lateralis and vastus intermedius
are divided in the direction of their fibres.

The upper and lower fragments of the fracture are exposed by retraction with bone
levers, and the fracture is reduced. The fracture is then disimpacted and the upper fragment elevated out of the wound. Some surgeons ream out the medullary canal with a
hand or power-reamer before inserting the nail to obviate a tendency for the nail to jam.
A clover leaf nail, slotted and pointed at both ends and of appropriate length, is inserted
into the upper fragment. This nail is driven through the trochanter into the buttock and
through a small skin incision made overlying, until the distal end is flush with the fracture surface. The fracture is then reduced and the nail driven from the upper end into the
lower fragment. The nail is inserted so that the slot at the upper end just projects above
the trochanter for removal of the nail at a later date.

The wound is closed in layers and the patient may be immobilised temporarily on a
Thomas splint.

Intramedullary fixation of tibial shaft fractures, Kuntscher nail

DEFINITION

Intramedullary fixation of tibial shaft fractures with a nail.

POSITION

Supine, with leg flexed over a triangular support (optional).

INSTRUMENTS

General set (Fig. 281)

Bone and fracture set (Fig. 338)

Kuntscher nail set (Fig. 343)

Power drill

9·6 mm ($\frac{3}{8}$ in) diameter twist drill

Intramedullary reamers, appropriate size

3(0) Plain catgut or Dexon for ligatures

4(1) Plain catgut or Dexon on a medium half-circle cutting or Mayo needle with a
   trocar point for muscle and fat sutures

2·5 (2/0) Silk or nylon on a medium curved or straight cutting needle for skin sutures.

OUTLINE OF PROCEDURE

Some surgeons perform this operation as a 'blind' procedure by inserting the nail into
the upper end of the tibia and controlling the position of the fracture and insertion

of the nail radiologically. However, the method generally used is to expose and reduce the fracture before 'nailing.'

A curved incision is made over the fracture site on either side of the anterior border of the tibia. The skin is reflected and the periosteum incised and retracted with bone levers. The fracture is reduced under direct vision and the reduction maintained with bone clamps.

A small incision is made medially at the upper part of the tibia and a 10 mm ($\frac{3}{8}$ in) hole is drilled with the drill pointing in the direction of the tibial tubercle. The nail is inserted and driven along the inside of the tibial shaft past the fracture and into the lower fragment. The nail may be bent slightly before insertion. The wounds are closed in the usual manner.

A useful bending tool can be fabricated from two lengths of tubular stainless-steel.

A splint is generally unnecessary until the patient commences weight bearing, and then a light plaster cast may be applied.

Osteotomy—McMurray's osteotomy of the femur

DEFINITION

Division of the upper shaft of the femur and displacement in order to alter the line of weight bearing of the extremity, e.g., in cases of osteoarthritis and certain femoral neck fractures.

POSITION

Supine, with leg abducted and supported by an assistant, or as Figure 73, Smith Petersen nail.

INSTRUMENTS

General set (Fig. 281)
Bone and fracture set (Fig. 338)
Power drill or hand drill
Twist drills, 3·2 mm ($\frac{1}{8}$ in) to 4·8 mm ($\frac{3}{16}$ in) diameter
Osteotomes 16 mm ($\frac{5}{8}$ in), 19 mm ($\frac{3}{4}$ in) and 38 mm ($1\frac{1}{2}$ in)
Bone punches (Smillie straight and angled), 2
(A high-speed airturbine and burr, e.g., the Hall Orthairtome, may be used for performing the osteotomy (Fig. 344)
3 (0) Plain catgut or Dexon for ligatures
4 or 5 (1 or 2) Plain or chromic catgut or Dexon on a medium half-circle cutting or Mayo needle with trocar point for muscle sutures
2·5 or 3 (2/0 or 0) Silk or nylon on a large curved or straight cutting needle for skin sutures.

Osteotomes, chisels and gouges generally are made from carbon or martensitic stainless-steel. Although carbon steel is the better material for a sharp edge, stainless-steel is less brittle, and there is less risk of a fragment breaking off during use (p. 424).

These cutting instruments are made in a variety of shapes and sizes as can be seen from Figure 345, but are classed according to the basic shape of the blade. An osteotome has two bevelled sides curving towards the cutting edge; a chisel has one flat side and one bevelled side; and a gouge has a curved cutting edge and is hollowed or grooved in section, being concave on one side and convex on the other.

Theoretically an osteotome is used for splitting as in the procedure of osteotomy, and a chisel for slicing; but many surgeons use a thick blade osteotome for splitting and a thin

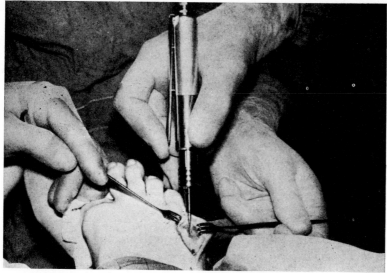

Figure 344   Hall Orthairtome (Howmedica U.K. Ltd.)

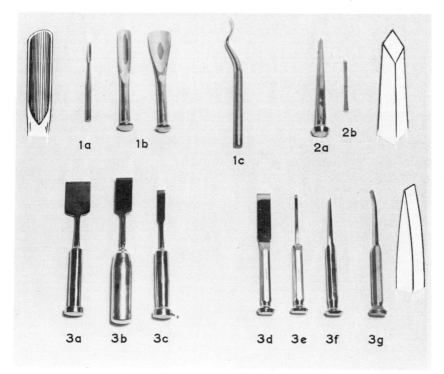

Figure 345   Gouges, chisels and osteotomes

1a. Hahn gouge.
1b. Jones gouges, medium and large.
1c. Smith Petersen hip gouge.
2a. MacEwan chisel, side view.
2b. Hahn chisel.
3a. Whitchurch Howell osteotome, large.

3b. Bristow osteotome, medium.
3c. Whitchurch Howell osteotome, small.
3d. MacEwan osteotome, medium.
3e. MacEwan osteotome, small.
3f. MacEwan osteotome, side view.
3g. Platt osteotome, curved on flat.

blade type for slicing. A gouge is used for grooving or hollowing and is of special use when saucering an osteomyelitis cavity or cyst.

If Plate Fixation is Contemplated
   Twist drill, No. 31 for 3·6 mm ($\frac{9}{64}$ in) screws, or 3·6 mm ($\frac{9}{64}$ in) for 4 mm ($\frac{5}{32}$ in) screws
   Set of bone screws
   Screw measure
   Plate and screw-holding forceps, 2
   Various bone clamps (Fig. 340)
   Automatic screwdriver (Williams or Burns)
   Plain screwdriver (Lane)
   Osteotomy plates (Wainwright, Wainwright-Hammond, Moore/Blount, etc., p. 658)
   Appropriate osteotomy driver/extractor.

OUTLINE OF PROCEDURE
   The trochanteric region of the femur is exposed as previously described for Smith Petersen nail.
   A hole is drilled across the shaft below the level of the trochanter but just above the level of the lesser trochanter. Sometimes this drill is left in position whilst a radiographic check is made. Several holes are then drilled in the line of the osteotomy and the femur is cleanly divided with an osteotome. Alternatively, the femoral shaft is divided with a high-speed turbine and burr, e.g., the Hall Orthairtome.
   The leg is abducted and pressure applied to the proximal portion of the lower fragment until the shaft is displaced inwards. If no plate is being inserted, the wound is closed and the patient immobilised in a double plaster of Paris spica.
   Some surgeons utilise metallic blade plates to fix the osteotomy, and these are driven into the upper fragment and screwed to the femoral shaft. The plate may incorporate a compression device to draw together the fragments on either side of the osteotomy, e.g., Wainwright-Hammond osteotomy plate. If this fixation is secure, the plaster spica is omitted.

Osteotomy of the tibia, with metallic fixation

DEFINITION
   Division of the shaft of tibia and excision of a wedge in order to alter the line of the shaft (especially performed for tibial deformities) and fixation with a plate or screws.

POSITION. Supine.

INSTRUMENTS
   General set (Fig. 281)
   Bone and fracture set (Fig. 338)
   Plating and screwing set (Fig. 340)
   Circular saws
   Osteotomes 16 mm ($\frac{5}{8}$ in), 19 mm ($\frac{3}{4}$ in) and 38 mm ($1\frac{1}{2}$ in)
   3 (0) Plain catgut for ligatures
   4 (1) Plain catgut or Dexon on a medium half-circle cutting or Mayo needle with a
      trocar point for muscle sutures
   2·5 (2/0) Silk or nylon or a medium curved or straight cutting needle for skin sutures.

OUTLINE OF PROCEDURE
   The area for osteotomy is exposed with minimal periosteal stripping. A wedge of bone

is excised, either with a circular saw or an osteotome, and the tibial shaft is re-aligned. The osteotomy is fixed by screws alone, or a plate contoured to the shape of the tibial shaft and secured with several screws.

The wound is closed in the usual manner; plaster of Paris may or may not be applied. This technique can be used for almost any bone shaft where it is necessary to excise a wedge of bone in order to alter the contour of the shaft.

Femoral and tibial epiphyseal arrest

DEFINITION

Arrest of epiphyseal growth by inserting staples across the epiphyseal line of the lower femur and upper tibia. This retards growth of a normal leg in a child so that the short leg is allowed to grow and the two are equal in length when maturity is reached.

POSITION. Supine.

INSTRUMENTS
    General set (Fig. 281)
    Bone and fracture set (Fig. 338)
    Staples, stainless-steel or Vitallium (Muller)
    Staple driver/inserter
    2·5 mm (2/0) Plain catgut or Dexon, for ligatures
    3 (0) Plain catgut or Dexon on a medium half-circle cutting needle for deep sutures
    2·5 (2/0) Silk or nylon on a medium curved cutting needle for skin sutures.

OUTLINE OF PROCEDURE

The epiphyseal lines of the lower end of the femur, upper end of the tibia and fibula are exposed through medial and lateral incisions which extend above and below the joint line on each side.

A 4 to 5 cm (1½ to 2 in) longitudinal incision is made along the central axis of the bone over the epiphyseal line, and the periosteum is reflected slightly. Two or more staples are inserted so that they bridge the epiphyses. This procedure is repeated on the other side of the femur and at both sides of the upper tibial epiphyses. The number of staples inserted, and whether femoral and tibial epiphyses are dealt with at the same operation, depends upon the degree of shortening required. The epiphyseal line of the proximal fibula may be curetted to obliterate the growth centre. This operation is generally performed under X-ray control.

The wound is closed in the usual manner. Growth of the bone continues after the staples are removed at a later date.

Bone grafts

Autogenous Bone Grafts (from the patient himself) are usually removed from either the tibia, fibular or ilium. These three provide cortical grafts, whole bone transplants or cancellous chips and strips respectively, although, of course, there is some of each type of bone in all.

Homogenous Bone Grafts (from another human donor) are obtained usually from non-infected amputated limbs and are stored in deep freeze, Merthiolate, or are freeze dried in pieces of a size suitable for grafting.

In deep freeze, grafts are stored at $-15°C$ and then thawed in warm saline just before use. A small fragment of bone must be cultured a few days before use to confirm sterility of the specimen.

In the case of freeze dried specimens these are reconstituted by submerging in sterile saline before use.

In the case of Merthiolated specimens, the graft is stored in an aqueous solution of Merthiolate 1 in 1000, with regular sampling and change of solution under aseptic theatre conditions. The changes are made every 6 weeks after an initial three negative cultures have been obtained during the first month of storage. Bone is then stored for periods of up to a year and is soaked in warm sterile saline for 15 minutes before use.

In all cases, before the bone is stored, all soft tissue and cartilage is removed from the specimen and a Wassermann reaction performed on the donor, together with a check on the medical history.

Autogenous onlay graft, tibia to other long bone

DEFINITION

The removal of a cortical bone graft from the anterior surface of the tibia for transplantation as an only graft, which is screwed into position to bridge a non-united fracture of another long bone. This type of graft may be used also for other procedures such as spinal fusion.

POSITION. Generally supine.

INSTRUMENTS
    General set (Fig. 281)
    Bone and fracture set (Fig. 338)
    Bone grafting set (Fig. 346)
    Bone clamps shown in Figure 340
    Twist drill of appropriate size
    Set of bone screws
    Screw measure
    Screw-holding forceps
    Automatic screwdriver (Williams or Burns)
    Plain screwdriver (Lane)
    2·5 or 3 (2/0 or 0) Plain catgut or Dexon for ligatures
    Appropriate size of catgut or Dexon and needles for muscle sutures in that area of the
        body
    2·5 or 3 (2/0 or 0) Silk or nylon on a medium curved or straight cutting needle for skin
        sutures
    Plaster of Paris.

OUTLINE OF PROCEDURE

The tibia is exposed through a curved incision and the periosteum is stripped off carefully from the graft area.

An oblong graft is removed from the anterior surface of the tibia with a circular or oscillary bone saw. Ordinarily the borders are not violated as this would considerably weaken the tibia. The circular saw is driven by a power drill, and may be a medium 38 mm ($1\frac{1}{2}$ in) to 40 mm ($1\frac{5}{8}$ in) single or twin blade for the sides, and a small 19 mm ($\frac{3}{4}$ in) to 20 mm ($\frac{3}{4}$in +) single blade for the ends. Saline irrigation provides lubrication for the saw, and the assistants must ensure that swabs and their hands are kept as far away from the blade as possible. In the first case, the gauze may foul the saw and become entwined with it; and in the second case, the saw may jerk during use with risk of injury to the assistant's hand. The use of an oscillatory bone saw reduces the danger of the blade 'jumping.' The oscillating movement of the blade from side to side permits cuts in either direction in bone but does not tear soft tissue, which if touched moves with the blade. Furthermore, it is considered that the amount of burning of the bone due to friction is reduced considerably.

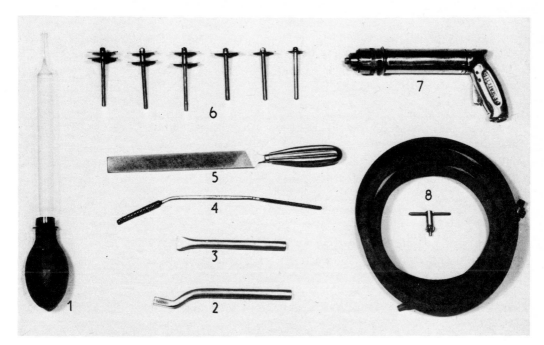

Figure 346   Bone-grafting instruments

1. Irrigation syringe.
2. Bone punch, angled (Smillie).
3. Bone punch, straight (Smillie).
4. Bone rasp (Tubby).
5. Bone file (Tubby).
6. Circular saws, twin and single.
7. Power drill (Desoutter compressed air).
8. Rubber air hose for power drill and chuck key.

The wound is closed in layers and the limb may be placed in a plaster cast. Sometimes if two teams are operating, one may cut the graft and the other insert it to reduce the operating time. In this case the instruments are split into two sets.

The non-united fracture area is exposed and the periosteum stripped off for the extent of the graft. The fracture ends are freshened, the bone re-aligned, and the cortical graft screwed in position on either side with two or more screws. The wound is closed in layers and a plaster cast applied.

Autogenous inlay or sliding graft

DEFINITION

Sliding an oblong-shaped graft cut from the affected bone itself across a non-united fracture.

POSITION. Generally supine.

INSTRUMENTS. As for onlay graft.

The fracture area is exposed and the periosteum stripped off for the extent of the graft. The fractured ends are freshened and fibrous tissue excised.

Using a twin saw, the surgeon cuts an oblong slot about 13 mm ($\frac{1}{2}$ in) wide, with one-third of its length at one side of the fracture line and two-thirds at the other. The grafts are levered from their bed and are re-inserted into the slot, but reversed so that the longer of the two bridges the fracture line. The two grafts are secured with screws and the wound is closed in the usual manner.

Either a plaster of Paris cast or a splint is applied.

Autogenous cancellous iliac grafts

DEFINITION

The removal of cancellous strips or wedges from the ilium as a bone graft for non-united fractures or in fusion procedures, e.g., spine.

POSITION. Supine.

INSTRUMENTS

General set (Fig. 281)
Bone and fracture set (Fig. 338)
Osteotomes, 16 mm ($\frac{5}{8}$ in), 19 mm ($\frac{3}{4}$ in) and 25 mm (1 in)
Diathermy leads, electrodes and lead anchoring forceps
Suction tubing, nozzles and tube anchoring forceps
Power saw may be required
Corrugated drainage tubing
4 (1) Plain catgut or Dexon for ligatures
4 or 5 (1 or 2) Plain or chromic catgut or Dexon on a large half-circle cutting or Mayo
  needle with a trocar point for muscle sutures
2·5 or 3 (2/0 or 0) Silk or nylon on a large curved cutting needle for skin sutures.

OUTLINE OF PROCEDURE

An incision is made along the subcutaneous border of the iliac crest and carried down to bone. The muscles are reflected off the bone subperiosteally to expose the graft area.

For sliver or chip grafts, these are removed with an osteotome parallel to the iliac crest. For wedge grafts, the graft is outlined with an osteotome and then peeled up with slight prying movements of a broad osteotome.

The wound is closed in the usual manner, occasionally with drainage. The graft is then transferred to the host area either as strips, chips, or a wedge which may be screwed into position.

Aspiration of a joint

DEFINITION

The removal of fluid from a joint by suction, using a syringe and hollow needle.

POSITION

Depends upon the joint being aspirated.

INSTRUMENTS. As Figure 347.

OUTLINE OF PROCEDURE

Basically the same set of instruments is required for the aspiration of any joint. Wide-bore aspirating needles are used with a syringe of at least 20 ml capacity.

The area is prepared and draped, and the needle attached to the syringe is inserted into the cavity. If the needle is large, a scalpel will be used to make a stab incision. The fluid is aspirated and a specimen sent to the laboratory for bacteriological examination. The puncture wound is sealed with cotton-wool and Nobecutane, and a pressure dressing may be applied in conjunction with a splint or guarding plaster.

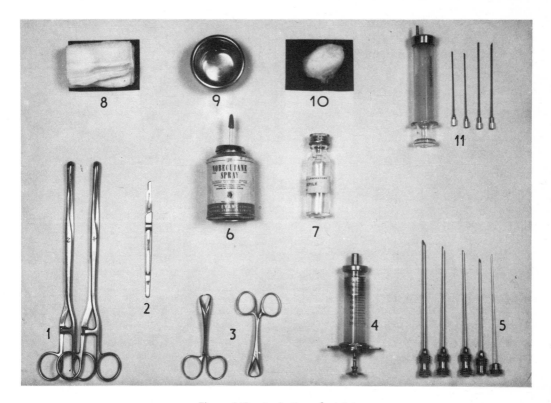

Figure 347　Aspiration of a joint

1. Sponge-holding forceps (Rampley), 2.
2. Scalpel handle No. 9 with No. 15 blade (Bard Parker).
3. Towel clips, 2.
4. Aspiration syringe (Martin).
5. Wide-bore needles for Martin aspiration syringe, 3 assembled needles and 1 dismantled to show needle and obturator.

6. Nobecutane for sealing puncture wound.
7. Specimen bottle.
8. Swabs.
9. Gallipot containing skin antiseptic.
10. Cotton-wool for sealing over puncture wound.
11. 20 ml syringe and aspiration needles.

Arthrotomy, meniscectomy or removal of loose bodies (knee)

DEFINITION

Removal of a torn semilunar cartilage, or removal of loose bodies which are usually osteocartilaginous in nature.

POSITION

Supine, with leg straight or flexed over the bottom section of the table, which is lowered or removed.

INSTRUMENTS

Sponge-holding forceps (Rampley), 5
Scalpel handles No. 4 with No. 20 blades (Bard Parker), 2
Dissecting forceps, toothed (Lane), 2
Dissecting forceps, non-toothed, 15 cm (6 in) 2
Scissors, straight, 15 cm (6 in) (Mayo)
Scissors, curved on flat, 15 cm (6 in) (Mayo)
Retractors, double hook, 2
Small retractors, single hook, 2
Artery forceps, curved on flat (Kilner), 5
Tissue forceps (Allis), 5
Needle holder (Kilner)
Meniscectomy set (Fig. 348)

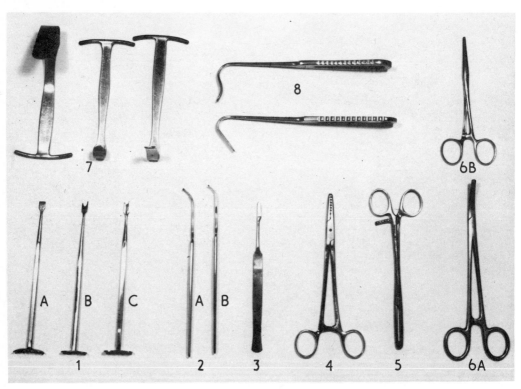

Figure 348   Meniscectomy

1. Cartilage knives (Smillie).
   A. Chisel-shaped blade.
   B. and C. With probe-shaped lateral projections.
2. Meniscectomy knives (Fairbank).
   A. Blade for cutting to the left.
   B. Blade for cutting to the right.
3. Cartilage knife (Munro).
4. Cartilage-holding forceps.
5. Cartilage-holding forceps (Martin).
6. A. Cartilage-holding forceps, curved on flat (Mayo-Oschner), 3.
   B. Cartilage-holding forceps, straight (Kocher), 2.
7. Cartilage retractors (Smillie), set of 3.
8. Cartilage retractors (Jackson Burrow).

2·5 (2/0) Plain catgut or Dexon for ligatures

3 or 4 (0 or 1) Plain catgut or Dexon on a medium half-circle cutting needle for deep sutures

2·5 (2/0) Silk or nylon on a medium curved cutting needle for skin sutures.

OUTLINE OF PROCEDURE

The long slender knives used for removing a torn cartilage need to be resharpened frequently. However, care must be taken to ensure that the knife is descarded when its dimensions and strength have been reduced considerably by grinding. A very thin, weak knife is dangerous in the knee joint, for if it breaks in the back of the knee, the surgeon may have to make an additional incision in order to remove the broken piece.

A curved or straight incision is made just medial or lateral to the patella, depending upon the location of the torn meniscus or loose bodies. Occasionally it may be necessary to make a posterior approach from the back of the knee. The incision is deepened through the fascia and the capsule and synovium is incised.

In the case of meniscectomy, the semilunar cartilage is detached from the tibial plateau, utilising the special clamps and cartilage knives. In the case of loose bodies, these are removed with forceps or a curetting spoon.

The wound is closed in layers and the knee is immobilised with a padded metal back back splint, wool and bandages.

Synovectomy (knee joint)

DEFINITION

Excision of a diseased synovial membrane.

POSITION. Supine.

INSTRUMENTS

General set (Fig. 281)

Tissue forceps, curved (Fagge), 5

Long scalpel, solid variety

Scissors, curved on flat 15 cm (6 in) (Mayo)

3 (0) Plain catgut or Dexon for ligatures

4 (1) Plain catgut or Dexon on a large half-circle cutting or Mayo needle with trocar point for capsule sutures

4 or 5 (1 or 2) Chromic catgut, Dexon or silk on a large half-circle cutting or Mayo needle with trocar point for muscle sutures

3 (0) Silk or nylon on a large curved cutting needle for skin sutures.

OUTLINE OF PROCEDURE

The joint is exposed through an anteromedial incision, which generally commences about 10 cm (4 in) above the knee joint on the medial border of the quadriceps tendon, curves round the inner border of the patella, and continues in the midline down to or below the tibial tubercle. The fascia is incised and retracted and the capsule exposed by dissection between the medial border of the quadriceps tendon and the vastus medialis muscle. The capsule and synovial membrane are incised and the patella retracted laterally.

The entire synovial membrane is excised by block dissection from the inner, outer and anterior aspects of the joint. The prepatellar pad of fat is excised and any other pathological tissue on the femoral condyles is removed with a scalpel or gauze swab.

Care is taken to avoid damage to the posterior capsule of the knee and the popliteal vessels in the midline.

After all the pathological tissue has been excised the wound is closed. If the ligaments have been divided they are apposed and sutured. The capsule is sutured, followed by the fascia and skin. The leg is immobilised either with a padded metal back splint, wool and bandages, or a plaster of Paris cast.

Patellectomy

DEFINITION
Excision of the patella for hypertrophic arthritis and fractures.

POSITION. Supine.

INSTRUMENTS
As for synovectomy
Bone-holding forceps (St Thomas')
Bone awl
Ligatures and sutures as for synovectomy.

OUTLINE OF PROCEDURE
A longitudinal or transverse incision is made over the patella and deepened down to the bone. The whole patella (or fragments in the case of a fracture) is dissected free from the tendon.

The knee is closed in the usual manner, repairing the defect in the quadriceps mechanism by overlapping the tendon with chromic catgut, Dexon or silk sutures. The leg is immobilised in a plaster of Paris cast.

Arthrodesis of toes

DEFINITION
Fusion of the proximal phalangeal joints of the toes.

POSITION. Supine.

INSTRUMENTS
Sponge-holding forceps (Rampley), 5
Towel clips, 5
Scalpel handles No. 3 with Nos 10 and 15 blades (Bard Parker), 2
Scalpel, solid variety
Fine dissecting forceps, toothed (Gillies), 2
Fine dissecting forceps, non-toothed (McIndoe)
Fine retractors, double hook, 2
Scissors, curved on flat, 13 cm (5 in) (Mayo).
Small bone cutting forceps (Liston)
Small bone nibbling forceps, curved
Bone levers (Trethowan ring spikes), 2
Small rugine (Faraboeuf)
Small gouges, 6 mm, 10 mm and 12 mm (Jenkins or Hahn), 3
Small mallet (Rowland)
Bone awl (optional)

Austenitic traction wires (Kirschner), 1·6 mm (0·062 in) diameter, 9 cm ($3\frac{1}{2}$ in) long, and sterile corks
Hand chuck or Kirschner wire drill, if wires are to be used
Wire-cutting forceps
Small needle holder
2 (3/0) Silk or nylon on a small curved cutting needle for skin sutures
Ribbon gauze and plastic dressing (Nobecutane) to form individual toe splints.

OUTLINE OF PROCEDURE

A transverse or longitudinal incision is made over the joint to be fused. The joint is exposed and the cartilage removed from the bone surfaces with bone cutters, gouges or the solid scalpel. Fusion is achieved either with a 'spike' arthrodesis or intramedullary wires.

With a 'spike' arthrodesis, the distal end of the proximal or middle phalanx is fashioned into the shape of a spike and a hole made with an awl in the proximal end of the middle or distal phalanx. This spike is wedged into the hole and the skin incision sutured before immobilising the toe with a Nobecutane splint.

For Kirschner wire fixation, the wire is drilled retrograde fashion from the joint through the distal phalanx and out through the toe pulp just below the nail, so that one end is flush with the joint surface being fused. The two bone ends are brought into apposition and the wire is drilled back across the joint surface and into the proximal phalanx. If an excess amount of wire is left protruding from the toe, this is cut short or turned over before attaching a cork to cover the point. The skin incision is sutured and the toe immobilised further with a Nobecutane splint.

Arthrodesis of ankle (sliding fibula graft)

DEFINITION

Fusion of the ankle utilising fibula graft.

POSITION

Supine, with a sandbag placed under the buttock on the affected side.

INSTRUMENTS

General set (Fig. 281)
Bone and fracture set (Fig. 338)
Plating and screwing set (Fig. 340)
Osteotomes, 13 mm ($\frac{1}{2}$ in), 16 mm ($\frac{5}{8}$ in) and 19 mm ($\frac{3}{4}$ in)
Gouges, 13 mm ($\frac{1}{2}$ in), 16 mm ($\frac{5}{8}$ in) and 19 mm ($\frac{3}{4}$ in)
Circular saws, medium and small, single blades
Wire saw and handles (Gigli or Olivecrona), optional
2·5 (2/0) Plain catgut or Dexon for ligatures
3 or 4 (0 or 1) Plain catgut or Dexon on a medium half-circle cutting or Mayo needle with a trocar point for muscle sutures
2·5 (2/0) Silk or nylon on a medium curved cutting needle for skin sutures.
Plaster of Paris.

OUTLINE OF PROCEDURE

An incision is made along the line of the fibula starting about 15 cm (6 in) above the ankle joint, curving slightly as it reaches the heel.

The superficial and deep sutures are incised to expose the fibula and ankle joint. The fibula is divided across about 13 cm (5 in) above the external malleolus and excised, and is placed in a sterile saline. The cartilage is excised from the joint surfaces of the tibia and talus. The lateral surface of the tibia adjoining the excised portion of the fibula is roughened and a groove cut in the lateral surface of the talus bone.

All periosteum and cartilage is removed from the fibula graft and the medial aspect is smoothed to ensure a close fit when the fibula is re-inserted below its original position. This graft is then screwed to the tibia and talus and any gaps which may be left are packed with cancellous bone chips which can be obtained either from the bone bank or the patient's iliac crest.

The wound is closed in the usual manner and the leg is immobilised in a plaster of Paris cast.

Triple Arthrodesis. Stabilisation of the foot

DEFINITION
Stabilisation of the foot by removing the cartilaginous surfaces of the subtaloid, calcaneocuboid and talonavicular joints.

POSITION
Supine, with a sandbag under the buttock on the affected side.

INSTRUMENTS
General set (Fig. 281)
Bone and fracture set (Fig. 338)
Osteotomes, 16 mm ($\frac{5}{8}$ in), 19 mm ($\frac{3}{4}$ in) and 25 mm (1 in)
Gouges, 16 mm ($\frac{5}{8}$ in), 19 mm ($\frac{3}{4}$ in) and 25 mm (1 in)
2·5 (2/0) Plain catgut or Dexon for ligatures
3 or 4 (0 or 1) Plain catgut or Dexon on a medium half-circle cutting or Mayo needle
    for deep sutures
2·5 (2/0) Silk or nylon on a medium curved cutting needle for skin sutures.

OUTLINE OF PROCEDURE
The subtaloid, talo-navicular and calcaneo-cuboid joints are generally exposed through a curved dorsolateral incision which is deepened through the fascia and ligaments. The foot is dislocated medially at mid-tarsal level.

The cartilage is removed from the joint surfaces in such a manner that the three bones can be brought in good contact with each other in the position chosen for fusion. The wound is closed and a plaster of Paris cast applied to the leg.

Some surgeons utilise metallic staples across the calcaneocuboid joint.

Arthrodesis of knee (Charnley's operation)

DEFINITION
Fusion of the knee joint by compression arthrodesis.

POSITION. Supine.

INSTRUMENTS
General set (Fig. 281)
Bone and fracture set (Fig. 388)

Amputation saw with detachable guard (Sergeant)

Large tissue forceps (Fagge or Lane), 4

Traction pins (Steinmann), 2 of size 4·8 mm ($\frac{3}{16}$ in) diameter by 20 cm to 25 cm (8 to 10 in) long, with diamond points and square or triangular chuck ends

Hand or power drill

Compression clamps (Charnley), 2

Pin caps or small corks, 2

3 (0) Plain catgut or Dexon for ligatures

4 and 5 (1 and 2) Plain catgut or Dexon on a medium half-circle cutting or Mayo needle with a trocar point for capsule, etc.

2·5 or 3 (2/0 or 0) Silk or nylon on a medium curved or straight cutting needle for skin sutures.

OUTLINE OF PROCEDURE

The joint is exposed through a longitudinal anterolateral incision or a transverse incision similar to patellectomy but with wider exposure.

The patella is either excised or the cartilage from the undersurface is removed with the amputation saw. The joint is flexed and a small amount of the upper end of the tibia and condyles at the lower end of the femur, together with the joint cartilage, are removed with the saw. The saw cuts are placed almost parallel to each other so that when the raw surfaces of the two bones are brought together, the knee is in the correct position for fusion (that is usually with about 10 degrees of flexion).

Two stout Steinmann's pins are inserted parallel to each other through the lower end of the femur and the upper end of the tibia. These are clamped together with Charnley's compression clamps on the medial and lateral aspect of the leg, with sufficient compression to maintain good contact between the two surfaces of raw bone.

The wound is closed and the leg is immobilised on a Thomas splint or in a plaster of Paris cast.

Arthrodesis of hip (Brittain extra-articular fusion)

DEFINITION

Extra-articular fusion of the hip by means of cortical bone graft which is driven through an osteotomy of the upper femur and into the ischium.

POSITION

As for Smith Petersen nail (Fig. 73).

INSTRUMENTS

General set (Fig. 281)

Bone and fracture set (Fig. 338)

Bone grafting set (Fig. 346)

Osteotomes, 13 mm ($\frac{1}{2}$ in), 25 mm (1 in) and 38 mm ($1\frac{1}{2}$ in)

Twin chisels (Brittain) for positioning of graft (optional)

Twist drills, 4·8 mm ($\frac{3}{16}$ in) and 6·4 mm ($\frac{1}{4}$ in) diameter, 13 cm (5 in) long

Bone punches (Smillie), angled and straight, 2

3 (0) Plain catgut or Dexon for ligatures

4 (1) Plain or chromic catgut or Dexon on a large half-circle cutting or Mayo needle with trocar point for muscle sutures

3 (0) Silk or nylon on a large curved or straight cutting needle for skin sutures.

OUTLINE OF PROCEDURE

The upper third of the femur is exposed through a lateral longitudinal incision as for Smith Petersen nail. A drill is introduced at a predetermined point through the femur and into the ischium. Its position is verified radiologically and, if correct, a number of holes are drilled along a transverse line each side of it.

Either a suitable piece of cortical bone about 13 mm ($\frac{1}{2}$ in) wide by 15 cm (6 in) long is cut from the tibia (see bone grafting) or removed from the bone bank. The graft is bevelled to a point at one end and denuded of any adherent soft tissue. An osteotomy of the femur is made in line with the drill holes and the osteotome is driven on until it has penetrated the ischium. A slot is created in the ischium by levering the osteotome backwards and forwards and the graft is inserted along the blade until it enters this slot. The osteotome is then removed and the graft is driven home. Some surgeons use the Brittain twin chisel to assist this manoeuvre but in either case the graft is inserted so that its endosteal portion lies distally.

The distal portion of the femur just below the osteotomy is then displaced inwards with the bone punch and the wound is closed in layers. The patient is immobilised in a double hip spica.

Arthrodesis of the hip (Charnley's central dislocation fusion)

DEFINITION

Intra-articular fusion of the hip by planing the head and neck of the femur into a tubular shape which fits into a corresponding size of hole in the acetabulum.

POSITION. Supine.

INSTRUMENTS

General set (Fig. 281)
Bone and fracture set (Fig. 338)
Artery forceps, curved on flat (Kelly Fraser), 20
Large tissue forceps (Fagge or Lane), 5
Large retractors (Hibb), 2
Scissors, heavy, curved on flat, 20 cm (8 in) (Mayo)
Long scalpel, solid variety
Osteotomes, 16 mm ($\frac{5}{8}$ in), 22 mm ($\frac{7}{8}$ in) and 38 mm ($1\frac{1}{2}$ in)
Osteotomes, 13 mm ($\frac{1}{2}$ in) and 16 mm ($\frac{5}{8}$ in) (curved)
Gouges, 13 mm ($\frac{5}{8}$ in), 22 mm ($\frac{7}{8}$ in) and 38 mm ($1\frac{1}{2}$ in)
Hip levers (Judet), 2
Reamers for shaping the femoral head (32 mm [$1\frac{1}{4}$ in] and 38 mm [$1\frac{1}{2}$ in]. Crawford Adam head shapers are suitable)
Perforator drills for acetabular hole (32 mm [$1\frac{1}{4}$ in] and 38 mm [$1\frac{1}{2}$ in])
Hip brace
Irrigation syringe and warm sterile saline
Suction tubing, wide nozzles and tube anchoring forceps
Diathermy leads, electrodes and lead anchoring forceps
3 and 4 (0 and 1) Plain catgut or Dexon for ligatures
4 or 5 (1 or 2) Chromic catgut or Dexon or silk on a large half-circle cutting needle for muscle sutures
3 (0) Silk or nylon on a large curved cutting needle for skin sutures.

There are several approaches to the hip joint, including anterior, lateral or posterior. Only one approach will be described to avoid confusion, and that is the anterolateral approach.

An incision is made commencing about 8 cm (3 in) below the trochanter, continuing to a point over the trochanter where it curves anteriorly to complete the flap. The fascia lata is incised in line with the longitudinal portion of the wound and the gluteus medius and minimus are divided transversely. The capsule of the hip joint is incised and the hip dislocated forwards.

The size of the femoral head is reduced to that of the femoral neck by gouging and planing away the cartilage and cortex of the bone. A hole of corresponding size is drilled in the acetabulum and all joint cartilage is removed. The cavity is irrigated to remove debris and the hip is returned to its normal position, but with the reconstructed head and neck jammed in the hole made in the acetabulum. Any gaps remaining in the joint cavity are filled with bone shavings obtained when drilling the acetabular hole.

The wound is closed with the leg supported in the optimum position for fusion, and a double hip plaster spica is applied for immobilisation.

Arthrodesis of shoulder (Smith Petersen trifin nail)

DEFINITION
Fusion of the shoulder joint with fixation obtained by the insertion of a Smith Petersen trifin nail across the joint.

POSITION
Supine, with a sandbag placed under the scapula on the affected side.

INSTRUMENTS
General set (Fig. 281)
Bone and fracture set (Fig. 388)
Artery forceps, curved on flat (Kelly Fraser), 20
Large tissue forceps, curved (Fagge), 5
Osteotomes, 13 mm ($\frac{1}{2}$ in), 16 mm ($\frac{5}{8}$ in) and 19 mm ($\frac{3}{4}$ in) (straight)
Osteotomes, 13 mm ($\frac{1}{2}$ in) and 16 mm ($\frac{5}{8}$ in) (curved)
Gouges, 13 mm ($\frac{1}{2}$ in), 16 mm ($\frac{5}{8}$ in) and 19 mm ($\frac{3}{4}$ in)
Scalpel, solid variety
Set of trifin nails (Smith Petersen)
Driver/extractor (Smith Petersen)
Guide wires, 20 cm (8 in), 2
Guide wire hand chuck (Watson-Jones)
Steel rule, 15 cm (6 in)
Twist drill 4·8 mm ($\frac{3}{16}$ in)
Hand drill
Diathermy leads, electrodes and lead anchoring forceps
Suction tubing, nozzles and tube anchoring forceps
2·5 and 3 (2/0 and 0) Plain catgut or Dexon for ligatures
3 or 4 (0 or 1) Chromic catgut, Dexon or silk on a small half-circle cutting or Mayo needle with trocar point for muscle sutures, etc.
2·5 (2/0) Silk or nylon on a medium curved cutting needle for skin sutures.

OUTLINE OF PROCEDURE

The chest portion of a shoulder spica is applied before operation. The shoulder joint is generally approached through an anterior incision which may curve laterally over the point of the shoulder.

The deltoid muscle is divided and the capsule exposed either by retraction or division of the muscle overlying the joint. The capsule is opened and the head of the humerus visualised by external rotation of the arm. Cartilage is excised from the head of humerus and glenoid cavity, and the arm is placed in the optimum position for fusion.

A hole is drilled just below the humeral neck and a guide wire is inserted into the glenoid and neck of the scapula. The position of this guide wire may be checked radiologically, and when correct, a Smith Petersen nail of appropriate length is driven across the joint and into the scapula. The guide wire is removed and the wound closed in layers. The acromium may be used to reinforce the fusion by being attached to the tubercle.

The plaster of Paris spica is completed to immobilise the arm until fusion takes place.

Arthrodesis of the wrist (Brittain fusion)

DEFINITION

Fusion of the wrist by inserting a bone graft between the lower end of the radius and the base of the third metacarpal bone.

POSITION

Supine, with affected arm extended on an arm table.

INSTRUMENTS

General set (Fig. 281)
Bone and fracture set (Fig. 338)
Bone grafting set (Fig. 346)
2·5 (2/0) Plain catgut or Dexon for ligatures
3 (0) Plain catgut or Dexon on a small half-circle cutting needle for deep sutures
2·5 (2/0) Silk or nylon on a medium curved cutting needle for skin sutures.

OUTLINE OF PROCEDURE

A longitudinal incision is made on the dorsal aspect of the wrist extending just distal to the base of the third metacarpal to about 8 cm (3 in) above the lower end of the radius. This incision is deepened and the tendons retracted to each side.

A circular saw is used to cut a longitudinal slot for the graft, extending from a point 5 cm (2 in) above the end of the radius to the proximal third of the third metacarpal bone. This graft bed, which is prepared about 13 mm ($\frac{1}{2}$ in) in width, includes the carpal bones between the radius and third metacarpal without respect to their identity. A small osteotome is introduced into each end of the bed of the graft to open the medullary cavity for about 10 mm ($\frac{3}{8}$ in).

A graft is taken from the bone bank or cut from the tibia and is the same width as the graft bed, but 13 mm ($\frac{1}{2}$ in) longer. This graft is pointed at both ends before introducing it into the radius for about 6 mm ($\frac{1}{4}$ in). Traction is exerted on the fingers and the other end of the graft is levered into the prepared hole in the third metacarpal bone. Release of traction will ensure a snug fit and good immobilisation of the graft.

The wound is closed in layers and a plaster of Paris cast is applied.

Arthroplasty of the hip (Austin Moore, Thompson, McKee Farrar, Howse and Charnley operations)

DEFINITION
The reconstruction of new joint surfaces in the hip by replacing the femoral head with a plastic or metallic prosthesis.

POSITION
Lateral or supine, with a sandbag under the buttock on the affected side.

INSTRUMENTS
General set (Fig. 281)
Bone and fracture set (Fig. 338)
Arthroplasty set (Fig. 349)

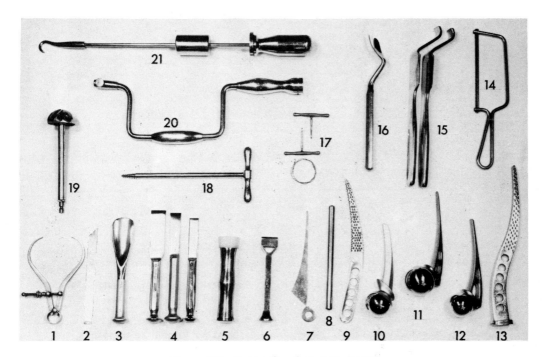

Figure 349   Basic arthroplasty instruments

1. Measuring calipers.
2. Steel rule 15 cm (6 in).
3. Large gouge or skid (for reductions of hip).
4. Straight osteotomes 16 mm ($\frac{5}{8}$ in), 19 mm ($\frac{3}{4}$ in), 25 cm (1 in).
5. Impactor (with nylon insert) for prosthesis.
6. Box chisel.
7. Template guide.
8. Tommy-bar for shaft of rasps.
9. Thompson rasp for femoral shaft.
10. Thompson prosthesis.
11. Austin Moore prosthesis, standard stem.
12. Austin Moore prosthesis modified, narrow stem.
13. Austin Moore rasp.
14. Hacksaw.
15. Hip Levers (Judet).
16. Femoral head skid (Smith Petersen).
17. Wire saw (Gigli) with handles.
18. Auger for extracting femoral head (Judet).
19. Acetabular reamer (Duthie).
20. Brace for acetabular reamer.
21. Extractor for Austin Moore heads.

Additional instruments for McKee Farrar operation if required (Fig. 350). Howse operation (Fig. 351) or Charnley operation (Fig. 352)
Artery forceps, curved on flat (Kelly Fraser), 20

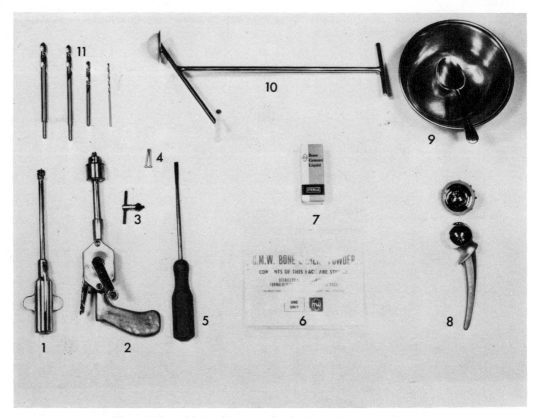

Figure 350   Additional instruments for McKee Farrer prosthesis.

1. Automatic screwdriver (Williams).
2. Pistol grip hand drill.
3. Key for Jacobs' chuck.
4. Sherman screws, Vitallium 32 mm ($1\frac{1}{4}$ in).
5. Ordinary screwdriver (Lanes).
6. Bone cement powder.
7. Bone cement liquid.
8. McKee Farrar prosthesis.
9. Mixing bowl and spoon for bone cement.
10. Instrument for holding acetabular cup in position during setting of bone cement.
11. Twist drills, No. 32 (for screws) 6·4 mm ($\frac{3}{8}$ in), 9 mm ($\frac{5}{16}$ in), 10 mm ($\frac{3}{8}$ in).

Large tissue forceps, curved (Fagge), 5
Deep retractors (Hibb), 2
Osteotomes, 16 mm ($\frac{5}{8}$ in), 19 mm ($\frac{3}{4}$ in) and 38 mm ($1\frac{1}{2}$ in) (straight)
Osteotomes, 16 mm ($\frac{5}{8}$ in) and 19 mm ($\frac{3}{4}$ in) (curved)
Gouges, 16 mm ($\frac{5}{8}$ in), 19 mm ($\frac{3}{4}$ in) and 38 mm ($1\frac{1}{2}$ in)
Wire saw and handles (Gigli or Olivecrona), optional
Femoral neck saw
Scissors, curved on flat 20 cm (8 in) (Mayo)
Long scalpel, solid variety
Diathermy leads, electrodes and lead anchoring forceps
3 and 4 (0 and 1) Plain catgut or Dexon for ligatures

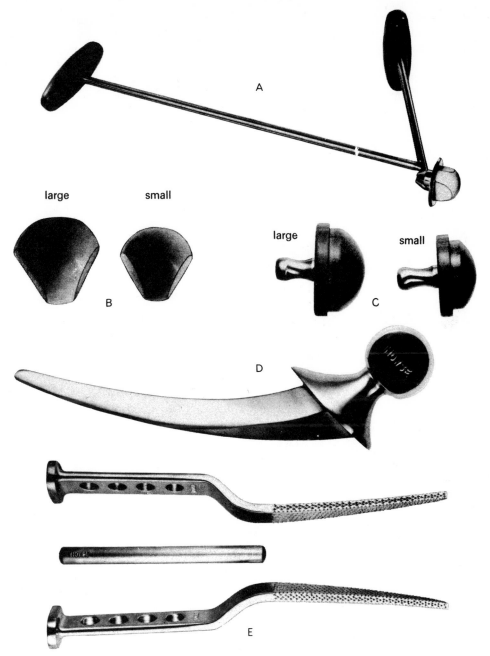

Figure 351   Additional instruments for Howse prosthesis.

A. Cup holder. Stainless steel. *TUFNOL* handle. Overall length 35 cm.

B. Adaptors. To screw on holder. Nylon (may be sterilised by autoclaving). The cup clips onto the adaptor and can be held firmly without fear of dropping off.

C. Socket size gauges. *TUFNOL*. With detachable heads for screwing onto cup holder if desired.

D. Test femoral stem. Stainless steel.

E. Left and right broaches with Tommy bar. Stainless steel. Overall length 25 cm.

4 or 5 (1 or 2) Chromic catgut, Dexon or silk on a large half-circle cutting needle for muscle sutures

3 (0) Silk or nylon on a large curved or straight cutting needle for skin sutures.

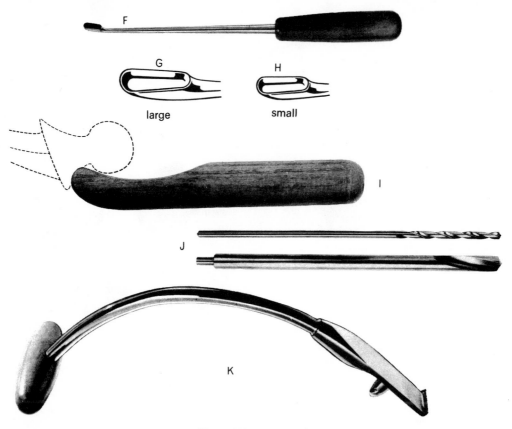

Figure 351   Continued

F. G. and H. Harris Bone curette. Stainless steel. *TUFNOL* handle. Overall length 29 cm.

I. Femoral pusher. *TUFNOL*. Overall length 15 cm.

J. Twist drills. Stainless steel.
6·6 mm × 250 mm long.
11 mm × 250 mm long.

K. Braddock retractor. Stainless steel handle. Overall length 28 cm. This retractor has a serrated claw edge that grips the back of the acetabulum. The protruding pin fits into the intramedullary cavity exposed by the removal of the femoral head. This enables the femur to be levered away from the acetabulum and held under control by an assistant, allowing the surgeon unrestricted access to the acetabulum.

OUTLINE OF PROCEDURE

The hip is exposed as described for central dislocation arthrodesis. Alternatively the approach may be more anterior for a McKee Farrar procedure, anterolateral for a Howse prostheses or lateral for a Charnley prosthesis. The surgeon may dislocate the hip and remove the femoral head with a hand saw or large osteotome, or may prefer to divide the femoral neck before dislocation and extract the head with a large corkscrew instrument. This latter method is applicable when a prosthesis is being inserted for the treatment of a subcapital fracture of the femoral neck which is not suitable for nailing, and when the head is separated and loose in the acetabulum.

The extent to which the acetabulum is prepared depends on whether a 'total hip replacement' is to be carried out; if not an Austin Moore or Thompson prosthesis is generally inserted. With this type of prosthesis, which is made from stainless steel or Vitallium, the stem projects along the femoral neck and curves into the femoral shaft. The femoral channel is made with a long curved rasp and small gouges.

The McKee Farrar total hip prosthesis. This consists of a two-part ball and socket appliance, the femoral part being basically similar to a Thompson prosthesis, and the acetabular part a hemispherical cup lapped to fit the head of the Thompson prosthesis thus forming a pair which should only be used as such. (Appendix page 652.) The outer surface of the cup is covered with small studs and the edge of the cup fashioned with a lip. The purpose of these studs is to provide a positive hold when the cup is embedded in acrylic cement in the acetabulum. Both parts of the prosthesis are manufactured from Vitallium.

The Howse total hip prosthesis. This is a ball and socket metal to plastic bearing prosthesis. (Appendix page 653.) The femoral part of the appliance is made from stainless steel and resembles a Thompson prosthesis; the acetabular cup is made from high density polyethylene (RCH 1000) incorporating a radio-opaque marker.

During manufacture the components are subjected to special optical lapping and polishing processes to ensure accuracy of fit. The acetabular cup is larger than a hemisphere and the depth of its internal surface, spherically-shaped, is greater than the radius of the sphere of the femoral head. This creates a vacuum effect which holds the prosthesis and reduces the risk of subsequent dislocation. The prosthesis has the characteristics of low friction and low wear. Both components are cemented in place with acrylic cement.

The Charnley total hip prosthesis. This also is a metal to plastic bearing prosthesis which was the original design of this type. It is manufactured from the same materials and to the same exacting standards as the Howse prosthesis.

The essential difference between this and the Howse is that the Charnley femoral head component is smaller and does not have the Thompson type extended seating area at the base of the neck.

During preparative stages the Charnley technique consists of detaching the great trochanter which subsequently is reattached after the prosthesis has been inserted. This together with the lateral approach to the hip is said to prevent dislocation after operation.

The acetabulum is prepared by removing all remnants of articular cartilage and roughening the walls with a gouge. Three or four 6 mm ($\frac{1}{4}$ in) to 10 mm ($\frac{3}{8}$ in) wide holes are made with a drill. These holes provide anchoring points for the acrylic cement. The outer cortex of the ilium immediately above the acetabulum is cleaned of soft-tissue attachments and in the case of the McKee Farrar procedure two screws are inserted parallel to the roof of the acetabulum. These are left projecting 6 mm ($\frac{1}{4}$ in) and provide further anchoring points for the acrylic cement.

The femoral neck is prepared in the usual way with gouges and a rasp although care is taken that the stem of the prosthesis lies accurately within the femoral shaft with adequate room for introduction of the acrylic cement.

The acrylic cement mix consists of two parts, a powder (the polymer) and a liquid (the monomer). These are available as a sterile pack containing the correct amount of each. They are mixed together in a metal bowl with a spoon until within 2 or 3 minutes the plastic assumes a soft, workable consistency and no longer sticks to the gloves. The dough mix is pushed into the prepared acetabulum and the cup inserted in the correct position. The cup is held firmly by a special dome-shaped instrument until the cement

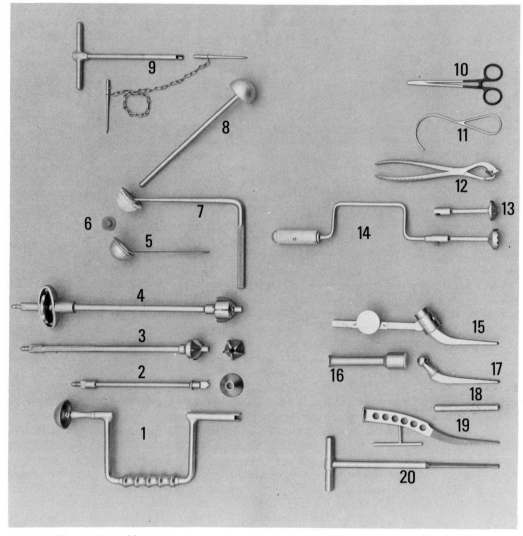

Figure 352 Additional instruments for Charnley low friction arthroplasty of the hip.

1. Brace, wide throw.
2. Starting drill, 12·5 mm ($\frac{1}{2}$ in) diameter with centering ring.
3. Deepening reamer, spigot is 12·5 mm ($\frac{1}{2}$ in) diameter and engages with the pilot hole made by the starting drill in the floor of the acetabulum. The reamer produces a concave surface of 25 mm (1 in) radius.
4. Expanding reamer, this completes the cutting of a 5 cm (2 in) hemisphere after the deepening reamer has thinned the floor of the acetabulum. The profile of the hemisphere is a circle of 2·5 cm (1 in) radius with a 6·25 mm ($\frac{1}{4}$ in) parallel section near the mouth.
5. Socket size gauge, small and large size gauges are used.
6. Cement restrictor.
7. Socket holder and guide, the plastic socket both small and large is held in position by an interference fit with three pins on the holder. The holder permits an orientation of 45° of the face of the socket to be made with precision. The plastic socket is clipped to the holder with the plane of the radiological marker in the same plane as the handle of the introducer. This enables the orientation of the radiological marker to be correct is an anteroposterior radiograph.

8. Socket pusher, is used to exert pressure in the centre of the socket holder where it engages in a depression. It enables the acrylic cement to be impacted in the cancellous bone by two blows of a mallet delivered through the socket pusher. This is done when the cement is nearly hard, and coins the cement to the cancellous bone and gets rid of any blood clot which may be interposed.
9. Pin retractor, used in the superior lip of the acetabulum to 'stake' back the abductor muscles improving the exposure of the acetabulum. Instruments used for reattachment of the trochanter (Nos. 10–14).
10. Wire holding forceps.
11. Wire passer.
12. Drill and wire guide forceps for trochanter.
13. Lightweight brace with female trochanter reamer.
14 Male trochanter reamer, used on the inner surface of the detached trochanter in preparation for reattachment in the correct position. Instruments required in the preparation of the acetabulum site and cementing of the plastic socket (Nos. 15–20).
15. Femoral prosthesis punch, designed to avoid damage to surface of head
16. Femoral prosthesis pusher.
17. Femoral prosthesis with standard prosthesis mounted.
18. Tommy bar for broach.
19. Femoral broach.
20. Taper reamer for medullary canal.

has set, usually about 5 minutes. Care must be taken to clean the mixing bowl immediately before the remnants of cement have set. A small quantity of acetone can be used for this purpose.

The femoral stem of the prosthesis is inserted and a trial reduction of the hip performed. After removing the prosthesis, a second mix of acrylic cement is made and inserted into the femoral shaft. The prosthesis is re-inserted and the cement allowed to set. The hip is then finally reduced.

Following insertion of the prosthesis the wound is closed in layers. Some surgeons may tie the legs together until the patient recovers consciousness. Russell traction of 3·2 to 4·5 kg (7 to 10 lb) may then be applied to the affected limb.

There are many types of arthroplasty but the reader will find that these are probably the ones used by most surgeons at present. It must be understood that only an outline of the procedures has been described. Each of the operations requires a special technique and the reader is recommended to consult the appropriate literature for further information.

Congenital dislocation of hip (shelf operation)

DEFINITION
To deepen the acetabulum by constructing a shelf of bone over the top of the femoral head.

POSITION
Lateral or supine, with a sandbag under the buttock on the affected side.

INSTRUMENTS
As for Charnley's central dislocation arthrodesis of the hip
As for skeletal traction, insertion of Steinmann pin or Kirschner wire (Fig. 336).

OUTLINE OF PROCEDURE
The hip joint is exposed through an anterolateral or lateral incision; the head of the femur is stripped of soft tissue structures which interfere with mobility.

(After shelf operations, it is essential that continuous traction be applied to the leg until the bone shelf has healed, as the femoral head tends to displace the grafts. This may be accomplished by skin or skeletal traction which is sometimes applied before operation.)

The shelf of bone on the acetabular rim may be constructed in several ways. The Albee technique involves the division of the acetabular rim with a thin blade osteotome in a semi-circular line following the natural curve of the acetabulum. This segment of bone is pried outward and downward and secured with triangular shaped cortical grafts from the tibia or bone bank.

The Gill operation is similar, but the shelf is made by turning down a bone flap from the outer table of the ilium, sufficiently wide to cover the portion of the femur which projects beyond the acetabulum. This flap is secured with bone wedges from the crest of the ilium or bone bank.

The wound is closed in layers and the patient is immobilised in a double plaster of Paris hip spica with traction on the affected limb.

Recurrent dislocation of the shoulder (Bankart's and Putti-Platt capsulorrhaphy)

DEFINITION

A plastic procedure on the capsule and ligaments of the shoulder joint to prevent recurrent dislocation.

POSITION

Supine, with a sandbag under the scapula on the affected side.

INSTRUMENTS
    General set (Fig. 281)
    Bone hooks, 2
    Small bone levers (Lane), 2
    Small mallet (Rowland)
    Small rugine, curved (Farabeouf)
    Osteotome, 13 mm ($\frac{1}{2}$ in)
    Bone awl
    Contra-angle dental drill (Bankart's operation only)
    Bone graft set. (Instruments as in Fig. 346 may be required for graft to deficient
        glenoid rim.)
    Staples and insertion punch, optional
    Diathermy leads, electrodes and lead anchoring forceps
    Suction tubing, nozzles and tube anchoring forceps
    2·5 and 3 (2/0 and 0) Plain and chromic catgut or Dexon for ligatures
    3 or 4 (0 or 1) Silk, etc., chromic catgut or Dexon on a small fish hook half-circle cutting
    6 or Mayo needle with trocar point for capsulorrhaphy, etc.
    3 or 4 (0 or 1) Chromic catgut or Dexon on a medium half-circle cutting needle for
        deltoid muscle sutures
    2·5 (2/0) Silk or nylon on a medium curved cutting needle for skin sutures.

OUTLINE OF PROCEDURE

Bankart Operation. An incision is made commencing at the outer border of the clavicle, curving medially to the coracoid process and continuing along the inner border of the deltoid muscle in line with the cephalic vein.

The interval between the deltoid and the pectoralis muscle is developed and the cephalic vein is retracted medially after dividing branches which may interfere with the exposure of the joint. The deltoid origin is reflected from the clavicle and the muscle retracted laterally. A hole about 3 mm ($\frac{1}{8}$ in) by 25 mm (1 in) deep may be drilled in the coracoid process with an awl or twist drill, to facilitate subsequent suture. The coracoid process is divided with an osteotome, and its tip, together with muscle attachments, is retracted medially and downwards.

The shoulder is then placed into external rotation and the subscapularis tendon is identified. A plexus of veins on the lower border of the tendon is usually ligated or diathermised and divided. Two silk sutures are placed in the medial part of the tendon and are left long for retraction. The tendon is incised, and medial portion of the tendon allowed to retract, and the capsule then opened by a vertical incision 6 mm ($\frac{1}{4}$ in) lateral to the glenoid rim.

The glenoid rim is freshened with a curette and three holes are drilled in it with an angled drill. The shoulder is placed in internal rotation and abduction, and the cartilaginous labrum which is invariably detached from the glenoid rim is sutured (or stapled) back to its original position, utilising the three holes in the bone. In order to reinforce this, the medial part of the capsule *may* be plicated over the area of repair as in the Putti-Platt procedure. The subscapularis tendon is approximated with sutures, the coracoid process is re-attached, and the rest of the wound closed in layers. The arm is immobilised to the chest with cotton-wool and crêpe bandages.

Putti-Platt Operation. The exposure is essentially the same as the Bankart's operation as far as the subscapularis tendon. This tendon is incised about 25 mm (1 in) medial to its insertion, and the joint is opened. The lateral portion of the subscapularis tendon is sutured either to the anterior rim of the glenoid cavity or the deep surface of the stripped capsule and subscapularis. The medial portion of the capsule is plicated over this lateral part of the subscapularis tendon, and finally the medial portion of the subscapularis tendon is plicated over all the previous suture lines, being attached to the bicipital groove or tendinous cuff over the greater tuberosity. This is in effect an overlapping of the medial and lateral parts of the capsule and subscapularis tendon so that a barrier to redislocation is formed.

The wound is closed as before, with immobilisation of the arm to the side.

Laminectomy

DEFINITION

Removal of laminae, usually to provide access to a prolapsed intervertebral disc which may be pressing on a nerve root.

POSITION

Knee/elbow, as Fig. 71, or lateral, or prone position of flexion.

INSTRUMENTS

General set (Fig. 281)
Laminectomy set (Fig. 353)
Diathermy leads, electrodes and lead anchoring forceps
Suction tubing, nozzles and tube anchoring forceps
Corrugated drainage tubing
2·5 (2/0) Plain catgut or Dexon for ligatures
1 (5/0) Silk on a small curved round-bodied non-traumatic needle for dural tears

4 or 5 (1 or 2) Chromic catgut or Dexon or silk, etc., on a large half-circle cutting needle for muscle sutures

3 (0) Silk or nylon on a large curved cutting needle for skin sutures.

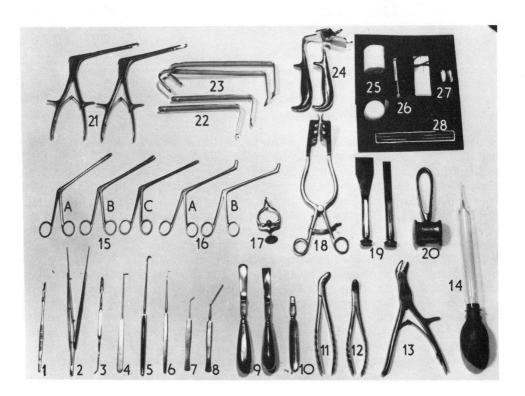

Figure 353   Laminectomy – removal of prolapsed intravertebral disc.

1. Scalpel handle No. 5 with No. 15; blade (Bard Parker).
2. Long fine dissecting forceps, toothed and non-toothed (Waugh), 2 of each.
3. Dissector (Macdonald).
4. Nerve hook, medium (Adson), 2.
5. Nerve hook, large (Love).
6. Nerve hook, small (Adson).
7. Seeker (Horsley).
8. Dura mater separator (Sergeant-Horsley).
9. Rugines, large (Mitchell), straight and round end.
10. Rugine, small (Faraboeuf).
11. Gouge or bone-nibbling forceps, angled on side.
12. Gouge or bone-nibbling forceps, angled on flat.
13. Gouge forceps, angled on side, compound action.
14. Irrigation syringe.
15. Pituitary forceps (Cairn Cushing).

A. Straight, small.
B. Straight, medium.
C. Straight, large.
16. Pituitary forceps (Cairn Cushing).
    A. Angled, small.
    B. Angled, medium.
17. Retractor, self-retaining (Little).
18. Retractor, self-retaining (Adson).
19. Broad osteotomes, 38 mm ($\frac{1}{2}$ in) and 25 mm (1 in).
20. Mallet (Heath).
21. Punch forceps (Duggan), forward and backward cutting.
22. Retractors, laminectomy (Charnley), 2.
23. Retractors, laminectomy (Hibb), 2.
24. Retractors, laminectomy (Penrose), 2.
25. Ribbon gauze 25 mm (1 in) and 50 mm (2 in).
26. Bone wax (Horsley).
27. Patties made from cottonoid, large and small.
28. Rubber or plastic corrugated drain.

OUTLINE OF PROCEDURE

A midline incision is made over the spines of the vertebrae from which the laminae are to be removed. This incision is deepened and the erector spinae muscles are reflected from the vertebrae with a rugine or broad osteotome.

The dura is exposed by excising the ligamentum flavum with a scalpel and the overlying lamina with bone-nibbling forceps. Retraction on the nerve root exposes the intervertebral disc which, if bulging, is incised with a fine scalpel and extracted with pituitary forceps. It may be necessary to expose a disc space above or below that selected if the findings are inconclusive in the first instance.

The wound is closed with or without drainage.

Laminectomy is performed also to obtain exposure for the removal of a spinal tumour. In this case, a wide exposure is made by removing several laminae and the spinous processes also (Chapter 21, Neurosurgery).

Spinal fusion

DEFINITION

Fusion of the spine in the treatment of tuberculosis, spondylolisthesis, scoliosis and some fracture dislocations.

POSITION

Knee/elbow, as Fig. 71, or prone position of extension similar to the application of a spinal jacket illustrated in Chapter 29.

INSTRUMENTS

As in laminectomy

Bone grafting set (Fig. 346)

Spinal rasps (Wheeler and Tubby), 2

Osteotomes, 13 mm ($\frac{1}{2}$ in), 16 mm ($\frac{5}{8}$ in), 19 mm ($\frac{3}{4}$ in) and 38 mm ($1\frac{1}{2}$ in) (straight)

Osteotomes, 13 mm ($\frac{1}{2}$ in), 16 mm ($\frac{5}{8}$ in) and 19 mm ($\frac{3}{4}$ in) (curved)

Gouges, 16 mm ($\frac{5}{8}$ in), 19 mm ($\frac{3}{4}$ in) and 25 mm (1 in)

For Wire Fixation

Wiring set (Fig. 340)

For Plating or Screw Fixation

Spinal plates (set of Wilson or Meurig Williams, small medium and large), 2 of each

Spinal bolts, nuts and washers (Wilson or Meurig Williams), various lengths

Angled awl or contra-angle drill

Set of suitable spanners for bolts

Plating and screwing set (Fig. 340), optional

Ligatures and sutures as for laminectomy.

OUTLINE OF PROCEDURE

The initial stages of the operation follow that for laminectomy, but with a wider exposure at both sides of the vertebrae. For disease of the spine, usually two vertebrae above and two below the lesion are fused.

Fusion is accomplished by a bone graft which can be taken from the patient himself or the bone bank. Cortical grafts, i.e., from the tibia, may be screwed or bolted in position either singly or as a twin graft on each side of the spine. The spinous processes and laminae are carefully prepared before the graft is inserted by removing periosteum and generally freshening the bone surfaces. Sometimes the spinous processes are removed completely and the area bridged with an 'H' bone graft. In addition to preparing the graft bed, the surgeon may perform a laminectomy and explore the intervertebral disc spaces.

Following the insertion of a cortical graft, the area is packed with cancellous bone chips or strips. Alternatively, especially in the treatment of fractures, metallic spinal plates may be used to bridge the affected vertebrae. These plates can be used as pairs, one on each side; or in combination with a cortical graft to stimulate osteogenesis. The plates are bolted or screwed in position and cancellous strips or chips inserted as before. Wire loops may be used also, in conjunction with cortical or cancellous bone grafts.

Another method of spinal fusion consists of removing soft tissue from the lamellae surfaces, excising the tips of the spinous processes and packing a large quantity of cancellous bone chips and shavings in the graft bed.

The wound is closed in the usual manner and the patient immobilised on a plaster of Paris bed which has been prepared to measurement before operation.

Hallux valgus (Keller's operation)

DEFINITION

Removal of an exostosis of the first metatarsal head and a portion of the proximal phalanx in the treatment of hallux valgus or bunions.

POSITION. Supine.

INSTRUMENTS

Sponge-holding forceps (Rampley), 5
Towel clips, 5
Scalpel handles No. 3 with No. 10 blades (Bard Parker), 2
Scalpel, solid variety
Dissecting forceps, toothed (Lane), 2
Scissors, curved on flat, 13 cm (5 in) (Mayo)
Scissors, straight, 13 cm (5 in) (Mayo)
Small retractors, double hook, 2
Artery forceps, curved on flat (Kilner), 5
Tissue forceps (Allis), 5
Bone levers (Trethowan), 2
Small rugine (Faraboeuf)
Bone-cutting forceps, compound action (Horsley)
Small bone-cutting forceps, single action (Liston)
Bone hook (Lane)
Mallet (Heath)
Osteotomes, 13 mm ($\frac{1}{2}$ in) and 16 mm ($\frac{5}{8}$ in)
Small needle holder (Kilner)
2·5 (2/0) Plain catgut or Dexon for ligatures
3 (0) Plain catgut or Dexon on a small half-circle cutting needle for subcutaneous structures
2 (3/0) Silk or nylon on a small curved cutting needle for skin sutures.

OUTLINE OF PROCEDURE

A curved incision is made over the medial aspect of the first metatarsophalangeal joint, and the skin reflected with bone levers placed on either side of the base of the proximal phalanx.

The base of the phalanx is divided with bone-cutting forceps and removed. The bursa which usually lies over the bunion is excised and the exostosis on the medial aspect of the first metatarsal is removed with an osteotome.

The subcutaneous structures are approximated with catgut or Dexon and the skin closed in the usual manner.

Hallux rigidus, arthroplasty procedure

DEFINITION

An operation for increasing the mobility of the first metatarsophalangeal joint which has restricted motion.

POSITION. Supine.

INSTRUMENTS
As for hallux valgus
Osteotome, 13 mm ($\frac{1}{2}$ in) (curved)
Bone file (optional).

OUTLINE OF PROCEDURE

An incision is made over the medial aspect of the metatarsophalangeal joint. The soft tissues may be divided by a U-shaped incision which has its base over the proximal phalanx. The joint is dislocated and the head of the metatarsal and base of the phalanx are refashioned to form a convex and concave surface respectively.

The soft tissue flap is inserted between the joint, and the wound closed in the usual manner.

Hammer toe (see arthrodesis of the toes page 446.)

Arthroplasty of the metacarpophalangeal and proximal interphalangeal joints (Calnan-Nicolle operation)

DEFINITION

Excision of the metacarpophalangeal joint or interphalangeal joint and replacement with an intramedullary prosthesis having an integral hinge joint.

INSTRUMENTS
Sponge-holding forceps (Rampley), 5
Towel clips, 5
Scalpel handles No. 3 with No. 10 blades (Bard Parker), 2
Scalpel handle No. 9 with No. 15 blade (Bard Parker)
Scalpel, solid variety
Dissecting forceps, toothed 13 cm (5 in) (Lane), 2
Dissecting forceps, fine toothed (Gillies), 2
Scissors, curved on flat 13 cm (5 in) (Mayo)
Scissors, curved on flat, 14·5 cm (5$\frac{3}{4}$ in) (Lahey)
Small retractors, double hook (Lane rake), 2
Skin hooks, single hook (Gillies), 2
Artery forceps, curved on flat (Kilner), 5
Tissue forceps (Allis), 5

Bone levers (Trethowan), 2
Small rugine (Faraboeuf)
Small bone-cutting forceps (Stamms)
Calnan-Nicolle reamers, set of 7 (Fig. 354)

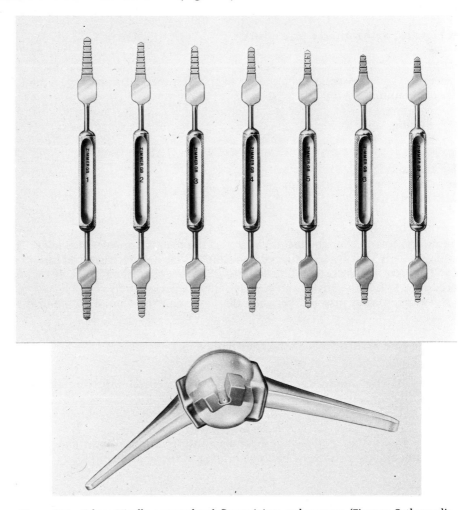

Figure 354   Calnan-Nicolle encapsulated finger joints and reamers (Zimmer Orthopaedic Ltd.). The prosthesis consists of two components; a polypropylene intramedullary integral hinged joint and a silicone-elastomer capsule. Seven sizes are available; four sizes for meta-carpalphalangeal joints and three sizes for proximal interphalangeal joints.

Set of 4 metacarpophalangeal or proximal interphalangeal Calnan-Nicolle joints (Pre-sterilised). (Fig. 354)
Power bone saw or Hall drill
Small needle holder (Kilner)
2·5 (2/0) or 2 (3/0) plain catgut or Dexon for ligatures
2 (3/0) or 1·5 (4/0) white braided nylon, Dacron or polyester on small curved cutting needle for extensor expansion and capsular tissues

1·5 (4/0) or 1 (5/0) silk, nylon or polyester on small curved cutting needle for skin
   sutures
2 ml syringe and needle for antibiotic
Malleable aluminium or plaster of Paris splints.

OUTLINE OF PROCEDURE

Metacarpophalangeal joint replacement. Longitudinal 40 mm ($1\frac{1}{2}$ in) incisions are made
over the mid-line of the joints being replaced. The skin is retracted, the extensor expansion is incised on the radial side of the common extensor tendon and the incision continued through the joint capsule and periosteum over the bone ends. The periosteum is
undermined around the neck of the metacarpal and the proximal end of the proximal
phalanx.

The bone ends are excised transversely with a power saw or drill removing 3 to 4 mm
($\frac{1}{8}$ in) of the proximal phalanx and 15 mm ($\frac{5}{8}$ in) of the metacarpal. The amount removed
will vary depending upon the size and shape of the bones and the degree of volar sub-
luxation and soft tissue shortening.

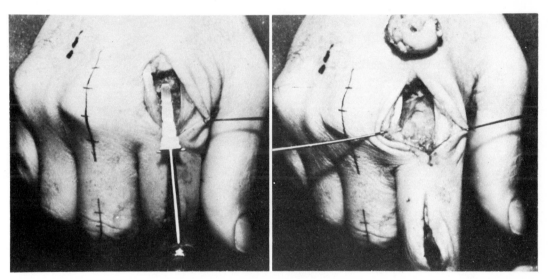

Figure 355   Calnan-Nicolle reamer *in situ*
Figure 356   Calnan-Nicolle encapsulated finger joints inserted.

(Zimmer Orthopaedic Ltd.)

Using the set of graduated reamers as intramedullary space is made in each bone. The
space so formed is tailored for a snug fit of the prosthesis to prevent rotation after
operation. The appropriate size of prosthesis is inserted with traction and flexion
applied to the finger and with the prosthetic joint flexed. Occasionally slight adjustment
may be required and if necessary careful trimming of the polypropylene intramedullary
stem of the prosthesis can be done with a scalpel.

Generally the capsules of the prosthesis are filled with a topical antibiotic such as
Neomycin 5 mg per ml and Bacitracin 500 units per ml. This is to prevent the accumulation of blood in the capsules in the immediate post-operative period. This fluid is introduced through the perforation in the capsule using a blunt needle and syringe.

The extensor expansion and capsular tissues are sutured with non absorbable material and finally the skin is closed in the normal manner. The hand is immobilised with a volar slab of Plaster of Paris or a malleable splint.

Proximal interphalangeal joint replacement. A longitudinal skin incision is again used, after which the central slip of the extensor tendon is divided by a 10 to 15 mm long 'V' shaped incision based distally on the insertion of the middle slip which is then preserved. The middle slip is then reflected distally and the lateral slips retracted to expose the bone ends. Space for the prosthesis is achieved by resection of an adequate amount of the proximal phalanx. Only a few millimetres of the middle phalanx is removed since the insertion of the middle slip must be preserved.

The joint prosthesis is then inserted as described previously and the 'V' shaped tendon incision is closed with interrupted non absorbable sutures. This allows adjustment of tension on the middle slip to restore correct balance between it and the lateral slips of the extensor mechanism. The skin is closed in the usual manner and the hand immobilised.

Exostosectomy

DEFINITION
The excision of an abnormal bony prominence.

POSITION
Dependent upon the location of the exostosis.

INSTRUMENTS
General set (Fig. 281)
Bone and fracture set (Fig. 338)
Osteotomes, 13 mm ($\frac{1}{2}$ in), 19 mm ($\frac{3}{4}$ in) and 25 mm (1 in)
Appropriate ligatures and sutures for that area of the body.

OUTLINE OF PROCEDURE
The exostosis is exposed and the periosteum elevated. An osteotome is used to excise the bony prominence and the wound is closed in the usual manner.

Osteomyelitis, drilling and saucerisation of cavity

DEFINITION
Drilling an osteomyelitis cavity for drainage in the acute stage of the disease; removal of sequestra and saucerisation of an osteomyelitis cavity in the cronic stage of the disease.

POSITION
Dependent upon the location of the lesion.

INSTRUMENTS
General set (Fig. 281)
Bone and fracture set (Fig. 338)
Aspiration syringe and wide-bore needles
Hand or power drill
Twist drills, 3·2 mm ($\frac{1}{8}$ in) and 4·8 mm ($\frac{3}{16}$ in)
Osteotomes, 13 mm ($\frac{1}{2}$ in), 16 mm ($\frac{5}{8}$ in) and 19 mm ($\frac{3}{4}$ in)
Gouges, 13 mm ($\frac{1}{2}$ in), 16 mm ($\frac{5}{8}$ in), 19 mm ($\frac{3}{4}$ in) and 25 mm (1 in)

Specimen tube for pus
Petroleum jelly ribbon gauze or similar
Appropriate ligatures and sutures for that area of the body.

OUTLINE OF PROCEDURE
Since the introduction of antibiotics, the operative treatment of this disease has become less frequent. Aspiration may be attempted initially, but the surgeon must have additional instruments available for evacuating pus from the abscess cavity.

Drilling. The affected area is exposed through a small incision, 8 cm (3 in) or so in length.

There may be an accumulation of pus underneath the periosteum and if this is found it is released by incising the periosteum. The periosteum is then elevated a little from the bone, and small drill holes are made into the medullary cavity. If purulent material exudes through these holes, either several more are drilled, or a small trap door about 13 mm ($\frac{1}{2}$ in) square is made through the bone with an osteotome to allow drainage.

The wound is usually closed and the limb immobilised either on a splint with wool and bandages, or in a plaster of Paris cast.

Saucerisation. The area is exposed through an incision which is sufficiently long to permit access to as many sinuses as possible. The periosteum is opened for the length of the incision and elevated for about 13 mm ($\frac{1}{2}$ in) on each side.

Multiple holes are drilled to outline the area of bone for removal, and a trap door is opened with an osteotome. Sequestra are removed and the cavity curetted, with excision of any sinuses which may connect the sequestra with the bone surface. The overhanging edges of the bone are excised and the bone cavity and wound are packed with petroleum jelly ribbon gauze or similar material.

The limb is immobilised either on a splint with wool and bandages, or in a plaster of Paris cast.

Bone tumours

The technique involved depends upon the location and extent of the lesion. If amputation of a limb is contraindicated, the surgeon may excise the tumour and replace the defect with a bone graft. This graft may be purely a question of filling in a cavity with cancellous chips, or may mean transplant of a large wedge of bone.

Instruments required vary but as a guide the surgeon will probably require a general set (Fig. 281); a bone and fracture set (Fig. 338); with the possible addition of instruments for bone grafting (Fig. 346) and instruments for plating and screwing (Fig. 340).

Amputation, forearm

DEFINITION
Amputation through the forearm, preferably at a level which is a few centimetres above the wrist.

POSITION
Supine, with the affected arm extended on an arm table.

INSTRUMENTS
General set (Fig. 281)
Rugine (Mitchell)
Bone-cutting forceps, compound action (Horsley)

Amputation saw (Sergeant)
Bone levers, small (Lane), 4
Fine rubber or plastic drainage tubing
Redivac suction drainage bottle, optional
2·5 and 3 (2/0 and 0) Plain and chromic catgut or Dexon for ligatures
3 (0) Silk, etc., for ligatures
2·5 (2/0) Silk or nylon on a medium curved cutting needle for skin sutures.

OUTLINE OF PROCEDURE

Equal anterior and posterior skin flaps are cut, together with the underlying fat and muscle fascia. These are reflected up and the radial and ulnar nerves are sectioned above the level for dissection of the bone.

The muscles are divided across just below the level of bone resection and are retracted proximally. The radius and ulna are divided across with a saw and the hand removed. The major vessels are identified and ligated with catgut, Dexon or silk and the two fascial flaps are approximated with catgut sutures. If the operation is being performed without a tourniquet, the major vessels are identified and clamped before transection of the muscles and bone.

A drain may or may not be inserted and the wound is closed.

Amputation through the humerus

DEFINITION

Amputation of the arm through the humerus.

POSITION

Supine, with affected limb extended on an arm table initially.

INSTRUMENTS

As for amputation of forearm.

OUTLINE OF PROCEDURE

Equal anterior and posterior skin flaps are cut, but may be modified in order to effect a plastic closure. These flaps are reflected with the fat and muscle fascia, and the anterior muscles are divided across just below the level for bone section. The major vessels are identified and clamped, and the posterior muscles are divided. The bone is divided with a saw and the arm removed.

The nerves are divided at the level of bone section and the major vessels are ligated with double ligatures. The muscles are bevelled to form a thin myofascial flap and are approximated with catgut or Dexon sutures. A drainage tube is inserted and the skin closed in the usual manner.

Amputation, forequarter

DEFINITION

Amputation of the entire arm, together with part of the clavicle and the whole scapula.

POSITION

Supine, with a sandbag under the thorax just below the scapula on the affected side and the patient well towards the edge of the operation table.

INSTRUMENTS

As for amputation of forearm
Artery forceps, curved on flat (Kelly Fraser), 40
Large tissue forceps, curved (Fagge), 6
Bone-holding forceps (St Thomas), 2
Wire saw and handles (Gigli or Olivercrona), optional
Diathermy leads, electrodes and Robin lead anchoring forceps
Ligatures and sutures as for amputation of the forearm.

OUTLINE OF PROCEDURE

An incision is made which starts at the lateral border of the sternomastoid muscle; follows the clavicle to the acromioclavicular joint and encircles the shoulder round the spine of the scapula and its angle; under the axilla and across the pectoral muscles to complete almost a circular incision.

The skin flaps are reflected, and starting at the front the pectoralis muscle is resected from its origin on the clavicle. The deep fascia is incised and the clavicle freed at its deep aspect. The external jugular vein is retracted or ligated, and the clavicle is divided with a Gigli saw, lifted upwards and removed by division of the acromioclavicular joint. The axillary vessels are exposed by division of the pectoralis major at its insertion on the humerus and the pectoralis at the coracoid. The subclavian artery and vein are doubly ligated and divided, and the soft tissues remaining which hold the shoulder girdle to the chest wall are divided.

The posterior part of the incision is now turned to, and the remaining muscles fixing the shoulder to the scapula are divided together with the muscles holding the scapula to the chest wall. The extremity is removed and the pectoralis major and other remaining muscular structures are sutured together over the lateral chest wall to form a pad.

A drain is inserted and the skin flaps are adjusted and sutured in the usual manner.

Amputation below the knee

DEFINITION

Amputation of the leg through the upper or middle tibia.

POSITION. Supine.

INSTRUMENTS

General set (Fig. 281)
Large tissue forceps (Fagge or Lane), 5
Rugine (Mitchell)
Bone-cutting forceps, compound action (Horsley)
Amputation saw (Sergeant)
Bone file (optional)
Wire saw and handles (Gigli or Olivercrona), or rib shears optional
Amputation knife
Bone-holding forceps (Fergusson lion)
Medium rubber or plastic drainage tubing
Redivac suction drainage bottle, optional
2·5 and 3 (2/0 and 0) Plain catgut or Dexon for superficial ligatures
3 and 4 (0 and 1) Chronic catgut, Dexon or silk for deep ligatures
4 (1) Plain catgut on a medium half-circle cutting needle for muscle sutures
2·5 (2/0) Silk or nylon on a medium curved cutting needle for skin sutures.

OUTLINE OF PROCEDURE

Unequal skin flaps are cut, with the anterior flap slightly longer than the posterior one at the selected level for amputation.

These incisions are carried down to muscle fascia and the flaps are reflected up on each aspect. The periosteum overlying the point for division of the bone is reflected and the anterior muscles are sectioned. During this stage the anterior tibial vessels are ligated and divided and the superficial peroneal and tibial nerves are divided at the level of bone section.

The tibia and fibula are sawn across about a quarter of an inch proximal to the divided anterior muscles. The posterior muscles are divided with an amputation knife and the posterior vessels identified, clamped and divided. The leg is removed and the vessels ligated. The fibula is exposed by subperiosteal dissection and is divided with bone-cutting forceps, a Gigli saw or rib shears at a point which is about 25 mm (1 in) to 40 mm ($1\frac{1}{2}$ in) above the level of the sectional tibia. The crest of the tibia is bevelled with a saw or file to prevent a sharp edge pressing on the skin. A flap of fascia is sutured over the stump, a drain is inserted and the skin closed in the usual manner.

Amputation, mid-thigh

DEFINITION

Amputation of the leg through the middle part of the femur.

POSITION

Supine, or with the knee flexed over the lower part of the table which is lowered or removed.

INSTRUMENTS

General set (Fig. 281)
Mid-thigh amputation set (Fig. 357)
Rugine (Mitchell)
Bone hook (Lane)
2·5 and 3 (2/0 and 0) Plain catgut or Dexon for superficial ligatures
3 and 4 (0 and 1) Chromic catgut, Dexon or silk for deep ligatures
4 (1) Chromic catgut or Dexon on a large half-circle cutting needle for muscle sutures
3 (0) Silk or nylon on a large curved or straight cutting needle for skin sutures.

OUTLINE OF PROCEDURE

Equal skin flaps are cut at the level for amputation and are reflected up with the fascia. If a tourniquet is in position, the muscles are severed by the circular sweep of an amputation knife which commences its cut on the anteromedial aspect of the thigh, cuts posteriorly, then laterally and finally anterolaterally. The muscles are then retracted with the amputation shield to a point about 25 mm (1 in) above the level for bone section. The femur is sawn across and the leg removed. The major vessels are picked up with forceps and ligated before release of the tourniquet. The tourniquet is released, hot packs applied and the smaller vessels picked up and ligated. The sciatic nerve is divided at the level of bone section.

If a tourniquet cannot be used, perhaps due to a high level of amputation, the femoral vessels are identified, ligated and divided before the muscles are cut across. The procedure then follows that described previously.

The muscles and fascia are sutured together over the end of the femur, a drain is inserted and the skin closed in the usual manner.

(Alternatively the limb may be amputated by disarticulation through the knee joint. In this procedure the skin flaps are fashioned at a lower level, but the basic technique is similar to that described.)

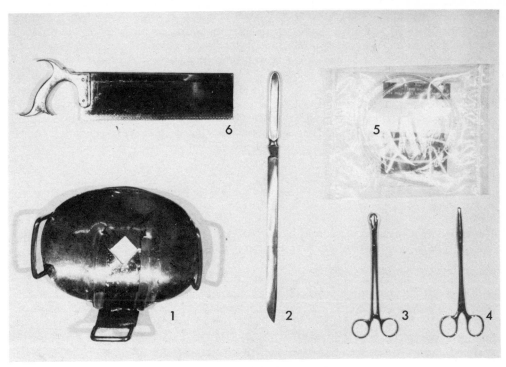

Figure 357   Mid-thigh amputation.

1. Amputation shield.
2. Amputation knife (Liston).
3. Tissue forceps (Lane or Fagge).
4. Artery forceps, straight, 20 cm (8 in) (Spencer Wells).
5. Long drainage tube, plastic, pre-packed sterile for use with Redivac or similar suction device.
6. Amputation saw.

Amputation, disarticulation of the hip

DEFINITION

Amputation of the leg in which it is severed from the trunk through the hip joint.

POSITION

Supine, with a sandbag under the affected side of the pelvis; or lateral position.

INSTRUMENTS

As for mid-thigh amputation, except stouter sutures (size 2) will be required
Artery forceps, curved on flat (Kelly Fraser), 35
Diathermy leads and electrodes.

OUTLINE OF PROCEDURE

An incision is made extending from just below the anterior superior iliac spine around the circumference of the thigh, just below the ischial tuberosity and about 10 cm (4 in) below the greater trochanter of the femur. The medial and lateral skin flaps are reflected widely and dissection is made down to the femoral artery, vein and nerve which are identified. These vessels are ligated and divided followed by the nerve which is divided only before being allowed to retract.

The limb is freed as follows: the sartorius and adductor muscles of the thigh are seoered near to their origin at the pelvis; the iliopsoas muscle is divided at its insertion on the lesser trochanter. The gluteus medius and minimus are severed from their insertion to the greater trochanter and the hamstring muscles are divided from the ischium. The sciatic nerve is identified and sectioned. (Some surgeons also ligate this large nerve.) The capsule of the joint is incised, the hip dislocated and the extremity removed.

A pad of muscle and fascia is made over the acetabulum by suturing the gluteal muscle flap to the origin of the pectineus and adductor muscles. A drain is inserted and the skin closed in the usual manner.

Tendon suture (end to end anastomosis and free grafts)

DEFINITION

The repair of a divided tendon either as an end to end anastomosis with or without tendon lengthening or transplant; free tendon grafts.

POSITION

Supine, with affected hand extended on an arm table.

INSTRUMENTS

Sponge-holding forceps (Rampley), 5
Scalpel handles No. 3 with No. 10 blades (Bard Parker), 2
Scalpel handles No. 9 with No. 15 blades (Bard Parker), 2
Fine artery forceps, straight, mosquito, 5
Fine artery forceps, curved on flat, mosquito, 10
Fine dissecting forceps, toothed (Gillies), 2
Fine dissecting forceps, non-toothed (McIndoe), 2
Fine scissors, curved on flat, 10 cm (4 in) (Kilner)
Fine scissors, straight, 10 cm (4 in) (Strabismus)
Scissors, stitch, 13 cm (5 in)
Fine tissue forceps (McIndoe), 6
Fine retractors, double end, 'rake' (Lane), 2
Skin hooks (Gillies or McIndoe), 4
Probe, malleable silver
Crocodile or tendon passing forceps
Fine bowl awl
Fine needle holder (West)
Lead hand splint or similar, for immobilisation of hand during operation
6 cm (2½ in) straight round-bodied needles for transfixion of tendon during operation (optional)
2 (3/0) Plain catgut or Dexon for ligatures
2 or 2·5 (3/0 or 2/0) Plain catgut or Dexon on a small half-circle cutting needle for subcutaneous sutures
33 SWG or 40 SWG stainless-steel wire or 1·5 (4/0) silk, polyester or polyethylene on a small curved non-traumatic needle for tendon sutures

Pearl button may be required for a 'pull through' suture

1·5 and 2 (4/0 and 3/0) Silk or nylon on small curved cutting needles for skin sutures

Malleable aluminium or plaster of Paris splint will be required.

OUTLINE OF PROCEDURE

For an end to end anastomosis, the cut tendon is exposed and fibrous tissue excised to effect mobility. The ends are approximated and straight round-bodied needles may be used to transfix the tendons and prevent the ends from retracting. The ends may or may not be trimmed with a knife, before suturing with stainless-steel wire or silk sutures, which are generally placed as modified mattress sutures.

Some surgeons use a 'pull through' wire technique in which a short strand of wire is included in the loop on one side of the anastomosis and is used to pull the wire suture out after the tendon has healed. This strand of wire is threaded on to a needle and passed through the skin at a point proximal to the anastomosis, and tied over a small pad of gauze. After the wire suture used for the anastomosis has been inserted in the distal part of the tendon, it is passed through the skin distal to this point (about 13 mm ($\frac{1}{2}$ in) to 25 mm (1 in) away) and is tied over a pearl button. This 'pull through' technique of Bunnell may be used also to take the tension off a suture line. In this case the tendon is approximated in the usual manner with fine stainless-steel wire or silk sutures, and a 'pull through' wire inserted proximal to the point of anastomosis being tied over a button, with slight tension. This relieves the strain on the anastomosis until healing is complete. The technique is applied mainly to the repair of extensor tendons although it may be used equally well for flexor tendons, especially transposition procedures.

In the case of injuries to flexor tendons in the fingers, it is generally preferable to make the anastomosis in the palm. Although an end to end anastomosis may be possible, a length of tendon is usually transplanted from the forearm or foot to bridge the gap between the palm and the distal phalanx of the finger.

A mid-lateral incision is made in the affected finger, the flexor tendons identified and removed completely, or leaving a small tag where the profundus is inserted into the terminal phalanx. The tendon pulleys are preserved if possible. The palm is incised and the proximal portion of the tendon identified and drawn into the palm with tissue forceps.

A tendon graft of suitable length is removed from the flexor aspect of the forearm and wrist (palmaris longus), or a plantaris tendon or extensor tendon to the toe and is threaded through the tendon tunnel from the palm and under the finger pulleys to the terminal phalanx. At this point it is either sutured to the remaining tag of tendon or a hole is drilled through the terminal phalanx and the tendon approximated to its insertion with a suture which passes through the bone. This suture is tied over a pearl button for subsequent removal. The skin wounds of the finger and forearm or foot are closed in the usual manner.

The finger is placed in the correct degree of flexion and an anastomosis made with the proximal tendon and graft in the palm. This is achieved either by simple side to side suture, or by interweaving the tendons before suturing. The palm wound is closed and the finger, as for all tendon sutures, is immobilised with a malleable splint or plaster of Paris back slab, wool and bandages.

24
Plastic Operations

Repair of harelip and cleft palate

DEFINITION

Closure of a harelip to establish continuity of muscle which is important for modelling the underlying bone and to produce a cosmetically acceptable lip; closure of a cleft palate and pushing back the soft palate so that it can approximate with the posterior pharyngeal wall.

POSITION

Harelip – supine. Cleft palate – supine, with sandbag between the shoulder blades and the neck in extension.

INSTRUMENTS

Cleft palate set (Fig. 358)
Sponge-holding forceps (Rampley), 2
Scalpel handles No. 9 with Nos. 11 and 15 blades (Bard Parker), 2
Scalpel handles No. 5 with Nos. 11 and 15 blades (Bard Parker), 2
Long fine dissecting forceps, toothed (Waugh), 2
Long fine dissecting forceps, non-toothed (Waugh), 2
Fine dissecting forceps, toothed (Gillies), 2
Fine dissecting forceps, non-toothed (McIndoe), 2
Angled tongue depressor
Suction tubing, fine nozzles and tube anchoring forceps
2 (3/0) Plain or chromic catgut or Dexon on cleft palate needles for cleft palate and harelip (mucosa)
1·5 or 1 (4/0 or 5/0) Silk or nylon on small curved non-traumatic cutting needles for harelip repair (skin).

OUTLINE OF PROCEDURE

Harelip. A Z-plasty type of incision is made, extending from the apex of the cleft to the mucosal edge of the lip. The tissues are undermined at each side of the cleft and if this extends up to the nose, the tissues of the cheek will be undermined towards the orbit in order to lessen tension when the wound is closed. The edges of the cleft are excised, drawn together and a fine silk suture inserted at the mucocutaneous junction in the centre. The muscles are approximated with catgut or Dexon sutures before completing the suture line with interrupted sutures of silk or nylon for the skin and fine plain or chromic catgut or Dexon for the mucosa. (Some surgeons apply Logan's bow to relieve the tension on the suture line.)

Cleft Palate. A suitable mouth gag is inserted, an incision made on each side of the cleft soft palate and the edges of the cleft are freshened. Two flaps of mucosa and muscle with their bases posteriorly are raised on each side from the underlying hard palate.

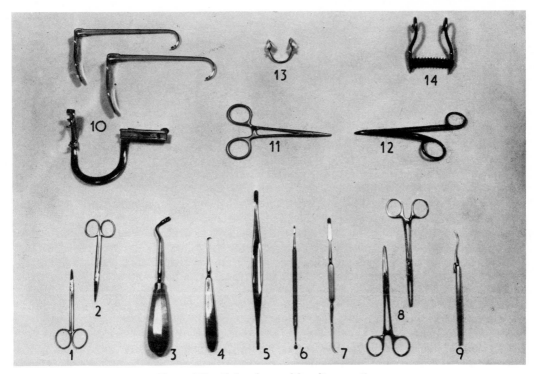

Figure 358   Cleft palate and harelip operation.

1. Fine scissors, curved on flat, sharp points.
2. Fine scissors, straight, sharp points.
3. Cleft palate raspatory, left and right patterns will be required, 2.
4. Cleft palate sharp hook; blunt hook may also be needed.
5. Raspatory (Howarth or Heath).
6. Cleft palate sharp hook and raspatory.
7. Dissector (Macdonald).
8. Fine tissue forceps (McIndoe), 2.
9. Cleft palate needle (Reverdin).
10. Mouth gag with appropriate size of blade (Dott).
11. Fine needle holder, fulcrum lever type with ratchet.
12. Fine needle holder (Gillies).
13. Harelip traction bow (Logan).
14. Mouth gag (Lane).

These two flaps are transposed and sutured together in the midline, thereby leaving a defect. This defect is filled temporarily with a gauze pack and will eventually epithelialise.

N.B.   Harelip cleft palate operations are rarely done as a combined procedure; the lip is repaired at about 12 weeks of age and the palate before the development of speech.

SKIN GRAFTS

Split-thickness Thiersch-type graft

DEFINITION

This is a graft which does not include all layers of the skin but only the epidermis and the tips of the papillae of the dermis. It is a useful type of graft which takes well and is therefore very widely used by surgeons. However, as healing takes place it contracts because it does not contain elastic fibres, does not have any sweat glands or hair, and may not, therefore, be cosmetically acceptable.

POSITION

This depends upon the location of the donor and recipient areas. In most cases where the graft is taken from the thigh for transference to an anterior area of the body, supine is suitable.

INSTRUMENTS. As Figure 359.

OUTLINE OF PROCEDURE

Unless it forms part of a fresh surgical defect, e.g., excision of tumour, debrided traumatic area, the recipient area is prepared by trimming excess granulation tissue to provide a smooth vascular bed for the graft. Haemostasis is secured by picking up blood-vessels and twisting them off or utilising diathermy.

The donor area is prepared by smearing lightly with sterile liquid paraffin or petroleum jelly and the graft is taken with a hand knife or dermatome.

A hand knife consists of a slender blade about 24 cm (9 in) long fitted to a handle. The knife may include also a guide, which is adjustable for various graft thicknesses. An example of the first type is the Blair-Bodenham knife, and of the second type, the Braithwaite knife (Fig. 359). When using a hand knife the skin is flattened by pressing a graft board at each end of the donor area.

There are two basic types of dermatome, the Paget's drum type and the mechanical oscillating blade type (Fig. 360). The Paget's dermatome is prepared by adjusting the 'depth of graft' mechanism and coating the half cylinder with skin graft adhesive. Adhesive is applied also to the donor area, and the edge of the cylinder is placed at the point on the skin selected for the commencement of the graft. As the cylinder is rotated slightly, the skin adheres and is lifted so that the graft may be taken by oscillating the cutting blade. This manoeuvre is continued until the whole surface of the cylinder is covered with skin. The graft is then detached from the donor area and removed from the drum.

The mechanical type dermatome is adjusted for depth of graft and is operated with a 'planing action' over the selected donor area. A small amount of lubricant may be applied to the skin and undersurface of the dermatome before taking the graft. If a very thin graft is required, sterile adhesive tape or polyvinyl can be applied to the skin, which is cut with the tape still attached. This provides support to aid manipulation of the graft afterwards.

The graft is applied as a sheet, sutured at its periphery to the skin around the recipient area.

Firm pressure is applied over the graft for a few minutes, and layer of petroleum jelly gauze is then placed over the whole area. A pad of polyurethane sponge or cotton-wool impregnated with proflavine emulsion is very useful for exerting localised pressure on the graft and the dressing is completed with gauze and wool and crêpe bandages applied firmly.

Some surgeons inject a solution of thrombin under the skin graft before applying pressure. This serves to encourage adherence of the graft to the underlying tissues and helps to avoid the accumulation of fluid which can prevent the graft taking. Finally, the operation is completed by dressing the donor area with petroleum jelly gauze, gauze, wool and bandages.

Unused portions of skin graft can be stored in a refrigerator at 1°C (34°F), spread on petroleum jelly gauze, and placed in a sterile container with a few drops of normal saline. The grafts are then available for application as required in theatre or ward without administering an anaesthetic. Normal storage is up to three weeks.

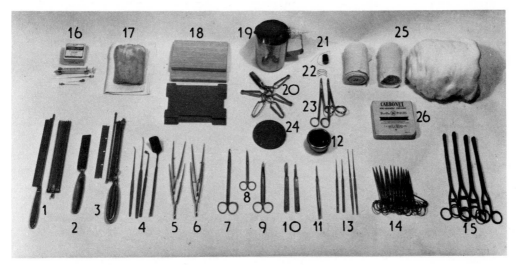

Figure 359   Skin grafting.

1. Skin graft knife (Blair-Bodenham), *or*
2. Skin graft knife (Thiersch), *or*
3. Hand dermatome (Braithwaite).
4. Graft manipulators.
5. Fine dissecting forceps, toothed (Gillies), 2.
6. Fine dissecting forceps, non-toothed (McIndoe), 2.
7. Long fine scissors, curved on flat (McIndoe).
8. Fine dissecting scissors, curved on flat, 10 cm (4 in) (Kilner).
9. Scissors, curved on flat 13 cm (5 in) (Mayo).
10. Scalpel handles No. 3 with Nos. 10 and 15 blades (Bard Parker), 2.
11. Skin pen.
12. Sterile ink, e.g., Bonney's blue.
13. Skin hooks (Gillies).
14. Fine artery forceps, straight or curved on flat, mosquito, 12.
15. Sponge-holding forceps (Rampley), 4.
16. Thrombin, 5 ml syringe and hypodermic needles.
17. Sterile gamgee tissue impregnated with proflavine emulsion.
18. Metal and wooden skin graft boards.
19. Saline and irrigation syringe.
20. Towel clips, 6.
21. 1·5 (4/0) or finer silk, braided nylon or Dexon.
22. Fine curved cutting needles, sizes 12 to 16.
23. Needle holders (Gillies), 2.
24. Stent impression material (optional; if used, bowl of hot sterile water or saline will be required to soften the material).
25. Cotton-wool and crêpe bandages.
26. Paraffin gauze dressing or similar.

Full-thickness Wolfe-type graft

DEFINITION

This is a free graft which includes all layers of the skin. Although it does not 'take' as easily as the Thiersch graft, it does not contract, contains sweat glands and hair and is therefore more cosmetically acceptable.

POSITION

This varies with the area to be grafted.

INSTRUMENTS

As for Thiersch graft
Sterile jaconet or polyvinyl sheet for patterns.

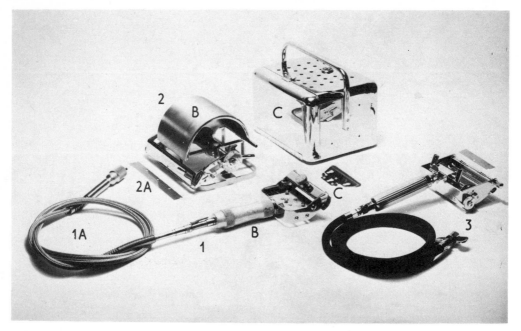

Figure 360   Dermatomes.

1. Electric dermatome.
   A. Flexible cable drive.
   B. Handpiece.
   C. Disposable blade.

2. Drum dermatome (Paget).
   A. Disposable blade.
   B. Drum dermatome.
   C. Sterilising case.

3. Pneumatic dermatome.

OUTLINE OF PROCEDURE

The recipient area is prepared as described previously by trimming granulation tissue. A pattern of the recipient area is made with a piece of sterile jaconet and this is used to outline the graft on the donor area with pen and ink.

An incision is made round this ink outline and deepened to the subcutaneous tissues. Starting at one end, the graft is undermined, held up with skin hooks and dissected free from the underlying fat. It is important that very little or no fat be included with the graft.

The graft is sutured at its periphery to the skin surrounding the recipient area. Fine silk or Dexon is used to obtain close approximation.

Pressure dressings are applied as for Thiersch graft.

Pedicle type flap

DEFINITION

This type of graft is a tube which includes skin and all subcutaneous tissue down to the muscle layer and is transferred to the recipient area with part of the tube still attached to the donor site. It is through this attachment to the donor site that the tube contains its blood supply and nourishment until it is established on the recipient area.

POSITION

This varies with the location of the donor and recipient areas.

INSTRUMENTS

As for Thiersch graft

Sterile jaconet or polyvinyl sheet for patterns.

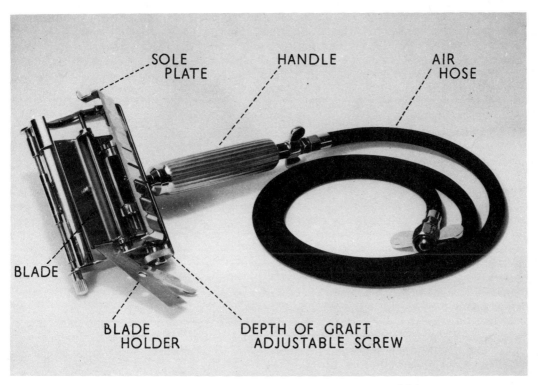

SOLE PLATE · HANDLE · AIR HOSE · BLADE · BLADE HOLDER · DEPTH OF GRAFT ADJUSTABLE SCREW

Figure 361   Pneumatic dermatome. (Eschmann Bros & Walsh.)

OUTLINE OF PROCEDURE

The number of stages necessary for this procedure depends upon the distance of the donor site from the recipient area and also whether the two areas can be brought together into direct contact with each other, e.g., hand to abdomen.

Two-stage operation, e.g., hand to abdomen and cross leg flap

Abdominal Flap. A large defect in the skin of the hand may be replaced by raising an abdominal skin flap and attaching it to the hand which is immobilised on the abdominal wall until healing is complete.

A pattern of the defect is made on a piece of sterile jaconet and the outline transferred to the selected abdominal area, e.g., inguinal region, with pen and ink. The outlined flap and underlying fat are raised on three sides and a Thiersch graft applied to the raw area beneath.

The hand defect is prepared in the usual manner and is approximated to the donor site and the flap sutured at its periphery to the skin surrounding the recipient area. Pressure dressings of petroleum jelly gauze, gauze, polyurethane sponge, proflavine wool, white wool and crêpe or adhesive bandages are applied.

Two or three weeks later, the fourth side of the flap is detached and sutured to the adjacent recipient skin edge. The donor site is trimmed at its periphery and if a defect remains where the flap has been detached, a further Thiersch graft is applied. Dressings are applied as before.

Cross Leg Flap. The recipient area, e.g., over the tibia, is prepared by excising excess granulation tissue and surrounding skin. A pattern of the defect, usually oblong in shape, is prepared on sterile jaconet. The outline of the pattern is transferred with pen and ink on to the calf of the other leg and an incision made round three sides of the outline. The base of the flap is always more anterior so that when the leg is crossed over the recipient site, the flap covers the defect without kinking.

The flap is sutured at its periphery to the skin surrounding the recipient area. The area underneath the raised flap on the donor leg is covered with a Thiersch graft from the thigh. Pressure dressings are applied in the usual way and the legs are immobilised with plaster of Paris bandages.

Three weeks later the flap is detached from its base and the fourth side sutured to the adjacent skin edge, followed by the application of dressings as before.

Multistage operation

If a pedicle graft needs to be transferred some distance, this is usually performed by raising a 'tubed flap' which can be moved in stages to the recipient area, e.g., abdomen to face.

A mobile area such as the inguinal region of the abdomen is selected and parallel incisions made for the entire length of tube required. The skin between these incisions is undermined and sewn together underneath to form a closed tube, the ends of which remain attached to the abdomen. The skin on each side of this raised tube is undermined and approximated with silk, nylon or Dexon sutures.

About 3 weeks later, one end of the tube is detached from the abdomen and sutured to a prepared area on the forearm. The wound caused by raising the tube on the abdomen is closed and the arm immobilised to the abdomnal wall with pressure dressings of gauze, wool and bandages or adhesive strapping.

After a further 3 weeks, the tube is detached from the abdomen and sutured to the prepared recipient area on the face. The arm is again immobilised whilst the facial attachment 'takes', and the wound caused when detaching the flap from the abdomen is closed with silk or Dexon sutures.

The final stage consists in severing the attachment of the tube from the hand and completing the suture of that end to the area on the face. The tube of skin is excised level with its attachment to the hand or forearm.

Rhinoplasty

DEFINITION

A special pedicle tube for correction of partial or complete loss of nasal covering. This is an operation which may be combined with correction of nasal deformities.

POSITION. Supine.

INSTRUMENTS

Scalpel handles No. 3 with Nos. 10 and 15 blades (Bard Parker), 2
Fine dissecting forceps, toothed (Gillies), 2

Fine dissecting forceps, non-toothed (McIndoe), 2
Fine artery forceps, straight, mosquito, 10
Fine artery, straight, mosquito, 10
Fine artery forceps, curved or flat, mosquito, 10
Fine tissue forceps (McIndoe), 5
Skin hooks (Gillies), 4
Fine scissors, curved on flat, 10 cm (4 in) (Kilner)
Scissors, curved on flat, 13 cm (5 in) (Mayo)
Dissector (MacDonald or Durham)
Small retractors, double hook, 2
Small retractors, double end, 'rake' (Lane), 2
Fine needle holder (Gillies or Kilner)
Stent composition material or plaster of Paris moulded into a splint
2 and 1·5 (3/0 and 4/0) Plain catgut or Dexon for ligatures
2 (3/0) Plain catgut or Dexon on a half-circle cutting needle for subcutaneous sutures
1·5 or 1 (4/0 or 5/0) Silk, etc., on a small curved cutting needle (preferably non-traumatic) for skin sutures.

If a bone graft is contemplated
Cancellous bone from the bone bank (with bone-cutting forceps, etc.)
or instruments for taking a bone graft (Fig. 346).

If nasal correction is contemplated
Nasal saw (Joseph)
Nasal rasp
Scissors, angled (Heyman)
Nasal septum forceps (Jansen Middleton)
Nasal raspatory (Hill or Howarth)
Nasal punch forceps, small and medium (Luc), 2
Nasal speculum, long (St Clair Thompson)
Dressing forceps, angled
Small gouges, 4 mm, 6 mm, 8 mm, 10 mm (Jenkins)
Small chisels, 4 mm, 6 mm, 8 mm, 10 mm.
Ribbon gauze impregnated with 1 in 10,000 adrenaline.

OUTLINE OF PROCEDURE
A pedicle tube is raised on the forehead with its base over one eyebrow. This pedicle is formed by making parallel incisions about 2 inches apart, which are curved towards the top of the flap. The flap is sutured underneath to form a tube, rotated and attached in position with fine silk sutures or Dexon to cover the nasal tissues.

The effect in the forehead is closed by a Thiersch graft. Pressure dressings are applied and held in position with the splint.

The pedicle is detached 2 or 3 weeks later and excess skin is excised.

Operation for protruding ears

DEFINITION
The removal of segments of aural cartilage and reconstruction of antihelix.

POSITION
Supine, with the head turned to one side.

INSTRUMENTS

Scalpel handles No. 9 with Nos. 10 and 15 blades (Bard Parker), 2
Fine dissecting forceps, toothed (Gillies)
Fine dissecting forceps, non-toothed (McIndoe)
Fine artery forceps, curved on flat, mosquito, 5
Skin hooks (Gillies), 2
Fine tissue forceps (McIndoe), 2
Fine scissors, curved on flat, 10 cm (4 in) (Kilner)
Small retractors, double end, 'rake' (Lane), 2
Dissector (MacDonald)
Fine needle holder (Gillies or Kilner)
1·5 (4/0) Plain catgut or Dexon for ligatures
1·5 or 1 (4/0 or 5/0) Silk, etc., on a small curved cutting needle (preferably non-traumatic) for skin sutures.

OUTLINE OF PROCEDURE

The operation consists essentially of removing a portion of auricular cartilage so that when an appropriate amount of post-auricular skin is excised, approximation of the wound tends to draw the ears into a more normal position. Small vessels are ligated or twisted off and the wound closed with fine silk sutures.

Mammaplasty (Cronin technique)

DEFINITION

Prosthetic breast restoration as an augmentation procedure or following subcutaneous mastectomy, using a seamless, thin walled, contoured breast prosthesis (SILASTIC ®).

POSITION

Sitting or supine possibly Trendelenberg.

INSTRUMENTS

General set (Fig. 281)
Local infiltration set (Fig. 271) with 0·5 per cent Lignocaine (Xylocaine) plus 1:200,000 adrenaline, optional.
Scissors, curved on flat, long, Metzenbaum
Retractors, Deaver, 25 mm (1 in) 2
Retractors, rake, medium 2
Special template (not heat sterilisable)
Diathermy leads, electrodes and anchoring forceps
Irrigation syringe and saline or topical antibiotic solution
Long drainage tube and Redivac
2 (3/0) Dermalon sutures on medium curved cutting needles for skins.

OUTLINE OF PROCEDURE

The SILASTIC ® Mammary Prosthesis features a seamless, thin walled silicone envelope designed to eliminate edge palpability of the prosthesis following augmentation procedures and subcutaneous mastectomy with prosthetic breast restoration. The uniquely contoured 'tear-drop' design closely simulates normal breast contour when implanted by providing desirable projection of the lower breast area with balanced upper area augmentation. In addition, thin, tightly woven Dacron net patches on the back of the prosthesis permit tissue ingrowth for positive fixation to the chest wall. Because body tissue or fluid will not invade the prosthesis itself, it retains initial softness when implanted while resisting absorption or degeneration.

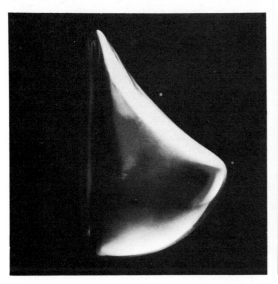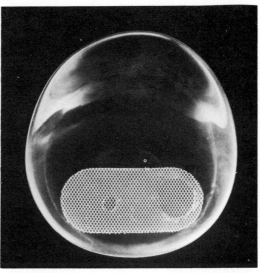

Figure 362   SILASTIC ® mammary prosthesis. (Dow Corning International.)

The SILASTIC ® Mammary Prosthesis is available in eight sizes to (1) meet the requirements of different operative procedures and patient conditions, (2) more adequately fulfil the demand for variations in tissue bulk, and (3) facilitate the achievement of symmetry. The extra-fill sizes are specifically designed for breast restoration following subcutaneous mastectomy.

The plastic template supplied with each prosthesis is designed to serve as a guide for both positioning of the implant and sharp or blunt dissection. A 13 mm ($\frac{1}{2}$ in) circumferential collar encircles each template.

In use, the template should be positioned over the breast to achieve the ultimately desired contour. A line is then marked on the skin around the edge of the template collar. This guide line provides the outer limits for the area requiring dissection.

With the patient in the sitting position, the inframammary fold is marked symmetrically beneath each breast. The small size can be inserted through a 6 cm ($2\frac{1}{2}$ in) incision, while shorter or longer incisions can be made for other sizes as appropriate. The line should be scratched in lightly with a needle prior to the skin prep. The template may be used as a guide to mark area of dissection.

Extending the patient's arms at right angles to her sides extends the pectoral muscles and facilitates dissection of the breast from the muscles. Bringing the arms to the sides of the body relaxes the skin and muscle and may ease the insertion of the implants. However, the complete operation can be done with the arms in either position.

Anaesthesia is usually general but the procedure is not infrequently performed under local anaesthesia. One half percent lignocaine with 1:200,000 adrenalin is infiltrated, fan-shaped between the breast and the pectoralis major muscle using a 22 gauge spinal needle.

The incision is made through the skin and subcutaneous tissue down to the loose superficial fascia over the rib cage. The upper edge of the wound is lifted with a rake retractor and with sharp dissection, the anterior surface of the fascia over the pectoralis major muscle is exposed. From this point, blunt dissection with a tonsil sponge in a ring forceps or the gloved fingers may be efficacious. Not infrequently, however, the use of long handled scissors will be needed. Dever or Harrington retractors are helpful and sometimes the Trendelenburg position may help the illumination of the cavity. Some surgeons have used a headlight.

Of greatest importance is that the cavity be made of *generous* size, directing particular attention to dissection of the anterior axillary fold and superiorly and medially. Forcing the implant into a small cavity will result in undue firmness of the breast due to the presure of the surrounding tissues. Hemostasis should be meticulous and is best accomplished by electrocoagulation. The space should be irrigated with saline, or, if preferred, with an antibiotic mixture such as Neomycin – 0·5 gm, or Bacitracin – 10,000 units.

The breast is lifted up with a Dever retractor. To facilitate sliding the Dacron spots over the floor of the cavity, a wide ribbon retractor or a piece of plastic, such as Vi-drape, is inserted first. The implant is then gradually forced through the small incision with a ring forceps and the fingers, the thin flattened part inserted first. The retractors and/or plastic film are then removed and the exact positioning of the implant is completed by the manipulation and inspection of the two inferior Dacron spots to detect any undesirable rotation.

The wounds are closed in layers, the final skin closure being with a continuous 2 (3/0) Dermalon intradermal suture which can be left in for 2 weeks without leaving suture marks.

As with any large wound, serum accumulation may sometimes be troublesome, and is indicated by enlargement, firmness and discomfort of the breast. After sterilising the skin, an 18 to 20 gauge needle is inserted obliquely (to avoid damage to implant) through the skin and subcutaneous tissues tissues inferiorly. Usually the fluid formation will subside after one to several aspirations. An alternative method is to insert a small polythene tube at the time of surgery and utilise Redivac.

Note. DOW CORNING ® Medical-Grade Silicone Elastomers are among the most non-reactive implant materials available, however, dust, lint, talc, skin oils and other surface contaminants deposited on the prosthesis in handling can evoke foreign body reactions with subsequent fluid and fibrous tissue buildup. Extreme care with strict adherence to aseptic techniques must be employed to prevent contamination of the prosthesis and the possible resultant complications.

If the prosthesis becomes contaminated before sterilisation, scrub thoroughly with a clean, soft-bristled brush in a hot water-soap solution to remove possible surface contaminants. *Use a non-oily cleaner or mild soap. Do not use synthetic detergents or oil-based soap, as these soaps may be absorbed and may subsequently leach out to cause a tissue reaction.* Rinse copiously in hot water and follow with a thorough rinse in distilled water.

To Sterilise: Autoclave by one of the following methods:

1. High speed instrument (flash) steriliser – Place on surgical towel in clean open tray. Sterilise 3 minutes at 130°C (270°F) at 28 p.s.i.

2. Standard gravity steriliser – Wrap in surgical towel and place in clean open tray. Sterilise 30 minutes at 120°C (250°F) at 15 p.s.i.

Do *not* use a prevacuum high temperature steriliser as this type of unit will cause the silicone gel to bubble and the prosthesis to swell.

Note: DOW CORNING ® Medical-Grade Silicone Elastomers are not deteriorated by repeated autoclaving, thus this method of sterilisation is strongly recommended. Ethylene oxide sterilisation may also be used although it is not recommended unless sufficient data is available regarding the time required for complete gas emission from the product with the specific system employed. (SILASTIC ® is the registered trade mark for Dow Corning's silicone elastomer products.)

Fasciectomy for Dupuytren's contracture

DEFINITION

Excision of hypertrophied palmar fascia which has contracted, thereby causing contracture of the fingers.

POSITION

Supine, with the hand extended on an arm table and the fingers separated by securing with a lead hand or similar splint.

INSTRUMENTS

Scalpel handle No. 3 with No. 10 blade (Bard Parker)
Scalpel handle No. 9 with No. 15 blade (Bard Parker)
Fine dissecting forceps, toothed (Gillies), 2
Fine dissecting forceps, non-toothed (McIndoe), 2
Fine scissors, curved (Kilner). Skin hooks (Gillies), 4
Small retractors, double end, 'rake' (Lane), 2
Fine artery forceps, curved on flat, mosquito, 10
Fine artery forceps, straight, mosquito, 10
Fine tissue forceps (McIndoe), 5
Dissector (MacDonald). Probe, malleable silver
2 (3/0) Plain catgut or Dexon for ligatures
2 and 1·5 (3/0 and 4/0) Silk on small curved cutting needles for skin sutures.
(Instruments for skin graft (Fig. 221) may be required.)

OUTLINE OF PROCEDURE

A tourniquet is always used for this operation (Chapter 23).

An incision is made in line with the mid-palmar crease from one side of the hand to the other. The skin on each side of the incision is undermined and freed from the palmar fascia, care being taken to avoid 'button holing'.

Beginning proximally, the hypertrophied fascia is dissected from the underlying blood-vessels, nerves and tendons which supply the fingers. If the scar tissue extends to the fingers themselves, a mid-lateral or straight incision is made and all the hypertrophied fascia excised.

Sometimes the fascia is so adherent to the skin that a segment must be excised, and in this case the defect may require skin grafting.

After fasciectomy is complete the tourniquet may be released and the divided blood-vessel ligated. Alternatively, the tourniquet remains inflated until a pressure dressing has been applied after wound closure.

The wounds are closed with fine silk sutures and petroleum jelly gauze applied followed by a pressure pad to the palm of sponge rubber, or wool impregnated with proflavine emulsion. The dressing is completed with wool and crêpe bandages applied firmly, so that the fingers are immobilised in the position of function.

Hypospadias operation (Denis Browne's procedure)

DEFINITION
The correction of a congenital abnormality where the urethral meatus lies at a point on the penis proximal to its normal position.

POSITION
Supine, with the legs separated.

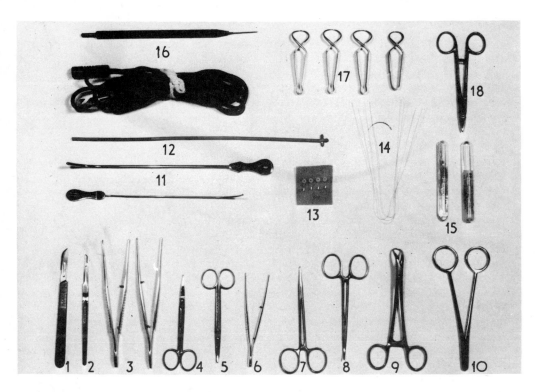

Figure 363 Hypospadias operation.

1. Scalpel handle No. 3 with No. 10 blade (Bard Parker).
2. Scalpel handle No. 9 with No. 15 blade (Bard Parker).
3. Fine dissecting forceps, toothed and non-toothed (Gillies and McIndoe).
4. Iris scissors, straight, sharp points.
5. Fine scissors, curved on flat, 10 cm (4 in) (Kilner).
6. Fine dissecting forceps, toothed, fixation.
7. Fine artery forceps, straight, mosquito, 6.
8. Fine artery forceps, curved on flat, mosquito, 6.
9. Towel forceps for penile holding.
10. Clamping forceps for aluminium collars (Denis Browne).
11. Catheter introducers, flexible and rigid (Denis Browne).
12. Catheter, self-retaining (Malecot), size 12 Charrière gauge.
13. Glass beads and aluminium collars (Denis Browne).
14. Size 5 (2) monofilament nylon and curved cutting needle.
15. 2 and 1·5 (3/0 and 4/0) chromic catgut or Dexon on 16 mm non-traumatic cutting needles.
16. Diathermy electrode and lead.
17. Towel clips, 4.
18. Fine needle holder (Kilner multiple joint).

INSTRUMENTS
 Sponge-holding forceps (Rampley), 5
 Hypospadias set (Fig. 363) and lead anchoring forceps.

There is usually a contracted undersurface of the penis in addition to a displaced meatus. The first stage of the operation consists of freeing this contraction before making a new urethra.

A transverse incision is made in the skin just below the glans and extended into the prepuce on each side. The rudimentary corpus spongiosum is then peeled away from the main erectile tissue and reflected towards the penile base. The short fibrous bands which exist on each side of the chordee are divided and the transverse skin incision is closed longitudinally with fine plain catgut or Dexon to effect a lengthening of the penis.

The second stage of the operation follows at a much later date. A fine Malecot's catheter is inserted into the bladder with a fine introducer. A more rigid sound is then passed along this catheter and used to press its mid-shaft towards the perineum. A diathermy knife is then used to cut down on to the catheter which, when seen, is thrust out with the sound. This diverts urine from the operative area until healing has taken place, i.e., perineal urethrostomy.

A U-shaped insertion is made, commencing at one side of the glans, continuing along the undersurface of the penis, around and proximal to the displaced meatus and finishing at the other side of the glans. The skin edges are reflected widely on each side, leaving a central strip of skin extending from the glans to the displaced meatus. The skin edges are brought together to cover the strip of skin in a manner similar to closing a single-breasted coat.

Approximation is achieved by using monofilament nylon tension sutures held with a lead stop and glass bead at each side of the wound. The procedure is as follows; a glass bead is threaded on to stout monofilament nylon at the end of which has been placed a short piece of crushed lead or aluminium tubing. The nylon is threaded on to a needle and introduced through both skin flaps to emerge on the opposite side. Another bead is threaded on to the nylon followed by an alluminium stop, and both are pushed down the nylon until the correct tension is achieved. The aluminium stop is crushed and excess nylon cut off. The skin edges are then sutured together with very fine catgut or Dexon on a non-traumatic needle, and a longitudinal relaxing incision is made down the whole of the dorsum of the penis to prevent tension to the suture line and swelling.

If the operation area involves the scrotum, it is usual to make a small incision or incisions on each side of it, leading down to the central wound, so as to allow drainage and prevent accumulation of fluid in the scrotal tissues.

25
Thoracic Operations

Oesophagoscopy

DEFINITION
Examination of the interior of the oesophagus by means of an endoscope which is passed along its lumen. The endoscope consists of a hollow tube with means of illuminating the tissues distal to its tip.

POSITION. See Chapter 4.

INSTRUMENTS. As Figure 364

OUTLINE OF PROCEDURE
This is an operation which may be performed under local or general anaesthesia.

When the procedure is to be performed under local anaesthesia, the patient dissolves a Desicaine tablet in his mouth before entering the theatre. The oropharynx is sprayed with a topical anaesthetic such as 4 per cent lignocaine (Xylocaine), and the patient placed in the position described in Chapter 4, with the head well extended.

The oesophagoscope is introduced into the pharynx with the patient's chin forward and head up anteriorly from the shoulders. The head is lowered and gradually moved to the right as the instrument is passed down the oesophagus.

The interior of the oesophagus is inspected and a biopsy taken if required. The pharynx and mouth are aspirated as the instrument is removed.

Sometimes oesophagoscopy will be followed with dilation of an oesophageal stricture by passing progressively larger sizes of dilators.

Bronchoscopy

DEFINITION
Examination of the trachea and main bronchi by means of an endoscope which is passed into their lumens. The endoscope consists of a hollow tube with means of illuminating the tissues distal to its tip. It is useful to repeat the point mentioned in earlier chapters, that the end of this endoscope has several side holes through which the patient is able to breathe, even if the end of the bonchoscope is obstructed.

POSITION. See Chapter 4.

INSTRUMENTS. As Figure 365.

OUTLINE OF PROCEDURE
Under general anaesthesia, (or local topical anaesthesia if indicated by the physical

condition of the patient), the patient is placed in the position described in Chapter 4, with the head extended.

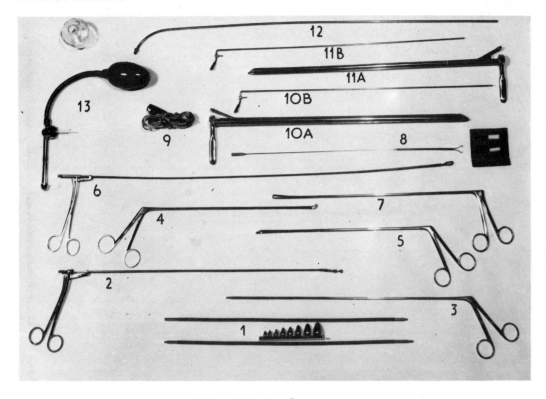

Figure 364   Oesophagoscopy.

1. Oesophageal dilators and flexible carriers.
2. Safety-pin closing forceps.
3. Grasping forceps (Chevalier Jackson).
4. Nodule forceps (Chevalier Jackson).
5. Specimen forceps, 'basket punch' (Chevalier Jackson).
6. Grasping forceps, fenestrated (Chevalier Jackson).
7. Rotation forceps (Chevalier Jackson).
8. Swab or mop holders (Coolidge), 2, and small mops.
9. Electric lead for light carriers.
10. A and B, Aspirating oesophagoscope, 9 mm, and light carrier (Chevalier Jackson).
11. A and B, Aspirating oesophagoscope, 7 mm, and light carrier (Chevalier Jackson).
12. Oesophageal aspirating tube.
13. Pharyngeal spray.

Not illustrated. Battery or transformer. Suction tubing and tube anchoring forceps.

The bronchoscope is passed into the pharynx, between the vocal cords into the larynx, and along the trachea. Both sides of the bronchial tree are examined by direct vision and with the telescope. Secretions are aspirated for histological examination and biopsies, if required, are taken with the appropriate forceps.

Thoracoscopy

DEFINITION

Examination of the interior of the chest cavity with an endoscope similar to a cystoscope, and which utilises a telescope for visualisation.

POSITION.
Lateral or sitting with support.

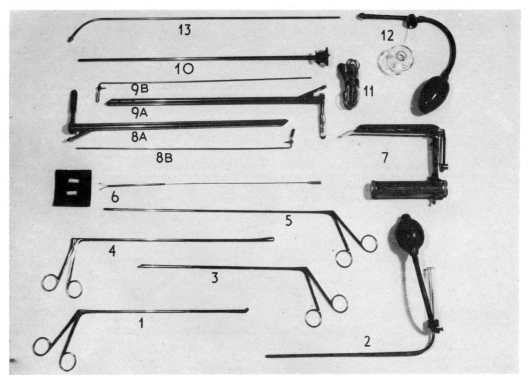

Figure 365   Bronchoscopy.

1. Nodule forceps (Chevalier Jackson).
2. Bronchus spray.
3. Specimen forceps, 'basket punch' (Chevalier Jackson).
4. Rotation forceps (Chevalier Jackson).
5. Grasping forceps (Chevalier Jackson).
6. Swab or mop holders (Coolidge), 2, and small mops.
7. Laryngoscope (Magill).
8. A and B, Aspirating bronchoscope, 5 mm, and light carrier (Chevalier Jackson).
9. A and B, Aspirating bronchoscope, 8 mm, and light carrier (Chevalier Jackson).
10. Telescope.
11. Electric cable for light carriers.
12. Pharyngeal spray.
13. Bronchus aspirating tube.

Not illustrated. Battery or transformer. Suction tubing and tube anchoring forceps.

INSTRUMENTS

Thoracoscope (Fig. 366)
Sponge-holding forceps, 5
Towel clips, 5
Scalpel handle No. 3, with No. 15 blade (Bard Parker)
Dissecting forceps, toothed, small
Dissecting forceps, non-toothed, medium
Scissors, curved on flat 13 cm (5 in) (Mayo)
Small needle holder (Kilner)
Cautery leads, electrodes and lead anchoring forceps
Suction tubing, long fine suction nozzles and tubes anchoring forceps

Tall jar containing hot sterile water for telescopes
Pneumothorax manometer
Local anaesthesia requisites (Fig. 271)
2 (3/0) Silk or nylon on small curved cutting needle for skin.

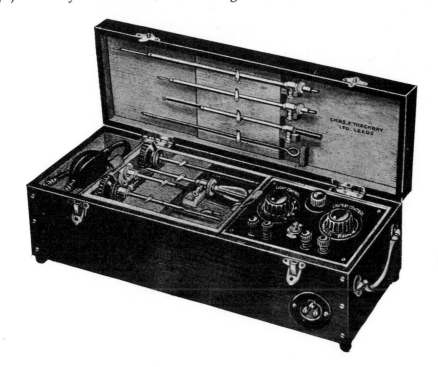

Figure 366   Thoracoscope. (Chas. F. Thackray Ltd.).

OUTLINE OF PROCEDURE

A double or single cannula thoracoscope may be used for this procedure, although the former method is the easier and this will be described.

Under local anaesthesia and a satisfactory premedication, a stab incision is made in the chest wall near to the lung adhesions. The thoracoscope is inserted into the chest through an intercostal space, and an examination of the lung made. (A pneumothorax must be present.) The lung adhesions are divided with a cautery point (which should be red hot and *not* white hot) passed along the instrument. A further examination is made to ensure that there are no more divisible adhesions. Effused blood or fluid is aspirated, and the pleural pressures are adjusted with the pneumothorax apparatus.

The thoracoscope is removed and the incision closed with one suture.

Intercostal tube drainage (for empyema or haemothorax)

DEFINITION

The insertion of a tube for the drainage of a collection of pus in the pleural cavity.

POSITION

Generally sitting with support.

INSTRUMENTS

   Sponge-holding forceps (Rampley), 5
   Towel clips, 5
   Scalpel handle No. 3 with No. 11 blade (Bard Parker)
   Trocar and cannula
   Catheter, self-retaining (De Pezzer or similar, size 28 Charrière gauge)
   Catheter introducer
   Syringe and wide-bore needles
   Underwater seal apparatus or pump
   Local anaesthesia requisites (Fig. 271)
   2 (3/0) Silk or nylon medium curved cutting needle *may* be required to secure the catheter.

OUTLINE OF PROCEDURE

   Under local anaesthesia, a stab incision is made in the chest wall, and a trocar and cannula introduced between two ribs into the empyema cavity or haemothorax. The trocar is removed and the catheter introduced through the cannula, which is then removed. To prevent collapse of the lung and to allow drainage of pus or blood the open end of the catheter is connected to an underwater seal apparatus and/or mechanical pump.

   One or two skin sutures are inserted, left untied and rolled up in a small piece of gauze. These are tied immediately when the tube is removed, so that a pneumothorax, possibly of 'tension' type, does not occur.

   An underwater seal apparatus consists of a sterile glass bottle, generally of 2 litres capacity, half filled with sterile water and closed with a cap which incorporates two tube connections. One tube connection terminates below the water level in the bottle and the other terminates just inside the cap. The former connection is coupled to the chest tube and the latter remains open to the atmosphere but protected with a gauze filter.

   The underwater seal apparatus reproduces the negative pressure which should be in the pleural cavity, and prevents air from entering from the atmosphere, but allows pus and air to escape from the expanding lung as the patient breathes out deeply. The pus collects in the bottle and the air bubbles out through the water. Any tendency for back suction will only result in the fluid being drawn slightly up the drainage tube connection.

   Alternatively, a suction machine creating a small amount of air displacement may be used, and in this case the drainage tubing is connected to the collection bottle fitted to the apparatus.

   Care must be taken that the drainage bottle is not elevated above the level of the patient. If this occurs, fluid may aspirate from the bottle and enter the patient's chest. During transportation of the patient, chest drains should be occluded with two clamps across each catheter.

Resection of a rib (for empyema)

DEFINITION

   The resection of part of a rib for inspection, evacuation and drainage of a collection of pus in the pleural cavity.

POSITION

   Depends upon the approach, but may be lateral.

INSTRUMENTS

General set (Fig. 281)

Small rugine (Faraboeuf or Sembs)

Rib raspatory (Doyen) for appropriate side

Rib shears (Costotome)

Aspiration syringe and wide-bore needles (Martin's)

Irrigation syringe, rubber catheter and warm sterile saline

Catheter, self-retaining (De Pezzer or similar, size 28 Charrière gauge) or 20 cm (8 in)
   length of size 12 rubber tubing and safety pin.

Catheter introducer (optional)

Suction tubing, suction nozzles and tube anchoring forceps.

Diathermy leads, electrodes and lead anchoring forceps

Underwater seal apparatus

Low vacuum suction apparatus

2·5 (2/0) Chromic catgut or Dexon for ligatures

4 (1) Chromic catgut or Dexon on a large half-circle cutting or Mayo needle for muscle

2·5 (2/0) Silk or nylon on a large curved cutting needle for skin.

OUTLINE OF PROCEDURE

Under general anaesthesia, the presence of pus is verified by aspiration. A vertical incision is made over the empyema cavity which is commonly accessible under the eighth rib in the posterior axillary line. A vertical wound is very useful for it allows the surgeon to resect a rib above or below the area selected, without making a separate incision.

The incision is deepened down to the rib and the periosteum and muscles are reflected. Two inches of rib is resected subperiosteally.

A small stab incision is made in the posterior periosteum and parietal pleura, and the pus is released gradually. The cavity is aspirated with a suction nozzle and the stab incision is then enlarged. Large clots of lymph are removed with sponge-holding forceps and the cavity may be irrigated with warm sterile saline.

A self-retaining catheter or rubber tubing is inserted, connected to the underwater seal bottle and the muscles and skin approximated loosely round the catheter. Low vacuum suction apparatus may be required also.

Decortication of the lung (for empyema or haemothorax)

DEFINITION

Stripping or peeling off the fibrin layer from the lung following empyema or haemothorax, to allow full pulmonary expansion and obliteration of the empyema cavity.

POSITION. Lateral chest (Fig. 63 or 64).

INSTRUMENTS. As for thoracotomy.

OUTLINE OF PROCEDURE

The approach is as for thoracotomy. All free clot is removed from the pleural cavity, and the fibrin layer peeled off the lung to allow full re-expansion. Drainage tubes are introduced at the apex and base of the chest, and are connected to underwater seals or suction apparatus. These drainage tubes are to allow the escape of air and exudate.

Thoracotomy

DEFINITION
Opening the chest cavity as a preliminary to surgery of the thoracic organs.

POSITION
Lateral chest (Fig. 63 or 64) or supine.

INSTRUMENTS
General set (Fig. 281)
Thoracotomy set (Fig. 367)
Suction tubing, nozzles and tube anchoring forceps
Diathermy leads, electrodes and lead anchoring forceps
2, 2·5 and 3 (3/0, 2/0 and 0) Silk on a small or medium half-circle round-bodied needle for transfixion sutures
4, 5 or 6 (1, 2 or 3) Chromic catgut, Dexon, silk or thread for ligatures
5 or 6 (2 or 3) Chromic catgut, Dexon or stainless steel wire or large half-circle round-bodied needles for rib closure
3 (0) Nylon or silk on large curved or straight cutting needles for skin.

OUTLINE OF PROCEDURE
The site of the incision depends upon which part of the chest contents is to be approached. The incision may be posterolateral, lateral or anterolateral, and may be placed overlying the upper or lower part of the thorax.

The incision is deepened through fascia and muscle down to the intercostal muscles. Haemostasis is secured with diathermy or ligatures, and the chest is entered either between two ribs or through the bed of an excised rib. In the former case an incision is made through the intercostal muscles, and the pleura opened with scissors. In the latter case the periosteum is reflected off the rib anteriorly with a Faraboeuf's, Sembs or Price Thomas rugine, and posteriorly by passing a Doyen's raspatory around and along the rib. The rib is excised, the pleura opened with scissors and a rib spreader inserted.

After the surgical procedure has been completed, an intercostal drain is inserted (see empyema) usually one apical and one basal. The drain is connected to the underwater seal and the wound is closed. Interrupted sutures of chromic catgut, Dexon or stainless-steel wire are inserted through the intercostal muscles above the upper rib of the wound into the chest cavity, and out again through the intercostal muscles below the lower rib. These sutures are left long until all have been inserted for the entire length of the wound. A rib approximator is used to approximate the ribs and the interrupted sutures are tied. Further interrupted sutures may be inserted to reinforce this suture line. If a drainage tube has been used, this is connected to an underwater seal apparatus and the anaesthetist inflates the lung or lungs.

Interrupted or continuous sutures of chromic catgut, Dexon or stainless steel wire are used to close the intercostal muscles and other chest muscles. The skin is sutured with interrupted silk or nylon.

Lobectomy or pneumonectomy

DEFINITION
Excision of a lobe of the lung or total removal of the lung.

POSITION
Lateral chest (Fig. 63 or 64)

INSTRUMENTS

As thoracotomy (Fig. 367).

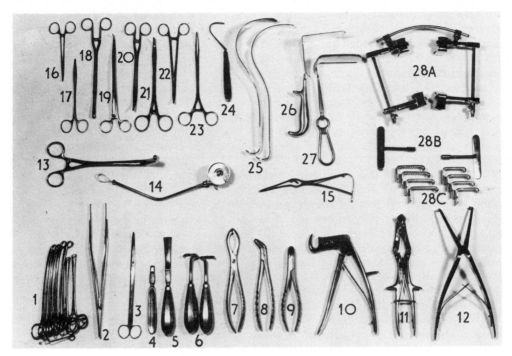

Figure 367   The thoracotomy set of instruments.

1. Tetra or skin towel forceps (Moynihan), 4 for sides of wound and 2 for ends of wound.
2. Long-toothed and non-toothed dissecting forceps, 25 cm (10 in).
3. Long scissors, curved (Nelson).
4. Small rugine (Faraboeuf).
5. Large rugine (Mitchell).
6. Rib raspatory (Doyen), left and right side.
7. Bone-holding forceps (Fergusson lion).
8. Gouge or bone-nibbling forceps, angled on side.
9. Gouge or bone-nibbling forceps, angled on flat.
10. Rib shears (Exner).
11. Rib shears (Price Thomas). (A variety of other rib shears may be required according to the site of thoracotomy.)
12. Rib approximator (Morriston).
13. Bronchus clamp (Thompson).
14. Lung tourniquet (Roberts-Nelson).
15. Long needle holder (Halstead).

16. Artery forceps, curved on flat (Kelly Fraser), 50.
17. Artery forceps, straight, 20 cm (8 in) (Spencer Wells), 12.
18. Sponge-holding forceps (Rampley), 4.
19. Lung artery forceps, right angled (O'Shaughnessy), 6.
20. Lung artery forceps, curved on flat (Roberts or Tudor Edward), 10.
21 and 22. Lung artery forceps, curved on flat (Moynihan (cholecystectomy) or Gordon Craig), 6.
23. Lung-holding forceps (Duval), 5.
24. Large aneurysm needle. Nelson right and left, 3 or each.
25. Lung retractors (Deaver or alternatively Allison 'fish slice' type), 2.
26. Deep retractor (Winsbury-White).
27. Deep retractor (Worrall).
28. A, Double-rib spreader (Tudor Edward), complete with one set of blades.
    B, Rib-spreader keys.
    C, Two sets of alternative sizes of blades.

Not illustrated. Sembs and Price Thomas rugines; Scapula retractor; Spinae erectus retractor.

OUTLINE OF PROCEDURE

The chest is opened as for thoracotomy, with a posterolateral incision usually over the sixth interspace. The sixth rib, or alternatively the fifth or seventh rib, is excised and the chest entered through the bed of the excised rib.

For lobectomy the affected lobe is held with lung forceps and any adhesions are freed with scissors or dissection swabs until the lobe is only attached by its main bronchus and vessels entering the hilum in the mediastium. The pulmonary artery and vein are isolated and clamped, divided and ligated. The bronchus is identified and clamped across with a special bronchus clamp. The rest of the chest is isolated with moist packs to prevent contamination as the lung is removed. Either the bronchus is divided by the cut and sew method, whereby sutures are inserted as the bronchus is divided; or a second clamp is applied and the bronchus divided between the two. With the latter method, the bronchus is oversewn before removing the clamp. In both cases a second and sometimes third layer of sutures (chromic catgut, Dexon, silk or stainless steel wire) are inserted to ensure a good closure. The stump of the bronchus is pleuralised, using interrupted silk, chromic catgut or Dexon.

For pneumonectomy the operative procedure is similar, but the dissection is more extensive, and the total lung is removed. The pericardium is incised and the dissection of the major vessels carried out through this opening in some cases.

If the pericardium has been opened, it is sutured with chromic catgut, Dexon or silk on a non-traumatic needle after haemostasis has been checked. The chest cavity *may* be irrigated with sterile saline, and chest drainage tubes inserted (usually one apical and one basal) and connected to the underwater seal. Low vacuum suction apparatus may be utilised for lobectomy, but not for pneumonectomy as this could cause mediastinal shift.

The chest is closed as for thoracotomy.

Thoraco-abdominal approach for oesophagogastrectomy

DEFINITION

Removal of part of the oesophagus and stomach for high gastric ulcer or tumour, oesophageal varices or oesophageal tumour. The operation is performed through a combined thoracic and abdominal incision. (Alternatively, laporatomy first to mobilise the stomach and perform a pyloroplasty followed by repositioning of the patient to make a thoracotomy incision to complete the resection.)

POSITION

Lateral chest (Fig. 63 or 64), with anterior supports well clear of the upper abdominal area.

INSTRUMENTS

As for thoracotomy (Fig. 367)
Intestinal occlusion clamps, straight (Doyen), 2
Intestinal occlusion clamps, curved (Doyen), 2
Intestinal occlusion clamps, right-angled (Finch), 2
Intestinal crushing clamps (Payr or Schoemaker), 2
Fine tissue forceps (McIndoe), 5
Long tissue forceps (Littlewood), 5
Nylon tape 6 mm ($\frac{1}{4}$ in) wide or No. 5 rubber tubing for retraction
Ligatures and sutures as for thoracotomy
2·5 and 3 (2/0 and 0) Chromic catgut or Dexon and silk on small half-circle non-traumatic needles for anastomosis
5 (2) Chromic catgut or Dexon on large half-circle round-bodied needle for peritoneum

5 (2) Chromic catgut, Dexon or silk or wire on a medium half-circle round-bodied needle for diaphragm

5 (2) Chromic catgut or Dexon on a large half-circle cutting needle for abdominal muscles.

OUTLINE OF PROCEDURE

A thoraco-abdominal incision is made, extending transversely across the epigastrium from the umbilicus, along the sixth or seventh intercostal space, to 5 cm (2 in) from the spine, i.e., behind the scapula. The sixth or seventh rib may be resected in the usual manner if insertion of a rib spreader indicates possible fracture of the ribs. The costal cartilage is cut across the diaphragm and peritoneum opened.

The tumour is palpated and resectibility determined. The oesophagus and upper end of the stomach are freed carefully, and vessels ligated with chromic catgut, Dexon or silk. Clamps are applied across the cardia of the stomach which is transected (if a tumour is present it would be distal to this point) and the lesser curvature narrowed by resection and closure with 2·5 or 3 (2/0 or 0) chromic catgut or Dexon on a non-traumatic needle.

Two occlusion clamps are applied across the oesophagus and the lesion is removed by dividing between the two clamps. The stomach is delivered into the chest and an end to end anastomosis made to the oesophagus with 'through and through' interrupted chromic catgut or Dexon non-traumatic sutures. The suture line is reinforced anteriorly and posteriorly with a serosa closure of interrupted silk sutures.

If the lesion is extensive, a total gastrectomy may be performed (Chapter 13) with oesophago-jejunostomy.

The diaphragm is closed with interrupted chromic catgut, Dexon or silk sutures, and the peritoneum with a continuous chromic catgut or Dexon suture. The chest cavity *may* be irrigated and an intercostal drainage tube is inserted through the eighth intercostal space. The chest muscles are sutured with interrupted chromic catgut, Dexon or wire, followed by interrupted silk or nylon for the skin.

The intercostal tube from the chest is connected to an underwater seal bottle.

Repair of diaphragmatic hernia (thoracic approach)

DEFINITION

The repair of an abnormal opening in the diaphragm (usually at the oesophageal hiatus), which allows a sliding hernia of stomach into the chest.

POSITION

Lateral chest (Fig. 63 or 64).

INSTRUMENTS

As for thoracotomy (Fig. 367)

Long tissue forceps (Littlewood or Vulsellum), 4

Ligatures and sutures as for thoracotomy

2·5 (2/0) Silk or stainless steel wire on a small half-circle round-bodied needle for diaphragm repair

Nylon tape or fine rubber tubing for oesophageal retraction.

OUTLINE OF PROCEDURE

A left posterolateral incision is made through the seventh intercostal space, and the chest opened as for thoracotomy. (A rib may, or may not be resected.) Rib spreaders are inserted, the mediastinal pleura opened, and the oesophagus mobilised and retracted with the nylon tape or rubber tubing.

The hernial orifice is identified, an incision made in the left dome of the diaphragm and the herniated organs returned to the abdomen. The edges of the orifice are grasped with tissue or Vulsellum forceps and the opening is repaired with interrupted silk or stainless steel wire sutures which are left long and are tied when all have been inserted. The incision in the left dome of the diaphragm is repaired in a similar manner.

The mediastinal pleura is approximated over the oesophagus and the chest closed in the manner usual for thoracotomy.

Sometimes the operation is performed through an abdominal or thoraco-abdominal incision, as described for oesophagectomy.

26

Cardiovascular Operations

This is a highly specialised and relatively new branch of surgery. The equipment and instruments used are extensive in range and often include many items which are of personal use only to a particular surgeon. In the following chapter it is possible only to cover those basic instruments for some cardiovascular procedures.

The reader is referred to Chapter 10 for a description of cardiac stimulant drugs, and Chapter 2 for the use of electric defibrillators and pacemakers which play an important part in heart operations.

A large proportion of heart and major blood vessel operations in the chest are performed under extracorporeal circulation (cardiopulmonary bypass) and/or hypothermia. With extracorporeal circulation the blood is diverted from the heart and the circulation maintained by means of a mechanical pump or pumps and oxygenator (heart/lung machine, e.g., the Melrose apparatus). With hypothermia, the patient's body temperature is lowered by physical cooling under anaesthesia to 30°C. At this temperature the metabolic rate and oxygen requirements are considerably reduced, and this allows the surgeon to stop the blood circulation for a period up to 7 minutes or so and thereby permit some intracardiac surgery.

During operation the patient lies on and is covered by special blankets which help to control the hypothermia. These blankets are made up of a series of rubber or plastic tubes through which fluid from a hypothermia machine circulates. The temperature of this fluid is adjusted to individual requirements and rewarming is started as soon as the patient is on the operation table.

Aortogram and cardiac catheterisation

DEFINITION

The introduction of a flexible catheter into the aorta or chambers of the heart, for the purpose of injecting a radio-opaque medium prior to radiological examination.

POSITION. Supine.

INSTRUMENTS
Aortogram
As Figure 368
Scalpel handle No. 9 with No. 15 blade (Bard Parker), optional
Radio-opaque medium, e.g., Hypaque 65 to 85 per cent
Sterile intravenous saline
Bowl with warm water for heating radio-opaque medium

Cardiac catheterisation
  As Figure 368
  Instruments for vein cut down may be required (Fig. 380)
  Radio-opaque medium, e.g., Hypaque 65 to 85 per cent
  Sterile intravenous saline
  Bowl with warm water for heating radio-opaque medium.

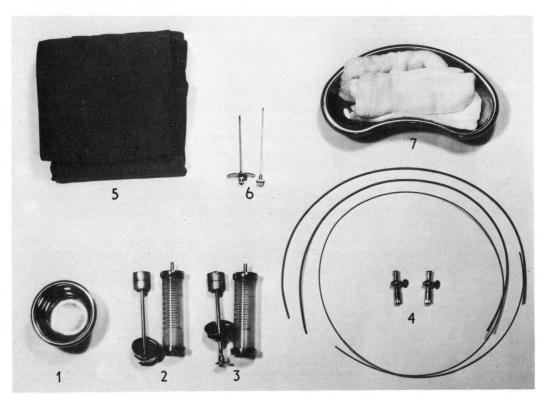

Figure 368   Aortogram and cardiac catheterisation.

1. Skin antiseptic.
2 and 3. 20-ml side-nozzle syringes. (Blunt or sharp-pointed drawing-up needle will be required, depending upon the presentation of the radio-opaque medium, either in a glass-capped or rubber-capped ampoule.)
4. Cardiac and aortic catheters, with connections for syringe.
5. Sterile towels.
6. Trocar and cannula for passing catheter.
7. Sterile swabs and kidney dish.

OUTLINE OF PROCEDURE

Aortogram. The procedure is performed under general anaesthesia so that the patient's respirations can be arrested during radiological examination. The groin is cleansed and draped in the usual manner and the trocar and cannula inserted through the palpated external iliac artery. The trocar is withdrawn, and the cannula is pulled back until its presence within the vessel is indicated by a flow of arterial blood. The guide wire is threaded through the cannula until it reaches the selected level in the aorta. (The guide wire has one end rigid and the other flexible; the flexible end is inserted into the catheter.) The catheter is then passed over the guide wire for the predetermined distance, and after confirmatory radiographs to check its position, the guide and cannula are withdrawn, leaving the catheter in place.

The patency of the catheter is maintained by periodic injections of heparinised sterile saline until the radio-opaque solution is ready for use. Hypaque tends to crystallise out in high concentrations and the ampoules must therefore be heated in warm water before use. A test dose injection of the radio-opaque solution is given to detect allergy. In addition, as radio-opaque solutions generally have a base of iodine the patient should always be patch tested. After the test dose the radio-opaque solution is injected rapidly and a series of radiographs taken immediately after. This procedure is suitable for investigating the vascular outline of the descending aorta and branch vessels leading off at the level of the catheter tip, e.g., for kidneys or liver. A pressure dressing is applied to the groin puncture site after the catheter has been removed.

Cardiac catheterisation. This is a similar procedure to aortogram, but the catheter is introduced into the median basilic vein in the antecubital fossa, and is passed into the chambers of the heart. When the radio-opaque medium is injected, the radiologist is able to take a series of radiographs which show an outline of the inside of the heart and major blood vessels (arch of aorta, pulmonary artery, etc.). The examination reveals also the blood flow in congenital abnormalities, e.g., patent ductus arteriosus, ventricular septal defect, etc.

It is not always possible to introduce the catheter through a cannula, especially in children, and in this case the vein is exposed by cut down procedure in the usual manner.

Intracardiac procedures

Although it has made great strides forward during the past few years, intracardiac surgery is still in the development era. There are many variations of technique for the same operation, each giving successful results in the hands of a particular team. Newer and more efficient prosthetic valve replacements are being designed and in the not too distant future, the use of auxiliary ventricles will become commonplace.

Cardiac surgery is complex and requires a specialised team of surgeons, anaesthetists, cardiologists, physiologists, technicians and nurses. Space will not permit more than a brief outline of surgical procedures for it would be easy to devote the entire book to describing these. In order to generalise the descriptions depart from the format of the book hitherto. Exceptions are the description of closed mitral valvulotomy (closed commissurotomy), a procedure which in many cases can be performed without the aid of cardiopulmonary bypass; coarctation of the aorta and patent ductus arteriosus.

Intracardiac lesions vary considerably in severity and in some cases the diseases overlap requiring several distinctly separate operative procedures during surgery. These lesions can be described as (a) acquired and (b) congenital, they are listed together with the corrective surgery required.

(A) ACQUIRED LESIONS

Mitral stenosis
1. Closed valvulotomy
2. Open valvulotomy (under direct vision)
3. Valve replacement.

Mitral insufficiency
1. Valvuloplasty
2. Valve replacement.

Tricuspid stenosis, and/or insufficiency
aortic stenosis, and/or insufficiency
1. Open valvulotomy

2. Valvuloplasty
3. Valve replacement.
Thoracic aortic aneurysm
1. Repair procedure
2. Replacement with a graft.

(B) CONGENITAL DEFECTS
Pulmonary stenosis
1. Valvulotomy.
Atrial septal defect
Ventricular septal defect
Tetralogy of Fallot
1. Repair procedure.
Patent ductus arteriosis
1. Ligation and division.
Coarctation of the aorta
1. Resection and end to end anastomosis
2. Resection and graft.

Mitral vulvulotomy

DEFINITION
Separation of fused commissures so as to mobilise the valve cusps in mitral stenosis.

POSITION
Lateral chest (Fig. 63 or 64), or supine.

INSTRUMENTS
As for thoracotomy (Fig. 367)
Auricular appendage clamp (Brock's), 2
Mitral valve dilators (Tubb's plus 15·2 cm (6 in) metal rule)
Wide Allis tissue forceps, 6
Long fine scissors (tonsil or McIndoe)
Long dissecting forceps, toothed, fine (Waugh)
Long dissecting forceps, non-toothed, fine (Waugh)
Long needle holders (Potts Smith or Holmes Sellor, etc.), 2
Irrigation syringe, rubber catheter and sterile warm saline
Routine thoracotomy ligatures and sutures
Sterile liquid paraffin
2·5 or 2 (2/0 or 3/0) Silk on a small curved non-traumatic needle for appendage purse-string suture
2 (3/0) Silk on a small curved non-traumatic needle for appendage closure
3 or 2·5 (0 or 2/0) Silk on a medium half-circle round-bodied needle for pericardium retraction and closure.

OUTLINE OF PROCEDURE
Generally a left posterolateral incision is made and the chest entered through the fourth interspace. The pleura is opened with scissors and a rib spreader inserted. It may be necessary to resect a rib.
The lung is retracted and the pericardium incised and retracted with interrupted silk

sutures. The left auricular appendage is identified and an appendage clamp applied. A purse-string suture may be placed in position beneath the clamp. An opening is made in the appendage tip and the clamp loosened to admit the surgeon's finger. (The purse-string suture may be tightened if there is a leak of blood.) If dilatation of the stenosed valve is impossible with the surgeon's finger, he withdraws it and inserts a dilator. After adequate dilatation has been accomplished, the dilator is removed and the appendage clamp reapplied. The opening in the appendage tip is closed with two rows of 2 (3/0) silk on non-traumatic needles.

Alternatively, a dilator may be passed from the ventricle. In this case the instrument is introduced through the ventricle wall, and after dilatation the opening in the myocardium is closed with 2 (3/0) silk on non-traumatic needles.

The pericardium is irrigated with warm saline and sutured with interrupted 2 (3/0) silk on a round-bodied needle. The chest is closed in the usual manner for thoracotomy.

Cannulation and cardiopulmonary bypass

Maintaining a patient's circulation by temporarily bypassing the blood from the heart enables protracted intracardiac procedures to be performed. Regardless of design the heart-lung machines, as they are known, consist of four basic parts, the oxygenator, arterial pump, heat exchanger and arteral filter.

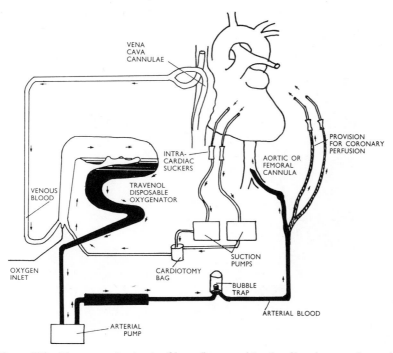

Figure 369   Diagrammatic circuit of heart/lung machine (cardiopulmonary bypass).

The Oxygenator takes the place of the patient's lungs, removing excess carbon dioxide from the venous blood and achieving oxygenation. It may consist of a screen, rotating discs or a bubbler, but basically separates the blood into a thin film which is then exposed to an atmosphere of oxygen where the interchange of gases takes place.

The Pump, usually a set of rollers rhythmically massaging the outside of the tubes conveying the blood, maintains the flow of blood back to the patient. The output of the pump depends on the speed of rotation and therefore the perfusion rate can be varied but should approximate the resting cardiac output.

The Heat Exchanger is used to lower or raise the temperature of the blood after it has passed through the pump/oxygenator. In conjunction with suitable drugs, the heat exchanger provides a means of rapidly inducing hypothermia if required.

The Arterial Filter is coated with a defoaming agent and acts as a bubble trap to remove any bubbles which may have been introduced during oxygenation. From this filter the blood passes directly back to the patient.

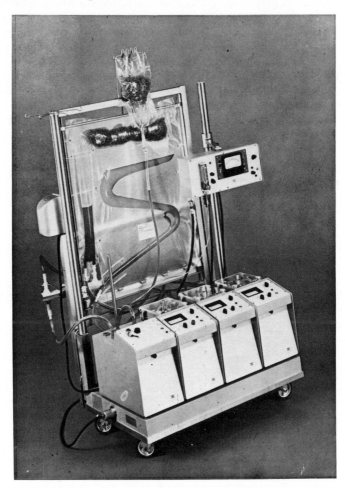

Figure 370   A heart/lung machine consisting of a Sarns modular pump console and disposable oxygenator. (Baxter Laboratories Ltd., Thetford, Norfolk.)

Cannulation is performed as a prelude to connecting the patient to the heart/lung machine. Venous blood is collected either from the superior and inferior venae cavae or the right atrium. If the venae cavae are cannulated Portex polyvinyl catheters 8 mm ($\frac{5}{16}$ in) are used; cannulation of the right atrium requires a larger size of catheter, 13 mm ($\frac{1}{2}$ in). A further plastic cannula is inserted into the left ventricle and connected to the venous blood reservoir on the heart/lung machine. This collects any blood pooling in the ventricular cavity, and is used to remove air from the heart immediately after bypass is stopped. A further suction line is also used to return aspirated blood into the venous blood reservoir.

Oxygenated arterial blood is returned either to a cannula inserted into the aorta or a cannulated femoral artery. The latter procedure is generally nowadays restricted to cardiopulmonary bypass for the repair of aortic aneurysms.

During cannulation the polyvinyl catheters are inserted with their obturators in position, an exception being the finer femoral catheters. After insertion, these obturators are removed and the proximal end of the catheter clamped shut. The catheters are then connected to the heart/lung machine with polyvinyl tubing. This is done carefully under a constant flow of sterile saline to ensure air free connections. All tubing is secured to the drapes with sutures or towel clips, to prevent accidental withdrawal of the cannulae.

Removal of the clamps on the tubing puts the patient on partial bypass, that is some blood still passes into the heart. Complete bypass is accomplished by passing tourniquets around the venae cavae where they join the heart. These consist of 6 mm ($\frac{1}{4}$ in) wide nylon tape passed around the venae cavae with both ends threaded through a 10 cm (4 in) length of No. 5 rubber tubing. Tightening the rubber tubing down on to the tape constricts the venae cavae and prevents blood entering the heart, the patient is then on total bypass.

INSTRUMENTS REQUIRED

General basic
As for thoracotomy (Fig. 367)
Various vascular clamps, Satinsky, Brock, Potts Smith, Blalock, Crafoord, etc. (Fig. 371)
Tissue forceps, Potts, 6
Long dissecting forceps, toothed, fine (Waugh)
Long dissecting forceps, non-toothed, fine (Waugh)
Long needle holders, (Potts Smith, Holmes Sellors, etc.), 2
Graduated jug for saline
Irrigation syringe and catheter
'Ether Hook' for flooding chest with CO_2 during bypass
Coronary suction tip 2, and tubing
Assorted stop cocks, connectors and needles, etc.
Recording catheters and insertion needles.

Cannulation and bypass
Polyvinyl catheters for cannulation
Connectors to attach catheters to heart/lung machine tubing
Nylon tape 6 mm ($\frac{1}{4}$ in) wide, 35 cm (14 in) long with 10 cm (4 in) lengths of No. 5 rubber tubing to act as tourniquets for major vessels.

Closure
2 or 2·5 (3/0 or 2/0) Silk, polyester etc. on medium half-circle round-bodied needle for pericardium retraction and closure sutures
2·5 to 1 (2/0 to 5/0) Silk, polyester, polyethylene or Dacron, etc., on small curved non-traumatic round-bodied or taper cut needle for vascular sutures, valve replacements and closure of the atrium. The size varies according to the vessel and surgeon's preference. A size 3 (0) may be used for closing ventricular incisions, combined with a Teflon felt reinforcing buttress. This may also be used as a purse-string suture for the cannulation sites.
Routine thoracotomy sutures.

Special instruments

  Valvulotomy

      Dilators, valvulotomes (Brock, etc.), various sizes

      Scissors, angled (Potts), set of 3

      Leaflet retractors.

  Valve replacement

      Prosthetic heart valve, e.g., Starr Edwards, homograft

      Valve holder

      Scissors, angled (Potts), set of 3

      Suture to secure valve, usually 2·5 (2/0) polyester etc. on double ended 25 mm taper
          cut non-traumatic needle.

  Septal defects

      Teflon or similar prosthetic repair material for patch

      Suitable sutures as detailed above.

PROCEDURES

Mitral valvulotomy. The chest is opened through a right posterior lateral incision or mediastinal split, the pericardium is opened and secured to the chest wall with 2 or 2·5 (3/0 or 2/0) silk or polyester etc. The 'Ether Hook' is secured to the chest wall with 3 (0) silk or polyester etc. This is used to flood the chest cavity with CO_2 during cardiopulmonary bypass. Carbon dioxide displaces air which is lighter and which may be trapped in the chest with danger of air embolism. If CO_2 becomes trapped in the open heart it is readily absorbed into the blood.

After the establishment of total bypass an incision is made into the left atrium. The mitral valve is opened under direct vision and the atrium then closed with 3 (0) silk or polyester etc. The patient is put onto partial bypass by releasing the venae cavae tourniquets, clamps are then placed on the tubing leading to the heart/lung machine and the bypass is discontinued. After removing the cannulae the incisions in the atrium are closed with 3 (0) silk or polyester and the chest closed in the routine manner.

Mitral valve replacement. Similar to the above except the valve is excised and a valve prosthesis inserted and secured with 2·5 (2/0) silk or polyester etc.

Mitral valvuloplasty. Similar to valvulotomy except the incompetent valve is plicated with sutures of 2 or 2·5 (3/0 or 2/0) silk or polyester etc.

Tricuspid valvulotomy, valvuloplasty, or valve replacement. Essentially the same as the mitral procedures described except the right atrium is opened to visualise the valve.

Aortic valvuloplasty or valve replacement. During this procedure which is performed under bypass, the normal coronary circulation will be compromised. It is essential to incorporate coronary perfusion in the bypass and this can be accomplished in several ways. A tube from the main arterial supply is split into two with a Y connection. The two tubes are then used to perfuse both coronary arteries one method being via hand-held metal suction ends.

The venous blood is collected from the right atrium via a 13 mm ($\frac{1}{2}$ in) Portex polyvinyl atrium catheter. Total bypass is accomplished by clamping the main pulmonary artery. Frequently the bypass is combined with hypothermia to minimise the hazards associated with interrupting the normal coronary blood supply.

After establishing complete bypass the aorta is clamped, incised and coronary perfusion started. Aortic valvulotomy, reconstructive valvuloplasty or valve replacement is then performed using 2·5 (2/0) polyester etc. on a 17 taper cut needle. After this has been completed the aorta is closed rapidly, for in order to do so the coronary perfusion has to be stopped. Saline 'slush' is often put into the chest cavity to produce some local hypothermia thereby protecting the myocardium until normal coronary circulation is started. Partial bypass is stated by unclamping the pulmonary artery and when the patient's condition is satisfactory this is discontinued and the chest closed in the normal manner. The sternum is generally approximated with stainless steel wire size No. 25 SWG.

Thoracic aortic aneurysm. This is performed through a left posteriolateral thoracotomy. The bypass required may be simply a shunt of blood from either the left atrium or left ventricle to a cannula in the femoral artery or as previously described for open mitral valvulotomy. In the former case the blood is oxygenated by the patient's own lungs, the cannulation of the atrium or ventricle is by a Portex polyvinyl 13 mm ($\frac{1}{2}$ in) right atrial cannula, the cannulation of the femoral artery is by a Portex 75 cm (30 in) intravenous cannula.

With the repair procedure, the distal portion of the aneurysm is clamped across both proximally and distally. The aorta is divided and sutured circumferentially back on itself to close the false channel. The aorta is then re-anastomosed.

Replacement with a graft or woven Dacron or aortic homograft is accomplished after excising the aneurysm between two aortic clamps. The graft is sutured with 2·5 (2/0) polyester etc.

After removing the cannula from the ventricle the incision is closed with 3 (0) silk or polyester etc., combined with two Teflon patches 25 mm by 6·3 mm (1 in by $\frac{1}{4}$ in) to prevent the sutures from cutting through the myocardium. If the cannula has been inserted into the atrium this is closed as described previously wthout a Teflon patch. The femoral artery is closed with 1 or 1·5 (5/0 or 4/0) silk or polyester etc. The chest is closed in the routine manner.

Pulmonary valvulotomy. This can be performed under hypothermia without cardiopulmonary bypass. The approach is through a sternal splitting incision with the patient supine. Tape tourniquets are placed in position round the major vessels (aorta, venae cavae and pulmonary vessels).

A Potts clamp (which constricts only one third of the vessel lumen) is placed on the pulmonary artery a few centimetres from the valve, and a longitudinal incision of about 2 cm is made in the segment held by the clamp. The heart is emptied of blood by tightening the tourniquets on the venae cavae, and when the chambers are empty the pulmonary artery and aorta are occluded. A careful note is made of the time that the tourniquets are applied. Pulmonary valvulotomy is then performed under direct vision after removing the Potts clamp. This is then reapplied to the pulmonary artery and the circulation started again, usually within 3 minutes or so of its cessation, by releasing the tourniquets. (First the venae cavae constrictions are released, then the pulmonary artery side clamp is applied, and finally the pulmonary artery and aorta tourniquets released.) The opening in the pulmonary artery is closed with 1 (5/0) silk or polyester etc. on a non-traumatic needle. If ventricular fibrillation is present, this is dealt with by electrical stimulation.

It should be noted that various arterial clamps may be used to occlude the major vessels as an alternative to tourniquets.

With the indirect Bourie procedure, a Bisch dilator (or Bisch knife) is passed into the right ventricle through the myocardium, pushed through the valve, opened 15 or 20 mm, thereby dilating the valve or cutting in two planes. The opening in the myocardium is closed with 2 (3/0) silk or polyester etc. on a non-traumatic needle.

Intraventricular pressures are reassessed, and the pericardium is irrigated and closed as described before.

The chest is closed as for thoracotomy.

Atrial septal defect. One of the most common of the congenital cardiac defects, it causes shunting of blood from the left to the right side of the heart. The gradual pressure build up and volume in the right heart and increased pulmonary resistance eventually causes a reverse of this shunt from right to left with consequent right heart failure. Surgical treatment of this condition consists of repairing the defect under direct vision, with complete bypass.

The approach is via a sternal splitting incision and the procedure approximates that for open mitral valvulotomy. The right atrium is opened and the intraseptal defect either sutured, or repaired with a Teflon patch. The atrioventricular valves may also require some reconstructive surgery. The atrium is closed with 3 (0) silk or polyester etc. bypass discontinued and the chest closed in the usual manner.

Ventricular septal defect. This again produced a left to right shunt of blood within the heart which may eventually 'balance' due to an increase in the right ventricular and pulmonary pressures. The reconstructive procedure is similar to repair of atrial septal defect except that the right ventricle is incised, and is closed with 3 (0) silk or polyester etc. combined with Teflon patches.

Tetraology of Fallot. This is a simultaneous occurrence of pulmonary stenosis; intra-ventricular septal defect; dextraposition of the aorta; and hypertrophy of the right ventricle. This results in increased pressure within the right ventricle due to pulmonary stenosis and a right to left shunt of blood via the ventricular septal defect with decreased oxygenation of the systemic blood.

The corrective procedure is similar to aortic valvulotomy under direct vision, and repair of the ventricular septal defect. The patient is placed on complete bypass.

During all open heart surgery it is generally necessary to arrest the heart beat by using a fibrillator which administers a constant D.C. shock. The effect is reversed with a defibrillator.

Correction of patent ductus arteriosus

DEFINITION

The ligation or division of a patent ductus which is a remnant of foetal circulation and allows blood to pass from the aorta into the pulmonary artery.

POSITION

Right lateral chest (Fig. 63 or 64).

INSTRUMENTS

As for thoracotomy (Fig. 367)
Ductus clamps (Potts), 3
Aortic clamp (Potts)
Large bulldog clamps (Potts), 3
Scissors, angled (Potts Smith), set of 3
Long needle holders (Potts Smith or Holmes Sellor, etc.), 2
Irrigation syringe, rubber catheter and sterile warm saline
Nylon tape or fine rubber tubing prepared for tourniquets
Routine thoracotomy ligatures and sutures
Sterile liquid paraffin
3 (0) silk or polyester etc. for ligation of ductus
2 (3/0) Silk or polyester etc. on a small half-circle round-bodied needle for mediastinal pleura
1 (5/0) Silk or polyester etc. on a small curved non-traumatic needle for ductus suture.

OUTLINE OF PROCEDURE

A left posterolateral incision is made and the chest entered through the fourth interspace or the bed of a resected fifth rib. A rib spreader is inserted and the lung retracted to expose the region of the ductus and the mediastinal pleura which is incised.

The aortic arch and pulmonary artery are dissected free on both sides of the ductus, using blunt and sharp dissection. In order to allow adequate mobilisation, some small vessels in the ductus region may require ligation. The vagus nerve is identified and retracted with tape or rubber tubing.

The ductus may be ligated with 3 (0) silk or polyester etc. ligatures which are placed at the aortic and pulmonary end of the ductus. Alternatively, the ductus may be divided after placing ductus clamps near to the pulmonary artery and aortic junction. With the latter method, the ductus is then divided and the ends closed with a continuous 1 (5/0) silk or polyester etc. on a non-traumatic needle, followed by an outer layer of interrupted sutures.

The clamps are then removed, haemostasis is secured and the mediastinal pleura sutured over the operation area with 2 (3/0) silk or polyester etc. The chest cavity is irrigated with saline and the thorax closed in the usual manner, with underwater drainage.

Correction of coarctation of the aorta

DEFINITION

Resection of a congenital narrowing of the arch or descending part of the aorta, and re-establishment of aortic continuity by end to end anastomosis.

POSITION

Right lateral chest (Fig. 63 or 64).

INSTRUMENTS

As for thoracotomy (Fig. 367)
Coarctation clamps, straight and curved (Crafoord, Potts, etc.), 2 or each
Clamps (Blalock), 2
Large bulldog clamps (Potts), 6
Various other arterial clamps (Blalock, etc.)
Long dissecting forceps, toothed, fine (Waugh)
Long dissecting forceps, non-toothed, fine (Waugh)
Long fine scissors (tonsil or McIndoe)
Long needle holders (Potts Smith or Holmes Sellor, etc.), 2
Irrigation syringe, rubber catheter and sterile warm saline
Nylon tape or fine rubber tubing prepared for tourniquets
Routine thoracotomy ligatures and sutures
Sterile liquid paraffin
2 (3/0) silk or polyester etc. on a small half-circle round-bodied needle for mediastinal
   pleura
1 (5/0) silk or polyester etc. on a small curved non-traumatic needle for anastomosis
Prepared homograft or fabric prosthesis may be required (Chapter 27).

OUTLINE OF PROCEDURE

A left posterolateral incision is made and haemostasis of the many collateral vessels is secured. The chest is entered through the fourth interspace or bed of a resected fifth rib. A rib spreader is inserted, the lung retracted, and the mediastinal pleura incised to expose the aortic arch. The aorta is freed by sharp and blunt dissection and tapes or rubber tubing passed above and below the stenosed area. Alternatively, arterial clamps may be employed.

Vessels which leave the aorta at the point of resection are ligated, and this may include the left subclavian artery which commonly rises at the stenosis.

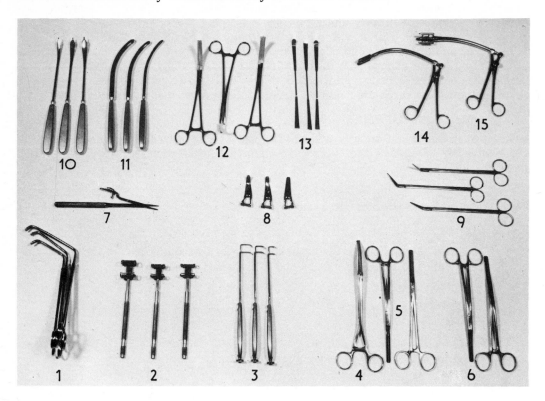

Figure 371   Instruments used for cardiovascular surgery.

1. Aorta clamps (Brock).
2. Aorta clamps (Potts Smith).
3. Aorta clamps (Blalock).
4. Clamps (Blalock).
5. Coarctation clamps (Crafoord).
6. Ductus clamps (Potts).
7. Long needle holder (Holmes Sellor).
8. Bulldog clamps (Potts).
9. Angled scissors (Potts Smith).
10. Pulmonary valvulotomes (Brock).
11. Pulmonary dilators (Brock).
12. Auricular clamps (Brock).
13. Aortic retractors.
14. Pulmonary dilator (Brock), closed.
15. Aortic dilator (Brock), open.

The vagus nerve is identified and retracted before applying coarctation clamps or Blalock clamps above and below the stenosed segment, which is then excised. The gap is closed either by end to end anastomosis with 1 (5/0) silk or polyester etc., or the interposition of a homograft or fabric (Teflon) tube prosthesis. The homograft or fabric prosthesis is anastomosed to each end of the cut aorta in the usual manner.

Haemostasis is secured and the mediastinal pleura sutured over the operation area. The chest cavity may be irrigated before closing in the usual manner, with underwater drainage.

27
Abdominal Vascular Operations

Excision and graft for aneurysm of the aorta

DEFINITION

Excision of a dilated portion of the abdominal aorta and insertion of a synthetic fabric prosthesis, e.g., Teflon, Dacron.

POSITION. Supine.

INSTRUMENTS

General set (Fig. 281)
Laparotomy set (Fig. 282)
Long fine dissecting forceps, toothed, 20 cm (8 in) (Waugh), 2
Lone fine dissecting forceps, non-toothed, 20 cm (8 in) (Waugh), 2
Dissecting forceps, toothed, 25 cm (10 in)
Dissecting forceps, non-toothed, 25 cm (10 in)
Long scissors, curved on flat, 23 cm (9 in) (Nelson)
Scissors, curved on flat, 18 cm (7 in) (Mayo)
Scissors, angled (Potts Smith), set of 3
Vena cava occlusion clamps, 2
Aortic clamps (Potts), 2
Large bulldog clamps, 6
Small bulldog clamps, 6
Long needle holders (Potts Smith or Holmes Sellor, etc.), 2
Polythene tubing or nylon tape
20 ml syringe, needles and blunt cannula
Heparin 10,000 units in 2 ml and protamine sulphate 100 mgm (*Note.* 1 mg of heparin is equivalent to 100 units, and for neutralisation the equivalent of 1 mg of protamine sulphate is given for each 100 units of heparin.)
Laparotomy ligatures and sutures
2 and 1 (3/0 and 5/0) Silk, etc., on small curved non-traumatic arterial needles for anastomosis
Occlusion cuffs (tourniquets) for both thighs.

OUTLINE OF PROCEDURE

A midline or left paramedian incision is made from the xyphisternum to the symphysis pubis. The bowel is retracted with moist packs and the posterior peritoneum opened over the aorta. The ureters are identified and retracted, and the inferior mesenteric artery is divided between ligatures.

The aorta is mobilised above the aneurysm and the aorta or the iliac vessels below, and polythene tubing or nylon tape passed round them. Other adjoining vessels are retracted in a similar manner, and after systemic heparinisation the aorta above the aneurysm (but below the renal arteries) is occluded with an occlusion clamp. The common iliac arteries are occluded with bulldog clamps and the aneurysm is mobilised and excised.

The aortic defect is bridged with a bifurcated fabric prosthesis (e.g., Teflon, Dacron, Fig. 372), and the anastomosis carried out with continuous non-absorbable sutures.

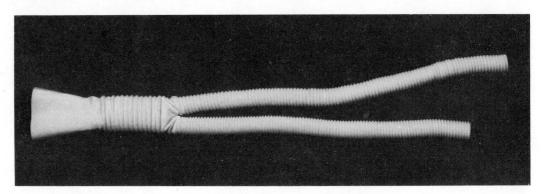

Figure 372   Bifurcated Teflon fabric prosthesis for the aorta. These crimped grafts may be obtained as knitted or woven types, the latter is less inclined to leak blood during the first few minutes after the clamps are removed.

Synthetic fabric prostheses of Teflon or Dacron are either of the knitted or woven type. The knitted type have a wider mesh and required 'pre-clotting'. This is done by immersing the graft for at least 20 min in 30 ml of patient's blood taken before heparinisation. After the anastomoses are completed, the clamps are carefully released one after another to test the integrity of the suture line. If necessary, the anastomoses may be reinforced with further interrupted sutures of non-absorbable material. Thigh occlusion cuffs are applied and inflated before release of the iliac occlusion clamps, and gradually released subsequently to avoid possible fall of blood-pressure. The action of the heparin is neutralised by the appropriate amounts of protamine sulphate.

Should occlusion of the aorta above the renal arteries be required for more than a very short time, hypothermia, a temporary bypass graft, or an extracorporeal circulation will be required.

The posterior peritoneum is closed with chromic catgut or Dexon sutures and the abdominal cavity aspirated free of blood before closure of the wound as described for laparotomy. Tension sutures are very important in the closure of this very long wound as paralytic ileus is frequent.

Splenorenal shunt

DEFINITION

Anastomosis between the splenic and renal veins to relieve hypertension in the portal venous system.

POSITION

Supine or right lateral chest for a left side approach.

INSTRUMENTS

Abdominal approach. As for laparotomy.

Thoraco-abdominal approach. As for thoracotomy.

Both routes

    Long fine dissecting forceps, toothed, 20 cm (8 in) (Waugh), 2

    Long fine dissecting forceps, non-toothed, 20 cm (8 in) (Waugh), 2

    Dissecting forceps, toothed, 25 cm (10 in)

    Dissecting forceps, non-toothed, 25 cm (10 in)

    Long scissors, curved on flat, 23 cm (9 in) (Nelson)

    Aorta clamps (Potts and Blalock), 2 of each, optional

    Large bulldog clamps (Potts), 6

    Small bulldog clamps, 6

    Long needle holders (Potts Smith or Holmes Sellor, etc.), 2

    Manometer, three-way tap, rubber or plastic tubing and exploration needle

    Polythene tubing or nylon tape

    20 ml syringe, needles and blunt cannula

    Heparin 10,000 units in 2 ml and protamine sulphate 100 mgm

    Laparotomy or thoracotomy ligatures and sutures

    1 and 0·75 (5/0 and 6/0) Silk or other non-absorbable material, etc., on small curved non-traumatic arterial needles for anastomosis.

OUTLINE OF PROCEDURE

For abdominal approach, a long, left paramedian incision with 'T' or 'L' extension as required is made and the peritoneum opened in the usual manner.

For thoraco-abdominal approach, the incision is made through the bed of the ninth rib which is resected, and extends across the epigastrium transversely. The left diaphragm is divided and a rib spreader inserted to obtain exposure.

The pressure in the splenic vein may be measured with a needle and manometer before mobilising the spleen, either directly from the vein or by splenic puncture. The spleen is freed and removed as described for splenectomy in Chapter 13, but leaving a maximum length of the vein by mobilising from the tail of the pancreas. The splenic vein is divided distal to the occlusion clamp applied close to the hilum of the spleen.

The left kidney is exposed and mobilised, and the renal vein is identified and marked with polythene tubing or nylon tape. Occlusion clamps or tubing tourniquets with rubber stops are applied to the renal vein to isolate a suitable segment for the anastomosis. It is wise to have temporary control of the renal artery with occlusion clamps at this stage also. The end of the splenic vein is trimmed before making an end to side anastomosis with 1 or 0·75 (5/0 or 6/0) non-absorbable sutures. Alternatively, a nephrectomy may be carried out to permit end to end anastomosis to the renal vein, but this method is avoided if at all possible. Heparin may be injected systematically before the clamps are applied and the anastomosis made, followed by an injection of the appropriate amounts of protamine sulphate after release of the clamps.

The wound is closed in the usual manner for laparotomy or thoracotomy.

Portacaval shunt

DEFINITION

Anastomosis between the portal vein and the inferior vena cava.

POSITION

Supine or left lateral chest for a right side approach.

INSTRUMENTS

As for splenorenal shunt except that the operation is on the other side.

OUTLINE OF PROCEDURE

The exposure is identical to that for splenorenal shunt but on the right side.

The portal vein and inferior vena cava are mobilised in the usual manner and either an end to side anastomosis or side to side anastomosis made. A laterally placed partial occlusion clamp on the inferior vena cava avoids obstruction to the venous drainage of the kidneys and lower part of the body during the formation of the shunt.

28

Peripheral Vascular Operations

Transfusion of blood and other intravenous fluids

Intravenous transfusions form a very important part of operative technique. If the patient is shocked, a pre-operative transfusion of blood or plasma becomes a life-saving measure. Blood transfusions are important also when the surgeon forsees the possibility of excessive haemorrhage occurring during operation, e.g., prostatectomy or craniotomy.

In most cases the patient will already have a transfusion started before he comes to the theatre but there are occasions when the surgeon has met with some unforeseen hazard and it becomes necessary for a transfusion to be set up during operation. Irrespective of the type of fluid to be transfused, the technique of administration in the theatre is almost identical. For details of blood groups, collection and storage, together with methods of cross-matching, the reader is referred to books dealing with this subject. Our main concern is the outline of procedures for setting up a transfusion, namely the insertion of a transfusion needle cannula (puncture method) or cannula (cut down method) in ward or theatre.

Puncture method

DEFINITION

The insertion of a pointed needle through the skin and into a vein for the purpose of transfusion of blood or other intravenous fluid.

POSITION

Supine, with the arm or leg extended. An arm is generally placed on a narrow arm table or board and may be splinted before or after insertion of the needle, depending upon whether the patient is conscious or under anaesthesia. Some conscious patients are sufficiently co-operative to defer application of the splint, but children are always splinted before the operation is commenced.

INSTRUMENTS

Bottle or disposable plastic container of fluid to be transfused (e.g., blood, plasma, saline, dextrose, etc.)
Transfusion cradle or bottle clip (some containers incorporate an eyelet for suspension without a cradle or clip)
Transfusion stand
Bandages, elastoplast and zinc oxide strapping, splint (if needle inserted into ante-cubital fossa or patient is restless)
Sterile disposable recipient set
Quick release tourniquet or blood-pressure cuff

Artery forceps
Antiseptic for skin and swabs.

OUTLINE OF PROCEDURE

If blood is being transfused, the patient's name and other details are checked against the cross-match label on the bottle. These details are checked again with the person putting up the transfusion.

The giving set is assembled aseptically in the manner illustrated in Figs. 373 to 375.

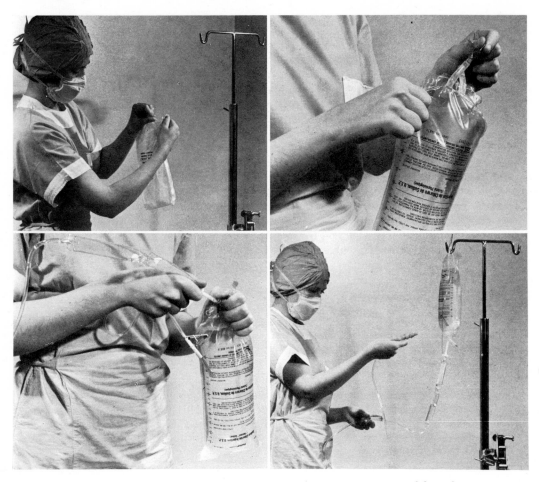

Figure 373   **Transfusion technique.** The outer protective cover is removed from the container of intravenous fluid.

Figure 374   **Transfusion technique.** The protective caps or sleeves are removed from the outlet tubes.

Figure 375   **Transfusion technique.** Inserting the plastic needle/connector of the recipient set.

Figure 376   **Transfusion technique.** The filter chamber is filled by gently squeezing and releasing. The control clamp is opened to allow fluid through the tubing thereby expressing any air contained.

A tourniquet is applied proximal to the vein, and either the patient is instructed to clench and unclench his fist several times, or the operator strokes the skin towards tourniquet in order to make the vein prominent. The area over the vein selected for transfusion is then cleansed with antiseptic.

Mounted on a syringe, the needle and cannula are inserted into the vein. The syringe is aspirated to ensure that the needle is in fact properly inserted in the vein. The needle is removed leaving the cannula in position. The transfusion set is connected and the screw control opened momentarily to allow the transfusion fluid to run rapidly for the first few seconds. The needle and tubing are secured with strapping (Fig. 376), a splint is applied if necessary, and the flow adjusted to the correct rate which generally lies between 20 to 40 drops per minute.

A vein at the dorsum of the forearm has been chosen for illustration and in this case a splint is not necessary (provided the point is not too near the wrist) for an adult, who is then able to move and use his hand to a certain extent. Alternatively the median basilic or cephalic vein can be used but this will require splintage of the arm. Transfusions may be administered also through a superficial vein of the foot, and this method is of special application in children where immobilisation of an arm is difficult.

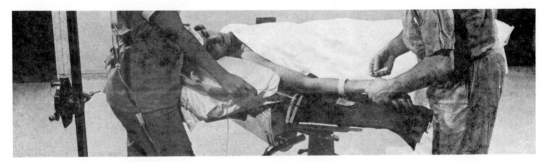

Figure 377 **Transfusion technique.** A tourniquet has been applied and the skin cleansed with antiseptic. The transfusion needle/cannula mounted on a syringe is inserted into the vein, and aspirated to check correct positioning.

As an alternative to using a Martin pump during rapid replacement of blood, the upper filter chamber can be rhythmically squeezed and released. Prolonged use of this method, however, will cause the drip chamber to be filled completely making it difficult to observe rate of fluid drip when normal administration is recommenced. This can be emptied by clamping off the tubing, inverting the transfusion bottle and squeezing *excess* fluid from the filter and drip chambers. The bottle is then resuspended. As the tubing was clamped off and remains filled with fluid, no air will enter the system during squeezing fluid out of the chambers. Another method used with plastic transfusion bags consists of a Fenwell bag which exerts pressure externally to the transfusion bag.

Cut-down method

DEFINITION

The direct exposure of a vein through an incision, for the insertion of a blunt cannula for the purpose of transfusing blood or other intravenous fluids.

POSITION

As for the puncture method.

INSTRUMENTS. As Figure 378.

OUTLINE OF PROCEDURE

The assembly of the apparatus is identical to that for the puncture technique except that a suitable cannula is connected to the luer fitting provided with the apparatus. The cannula may be made of metal but generally are of nylon or polythene which fit directly to the luer fitting of the giving set.

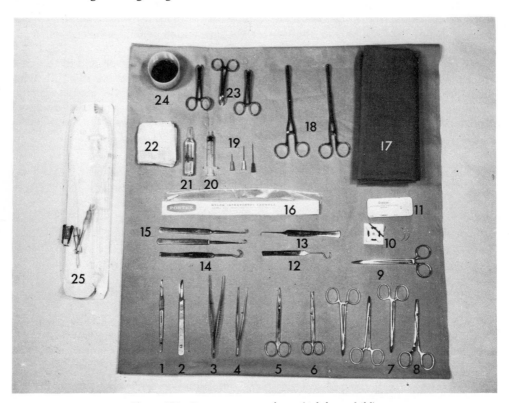

Figure 378   Intravenous cut-down (Adult or child).

1. Bard Parker scalpel No. 9 with No. 15 blade.
2. Bard Parker scalpel No. 3 with No. 10 blade.
3. Dissecting forceps, fine toothed, Gillies.
4. Dissecting forceps, fine toothed, fixation.
5. Scissors, straight, fine pointed iris.
6. Scissors, curved, fine dissecting points, Kilner.
7. Artery forceps, curved, mosquito.
8. Artery forceps, straight, Spencer Wells.
9. Needle holder, fine, West's.
10. 2·5 (2/0) silk or nylon and curved cutting needles for skin.
11. 2·5 or 2 (2/0 or 3/0) chromic catgut or Dexon.
12. Medium aneurysm needle.
13. Fine aneurysm needle.
14. Single hook, blunt.
15. Double hook retractors, fine.
16. Intravenous nylon cannula, Portex.
17. Sterile towels.
18. Sponge holding forceps, Rampley.
19. Hypodermic needles, disposable, sizes 20, 12 and 1.
20. Hypodermic syringe, disposable, 2 ml.
21. Lignocaine (Xylocaine) 1 per cent.
22. Sterile green swabs.
23. Towel clips.
24. Skin Antiseptic.
25. Disposable recipient set.

Under local or general anaesthesia, an incision is made over the vein selected, which is then freed by blunt dissection. Two ligatures of catgut are passed around the vessel about one centimetre apart, and the distal one is tied and left long. An incision is made in the vein between these ligatures and the cannula is introduced. The proximal ligature is tied to secure the cannula in the vein and to prevent leaks. The distal ligature is also tied round the cannula to prevent movement and the wound is sutured with interrupted nylon or silk. The tubing is secured in the manner illustrated and a splint applied if necessary.

Cannulae can be introduced without the necessity of cutting down on the vein. Some cannulae, such as the Braunula or Frankis Evans type, incorporate an inner hollow trocar which can be connected to a syringe, and acts as a standard puncture needle with the advantage of aspiration to check that it has entered the vein properly. The trocar is then removed, thereby leaving a blunt cannula in the vein which may be connected to the transfusion tube in the usual manner (as described under the puncture technique).

There are ready-sterile plastic cannulae such as Bardic intracath which can be threaded through a special wide-bore needle after they have been inserted into the vein. This needle is then removed by pulling it back over the cannula to the proximal end. The proximal end is made slightly bulbous and wedges in the hilt of the needle, which can then be connected to the standard luer fitting on the giving set. This obviates the need for cutting down and ensures minimal handling of the cannula which remains in the plastic tube-like pack until it is threaded into the vein.

Operations for varicose veins (Trendelenburg's operation and vein stripping)

DEFINITION

Ligation and division of the long saphenous vein at the point where it joins the femoral vein and of the terminal long saphenous vein tributaries. In the stripping operation, a flexible stripper is used to remove a length of the diseased vein from the leg.

POSITION

Supine, with the legs slightly abducted.

INSTRUMENTS

General set (Fig. 281)
Vein stripper, if stripping operation is to be performed (see Appendix)
2·5 and 3 (2/0 and 0) Chromic catgut, Dexon or silk for ligatures
3 (0) Chromic catgut or Dexon on a small half-circle round-bodied needle for deep
   sutures
2·5 (2/0) Silk or nylon on a medium curved or straight cutting needle for skin sutures.

OUTLINE OF PROCEDURE

For Trendelenburg's Operation an incision is made in the upper thigh, parallel to the crease in the groin over the saphenous opening. Dissection is made through the fat down to the point where the saphenous vein joins the femoral vein. (Small tributaries are ligated as the dissection proceeds.) The saphenous vein is isolated, divided, and both ends ligated at the femoral junction. The wound is closed in layers. The operation may require to be supplemented by ligation of the deep perforating veins, or stripping.

For the Stripping Operation, before the groin wound is closed, an incision is made at the ankle and a stripper threaded up the saphenous vein to the groin. The lower part of the divided saphenous vein in the ankle is secured to the bulbous end of the stripper by a ligature, and the whole withdrawn through the groin incision, thereby pulling the saphenous vein out of the leg. The short saphenous vein is treated by division and ligation at the sapheno-popliteal junction and stripped between there and an incision on the outer side of the tendino Achilles. A crêpe bandage is applied after the wounds have been closed. The patient has the foot of his bed elevated on blocks after operation, but is mobilised as soon as possible.

Arterial and venous embolectomy

DEFINITION

Removal of a blood clot which has become impacted in an artery or vein and is interfering with the circulation below that point. The most common sites for an arterial embolism to occur are at the arterial bifurcations, such as that of the abdominal aorta, the femoral and popliteal arteries. Similarly, venous emboli are also common at venous bifurcations such as the junction of the vena cava with the common iliac vessels. This is an emergency operation.

POSITION

Depends upon the site of the embolus.

INSTRUMENTS

General set (Fig. 281)
Peripheral vascular anastomosis set (Fig. 379)
Scalpel handle No. 9 with No. 15 blade (Bard Parker)
Fine dissecting forceps, toothed (Gillies), 2
Fine dissecting forceps, non-toothed (McIndoe), 2
Fine scissors, curved on flat, 10 cm (4 in) (Kilner or iris)
Fine needle holders, 2
Suction tubing, fine nozzles, rubber catheter with connection
Irrigation syringe, rubber catheter and non-pyrogenic saline
20 ml syringe, needles and blunt cannula
Fogarty embolectomy catheters 3FG to 7FG (Balloon inflation according to catheter size, i.e., 0·5 ml to 2·5 ml)
Fogarty irrigating catheters 4FG to 6FG (Balloon inflation according to catheter size, i.e., 0·5 ml to 2·5 ml)
Heparin 10,000 units in 2 ml protamine sulphate 100 mgm
Local anaesthetic requisites may be required (Fig. 271)
2·5 and 3 (2/0 and·0) Chromic catgut, Dexon or silk for ligatures
1·5, 1 or 0·75 (4/0, 5/0 or 6/0) Silk or polyester etc. on a small curved non-traumatic arterial needle for vascular suture
Appropriate sutures for that area of the body.

OUTLINE OF PROCEDURE

Method 1. An incision is made over the point at which the embolus has lodged. Dissection is made down to the vessel and an adequate exposure obtained. Polythene tubing or nylon tape is passed round the vessel and any immediate branches above and below the clot. This tubing or tapes can be threaded through short pieces of rubber or plastic tubing, as shown in Fig. 379, which can be slid down to occlude the vessel. Alternatively, bulldog or other vascular occlusion clamps (e.g., Carrel's) are applied to occlude the vessels. Heparin solution may be injected systemically before the application of clamps. An incision is made in the vessel wall and the clot milked or suctioned out. After as much of the clot as can be seen and palpated has been removed, the patency of the vessels below the thrombosed section is checked by momentarily releasing the constrictions and allowing the blood to flow. When the surgeon is satisfied that all the thrombus has been removed, the vessel incision is closed with 1 (5/0) silk or polyester and if the heparin has been injected, it is neutralised with protamine sulphate (or polybrene), following which the blood circulation is recommenced.

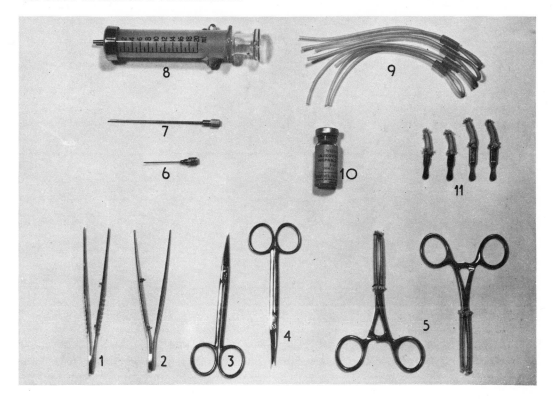

Figure 379 Peripheral vascular anastomosis.

1. Fine dissecting forceps, toothed, fixation, 2.
2. Fine dissecting forceps, non-toothed, fixation, 2.
3. Iris scissors, straight, sharp points.
4. Iris scissors, curved, sharp points.
5. Vascular occlusion clamps (Carrel), 2 or more.
6. Hypodermic needle, size 14.
7. Drawing-up needle.
8. 10 ml syringe.
9. Plastic or rubber tube tourniquets.
10. Heparin. (If used protamine sulphate (or polybrene) will be needed also.)
11. Vascular occlusion clamps (bulldog type), up to 12 will be needed.

The wound is closed in layers.

Method 2. Using the Fogarty embolectomy balloon catheter for saddle emboli, iliac artery and peripheral artery emboli.

Bilateral incisions are made over the common femoral arteries and the superficial and deep femoral arteries are isolated. After applying suitable arterial clamps, incisions are made at the junction of the superficial and deep femoral arteries. Appropriate sizes of embolectomy catheters are threaded distally as far as they will go, inflated with fluid and withdrawn to remove the distal thrombus. After removal 20 mg of heparin in 50 ml of saline is injected into the distal arterial tree via irrigation catheters.

This procedure is repeated by passing a catheter through the common femoral artery and into the aorta, inflating the balloon with fluid and withdrawing to extract the thrombus.

The incisions in the vessels are then closed with 1 or 0·75 (5/0 or 6/0) silk or polyester etc. and the groin incision is closed in the usual manner.

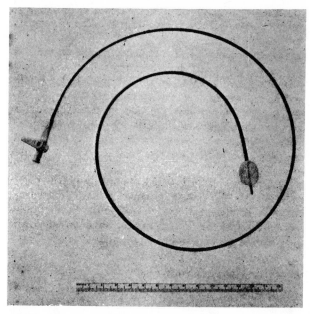

Figure 380   Fogarty embolectomy catheter. (Genito-Urinary Mfg. Co.)

Method 3. Vein emboli. Using the Fogarty embolectomy balloon catheter for ileo-femoral embolii. An incision is made over the sapheno-femoral junction on the unaffected side. The largest major tributary is isolated, ligatured distally and its stump utilised to introduce an embolectomy catheter. The catheter is passed up the iliac vein to the vena cava where it is left uninflated.

An incision is then made in the femoral triangle on the affected side and the common, superficial and deep femoral vessels identified. If dissection is difficult the balloon catheter already inserted in inflated with fluid to prevent movement of emboli up the vena cava.

Through a venotomy at the junction of the superficial and deep femoral veins on the affected side a further balloon is introduced until it is obstructed by the previously inflated catheter. It is then inflated and withdrawn until it lies within the proximal iliac vein segment – the first catheter is then deflated.

A second catheter is then inserted proximally into the affected side and when it reaches the inflated balloon, is itself inflated with fluid. Withdrawal of this catheter extracts the thrombus. Further catheters may be inserted distally into the limb to extract distal thrombus after which 20 mg of heparin in 50 ml of saline is injected.

Femoral popliteal bypass graft

DEFINITION
The creation of a channel for arterial blood to bypass an occluded segment of the femoral artery. The patient's long saphenous vein is generally used as a graft but if unsuitable, thrombo endartectomy may be performed as an alternative procedure (page 525).

POSITION
Supine, with the leg slightly abducted and flexed.

INSTRUMENTS
As arterial embolectomy, minus embolectomy catheters
Graft introducing tube and obturator
Long crocodile forceps
Solution for inflating vein graft which is made up at commencement of operation as
   follows:
      Normal saline 500 ml
      Heparin 5,000 units in 1 ml
      Procaine hydrochloride 2 per cent, 10 ml.

OUTLINE OF PROCEDURE
Longitudinal incisions, separated by small skin bridges, are made over the course of
the long saphenous vein from the groin crease to behind the knee. (This relieves tension
from the suture line and preserves skin vitality.) The long saphenous vein is exposed and
inspected. If found suitable it is removed at a later stage in the operation.

Systemic heparinisation with 10,000 units in 2 ml is now carried out. The common
femoral artery and its branches in the femoral triangle are exposed and isolated with tapes
or polythene tubing. The popliteal artery is also exposed and mobilised so that it may be
brought up into the superficial part of the wound. In order to select a patent length of
healthy artery suitable for receiving the distal end of the graft, it may be necessary
to divide both the tendon of adductor magnus and the medial head of the gastrocnemius
muscle. Small arterial branches are controlled either with small bulldog clamps or
double-looped slings of strong silk or polyester.

After ligating its tributaries, the vein is removed and cleaned of adventitia. To test for
leaks and size, the proximal end of the vessel is clamped and a suitable arterial cannula
tied into the distal end. Using a 20 ml syringe the vein is 'blown up' with a solution of
saline/heparin/procaine. Sections of the vein which appear narrow may be due to spasm
or constricting adventitia; removal of the latter will allow it to dilate.

The graft introducing tube is inserted, with gentle pressure, from the popliteal fossa,
through the adductor canal to emerge in the groin incision. The vein graft is reversed and
pulled through the tube with long forceps. The tube is then removed and the proximal
end of the vein anastomosed (only three-quarters of the anastomosis being completed at
this stage) end-to-side to the popliteal artery using 1 or 0·75 (5/0 or 6/0) silk or polyester
as a continuous running suture. The proximal anastomosis of the narrow (distal) end of
the vein to the common femoral artery, also end-to-side is completed. Distal, then
proximal clamps are released to test for distal reverse flow and to wash out any clots from
the graft. The clamps are then re-applied, the distal anastomosis completed and the
clamps removed for a second time.

Surgicel may be applied locally to control small leaks, but larger ones will require
insertion of further sutures. Heparinisation is reversed with appropriate amounts of
protamine sulphate.

Wounds are closed with interrupted skin sutures only with closed Redivac suction
drainage.

Disobliteration (Re-bore thrombo endarterectomy)

DEFINITION
Removal of a central atheromatous obstructive core of an artery leaving an outer

layer which is free from disease, usually performed on the aorta, iliac, femoral, or popliteal arteries, also the vertebral, subclavian and carotid arteries.

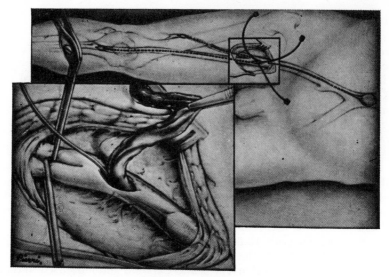

Figure 381   The atheromatous core after it has been stripped out of the femoral artery.
(Genito-Urinary Mfg. Co.)

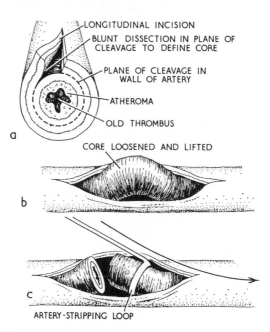

Figure 382   Disobliteration of 'rebore': (a) is the cross-section of the diseased artery. The dotted line shows the plane of cleavage within the wall of the artery around the atheromatous inner layer and the solid centre of old thrombosis. In (b) the core has been lifted out and in (c) the core has been divided and an artery stripping loop threaded over it, preparatory to being thrust up the affected length of artery. (Figures 382 and 383 by kind permission of Prof. A. Harding Rains and the Nursing Times, published May 1964.)

POSITION AND INSTRUMENTS

As femoral popliteal bypass graft
Cannon's endarterectomy ring strippers or similar.

OUTLINE OF PROCEDURE

A long thrombo endarterectomy may be performed if the long saphenous vein is not suitable as a graft (see previous operation). This may occur if the vein is too narrow, or has been thrombosed, or is varicose, or absent.

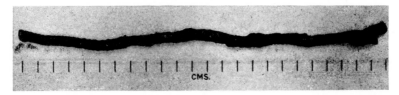

Figure 383   The atheromatous core after it has been stripped out of the femoral artery (the mark indicates 1 cm.)

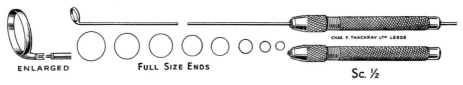

Figure 384   Cannon endarterectomy ring strippers.

The thrombo endarterectomy is carried out from patent artery above to patent artery below, through multiple arteriotomies. These are repaired using patches of vein graft or Dacron to prevent narrowing.

Through the arteriotomies, the atheromatous core is divided and the loop of the instrument is threaded over one end of the core. Holding this core with artery forceps, the loop is pushed along the plane of cleavage between the core and the vessel wall thereby affecting separation.

At the most distal arteriotomy, the intima is tacked down to the subjacent media by 3 or 4 0.75 (6/0) silk or polyester sutures tied on the outside. This prevents flap formation or 'dissection' which results in occlusion.

There are a number of ring strippers and dissectors in use including Cannon's ring strippers and Macdonald's dissector. A method has been developed using high pressure CO_2 gas which acts in a similar manner.

Short occlusions are treated by localised thrombo endarterectomy and the arteriotomy is repaired by vein or Dacron patches.

29

Plaster of Paris Technique

For further details of plaster techniques, the reader is referred to *Gypsona Technique* by Smith & Nephew, and to English, M. (1957). *Plaster of Paris Technique*. Edinburgh: Livingstone.

Although metal and wooden splints are still used for the immobilisation of some fractures, plaster of Paris has almost entirely superseded these. Gone are the days when theatre or plaster room staff had to prepare their own bandages, for manufacturers now make ready prepared bandages which have all the advantages of the hand-made articles. The basic constituent of plaster of Paris is gypsum or calcium sulphate which is quarried in rock form. The gypsum is ground into a fine powder and heated to evaporate most of the water content to form plaster of Paris. The powder is mixed with chemical solvents and cellulose. Combined with a heating process, the liquid is impregnated on to an open woven, interlocked fabric which holds the plaster uniformly. The impregnated fabric can then be fashioned into bandages and slabs of various sizes. The addition of resin to the basic process of manufacture helps to minimise plaster loss after moistening the bandage, thereby reducing the number of bandages needed for each cast.

Gypsona, manufactured by Smith & Nephew Ltd., is a brand of plaster of Paris which is used extensively in orthopaedics today. The booklet *Gypsona Technique* provides an excellent treatise on all aspects of the 'art and craft' of plastering. This chapter provides a basic outline of plaster procedure related to the operating theatre and readers are referred to *Gypsona Technique* for a more extensive exposition.

Requirements for plaster of Paris application

A deep pail or bowl for soaking the plaster bandages. (This should be three parts filled with tepid water 25 to 35°C (77 to 95°F).)

Plaster bandages of various widths.

Prepared slabs in Gypsona dispenser.

Cotton bandages 5 cm and 7·5 cm (2 in and 3 in).

Crepe bandages of various widths.

Macintoshes, or disposable paper towels.

Plaster wool and orthopaedic felt for padding.

Tubular stockinet of various widths.

Plaster scissors (usually of the Böhler type).

Heavy angled dressing scissors.

Plaster shears.

Plaster benders.

Plaster knife.

Tape measure and marking pencil.

A suitable table top or glass sheet for the preparation of slabs.

Dusting powder or olive oil may be needed for application to the patient's skin before plastering is commenced, especially if a tight plaster cast is being applied.

An electric plaster saw may be required for the removal of a dry cast.

Application of plaster of Paris

Some surgeons prefer to apply their own plaster casts but this may be left to experienced plaster staff who specialise in the art.

The person applying plaster usually wears rubber boots and apron. Rubber gloves may be worn although this is a matter for individual preference.

Plaster slabs

Some operations such as tendon suture of the hand and certain fresh fractures require only the application of a plaster slab for immobilisation, followed by a gauze or crêpe bandage. This provides a well-fitting splint which is quick to prepare and easy to remove for dressings, etc.

There are four methods of preparing plaster slabs:

(a) By unrolling dry plaster bandages,
(b) By unrolling wet plaster bandages,

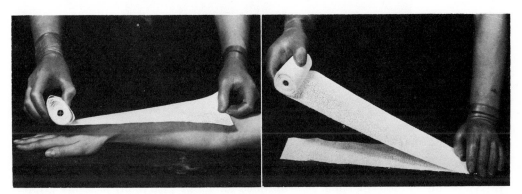

Figure 385   Dry method of preparing plaster slabs.

(c) By using 5 or 6 thickness plies material from a dry plaster dispenser,
(d) The pattern technique.

(a) The slab is prepared from either dry or wet Gypsona plaster bandages folded out on a smooth surface. The most usual way is to use dry plaster bandages, for the operator may measure and cut the slab at his own speed without fear of the plaster setting before this has been completed.

The dry bandage is placed alongside the limb and the length required marked with a pencil or cut. Alternatively, a tape measure may be used and the length required marked on a bandage which has been unrolled sufficiently on the table-top. The necessary thickness, usually four to six layers, is obtained by unwinding the bandage 'to and fro'. Care must be taken to ensure that all layers extend for the same distance and short ends are discarded.

To apply, the slab is lightly folded from each end to the centre, immersed in water and immediately removed. After submergence, surplus water may then be removed by compression, which must be moderately light, for strong squeezing will cause quick setting and vice versa.

After extending the squeezed slab, it is placed on the table-top and carefully smoothed out to remove air bubbles. Failure to do this may cause the finished slab to crack or crumble after application.

Widths of slabs vary according to the individual surgeon's requirements, but the nurse will find generally that a 10 to 15 cm (4 to 6 in) wide slab is suitable for the forearm or a child's leg, but a 15 to 20 cm (6 to 8 in) wide slab will be needed for the lower limb. A larger cast such as a spica may incorporate wider slabs described in the pattern technique.

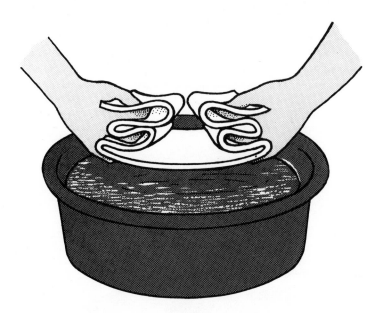

Figure 386   Method of wetting a plaster slab. (From *Gypsona Technique*.)

(b) With this method the bandage is unrolled for about 5 cm (2 in), *held* (not gripped) in the hand and lowered into the water until all bubbling has ceased, usually 5 to 10 seconds. Gripping of the bandage should be avoided because it tends to force plaster out of the fabric. The bandage is then lifted out of the water, and the two edges squeezed towards the centre and each other with the thumb and forefinger of each hand. This will allow excess moisture to run out of the bandage, but will retain the greater part of the plaster.

The slab is made by pressing the end of the bandage on to the table-top and holding it there with the left hand. The bandage is then unrolled with the right hand, 'to and fro,' to form the correct length and thickness of slab. The air bubbles are smoothed out and the slab applied immediately. The nurse will find it useful to place a stout rod through the centre core of the bandage before unrolling during the preparation of a slab.

(c) The required length of 6 thickness plies (5 thickness low plaster loss) is withdrawn from a dry plaster dispenser. This is quicker and more reliable than the unrolling method. The slab is applied as described under (a).

(d) Another method is the pattern technique by which standard dry plaster slabs are prepared before they are required, using wide Gypsona material.

The patterns described in this chapter are for hip, shoulder and spinal jacket.

The patterns allow for shrinkage after the slabs have been moistened. If the slabs are cut to individual measurements and not the patterns, 10 per cent should be added to these measurements to compensate for this shrinkage.

The slabs are moistened by submerging flat in a sink filled to a depth of 8 to 10 cm (3 to 4 in). The surplus water is removed by drawing the slab over the edge of the sink as it is lifted out. Air bubbles are expressed by smoothing the slab on the table-top, after which it is applied immediately, moulded to the part, and held in place by open wove or Gypsona bandages.

Any slab may be reinforced to withstand additional stress by ridging or girdering. Ridging consists of raising the centre of the slab for 10 mm ($\frac{3}{8}$ in) along its length, after which it is applied carefully to the cast. Girdering is accomplished by superimposing a ridged slab which is about 10 cm shorter than the underlying one.

If the cast has dried, the surface should be roughened and moistened before the application of further slabs.

Application of plaster bandages

Plaster bandages may be used either to make a cast or to complete one after slabs have been applied.

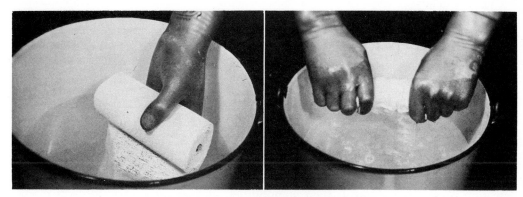

Figure 387   Method of wetting a plaster bandage.

Bony prominences are padded with plaster wool or felt after applying tubular stockinet if required. The stockinet should be longer than the completed plaster to allow turning back for 2·5 cm (1 in) or so just before the final bandages are applied.

The bandages are submerged in tepid water in the manner described for the preparation of wet slabs. They are applied, using even circular turns with no reversing and with a rolling action, not as an ordinary bandage. Any threads which work free from the bandage as it is applied should be cut away, otherwise tightening may occur afterwards. Each turn of the bandage should cover approximately two-thirds of the previous turn. Smooth pleats can be made in the upper or lower edges of the bandage, to allow it to 'sit' evenly when following the contour of a limb. A pause is made after each bandage has been applied, to mould the plaster to the part and allow the layers to set. As the finished plaster cast should be an homogenous mass rather than a series of layers, the moulding is very necessary, together with the exclusion of air between each plaster bandage.

The nurse holding the limb should support it with extended palms to avoid indentations from her finger tips which can cause pressure sores at the point of indentation. She should be very careful to maintain the correct position during the whole period of application.

After application, the plaster cast should be supported on macintosh covered pillows until it has dried. Drying may be hastened in the ward with a heat cradle, but care must be taken to protect exposed areas of the patient's skin from burns, especially if he is unconscious.

An unpadded plaster is very rarely applied to fresh fractures due to the subsequent swelling which always occurs. Even with padding, it may be necessary to bi-valve or cut the plaster along its entire length to allow for this swelling. As the swelling subsides and the plaster becomes loose, it may need to be reapplied (with little padding) to ensure immobilisation.

If it is known that a plaster cast may require splitting, a greased rubber or plastic tube should be placed anteriorly along the length of the limb before plastering is commenced. This tube may be pulled out of the completed plaster easily, leaving a channel inside which simplifies cutting afterwards.

Control of setting time

Normally tepid water (25 to 35°C (77 to 95°F)) should be used for moistening plaster bandages; cold water may cause involuntary muscular contractions if the patient is conscious, and hot water will cause the plaster to set too quickly.

Gypsona bandages set in four to six minutes using tepid water. It is possible to retard this setting time by adding borax to the water.

The setting may be retarded for 1 minute by adding two heaped teaspoonfuls of borax to 1 gal (0·5 per cent); for 7 minutes by adding four level dessertspoonfuls of borax to 1 gal (0·75 per cent); and for 15 minutes by adding one heaped tablespoonful of borax to 1 gal.

TYPES OF PLASTER CASTS

Arm

Colles' fracture

After reduction, the hand is maintained in a position of full pronation and ulnar deviation. A simple fracture is then immobilised with an incomplete forearm plaster, and a severe fracture is immobilised with a mid-arm pronation plaster.

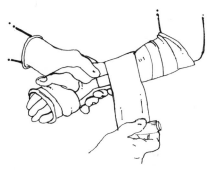

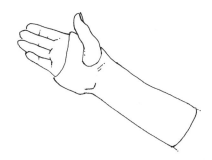

Figure 388   Colles fracture. Slab bound with
            wet gauze bandage.

Figure 389   Colles fracture plaster completed.

For an incomplete plaster, the elbow is flexed to 90 degrees and the arm is covered with stockinet or a thin layer of plaster wool bandage. A dorsal slab is made from 15 cm (6 in) wide 5 or 6 ply plaster bandage, the length of the slab being 15 cm (6 in) more than the measurement from the elbow to the metacarpal heads. The slab is applied and extends 2·5 cm (1 in) from the olecranon process (where it is folded obliquely to avoid pressing into the antecubital fossa when the elbow is flexed) to 13 mm ($\frac{1}{2}$ in) proximal to the meta-carpal heads. The slab must be well moulded and extend round the ventral surface of the radius and base of the first metacarpal to prevent radial deviation. The slab is fixed to forearm with a *wet* gauze bandage or a crêpe bandage which is applied from the elbow to the wrist where it is carried across the palm.

For a complete plaster, stockinet is applied and the elbow flexed to 90 degrees with full pronation of the hand. Plaster wool bandage is used at the elbow and at mid-arm. A short Colles' plaster is applied as previously described, followed by a U-slab made from 10 cm (4 in) wide 5 or 6 ply plaster bandage which is applied to the upper arm. This slab is secured with a wet gauze bandage or crêpe bandage, followed by a 10 cm (4 in) wide by 2·74 m (3 yd) plaster bandage, which extends below for one turn only.

Both these plasters may be completed after swelling has subsided by applying plaster bandages circular fashion round the forearm and upper arm.

Alternatively, a completed plaster cast may be applied over plaster wool bandage and is changed for a skin-tight plaster when swelling has subsided.

Scaphoid fracture

The wrist is maintained in a position of radial deviation and dorsiflexion. A modified short arm Colles' plaster which incorporates the thumb up to the distal joint is applied.

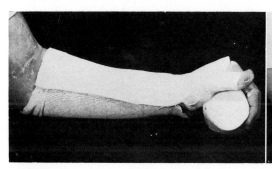 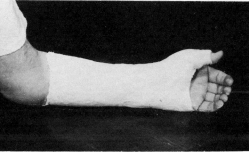

Figure 390   Scaphoid fracture. Dorsal slab applied.   Figure 391   Scaphoid fracture. Plaster completed.

The slab is prepared by cutting a notch to accommodate the thumb, and it is then bound to the dorsum of the arm and hand with a *wet* gauze bandage in the usual manner.

When the swelling has subsided, the plaster is completed with circular turns of two 10 cm (4 in) wide by 2·74 m (3 yd) plaster bandages. Alternatively, a completed padded cast may be applied at first and renewed when it becomes loose.

Fractures of the radius and ulna

There are two types of plasters – full flexed elbow and straight arm. The flexed elbow plaster is most generally used unless contraindicated by the position of the fracture, as straight arm plasters tend to cause a stiff elbow joint, especially in adults.

For a flexed arm plaster, the forearm is generally in a position of mid-pronation, although some fractures may require full pronation or supination. The fracture is reduced with counter-traction applied by means of a sling round the upper arm. Stockinet is applied, followed by plaster wool bandage round the wrist, elbow and upper arm. A U-slab is prepared from 10 cm (4 in) 5 or 6 ply wide 2·74 m (3 yd) plaster bandage and is applied along the dorsal aspect of the forearm, extending from 13 mm ($\frac{1}{2}$ in) behind the knuckles, round the elbow and along the palmar aspect to finish at the wrist crease. This slab is retained with a few turns of a circular plaster bandage and after it has set the counter-traction sling is removed.

A second U-slab is prepared from 10 cm (4 in) 5 or 6 ply wide by 2·74 m (3 yd) plaster bandage sufficiently long to extend from the axilla round the elbow and up the outer

Figure 392   Forearm fractures, flexed elbow plaster. U-slab applied to forearm and secured with a few turns of a circular plaster bandage.

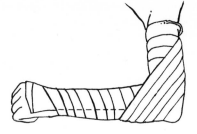

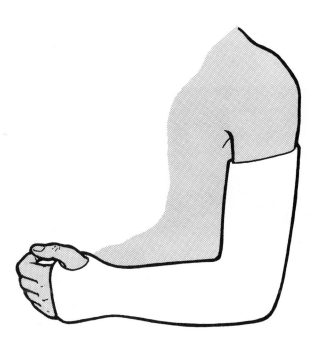

Figure 393   Full arm plaster cast completed. (From *Gypsona Technique*.)

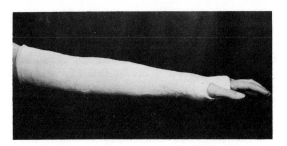

Figure 394   Forearm fractures. Straight arm plaster cast completed.

aspect of the arm to just below the shoulder. This slab is retained with a few turns of a circular plaster bandage in the usual manner, and the elbow section is strengthened with one 10 cm (4 in) wide by 2·74 m (3 yd) plaster bandage applied obliquely from upper to lower arm round the elbow.

If swelling increases, the gauze bandage is cut and a fresh one applied. As swelling decreases, fresh or additional gauze bandages are applied to take up the 'slack'. When swelling has completely subsided, the cast is completed with circular turns of one or two plaster bandages.

Alternatively, a complete padded plaster may be applied at first, and changed when it becomes loose.

For a straight arm plaster, the elbow is extended and stockinet applied, followed by plaster wool bandages to the wrist, elbow and upper arm. The wrist is placed in a position of pronation and a dorsal slab made from 10 cm (4 in) 5 or 6 ply plaster bandage is applied. This should extend from the axilla to the wrist for olecranon fractures, and from just below the axilla to 13 mm ($\frac{1}{2}$ in) proximal to the metacarpal heads for all forearm fractures. The slab is held in position by a wet gauze bandage, and when swelling has subsided the cast is completed with plaster bandages in the usual way.

Fractures of the humerus

Middle and Upper Third. The patient stands or sits with his trunk inclined towards the injured side and his upper arm hanging vertically. The forearm is supported with the elbow flexed to 90 degrees and adhesive felt is applied to pad the outer end of the clavicle and acromium process. A thin layer of plaster wool bandage may be applied from the elbow to the axilla and any tendency to outward angulation of a high shaft fracture is countered with a pad of wool placed to keep the elbow away from the body.

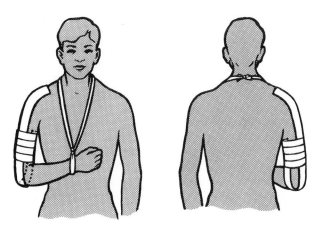

Figure 395   Upper and middle third fractures of the humerus. Slab applied and secured with wet gauze bandage or crêpe bandage and arm supported with collar and cuff sling. (From *Gypsona Technique*.)

A slab is made from 15 cm (6 in) 5 or 6 ply plaster bandage, and is applied from the axilla, along the inner aspect of the arm, round the elbow, up the outer aspect of the arm and over the shoulder where 15 cm (6 in) excess (allowed in the slab length) is turned back and secured with strapping. The slab is bound to the arm with a *wet* gauze bandage or a crêpe bandage, and the forearm is supported with a collar and cuff sling.

Lower Third. A U-slab is applied in the manner just described, and a strip of wet lint is placed over the forearm and lower part of the U-slab. A short slab about 40 cm (16 in) long is prepared and applied to the dorsal aspect of the forearm. This slab extends from the wrist to just above the elbow, and is secured with a *wet* gauze bandage or crêpe bandage. The wet lint prevents adherence of the two slabs so that the lower slab can be removed after an interval of two weeks or so.

Alternatively, a padded complete plaster may be applied at first and renewed if necessary.

Shoulder

Shoulder abduction spica

This is used for some upper humeral or shoulder fractures and post-operative immobilisation for shoulder arthrodesis.

The cast is applied with the patient seated on a backless stool or supported sitting up on the operation table. The arm is abducted about 60 degrees from the side, being carried well forward in front of the coronal plane and with some 15 degrees lateral rotation. The correct position for ankylosis should enable the hand to reach the mouth by flexion of the elbow alone. An assistant supports the elbow and forearm.

A stockinet lining is applied followed by adhesive felt pads over the iliac crests, either side of the spinous process, across the clavicle on the affected side and under the elbow with a small hole to accommodate the medial epicondyle. Plaster wool bandages are then applied to cover the area to be enclosed.

A light layer of plaster bandage is applied over the plaster wool. Plaster slabs, 15 cm (6 in) wide, are applied from the iliac crests under the axilla to the elbow; from the axilla on the soundside across the affected shoulder and upper arm, anteriorly and posteriorly (Fig. 396). In addition 15 cm (6 in) wide slabs can be applied from the suprasternal notch to the symphysis pubis and posteriorly from the seventh cervical vertebra to the sacrum. The cast is completed with circular plaster bandages.

Using the pattern technique, identical posterior and anterior body sections are prepared from six layers of 90 cm (24 in) wide plaster material. A combined shoulder, arm and forearm slab is made in a similar manner, using the pattern technique as illustrated. The length A-B equals the distance (plus 10 per cent) between the base of the neck and upper aspect of the flexed elbow joint (point E), plus half the circumference of the forearm. The length C-D is the distance from the same point E to the knuckles, plus half the circumference of the arm. The distances M-L and B-N are the circumference of the arm and of the forearm respectively. The distance A-S usually equals that between the base of the neck and the point of the shoulder. The shaded portions are cut away and reserved for reinforcement of the cast.

Stockinet and felt padding is applied as previously described followed by the anterior and posterior body sections which are moulded carefully and secured with one or two 10 cm (4 in) wide by 2·74 m (3 yds) plaster bandages. The arm section is then applied, moulded and secured with plaster bandages in a similar manner, and the axilla is strengthened with the surplus plaster material remaining from the wide pieces.

If a strut is desired, this may be made from the cores of the bandages, cut to length, covered with plaster material and fixed between the body and arm with a few turns of plaster bandage.

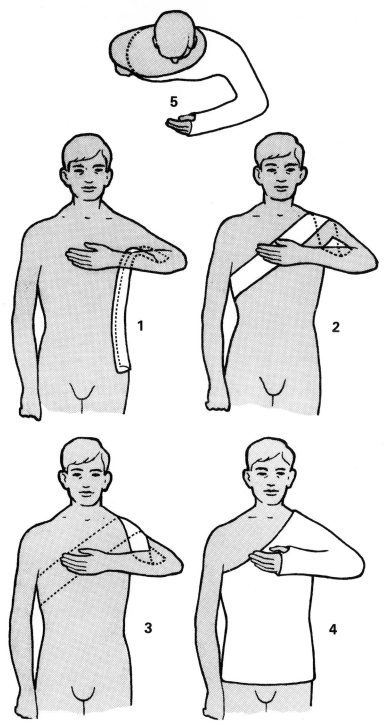

Figure 396 Method of applying slabs for shoulder abduction spica and completed spica cast. (From *Gypsona Technique.*)

The cast is trimmed as indicated in Figure 396 and the edges made neat by turning back and securing the edges of the stockinet lining.

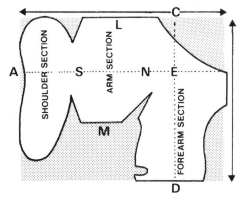

Figure 397   Shoulder abduction spica. Pattern for shoulder and arm section.

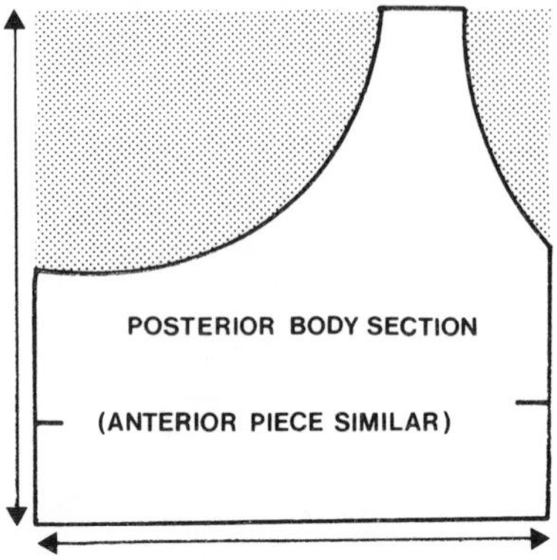

Figure 398   Shoulder abduction spica. Pattern for anterior and posterior body sections.

Leg

Fractures of the tarsus, metatarsus, internal and external malleoli, and stable Potts fractures

These fractures are immobilised with below-knee casts. The fracture is reduced (if necessary) and the knee flexed as shown in the illustration, with the foot dorsiflexed. Alternatively, a padded knee rest may be used and the leg supported by an assistant. Stockinet and plaster wool bandage are then applied from just below the knee to the toes.

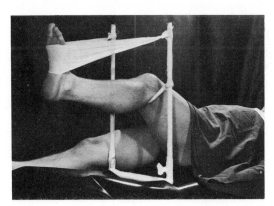

Figure 399   Below-knee plaster cast. Leg supported with foot dorsiflexed.

A plaster stirrup may then be prepared from 10 cm (4 in) plaster bandages and applied commencing just below the knee, continuing down the leg, round the heel, to finish just below the knee on the outer side where any excess is turned back. This stirrup is bound loosely in place with a plaster bandage.

A back slab is prepared from 15 cm (6 in), 5 or 6 ply plaster bandage (10 or 12 ply if the plaster stirrup has not been used) and is applied extending from just below the knee, round the heel (where a cut is made to accommodate the ankle) and along the sole of the foot where excess slab is temporarily dropped over the toes, or in front of the surgeon's knees if the plaster is being applied with the leg flexed over the end of the table. The slab is secured with two 15 cm (6 in) wide by 2·74 m (3 yd) plaster bandages from just below

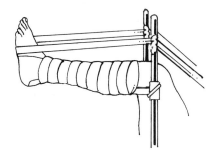

Figure 400   Below-knee plaster cast. Stirrup applied and secured with plaster bandage.

the knee to include the ankle. The excess slab is turned back to make a double thickness of plaster which extends just beyond the toes (toe platform). This foot portion of the slab is secured with one or two 10 cm (4 in) wide by 2·74 m (3 yd) plaster bandages and another similar bandage is applied round the ankle to provide reinforcement. The toe platform portion of the slab must not be bent upwards, as contracture of the extensor tendons may occur.

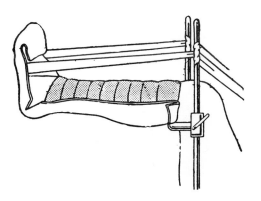

Figure 401   Below-knee plaster cast. Back slab applied and excess turned over toes temporarily.

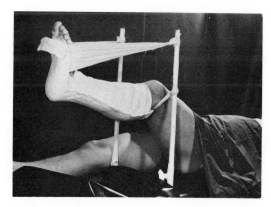

Figure 402   Below-knee plaster cast. Showing how toe platform is made by turning back slab.

Severe Potts fractures; fractures of the lower third of the tibia; and fractures of the upper tibia when the patient is immobilised in bed.

These fractures are immobilised with mid-thigh casts. If the fracture is comparatively stable, the below-knee portion of the cast is applied first as described previously, but with the stockinet extended to mid-thigh. Plaster wool bandage is then applied round the knee joint and thigh.

Anterior and posterior slabs 76 cm (30 in) long are each prepared from two 15 cm (6 in) wide by 2·74 m (3 yd) plaster bandages. These are applied from a point 20 cm (8 in) below the knee joint to mid-thigh, where any excess bandage is turned back. The slabs are secured to the limb in the usual manner with two 15 cm (6 in) wide by 2·74 m (3 yd) plaster bandages.

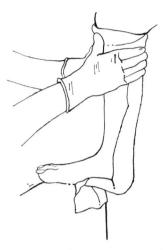
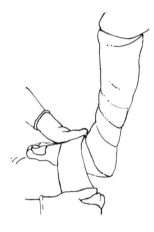

Figure 403   Below-knee plaster cast, alternative method. Back slab applied and excess turned back in front of surgeon's knees temporarily.

Figure 404   Below-knee plaster cast, alternative method. Plaster bandages applied spirally to secure back slab. Note how toe platform is made.

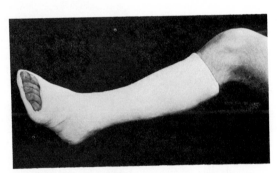

Figure 405   Below-knee plaster cast completed.

If the fracture is unstable, it is usually easier to apply the upper and lower portions of the cast in one operation. A thin layer of plaster wool is applied to the limb and the fracture is reduced. The limb is supported by two padded wedges, as illustrated, one under the knee joint and one under the fracture, or alternatively, this second wedge is dispensed with and the fracture area supported by an assistant.

Two anterior slabs are prepared from six layers of wide plaster material, or alternatively, from 15 cm (6 in) wide by 2·74 m (3 yd) plaster bandages. These slabs are applied on each side, from mid-thigh along the anterolateral aspect of the limb, and round the sole of the foot. They are moulded carefully and secured with two 15 cm (6 in) wide by 2·74 m (3 yd) plaster bandages, leaving two small gaps where the limb is supported by the wedges or assistant.

When the anterior slabs have set, the lower wedge or support is withdrawn and a back slab made from two 15 cm (16 in) wide by 2·74 m (3 yd) plaster bandages is applied from behind the knee to the toes, where it forms the toe platform. The slab is secured with two 15 cm (6 in) wide by 2·74 m (3 yd) plaster bandages applied spirally.

The knee wedge is removed and another back slab prepared from two 15 cm (6 in) wide by 2·74 m (3 yd) plaster bandages. This slab is applied to the back of the thigh, extending down beyond the knee, and is secured with two 15 cm (6 in) wide by 2·74 m (3 yd) plaster bandages.

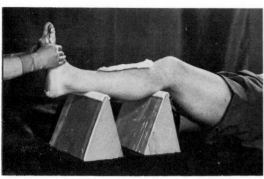 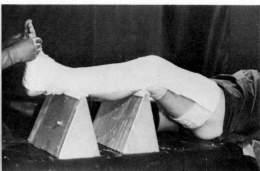

Figure 406   Mid-thigh plaster cast for unstable fractures of the lower leg. Supporting wedges in position.

Figure 407   Mid-thigh plaster cast for unstable fractures of the lower leg. Anterior lateral slabs applied.

When the swelling has subsided and the plaster becomes loose, it will be changed to a full length tuber bearing plaster, which is in effect a mid-thigh cast extended to the tuber ischii where it is padded similarly to a walking caliper.

Hip

Hip spica

This is used for immobilisation of infective conditions of the knee, femur and hip; fractures of the femur and hip; osteotomy of the femur; pelvic injuries and arthrodesis of the hip. The double hip spica is the cast most frequently applied in theatre and this will be described.

The patient is placed on extension apparatus as illustrated, and all bony prominences are padded with adhesive felt, i.e., the anterior superior iliac spines, the sacrum, head of the fibula, both malleoli and the tendo achillis. Stockinet is applied to the trunk and legs. Other padding depends upon the type of patient. A thin patient will require a good deal of padding in the form of plaster wool, whereas a stout patient will require very little.

The cast consists of a series of circular bandages and reinforcing slabs, 15 cm (6 in) wide applied as illustrated in Fig. 408. The hip section is reinforced by slabs positioned anteriorly and posteriorly from the lower ribs on each side around the hip to the groin and also from the lower ribs down to the lateral side of the knee. The cast is completed by circular bandages; 20 cm (8 in) used in a figure of eight manner around the pelvis and the hip, and 15 cm (6 in) bandages from the hip joint to the knee joint. Using the pattern technique the main part of the spica consists of slabs which are made from wide plaster material. For a double hip spica five slabs are required: a posterior section of seven or eight layers, two anterior sections of four layers, a complete long leg section of eight layers, and a thigh and pelvic section of eight layers. One heaped tablespoonful of borax may be added to a sink filled with tepid water to a depth of about 8 cm (3 in), and this retards setting of the plaster and allows time for adequate moulding.

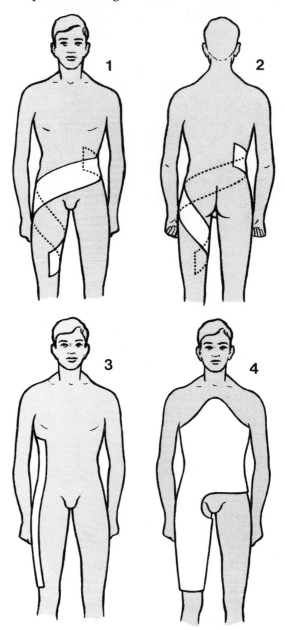

Figure 408 Hip spica. Method of applying reinforcing slabs to right hip. This manoeuvre is repeated for the left side in a double hip spica. (From *Gypsona Technique*.)

The posterior body section is soaked, drained, smoothed and applied. The slab is moulded carefully and secured with a few turns of a 20 cm (8 in) wide by 2·74 m (3 yd) plaster bandage.

The first anterior body section is then soaked, drained, smoothed and applied, followed by the second anterior section which is reversed so that each thigh section can be moulded carefully round the upper part of the leg.

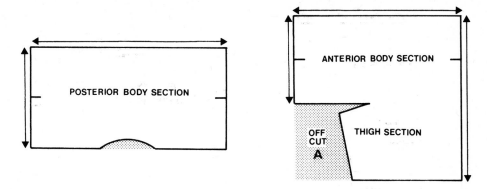

Figure 409 Hip spica. Pattern for posterior body section.

Figure 410 Hip spica. Pattern for anterior body section.

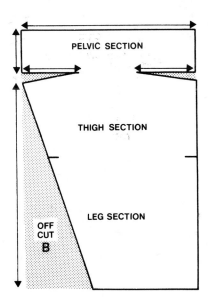

Figure 411 Hip spica. Pattern for leg sections.

The long leg section is then soaked, drained, smoothed and applied to the lateral aspect of the body, thigh and lower leg, so that the pelvic section stretches roughly from the opposite anterior superior iliac spine to the tuber ischii on the slab side, and the leg section extends down to the foot stirrup. The thigh and leg sections are carefully moulded and the back of the hip is reinforced with the surplus material remaining from the cut slabs.

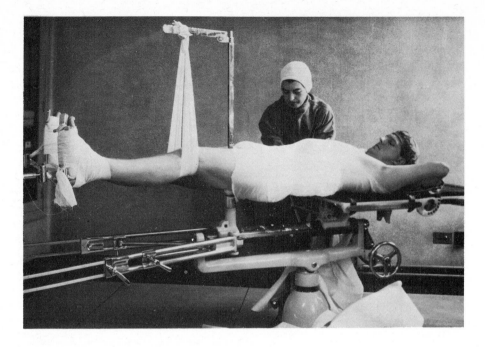

Figure 412   Hip spica, pattern technique. Posterior body section applied.

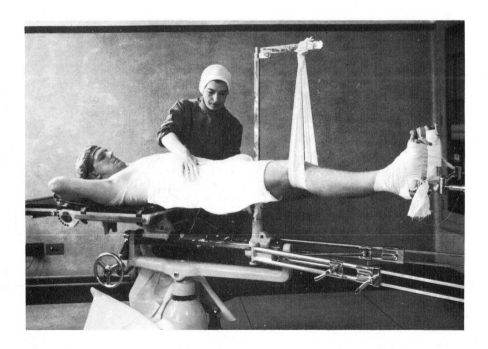

Figure 413   Hip spica, pattern technique. Anterior body section applied.

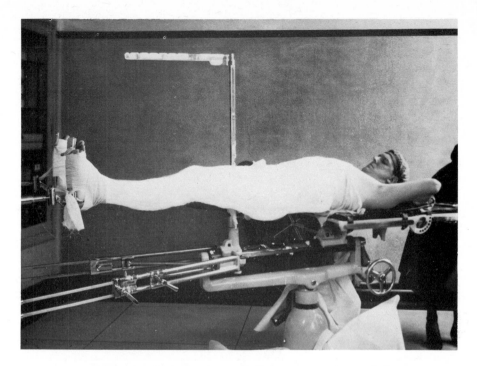

Figure 414   Hip spica, pattern technique. Leg section applied.

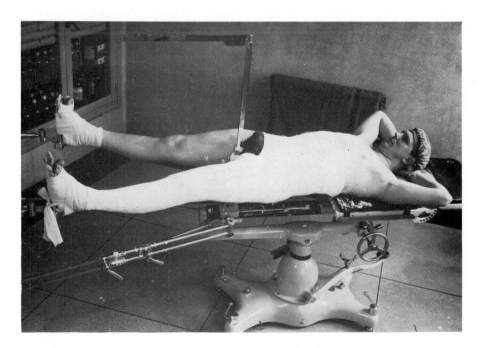

Figure 415   Hip spica completed.

The short thigh section is soaked, drained, smoothed and applied to the opposite pelvis and thigh. This section is finished just proximal to the knee joint so that full flexion is possible afterwards. The ankle section is completed with 10 cm (4 in) wide by 2·74 m (3 yd) plaster bandages and this may be extended to include the foot if required.

The whole spica is secured firmly with several 15 and 20 cm (6 and 8 in) wide plaster bandages and the stockinet is turned back at the upper and lower limits of the plaster in the usual manner. If the spica is required to incorporate the upper ribs, the depth of body sections must be increased accordingly.

Spine

Spinal jacket

This is used for immobilisation of a fractured spine. The patient is placed in a position of hyperextension between two tables as illustrated or standing erect. Cervical traction may

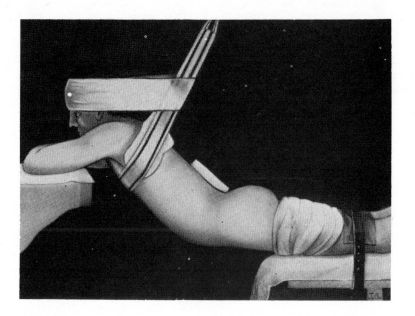

Figure 416   Plaster spinal jacket. Position of patient.

be used if standing, to give extension to the spine and to overcome spasm of the erector spinae muscles. Stockinet is applied to the trunk and leg and adhesive felt pads are applied to the manubrium sternum, the symphysis pubis and over the fracture area.

Stockinet is applied followed by felt padding over the iliac crests and down either side of the spinous processes. The whole area is covered with plaster wool compressed with a light covering of plaster bandages. Plaster slabs 15 cm wide (6 in) are applied (as illustrated in Fig. 417) followed by 15 or 20 cm (6 or 8 in) plaster bandages to complete the cast (Fig. 419). Using the pattern technique, two slabs are made from six layers of wide plaster material and are soaked, drained, smoothed separately and applied to overlap as illustrated. The overlap anteriorly should be 15 cm (6 in) and the slab extends from the manubrium sternum to the symphysis pubis. Posteriorly the shorter edges overlap in the lumbar region. The slabs are secured with several 15 cm (6 in) wide plaster bandages and the edges turned over where necessary to avoid trimming. The stockinet is turned back at the periphery of the jacket in the usual manner.

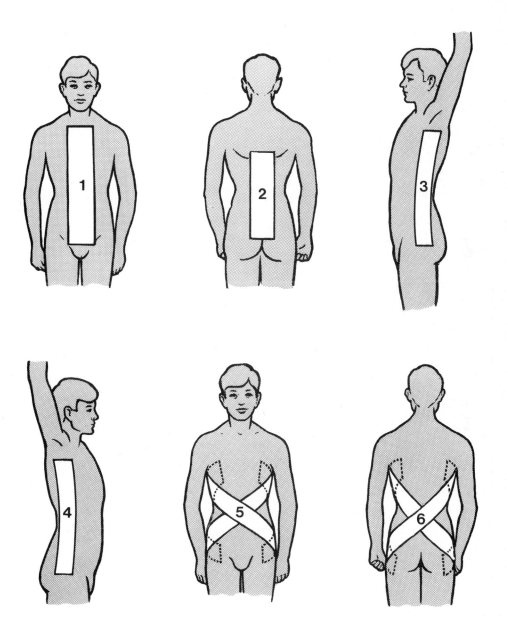

Figure 417   Plaster spinal jacket. Application of plaster reinforcing slabs. (From *Gypsona Technique*.)

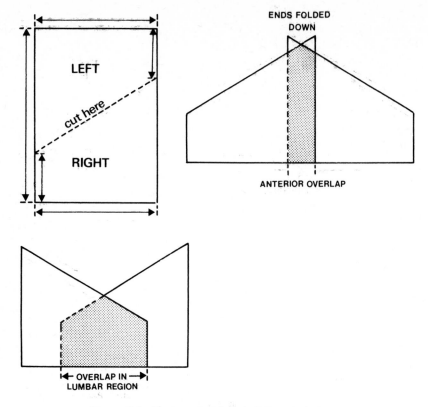

Figure 418   Plaster spinal jacket. Pattern technique.

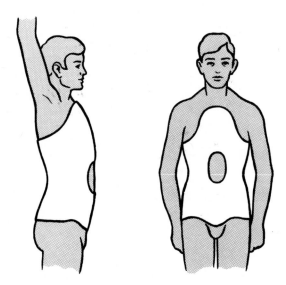

Figure 419   Plaster spinal jacket. Completed cast. (From *Gypsona Technique*.)

30

Radioactive Materials in the Theatre

Radium is an element emitting powerful rays which are used for the destruction of malignant or other abnormal tissue.

These rays are energy liberated as a result of constant disintegration of the element, and consist of three forms: alpha, beta and gamma radiation. It is gamma rays which are utilised for therapeutic purposes, the alpha and beta rays generally being excluded by using metal screens made of platinum 0·5 to 1·0 mm thick, although beta rays are sometimes used therapeutically.

Radium is generally used in the form of radium sulphate and is virtually indestructible, for its 'half-life' is about 1,700 years.

Over-exposure to the radiation from radium or radioactive products is dangerous, and care must be taken to ensure that this does not occur, either to the patient or staff.

Radium needles and tubes

Practically all the radium used medically today is prepared as needles or tubes. The needles, made from platinum, are hollowed to contain the radium salt and have a trocar point and an eye to which thread may be attached. Radium for use in gynaecology is in tubes, having no trocar and sometimes an eye. There are varying sizes of needles and tubes containing from 0·5 to 50 mg of radium salt.

If needles are used individually, they are threaded with strong silk, tying the thread near but not on the eye, and leaving it about 15 cm (6 in) long. The silk threads may be of different colours, according to the strength of radium packed in the needle and help in the sorting and handling of various types, although the needles are engraved accordingly and vary in length. The knot should not be tied actually on the eye for it may break during or after insertion into the tissues.

Larger amounts of radium may be prepared by packing various sizes of needles or tubes into a silver or plastic box or tubes, making applicators which are covered with plastic or rubber before disinfection and insertion.

The needles and applicators are disinfected by pasteurisation in a suitable container, care being taken to avoid tangling of the threads. These should be clipped individually with artery forceps or arranged in slots incorporated in the container.

Other radioactive products for therapeutic use

Radium is being superseded by isotopes prepared by treating elements in the atomic reactor.

Radioactive cobalt, Co 60, 'half-life' of 5·3 years, and *radioactive caesium 137*, 'half-life' 30 years, has replaced radium to some degree. The cobalt/caesium element is placed in the atomic reactor and after radio-activation is prepared as needles and tubes in a similar manner to radium. Large amounts of radioactive cobalt Co 60 or caesium 137 are also incorporated in the beam unit for teletherapy.

Radioactive tantalum wire and radioactive gold-198 seeds 'half-life' 2·7 days are often used therapeutically, the radioactive gold seeds having superseded radon. As the emanation is for a limited time, these seeds may be left buried in the tissues, but are sometimes removed owing to the value of the containers.

All these radioactive isotopes require very careful handling as the radiation may be equally lethal to that of a similar amount of radium or radon.

Methods of radium application

1. *Surface application* is made by embedding the needles or applicators in a mould made from plaster of Paris, Stent composition, Acrylic, or sorbo rubber, etc. These moulds are placed in position over the area being treated for the requisite period.

2. *Teletherapy* is a form of treatment with a large amount of radioactive cobalt Co 60 or caesium 137 which is enclosed in a thick lead-walled chamber having an aperture through which the rays may be directed on to the area being treated. This is often called the radium or cobalt beam unit, but alternatively deep X-rays are used, generated by machines using several million volts of electricity.

3. *Interstitial irradiation* is applied by inserting radium needles, radioactive tantalum wire or radioactive gold seeds into the tissues.

4. *Cavitary irradiation* is applied by inserting applicators into the natural cavities of the body, e.g., the vagina or cervical canal.

Of the four methods of radium or radioactive isotopes application, only the last two are generally performed in the theatre. Surface application and teletherapy are performed on patients in the radiotherapy department either as inpatients or outpatients.

Precautions during the handling of radioactive products

1. All radioactive needles, applicators, wires, seeds are manipulated with long-handled forceps, the jaws of which are covered with rubber or plastic. *On no account should they be picked up by hand.*

2. All radioactive products must be carried in a special lead-lined container during transport between radium safe and the theatre. This container should be carried by the long handle or strap provided.

3. Any preparation of needles, wires or applicators must be performed behind special lead screens, using the long manipulation forceps.

4. Proximity to radioactive products should be minimal. All persons coming into regular contact with these are issued with personal monitoring films from which the physicist can determine the radiation dose received by the person concerned. Blood tests may be made regularly to ensure that the white cell-count remains within normal limits, especially if a suspected high dose has been recorded on the monitoring film.

5. The theatre sister or nurse is responsible for checking the radium, etc., when it arrives at the theatre and after disinfection.

Used needles and applicators are entered on the record sheet, and unused ones checked and placed in the transport container for immediate return to the radium custodian. If it is necessary to keep radioactive materials in the theatre for any length of time, a special lead-lined safe must be provided and the key retained by the person accepting responsibility for the materials.

6. The success of the treatment is dependent upon a carefully calculated dosage. The time at which the radium treatment is due to start and terminate must be carefully noted and strictly adhered to, for the time of contact with the tissues is one factor which affects dosage.

It is usual to use special record charts for the guidance of ward staff and others responsible during the course of treatment. In theatre on this card or chart is entered all relevant details, including the number, strength and position of needles, applicators, wires or seeds. The time inserted and time due for removal is also entered on this record chart, a sample of which is illustrated. This record is sent to the ward when the patient returns. There may also be a duplication which is returned to the radium custodian after the radioactive products have been inserted.

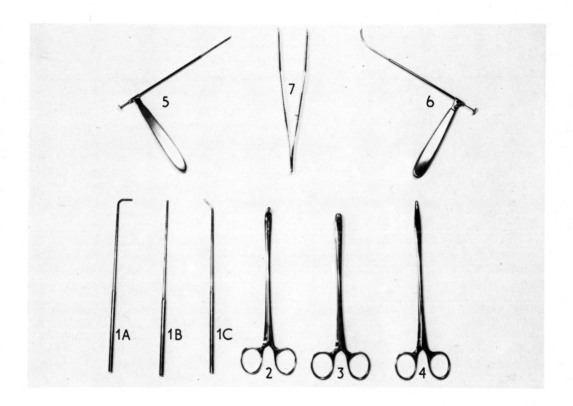

Figure 420   Radium insertion instruments.

1. A, B, C, Radium needle probes.
2., 3., 4., Radium needle insertion forceps (Finzi).

5., 6. Radon seed introducers (Christie Cancer Hospital).
7. Radium needle-holding forceps (Chester Williams).

Radium, cobalt and other products are very valuable as well as very dangerous. Careful checking at each stage of handling is important to avoid accidental loss. Radium containers left lying about the wards or departments, or radium needles, etc., which may have slipped out of their proper place and are lying in contact with healthy tissues are in the first case a danger to the staff, and in the second case a danger to the patient.

Misplacement or loss of any radioactive element must be reported immediately either to the radiotherapist or to the physicist. Strict observance of the instructions regarding handling of the radioactive materials makes this work completely safe nowadays.

COVENTRY & WARWICKSHIRE HOSPITAL
PHYSICS DEPARTMENT

DOSAGE FOR INTERSTITIAL RADIUM

PATIENT'S NAME Mr. R.J. SMITH

REG. No   XY 1234

SKETCH AND DETAILS:—

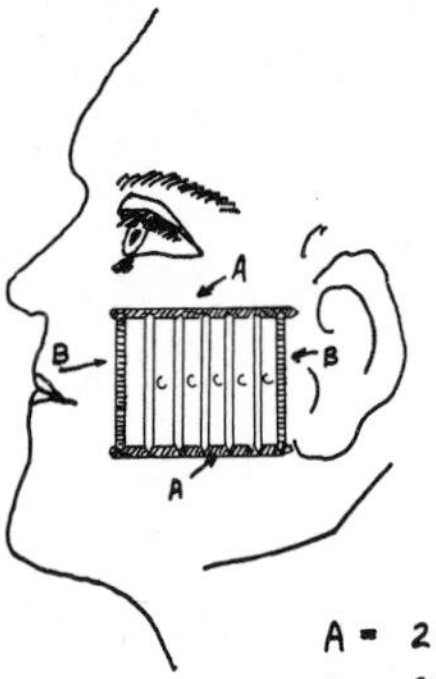

Surface lesion of cheek. Plane implant area approximately 2 × 3 cm, for lesion;— 4 × 5 cm, for implant.

Above area needs 2390 mg hrs of Radium (of filtration 0·5 mm Pt) ie: 168 hrs treatment requires 14 mg Ra.

Radium to be distributed as in sketch Effective Radium = 14·3 mg. Treatment time = ·167 hrs.

A = 2 of 3 mg (5·8 cm)
B = 2 of 2 mg (4·2 cm)
C = 5 of 1 mg (4·2 cm)

PROVISIONAL DOSAGE PRESCRIBED: 6500 RADS TO: 0·5 cm
PROVISIONAL DOSE RATE: 38·5 R/HR
PROVISIONAL DURATION OF IMPLANT: 168 HOURS
PROVISIONAL DATE & TIME FOR REMOVAL: 7 Days from time of implant

CORRECTED DOSE [ ]

SIGNATURE OF RADIOTHERAPIST

CORRECTED DOSE RATE: 40·5 R/HR
(METHOD OF DETERMINATION): Stereoscopic Reconstruction of implant from X-Rays.

CORRECTED DURATION OF IMPLANT: 150 hrs (6 days 6 hrs) HRS
CORRECTED DATE & TIME FOR REMOVAL [ ]

SIGNATURE OF PHYSICIST

Figure 421 Radium insertion record.

FURTHER READING

DHSS (1972) *Code of Practice for the Protection of Persons Against Ionizing Radiations Arising From Medical and Dental Use.* London: HMSO.

DHSS (1973) *The Safe Use of Ionizing Radiations – A Handbook for Nurses.* London: HMSO.

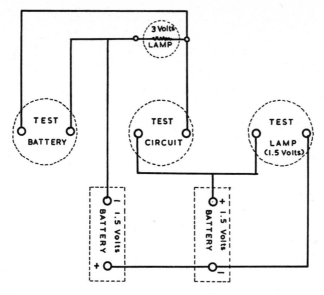

VOLT/AMP METER MAY BE SUBSTITUTED FOR LAMP

Figure 422   Voltage Diagram

Appendix I

TABLE I

SHOWING THE PRESSURE/TEMPERATURE RELATIONSHIP OF PHASE BOUNDARY STEAM AND THE ACTUAL TEMPERA-
TURES ACHIEVED IN AN AUTOCLAVE CHAMBER WITH PARTIAL AIR DISCHARGE

lb p.s.i.	Pure steam and complete air discharge		Two-thirds air discharge 20 in vacuum		One-half air discharge 15 in vacuum		One-third air discharge 10 in vacuum	
	Degrees C	Degrees F	Degrees C	Degrees F	Degrees C	Degrees F	Degrees C	Degrees F
15	121	250	115	240	112	234	109	228
20	126	259	121	250	118	245	115	240
25	130	267	126	259	124	254	121	250
30	135	275	130	267	128	263	126	259

This chart indicates the importance of temperature, as pressure which is a mixture of air and steam has a much lower temperature than that of pure steam. Partial air discharge means a much longer sterilisation period than if complete air discharge had been achieved from the chamber.

TABLE II

MEDICAL GAS CYLINDER CAPACITIES AND PRESSURES

Gas	Pressure of a full cylinder (lb p.s.i.)	Capacities of cylinders in common use	
		Boyle's machine	Transportable circle circuit machines
Oxygen, O_2	1,500/2,000	24 cubic feet	36 or 72 gallons
Nitrous oxide, N_2O	600/700	200 gallons	100 or 200 gallons
Carbon dioxide, CO_2	1,000	2 pounds weight	2 pounds weight
Cyclopropane, C_3H_6	90	40 or 80 gallons	40 or 80 gallons

TABLE III

CALIBRATIONS OF ROTAMETERS ON ANAESTHETIC MACHINES

Gas	Calibration	Maximum measurable flow per minute
Oxygen, O_2	In 100 ml divisions	2,000 ml or 2 litres
Carbon dioxide, CO_2	...	...
Nitrous oxide, N_2O	In 1,000 ml or 1 litre divisions	10 litres
Cyclopropane, C_3H_6	In 50 ml divisions	750 ml

NOTE. A bypass is usually incorporated adjacent to the flowmeter bank whereby an increased flow of oxygen (and sometimes nitrous oxide also) can be obtained. This increased flow is not measurable without additional instruments, but in the case of oxygen is probably in the region of about 6 to 8 litres per minute.

BRITISH STANDARD COLOURS FOR MEDICAL GAS CYLINDERS

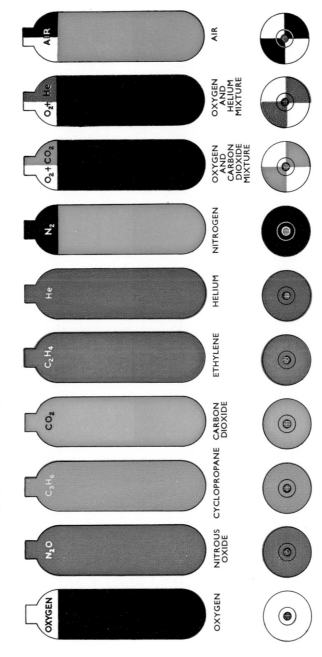

AIR

OXYGEN AND HELIUM MIXTURE

OXYGEN AND CARBON DIOXIDE MIXTURE

NITROGEN

HELIUM

ETHYLENE

CARBON DIOXIDE

CYCLOPROPANE

NITROUS OXIDE

OXYGEN

TABLE IV
RECOMMENDED SIZES OF TWIST DRILLS TO BE USED FOR VARIOUS SCREWS OR BOLTS

SCREW OR BOLT, OUTSIDE DIAMETER	DRILLS, OUTSIDE DIAMETER
Finger screws, 1·6 mm ($\frac{1}{16}$ in)	No. 55 1·2 mm ($\frac{3}{64}$ in)
Wood screws, 2·8 mm ($\frac{7}{64}$ in)	2·3 mm ($\frac{3}{32}$ in)
Wood screws, 3·6 mm ($\frac{9}{64}$ in)	2·8 mm ($\frac{7}{64}$ in)
Sherman, Phillips, or cruciform screws – 3·6 mm $\frac{9}{64}$ in	No. 31 (3·0 mm)
4·0 mm ($\frac{5}{32}$ in)	3·6 mm ($\frac{9}{64}$ in), or 3·2 mm ($\frac{1}{8}$ in)
Transfixion screws, 4·4 mm ($\frac{11}{64}$ in) . .	3·6 mm ($\frac{9}{64}$ in), cancellous bone; 4·0 mm ($\frac{5}{32}$ in), cortical bone
Wilson bolts, 3·6 mm ($\frac{9}{64}$ in) . . 7	3·6 mm ($\frac{9}{64}$ in)
Barr bolts, 4·3 mm ($\frac{11}{64}$ in)	4·0 mm ($\frac{5}{32}$ in)
Johannson lag screws, 4·0 mm ($\frac{5}{32}$ in) (shaft diameter)	4·8 mm ($\frac{3}{16}$ in) for 3·2 mm ($\frac{1}{8}$ in) depth, followed by 4·0 mm ($\frac{5}{32}$ in) for total depth of screw
Venable hip screws, 6·4 mm ($\frac{1}{4}$ in) . .	No. 4 (5·3 mm)
Venable hip screws, 5·5 mm ($\frac{7}{32}$ in) . .	4·8 mm ($\frac{3}{16}$ in)

METHOD OF REPROOFING VENTILE OR SCOTCHGUARD IN THE LAUNDRY*
(Based on a 250-lb load)

After washing and rinsing the material three times, the machine is filled with cold water to a 30 cm (12 in) dip.

Add 3¼ pints of 50 per cent acetic acid previously diluted with an equal amount of cold water and rotate the machine for 3 minutes.

Add 25 lb of Mystolene M.K.7† previously diluted with its own weight of cold water and raise the temperature slowly to 49°C to 54·5° C (120° F to 130° F), when the milky liquor should have cleared. Turn off the heat and continue running the machine for a further 2 to 3 minutes.

Run the liquor to waste and add cold water until the materials are cool enough to handle when they can be removed, hydro-extracted and finished in the usual way.

This method produces a reproofed dense fabric which possesses more advantages than most disposable products yet available. It is a method which can easily be absorbed into the normal hospital laundry service and has the advantage that larger pieces than one square yard can be used. (The average size of a disposable drape). The latter are useful as water-repellent layers in theatre packs or perhaps as drapes for lotion bowl stands.

There is no reason why the material should not be used as ordinary drapes, and it is particularly suited to making up abdominal 'slit' sheets. Used over the incision area in conjunction with Vi-Drape or similar plastic, the water-repellent sheet is ideal, particularly where excessive soiling is likely to occur, as in Caesarean section.

* Published in the *Nursing Times*, 11th December 1964.
† Mystolene M.K.7 is obtainable from Catomance Ltd., 94 Bridge Road, Welwyn Garden City, Herts.

Appendix II

Pre-set Trolley Top Trays (Edinburgh system)

The trays are of three sizes to conform with the width 66 cm (26 in) and depth 66 cm (26 in) of British Standard high vacuum rectangular dressings sterilisers. The dimensions are: full size 60 cm by 60 cm (24 in by 24 in) half size 60 cm by 30 cm (24 in by 12 in), and quarter size 30 cm by 30 cm (12 in by 12 in).

In order to provide adequate residual heat to vaporise condensate trapped during the steaming period within trays loaded with metal instruments, the two larger trays are constructed from 12 S.W.G. aluminium sheeting (99·5 per cent aluminium and 0·5 per cent manganese) and weigh 4 kg and 2 kg respectively. For the quarter size tray, 14 S.W.G. aluminium is used and the tray weighs less than 1 kg. All joints are aluminium welded.

The inner aspect of all four sides of each tray measures 41 mm ($1\frac{5}{8}$ in) in height and the upper edge is turned outwards to form a 13 mm ($\frac{1}{4}$ in) flange lip. On the outer aspect of each side and at a distance of 16 mm ($\frac{5}{8}$ in) below the flange, a second 13 mm ($\frac{1}{2}$ in) wide flange is welded into position in order to provide a 16 mm ($\frac{5}{8}$ in) wide gutter round the upper outer aspect of the tray. Two simple turn-down handles protrude from the lower flange on one end of the tray so that the overall dimensions of the tray are as follows:

Full size tray 63·5 cm (25 in) × 61·5 mm ($24\frac{1}{2}$ in) breadth.
Half size tray 63·5 cm (25 in) length × 30 cm (12 in) breadth.
Quarter size tray 31·75 cm ($12\frac{1}{2}$ in) length × 30 cm (12 in) breadth.

The handles are needed to facilitate the unloading of the trays while still hot from the steriliser. They also act as the guide in positioning the covered sterile tray upon the instrument trolley in the operating theatre – the handles should point away from or to the side of the scrub nurse. The gutter round the upper outer aspect of the tray is required for the retaining spring cord holding the covers in position, relative to the tray and trolley.

The above is extracted from the 'Theatre Service Centre' report, published by the South-Eastern Regional Hospital Board, 11 Drumsheugh Gardens, Edinburgh, 3. The trays are patented and can be obtained from Matburn Surgical Equipment Ltd.

Appendix III

VENTILATORS—A METHOD OF DECONTAMINATION—THE CAPE VENTILATOR IN PARTICULAR
(Based on an article by Mr D. I. Ankrett, Dudley Road Hospital, Birmingham,
reproduced by kind permission of NATNews)

Freshly prepared 20 volume hydrogen peroxide should be used each time. This should be made by diluting a solution of 100 volume hydrogen peroxide 1 in 5 with distilled water or freshly drawn tap water in areas supplied by high quality soft mains water.

A flow rate of 15 litres per minute is required to drive a suitable nebuliser (e.g. Ohio). A direct oxygen supply can be used if the pressure is sufficient; the valve on the top of the nebuliser set at 60 per cent to prevent build-up of pressure and possible release of peroxide through the safety valve. (Alternatively a De Vilbiss or LKB NB 100 nebuliser may be used as described on page 251, Chapter 10.)

The ventilator should be running with the respiratory volume set at 1000 mls per respiration; the respiration rate is adjusted to 25 per minute and expiratory assistance set exactly in the midway position between minimum and maximum. Failure to do this will cause a section of the expiratory circuit to remain unexposed to the aerosol. The oxygen inlet must be closed with a plug or cap during the process.

(Cape ventilator: the three drainage taps should be opened and left open with the machine running for 2–3 minutes, then closed and the drain tap cover door closed. This is to remove any moisture which may have accumulated and could neutralise nebulised hydrogen peroxide.)

Nebulised hydrogen peroxide is introduced at the air intake and allowed to escape directly into the atmosphere at the inspiratory port. This is continued for a period of 60 minutes and its effectiveness monitored by a potassium iodide indicator paper placed by the inspiratory port. The indicator paper should turn deep brown within 5 minutes of the process commencing.

The same procedure is then carried out by introducing nebulised hydrogen peroxide for 60 minutes into the expiratory port, the aerosol emerging at the air outlet. This should be similarly monitored with the potassium iodide indicator placed at the air outlet. To save time two nebulisers can be used simultaneously.

This method will not decontaminate the length of tubing from the valve block to the spirometer outlet. If a spirometer has been used, decontamination can be achieved by an additional 10 minutes nebulisation on the expiratory side with the spirometer control held in the 'in' position.

The ventilator should be adequately aired after this process. After removing the nebuliser, drainage taps are opened and the ventilator allowed to run for 10 minutes. The drainage tubes are then closed and the ventilator allowed to run until peroxide can no longer be detached in the air passing through inspiratory port, air outlet or respirometer outlet; a period of 2–4 hours will be required in some instances. At the end of the airing process, drainage taps should again be opened for 10 minutes. If the respirometer has been decontaminated, at least 30 minutes venting will be required with the spirometer control held in the 'in' position.

Detection of residual peroxide vapour: if potassium iodide indicator strips held at the outlets described do not show detectable brown discoloration, the ventilator may be considered free of peroxide vapour. These indicator strips are prepared by the immersion of filter papers in a saturated solution of potassium iodide in distilled water followed by drying in a peroxide-free atmosphere.

Appendix IV

The Lewin Report* included guides to job descriptions for nurses and operating department assistants. Although it was accepted that these may need modification in accordance with local policy, it was thought useful to include them in the Report to facilitate the understanding of the type of organisation in the operating department envisaged by the Committee.

The job descriptions are outlined here, although readers are advised to consult the Lewin Report in full in order not to read them out of context.

Guide to Job Description: Nursing Officer: Operating Department Superintendent

Role. Programming and implementing policies formulated by Senior Nursing Officers. Formulating and programming, as a member of the Operating Department Committee, departmental policies within the overall framework of the Regional Health Authority, Area Health Authority and District Management policies. Ensuring that operational policies aimed at a high standard of patient care, staff welfare and training are implemented. As a registered nurse the operating department superintendent has responsibilities involving the storage, checking and administration of drugs.

Experience. Charge Nurse/Operating Department Sister.

Minimum Qualifications. State Registered Nurse
Middle Management Course
Successful assessment following operating department training

Functions

Management of the Operating Department

1. Controlling and co-ordinating the work of non-medical staff within the operating department, allocating staffing according to need, applying maximum delegation compatible with safety, and ensuring that high standards of service and good order are provided and maintained.

2. Reporting to the Senior Nursing Officer and the hospital administrator (in the case of ancillary staff) on current staffing situations and future requirements, staffing difficulties and problems; co-ordinating annual leave arrangement.

3. Reviewing the organisation and management of the department and reporting to the appropriate personnel, the efficiency of existing operational policies particularly in relation to:

    A. the allocation of theatres
    B. provision for emergency surgery
    C. length of operating sessions.

* The Organisation and Staffing of Operating Departments (1970). A report of a Joint Subcommittee of the Standing Medical Advisory and Standing Nursing Advisory Committee. London: HMSO.

4. Initiating and developing new ideas and controlling the introduction of new methods in consultation with senior nursing officers, the operating department committee and departmental staff, within the limits of Regional Health Authority, Area Health Authority and District Management policies.

5. Maintaining and updating procedure manuals in consultation with teaching staff.

6. Maintaining responsibility for the custody and registration of all scheduled drugs used in the operating department. Supervising custody and stock levels of drugs, lotions, and anaesthetic agents held in the department in co-operation with the hospital pharmacist.

7. Exercising responsibility for the control of stock levels within the department and ordering new equipment in consultation with medical and administrative staff.

8. Receiving and recording details concerning mishaps, complaints and defects in supplies and equipment; investigating the circumstances in collaboration with appropriate staff and reporting findings to a senior nursing officer and other staff in accordance with hospital policy.

9. Ensuring that policy relating to operating department record-keeping is followed.

10. Co-operating with medical and other staff in research procedures, including clinical trials and evaluation of equipment and supplies.

11. Arranging and participating in programmes for professional visitors to the operating department.

Communication and Liaison

12. Controlling alterations to operating lists, informing all relevant personnel in the operating department, other hospital departments and ward units of proposed list changes.

13. Ensuring that ward and recovery room staff receive the necessary information on which to base nursing care and in emergency situations reporting details of the patient's condition to appropriate hospital staff.

14. Conferring with ward staff and representatives of other departments, e.g. Theatre Sterile Supply Units/Central Sterile Supply Departments, education, supplies, pharmacy, pathology, X-ray, medical photography, hospital administration and housekeeping services.

15. Conferring with, and co-ordinating the work of medical and paramedical staff concerned with procedures in the operating department from time to time (e.g. radiological Protection Officer, Control of Infection Officer, Microbiologist.)

16. Attending operating department and procedure committee meetings, hospital and area (hospital) nursing meetings, to report on the work of the department.

17. Conferring with representatives of surgical firms to obtain information on new products and to report on products currently in use.

18. Collaborating with senior nursing officers to provide operating department planning guidance for building project team.

Safety

19. Ensuring that agreed safety procedures are known and followed by theatre staff especially measures concerning swab, instrument and needle counts; the storage and administration of blood and drugs; ionising radiation; static electricity/explosion hazards; fire; departmental cleaning.

20. Checking, receiving and relaying to the appropriate staff information concerning environmental conditions; interior fabric maintenance; planned maintenance and the integrity of piped gas supplies.

Education

21. Organising and participating (in consultation with the teaching division and other appropriate staff) in training programmes for post qualification, student and pupil nurses and operating department assistants.

22. Organising in-service training (in consultation with appropriate staff) for nursing and ancillary staff. Participating in collaboration with the medical staff as appropriate in instruction for medical students within the department.

23. Participating in general hospital staff training programmes in the Hospital Education Centre by lecturing on subjects such as theatre techniques and procedures.

24. Arranging visits by departmental staff to operating departments in other hospitals.

Personnel

25. Participating with appropriate staff in the recruitment and selection of operating department staff.

26. Organising and participating in the orientation of new staff in consultation with appropriate nursing and administrative staff.

27. Counselling staff on professional and personal problems.

28. Preparing reports and discussing the progress of operating department staff in training with appropriate officers; compiling reports on operating department staff in accordance with hospital policy.

29. Encouraging staff to pursue further studies and discussing with senior nursing officers or the hospital administrator where appropriate the suitability of staff for further courses of study.

30. Ensuring that procedures to safeguard staff health and welfare during working hours are implemented.

31. Participating as an assessor in the selection of operating department staff in other hospitals.

32. Attending professional conferences, careers conventions and making contacts with professional colleagues in other hospitals.

Guide to Job Description: Charge Nurse: Operating Department Sister

Role. Management of an operating suite or a small operating department according to local policy. Implementing policy formulated by Nursing Officer in consultation with the Operating Department Committee, directed towards high standards of patient care, staff welfare, and staff training in the operating department. As a registered nurse the Operating Department Sister/Charge Nurse has responsibilities involving the storage, checking and administration of drugs, and may also at times act as a scrubbed assistant in surgical procedures. The Sister/Charge Nurse may carry out the duties of the Nursing Officer in her absence.

Experience. Operating department staff nurse.

Minimum Qualifications. State Registered Nurse.
Successful assessment following operating department training, including first-line management course.

Functions

General

1. Supervising the work of all staff in the area under her control. Checking that work is

carried out in accordance with agreed policy and ensuring that high standards of service and good order are provided and maintained.

2. Reporting to Nursing Officer on the current state of staffing, seeking or offering support as available. Advising Nursing Officer of likely future alterations in staffing requirements or special off-duty or 'time off in lieu' requests. Submitting annual leave requests to Nursing Officer for approval and reporting problems associated with the health of operating department staff (e.g. infected lesions).

3. Reviewing the efficiency of departmental operational policies and reporting on matters affecting policy to Nursing Officer. Communicating policy changes to relevant staff.

4. Developing and discussing with Nursing Officer new ideas and methods of procedure.

5. Participating in the maintenance and review of procedure manuals in consultation with teaching staff.

6. Maintaining the custody and register of scheduled drugs used in the area under her control. Checking and witnessing the administration of drugs in accordance with hospital policy.

7. Maintaining or delegating responsibility for levels of supplies in accordance with departmental policy.

8. Reporting to Nursing Officer incidence of accidents, complaints, and defects in drugs, supplies or equipment.

9. Supervising maintenance of the operations register in co-operation with appropriate staff.

10. Co-operating with medical and other staff in research procedures, including clinical trials and evaluation of equipment and supplies.

11. Advising Nursing Officer of proposed changes in the operating list order.

12. Participating in discussions with Nursing Officer concerning the repair or renewal of major equipment.

13. Establishing personal contacts with patients through ward and/or anaesthetic room visits in accordance with hospital policy.

14. Participating as a scrubbed assistant in surgical procedures.

15. Arranging for the care of patient's property in emergency situations.

16. Carrying out duties of Nursing Officer (operating department superintendent) in an 'acting up capacity', in the absence of the former.

17. Reporting on the work of the operating suite to Nursing Officer.

18. Participating in programmes for professional visitors to the operating department.

Liaison and Communication

19. Relaying to ward and recovery room staff details of the patient's physical condition and other information affecting nursing care of the patient.

20. Co-operating with medical, receptionist and ward staff in calling patients to the operating department when required, in accordance with hospital policy.

21. Co-operating with medical and paramedical staff from other departments in procedures carried out in the operating department from time to time, e.g. radiological protection officer, control of infection officer, microbiologist.

22. Participating in regular meetings of operating department staff and hospital nursing staff meetings at the appropriate level.

23. Co-ordinating the arrival and departure of patients, and staff from departments such as X-ray of laboratory, in co-operation with medical and receptionist staff.

Safety

24. Ensuring the implementation of safety measures concerning swabs, instrument

and needle counts, the storage and administration of blood and drugs, ionising radiation, static electricity/explosion hazards, fire, and departmental cleaning.

25. Checking, receiving and relaying to Nursing Officer reports concerning the state of the following within the department:

> Heating
> Lighting
> Ventilation
> Fabric maintenance
> Routine maintenance
> The integrity of piped gas supplies.

Education

26. Implementing and participating in training programmes (including in-service training) for all grades of staff.

27. Instructing staff in new procedures as these are introduced.

Personnel

28. Introducing new members of staff to their duties.

29. Counselling operating department staff on personal and professional matters.

30. Discussing reports, on operating department staff and nursing progress reports on staff in training with Nursing Officer in accordance with hospital policy.

31. Taking all possible steps to safeguard the welfare and safety of staff in the operating theatre during working hours.

32. Encouraging staff to pursue further studies.

33. Attending professional conferences, careers conventions, and making contact with professional colleagues in other hospitals.

Guide to Job Description: Operating Department Staff Nurse

Role. To provide nursing care in the operating department and as a skilled member of the theatre team, to act as the scrubbed or circulating assistant during surgical procedures. As a registered nurse the Staff Nurse has responsibilities involving the storage, checking and administration of drugs. The Staff Nurse may carry out duties of Charge Nurse in her absence.

Experience: Post-registration training course and operating department experience.

Minimum Qualifications: State Registered Nurse.

> Successful assessment following operating department training.

Functions

General

1. Providing nursing care for patients within the operating department.
2. Performing operating department work in accordance with agreed policy, e.g.
   A. Participating as a scrubbed member of the theatre team and carrying out safety checks of swabs, instruments and needles, in conjunction with a second person, and reporting on the same to the surgeon.
   B. Acting as a circulating member of the theatre team.
   C. Assisting with other members of the team in the preparation and clearing of theatres.
   D. Assisting in compiling the operations register.
   E. Checking and labelling and despatch of laboratory specimens.

F. Providing assistance to the anaesthetist and surgeon as required.

G. Checking, witnessing and administering dangerous drugs.

H. Co-operating with appropriate departmental and ward staff in sending for patients to the operating department.

I. Advising Charge Nurse of proposed changes in the order of operating lists.

3. Participating in the supervision of junior staff and staff in training.

4. Discussing departmental policies and developing and discussing new procedures with Charge Nurse. Communicating policy changes to relevant staff.

5. Assisting in the compilation of procedure manuals.

6. Ensuring that appropriate stock levels are maintained in the operating suite if required to do so.

7. Reporting to Charge Nurse incidents of accidents, complaints, defects in drugs, supplies or equipment.

8. Participating in clinical trials of new equipment and supplies and the evaluation and serviceability of existing equipment.

9. Co-operating with medical or other staff in research procedures.

10. Assisting when required in bacteriological investigations in the operating department.

11. Assisting medical and paramedical staff from other departments with procedures carried out in the operating department as required.

12. Participating in programmes for professional visitors to the department.

13. Carrying out the duties of Charge Nurse in her absence.

Liaison and Communication

14. Ensuring the maintenance of good relationships, communications and teamwork with all disciplines within the department and other departments of the hospital concerned with operating department work.

15. Participating in regular meetings of operating department staff.

16. Implementing safety measures in relation to:

> Swabs, instruments and needle count
> Storage and administration of blood and drugs
> Ionising radiations
> Static electricity/explosion hazards
> Fire.

Education

17. Participating in teaching programmes for staff in training.

Personnel

18. Assisting with the orientation of new staff.

19. Assisting Charge Nurse in the assessment of nurses in training and a compilation of staff progress reports.

Guide to Job Description: Operating Department State Enrolled Nurse

Role. To provide nursing care for the patient in the operating department and to act as a scrubbed or circulating member of the theatre team. The responsibility accorded to her and the degree of supervision under which she carries out her work is a matter for local professional assessment.

Experience. Two months' appraisal if no pupil nurse training in operating department.

Post-enrolment training course and operating department experience.

Minimum Qualifications. State Enrolled Nurse.

Successful completion of operating department state enrolled nurse training.

Functions

General

1. Providing nursing care for patients within the operating department.

2. Performing operating department work in accordance with agreed local policy including:

    A. Participating as a scrubbed member of the theatre team and carrying out safety checks of swabs, instruments and needles in conjunction with a second person and reporting on the same to the surgeon if in accordance with agreed local policy.

    B. Acting as a circulating member of the theatre team.

    C. Assisting with other members of the team in the preparation and clearing of theatres.

    D. Assisting in compiling the operation register.

    E. Assisting in the labelling and despatch of specimens for laboratory examination.

    F. Providing assistance to the anaesthetist and surgeon as required.

    G. Checking, witnessing and administering dangerous drugs in agreed circumstances.

3. Discussing departmental policies and new procedures with staff nurse or Charge Nurse in appropriate circumstances.

4. Assisting in the compilation of procedure manuals.

4. Ensuring where appropriate that stock levels are maintained if required to do so.

6. Reporting to the staff nurse or Charge Nurse incidents of accidents, complaints, defects in drugs, supplies or equipment.

7. Participating in clinical trials of new equipment and supplies and the evaluation and serviceability of existing equipment.

8. Co-operating with medical or other staff in research procedures.

9. Advising staff nurse or Charge Nurse of proposed changes in the order of operating lists.

10. Assisting medical and paramedical staff from other departments with procedures carried out in the operating department as required.

11. Participating in programmes for professional visitors to the department.

Liaison and Communication

12. Ensuring the maintenance of good relationships, communications, and teamwork with all disciplines within the department and other departments of the hospital concerned with operating department work.

13. Participating in regular meetings of operating department staff.

Safety

14. Implementing safety measures, in accordance with agreed local policies in relation to:

Swab, instrument and needle counts
Storage and administration of blood and drugs
Ionising radiations
Static electricity/explosion hazards
Fire.

Education

15. Participating in in-service training programmes.

Personnel

16. Assisting with the orientation of new staff.

Guide to Job Description: Operating Department Assistant

Role. To provide skilled assistance in the operating department and act as a member of the theatre team. To care for specified equipment relevant to his skills.

Experience. Two years' operating department training.

Minimum Qualifications. Successful assessment following operating department training.

Functions

General

1. Performing operating department work in accordance with agreed operational policies.

2. Participating as a scrubbed member of the theatre team in surgical procedures and carrying out safety checks on swabs, instruments, and needles in conjunction with a second person and reporting on the same to the surgeon.

3. Providing assistance as a circulating member of the theatre team including:
    A. Positioning and any preparation of a patient on the operating table as required by the surgeon and anaesthetist.
    B. Assisting the anaesthetist and surgeons as required, including assistance with blood transfusions and intravascular procedures.
    C. Assisting, with other members of the team, in the preparation and clearing of operating theatres, e.g. moving apparatus and lights and cleaning up during and after an operation.
    D. Preparing splints and plasters in the operating department.

4. Assisting in movement of patients in the operating department.

5. Acting as a member of the resuscitation team.

6. Cleaning, preparation and minor maintenance of instruments where appropriate.

7. Maintaining in an effective condition anaesthetic, inhalation and resuscitation equipment in accordance with local policies.

8. Cleaning, care and day-to-day maintenance of all equipment in general use in the operating department.

9. Operating autoclaves within the operating department where appropriate.

10. Assisting in the care, labelling and despatch of specimens for laboratory examination.

11. Assisting in compiling the operations register in co-operation with other staff.

12. Maintaining appropriate stock levels if delegated this task within the suite or department.

13. Reporting to Charge Nurse or Senior Operating Department Assistant, as appropriate, accidents, complaints, defects in drugs, supplies or equipment.

14. Participating in clinical trials of new equipment and supplies and the evaluation of existing equipment in collaboration with medical and nursing staff.

15. Assisting as required in research procedures.

16. Reporting to Charge Nurse and/or Senior Operating Department Assistant on the state of fabric maintenance and any deviation from accepted standards of operating department cleaning.

17. Proposing new ideas and procedures for discussion with Senior Operating Department Assistant or Charge Nurse.

18. Such other duties as may be determined by the Operating Department Superintendent and the Operating Department Committee.

Liaison and Communication

19. Attending departmental staff meetings.

20. Ensuring the maintenance of good relationships, communications, and teamwork with all disciplines within the department and other departments in the hospital concerned with operating department work.

Education

21. Participating in in-service training programmes.

Personnel

22. Assisting with the orientation of new staff.

Safety

23. Ensuring that safety procedures agreed by the Operating Department Committee are carried out in relation to swab, instrument and needle counts and in relation to hazards from ionising radiation, static electricity/explosion, and fire.

Guide to Job Description: Senior Operating Department Assistant

Role. To perform all the duties of an operating department assistant and in addition duties requiring special skill and ability in at least one particular branch of work including in appropriate circumstances the supervision of an operating suite. To implement agreed policies directed towards high standards of patient care, staff welfare and staff training.

Experience. Two years' experience in qualified grade (or possibly less according to educational qualifications).

Minimum Qualifications. Successful assessment following one year's training for the senior grade.

Functions

General

1. Co-ordinating the work of operating department assistants where this is appropriate:

2. Participating as a scrubbed assistant in general and specialised surgical procedures including responsibility for carrying out safety checks in conjunction with a second person.

3. Providing specialised assistance to the anaesthetist and acting as a member of the resuscitation team.

4. Exercising responsibility for effectiveness of anaesthetic and resuscitation equipment in the department, and dispersed throughout the hospital, if in accordance with local policy.

5. Exercising responsibility for the care, cleanliness and day-to-day maintenance of specialised equipment and assisting with their use in the theatre, e.g., pressure transducers, blood gas analysers within the department and hospital, if in accordance with local policy.

6. Advising Charge Nurse or Nursing Officer of proposed changes in the order of operation lists.

7. Ensuring the correct care, labelling and despatch of laboratory specimens.

8. Supervising the work of operating department assistants in training.

9. Ensuring if appropriate, or if required to do so, that stock levels (except drugs) are maintained in the operating suite or department.

10. Reporting to Nursing Officer or Charge Nurse as appropriate, accidents, complaints, defects in drugs, supplies or equipment.

11. Co-operating with medical or other staff, in consultation with Nursing Officer, in research procedures, including clinical trials and the evaluation of equipment and supplies.

12. Assisting when required in routine bacteriological investigations in the operating department under the direction of a microbiologist.

13. Discussing with Nursing Officer or reporting to Nursing Officer the current state of operating department assistant staffing and possible future staffing requirements and consulting with nursing officer in charge in respect of annual leave or time off 'in lieu' requests for operating department assistants.

14. Discussing departmental policies with Charge Nurse or Nursing Officer. Communicating policy changes to relevant staff.

15. Developing and discussing with Nursing Officer or Charge Nurse new ideas and methods of procedures.

16. Assisting in the compilation of procedure manuals, in consultation with teaching staff.

17. Encouraging the development of managerial skills in operating department assistants by the delegation of tasks.

18. Participating in programmes for professional visitors to the operating department.

Liaison and Communication

19. Co-operating with medical, receptionist and ward staff in appropriate circumstances in calling patients to the operating department when required according to local policy.

20. Assisting medical and paramedical staff from other departments with procedures carried out in the operating department from time to time, e.g. radiological protection officer, control of infection officer, microbiologist.

21. Reporting on the work of the suite (if appropriate) to Nursing Officer.

22. Ensuring the maintenance of good relationships and teamwork between other disciplines and staff under his supervision.

23. Participating in regular meetings of operating department staff.

24. Organising meetings of operating department assistants.

25. Co-ordinating, in appropriate circumstances, the arrival and departure of patients, and staff from other departments such as X-ray or laboratory.

Safety

26. Ensuring, in appropriate circumstances, the implementation of safety measures in relation to swab, instrument and needle counts; the storage and administration of blood and drugs, ionising radiation, static electricity/explosion hazards, fire and departmental cleaning.

27. Checking, receiving and relaying to Nursing Officer reports concerning the state of the following within the department:

> Heating
> Lighting
> Ventilation
> Fabric maintenance
> Routine maintenance
> The integrity of piped gas supplies.

28. Participating in discussions with Nursing Officer or Charge Nurse concerning the repair or renewal of major equipment.

29. Reporting to Nursing Officer or Charge Nurse as appropriate (a) the need for fabric or plant maintenance and (b) the satisfactory implementation of the planned maintenance programme.

Education

30. Assisting Nursing Officer in the compilation of training and teaching programmes for operating department assistants.

31. Participating in training and teaching programmes for all operating department staff.

32. Instructing staff in accordance with agreed policies, in new procedures and the use of new equipment.

Personnel

33. Encouraging operating department assistants and other ancillary staff to pursue further studies.

34. Counselling operating department assistant staff.

35. Discussing progress reports on trainee operating department assistants with Nursing Officer and with the staff concerned.

Guide to Duties: Operating Department Receptionist/Clerk Typist

To receive patients and direct their escorts on arrival in the operating department; to co-ordinate communications within the operating department and with wards and other departments. Staff in these grades should have clerical and typing experience and receive in-service training. Whether the duties of receptionist and clerk typist are separated will depend upon the size of the department. Normally the following duties will be involved:

Communications

1. Receiving and relaying messages.

2. Maintaining communication and liaison with other hospital departments and with outside callers.

3. Providing information regarding location of departmental staff.

Reception

1. Receiving and directing patients and escorts on arrival at the operating department.

2. Receiving and directing visitors to the operating department.

Clerical

1. Maintaining appropriate departmental records in accordance with local policy.
2. Dealing with departmental correspondence in association with Nursing Officer in charge.
3. Typing departmental information including:

> Off-duty and emergency rosters
> Departmental procedures
> Notices
> Operating lists where appropriate
> Study programmes
> Visitors' programmes.

4. Preparing requisitions for equipment, supplies, stationery in consultation with relevant staff.
5. Such other duties as may be determined by operating department superintendent.

Guide to Duties: Domestic Assistant

1. Clearing and cleaning scrub-up and changing rooms as required during working hours.
2. Checking and clearing or cleaning as required wash hand basins, W.C.'s and showers.
3. Receiving and sorting clean non-sterile linen and topping up to pre-determined levels.
4. Topping up changing room linen.
5. Checking and topping-up supplies of cleaning materials, disposal bags, hand towels.
6. Serving refreshments.
7. Clearing and washing up crockery.
8. Cleaning pantry.
9. Assisting in the preparation of patients' trolleys.
10. Removing waste materials, i.e. changing room linen bags and pantry waste to the appropriate disposal area within the operating department.
11. Such other duties as may be determined by the Nursing Officer and Domestic Superintendent not demanding a higher level of responsibility than those listed above.

Guide to Duties: Operating Department Orderly

Role. To carry out portering and general duties in the operating department.

Duties

1. Lifting patients and moving them between beds, trolleys and special tables.
2. Preparing patients' trolleys.
3. Receiving and sorting stores.
4. Moving and storing equipment.
5. Assisting in the maintenance of stock levels.

6. Clearing theatre and assisting with cleaning within the department.

7. Caring in general way for theatre equipment, e.g. operating table, lights, etc.

8. Changing of medical gas cylinders.

9. Operating autoclaves within the operating department, where appropriate.

10. Providing messenger service within the operating department.

11. Cleaning theatre footwear.

12. Such other duties as may be determined by the operating department Superintendent and the Operating Department Committee.

Appendix V

Artery Forceps

CHAS. F. THACKRAY LTD.

The scales given are approximate only.

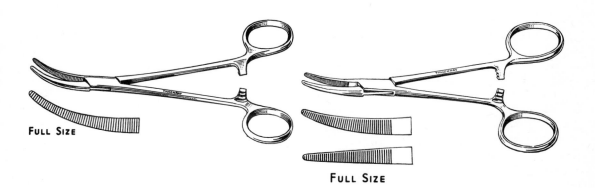

Crile Artery Forceps (Sc. $\frac{2}{3}$)   Dunhill Artery Forceps (Sc. $\frac{2}{3}$)

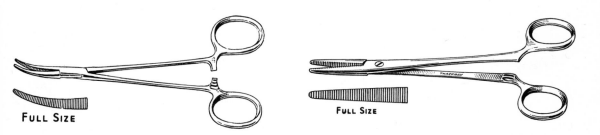

Halstead Mosquito Artery Forceps (Sc. $\frac{1}{2}$)   Spencer Wells Artery Forceps (Sc. $\frac{1}{3}$)

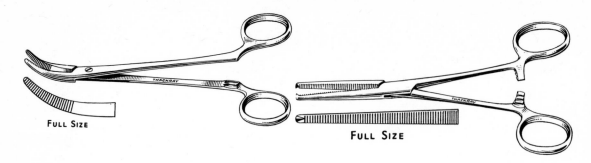

Moynihan Cholecystectomy Forceps (Sc. $\frac{1}{3}$)   Kocher Artery Forceps (Sc. $\frac{1}{3}$)

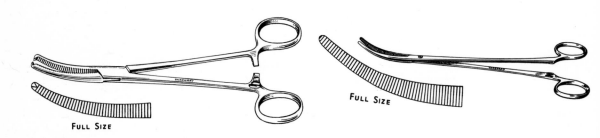

Mayo-Ochsner Artery Forceps (Curved) (Sc. $\frac{1}{3}$)   Roberts Artery Forceps (Sc. $\frac{1}{4}$)

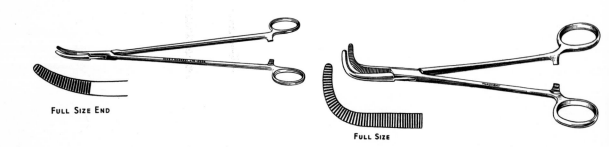

Dudfield Rose Lung Artery Forceps (Sc. $\frac{1}{4}$)   O'Shaughnessy Lung Artery Forceps (Sc. $\frac{1}{3}$)

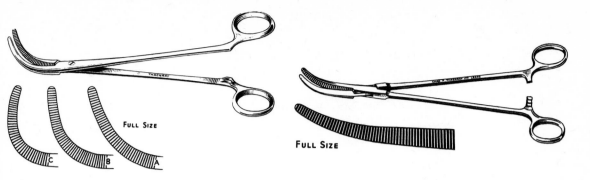

FULL SIZE

Ronald Edwards Artery Forceps (Sc. $\frac{1}{3}$)

FULL SIZE

Lloyd Davies Artery Forceps (Sc. $\frac{1}{3}$)

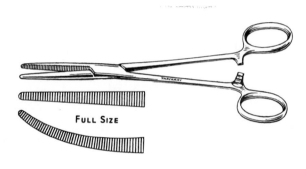

FULL SIZE

Rochester Pean Artery Forceps (Sc. $\frac{1}{2}$)

Dissecting Forceps

CHAS. F. THACKRAY LTD.

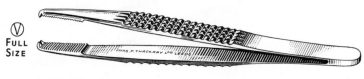

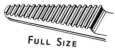

Bonney Toothed Dissecting Forceps (Sc. $\frac{1}{2}$)

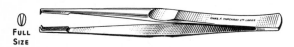

Lane Toothed Dissecting Forceps (Sc. $\frac{1}{2}$)

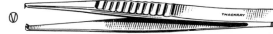

Treves Toothed Dissecting Forceps (Sc. $\frac{1}{2}$)

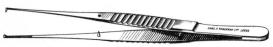

Waugh Toothed Dissecting Forceps (Sc. $\frac{1}{3}$)

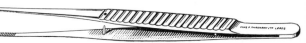

Gillies Toothed Dissecting Forceps (Sc. $\frac{1}{2}$)

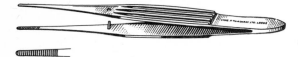

McIndoe Non-Toothed Dissecting Forceps (Sc. $\frac{1}{2}$)

Non-Toothed Dissecting Forceps (Sc. $\frac{1}{3}$)

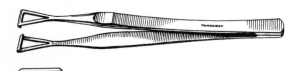

Duval Dissecting Forceps (Sc. $\frac{1}{2}$)

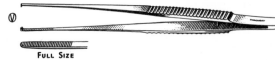

St Marks Dissecting Forceps (Sc. $\frac{1}{4}$)

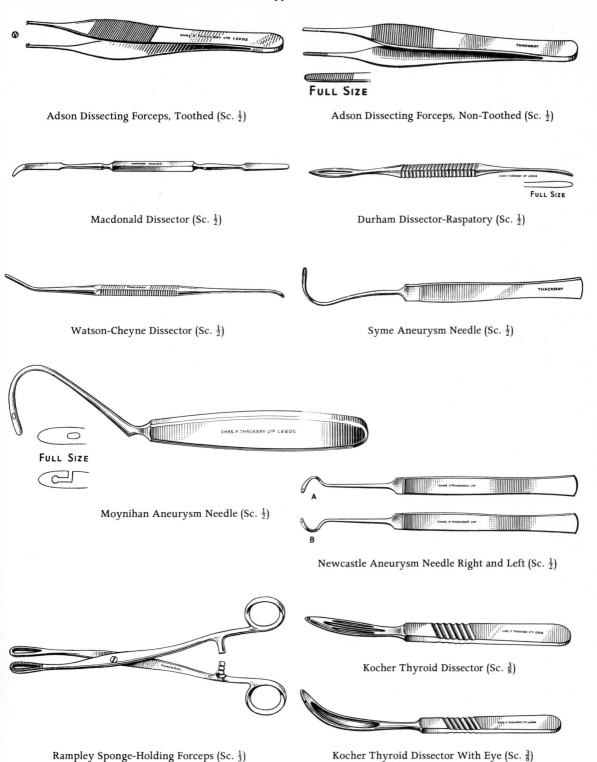

Adson Dissecting Forceps, Toothed (Sc. $\frac{1}{2}$)

Adson Dissecting Forceps, Non-Toothed (Sc. $\frac{1}{2}$)

FULL SIZE

Macdonald Dissector (Sc. $\frac{1}{2}$)

Durham Dissector-Raspatory (Sc. $\frac{1}{2}$)

FULL SIZE

Watson-Cheyne Dissector (Sc. $\frac{1}{2}$)

Syme Aneurysm Needle (Sc. $\frac{1}{2}$)

FULL SIZE

Moynihan Aneurysm Needle (Sc. $\frac{1}{2}$)

Newcastle Aneurysm Needle Right and Left (Sc. $\frac{1}{2}$)

Kocher Thyroid Dissector (Sc. $\frac{3}{8}$)

Rampley Sponge-Holding Forceps (Sc. $\frac{1}{3}$)

Kocher Thyroid Dissector With Eye (Sc. $\frac{3}{8}$)

Needle Holders

CHAS. F. THACKRAY LTD.

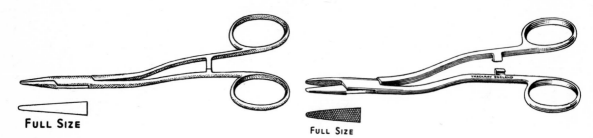

FULL SIZE

Kilner Needle Holder, Simple Pattern (Sc. ½)

FULL SIZE

Micron Kilner Needle Holder (Sc. ½)

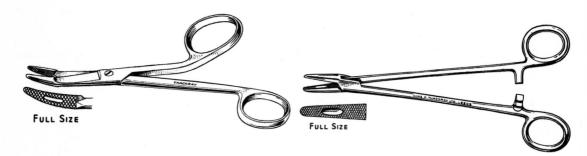

FULL SIZE

Gillies Needle Holder and Scissors (Sc. ½)

FULL SIZE

Mayo Needle Holder (Sc. ⅓)

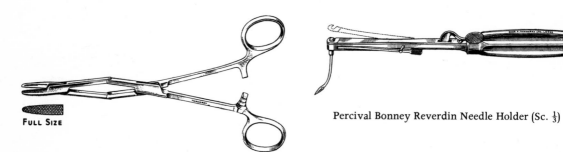

FULL SIZE

Percival Bonney Reverdin Needle Holder (Sc. ⅓)

Naunton Morgan Needle Holder (Sc. ⅓)

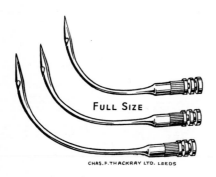

FULL SIZE

Bonney-Reverdin Needles (Full Size)

CHAS. F. THACKRAY LTD. LEEDS

Retractors

CHAS. F. THACKRAY LTD.

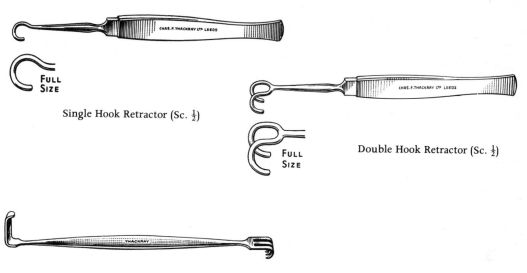

Single Hook Retractor (Sc. $\frac{1}{2}$)

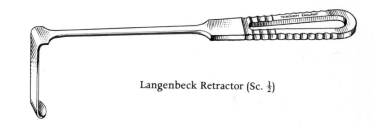

Double Hook Retractor (Sc. $\frac{1}{2}$)

Kilner Skin Retractor (Sc. $\frac{1}{3}$)

Langenbeck Retractor (Sc. $\frac{1}{2}$)

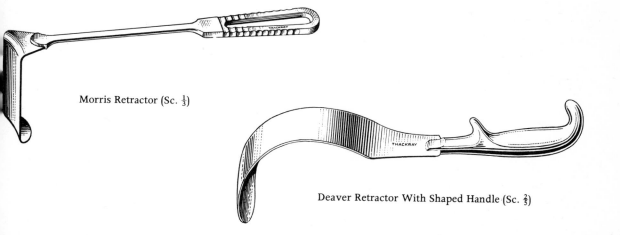

Morris Retractor (Sc. $\frac{1}{3}$)

Deaver Retractor With Shaped Handle (Sc. $\frac{2}{5}$)

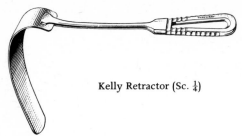

Kelly Retractor (Sc. $\frac{1}{4}$)

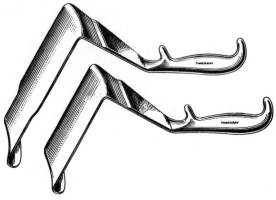

St Marks Hospital Pattern Retractor (Sc. $\frac{1}{3}$)

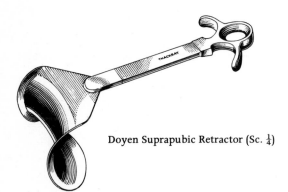

Doyen Suprapubic Retractor (Sc. $\frac{1}{4}$)

Weight For Use With Retractor (Sc. $\frac{1}{2}$)

Self Retaining Retractors

CHAS. F. THACKRAY LTD.

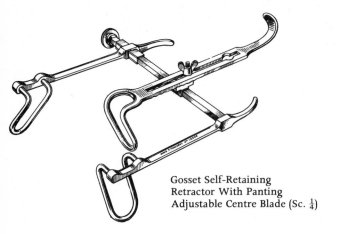

Gosset Self-Retaining
Retractor With Panting
Adjustable Centre Blade (Sc. $\frac{1}{4}$)

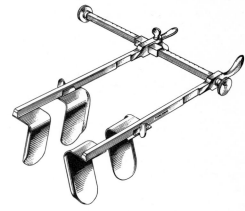

Comyns Berkeley Self-Retaining Retractor (Sc. $\frac{1}{4}$)

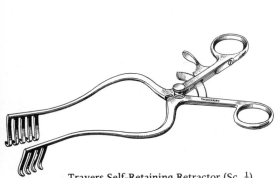

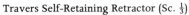

Travers Self-Retaining Retractor (Sc. $\frac{1}{3}$)

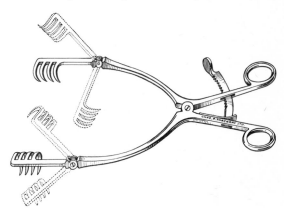

Mayo Self-Retaining Retractor (Hinged) (Sc. $\frac{1}{4}$)

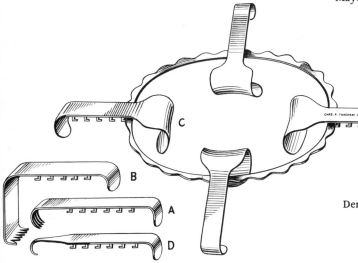

Denis-Browne Retractor Set (Sc. $\frac{1}{4}$)

Scalpels

CHAS. F. THACKRAY LTD.

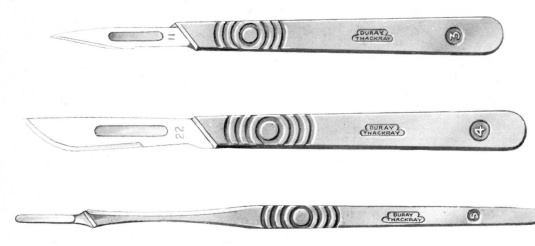

Duray Scalpel Handles Sizes 3, 4 and 5 (Full Size)

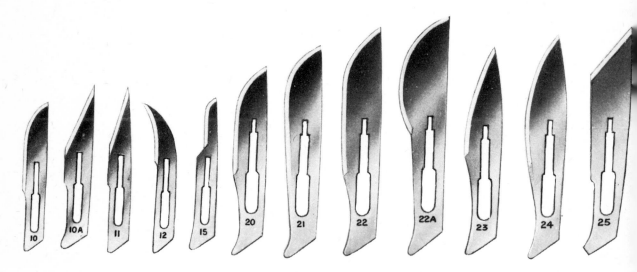

Disposable Scalpel Blades Sizes 10–25 (Full Size)

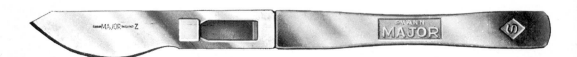

Major Scalpel Handle (Full Size)

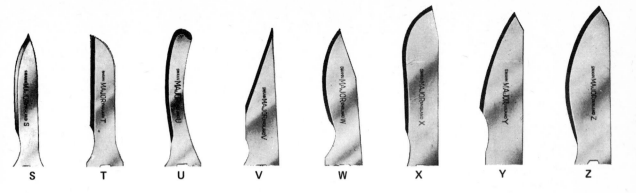

| S | T | U | V | W | X | Y | Z |

Major Scalpel Blades Sizes S–Z (Full Size)

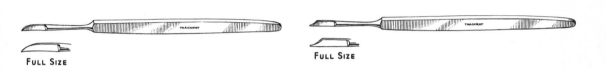

FULL SIZE   FULL SIZE

Robert Jones Tenotomy Knives (Sc. $\frac{1}{2}$)

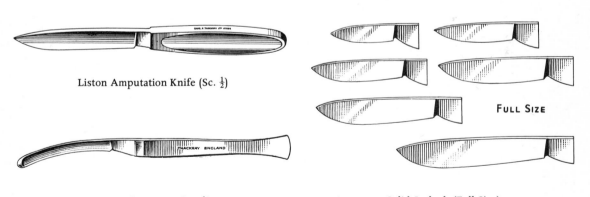

Liston Amputation Knife (Sc. $\frac{1}{2}$)

FULL SIZE

Curved Bistoury (Sc. $\frac{1}{3}$)

Solid Scalpels (Full Size)

Scissors

CHAS F. THACKRAY LTD.

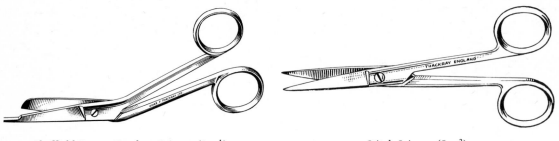

Sheffield Pattern Bandage Scissors (Sc. ⅓)   Stitch Scissors (Sc. ⅔)

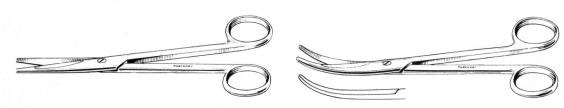

Mayo Scissors (Straight) (Sc. ⅓)   Mayo Scissors (Curved) (Sc. ⅓)

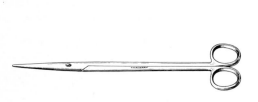

Metzenbaum Dissecting Scissors (Curved) (Sc. ⅓)

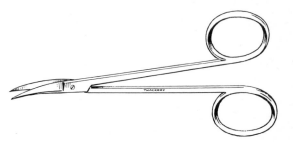

Iris Scissors (Curved) (Sc. ⅔)

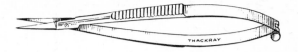

Micro Dissecting Scissors (Sc. $\frac{2}{3}$)

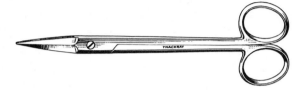

Cartilage Scissors (Sc. $\frac{1}{2}$)

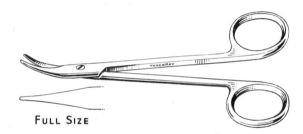

Strabismus Scissors (Curved) (Sc. $\frac{2}{3}$)

FULL SIZE

Tissue Forceps

CHAS. F. THACKRAY LTD.

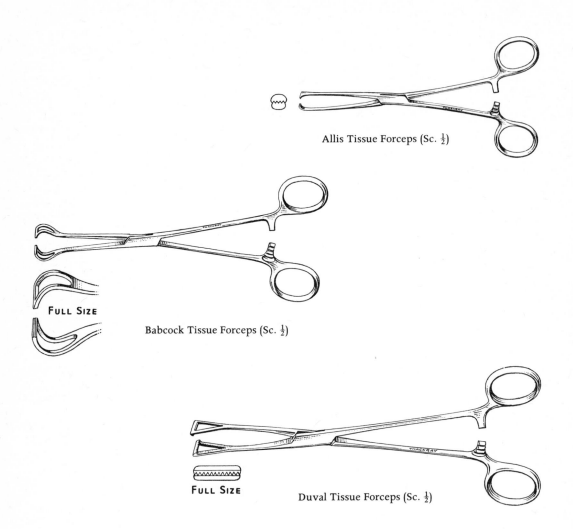

Allis Tissue Forceps (Sc. $\frac{1}{2}$)

FULL SIZE

Babcock Tissue Forceps (Sc. $\frac{1}{2}$)

FULL SIZE

Duval Tissue Forceps (Sc. $\frac{1}{2}$)

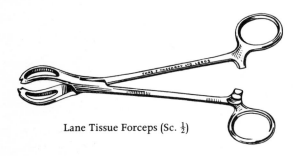

Lane Tissue Forceps (Sc. $\frac{1}{2}$)

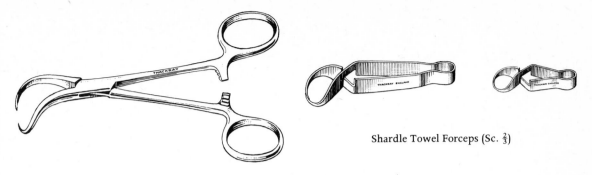

Mayo Backhaus Towel Forceps (Sc. $\frac{1}{2}$)

Shardle Towel Forceps (Sc. $\frac{2}{3}$)

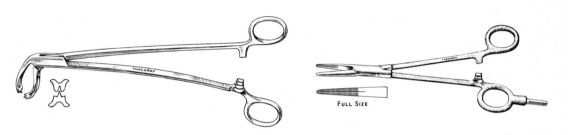

Fagge Tissue Forceps (Sc. $\frac{1}{3}$)

Wilson-Hey Diathermy Forceps (Sc. $\frac{1}{3}$)

FULL SIZE

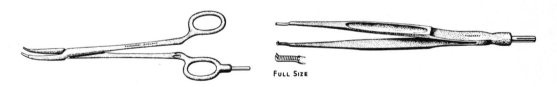

Riches Diathermy Forceps (Sc. $\frac{1}{3}$)

Diathermy Dissecting Forceps (Sc. $\frac{1}{3}$)

FULL SIZE

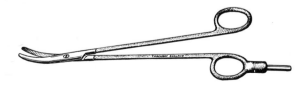

Turner-Warwick Diathermy Forceps (Sc. $\frac{1}{3}$)

E.N.T. Endoscopic Instruments

DOWN BROS. LTD.

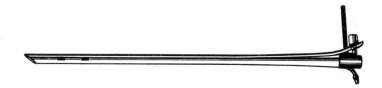

Negus Aspirating Bronchoscope, Fibre Light (Sc. $\frac{1}{4}$ approx)

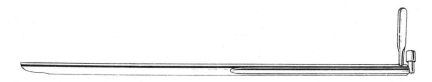

Negus Oesophagoscope, Fibre Light (Sc. $\frac{1}{4}$ approx.)

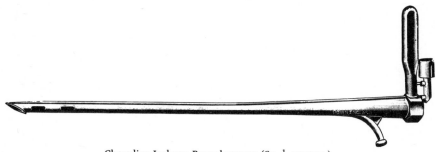

Chevalier Jackson Bronchoscope (Sc. $\frac{1}{4}$ approx.)

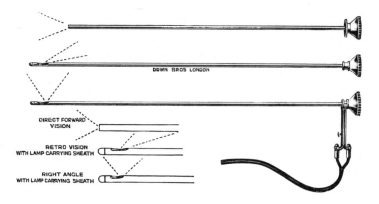

DOWN BROS LONDON

DIRECT FORWARD VISION

RETRO VISION WITH LAMP CARRYING SHEATH

RIGHT ANGLE WITH LAMP CARRYING SHEATH

Poppers Telescope (Sc. $\frac{1}{4}$ approx.)

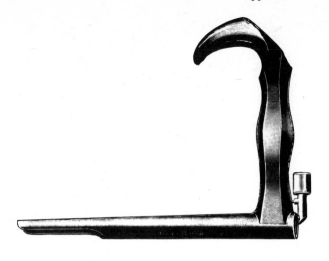

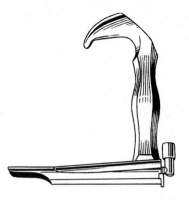

Negus Laryngoscope (Sc. $\frac{1}{3}$)
Fitted with fibre light carrier.

Chevalier Jackson Oesophageal Speculum (Sc. $\frac{1}{2}$)
Fitted with fibre light carrier.

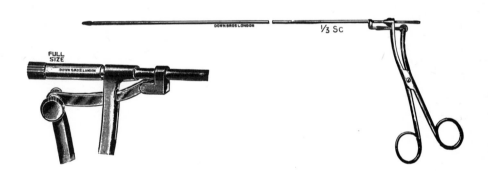

Chevalier Jackson Grasping Forceps with Negus Handle (Sc. $\frac{1}{3}$)

Chevalier Jackson Grasping Forceps continued

A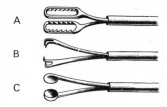

B

C

F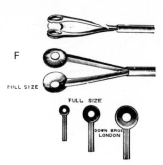

FULL SIZE

D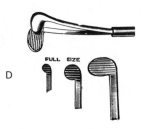

G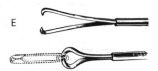

E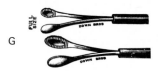

A. Forward grasping forceps.
B. 2/2 teeth claw forceps (Brünings).
C. Scoop cutting biopsy forceps (Brünings).
D. Side grasping forceps.
E. Rotation forceps.
F. Bronchial fenestrated biopsy forceps
   (Brünings).
G. Round foreign body forceps.

E.N.T. Aural Instruments

DOWN BROS. LTD.

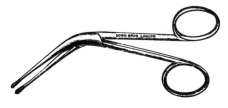

Tilley Dressing Forceps (Sc. $\frac{2}{3}$)

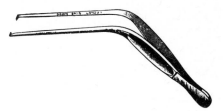

Wilde Aural Forceps (Sc. $\frac{2}{3}$)

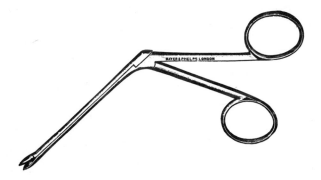

Henckel Aural Forceps (Sc. $\frac{2}{3}$)

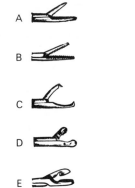

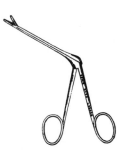

Hartman Aural Forceps (Sc. $\frac{1}{4}$)

A. Serrated jaws.
B. Extra fine jaws.
C. Fine tenaculum points.
D. Round cutting jaws.
E. Grunwald punch action jaws.

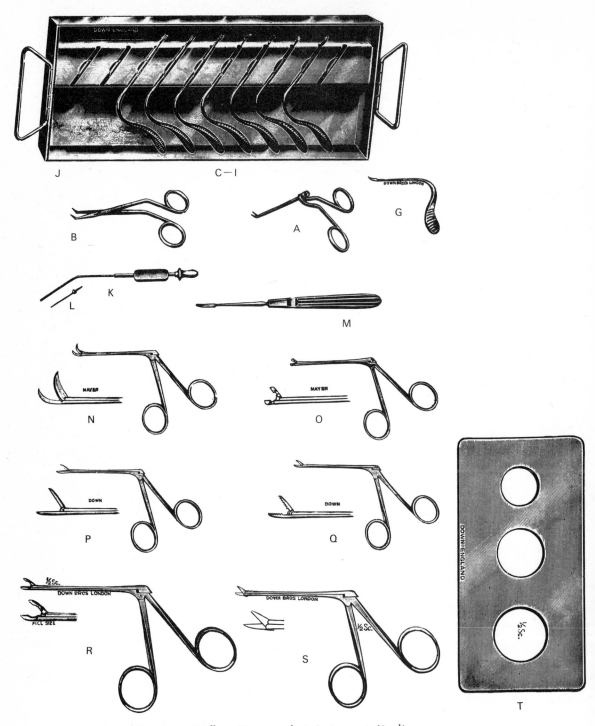

Zoellners Tympanoplasty Instruments (Sc. $\frac{1}{2}$)

As used at the Royal National Throat, Nose and Ear Hospital, London.

A. Zoellner's scissors, bayonet shaped, tubular model, with upward cut, lateral action.

B. Zoellner's scissors, angular, with upward cut, lateral action, screw joint.

C. Zoellner's fine raspatory, curved to right, with thumb grip, matt finish.

D. Ditto, curved to left, with thumb grip, matt finish.

E. Zoellner's fine spear-pointed needle, curved to right, with thumb grip, matt finish.

F. Ditto, curved to left, with thumb grip, matt finish.

G. Zoellner's knife, upward cutting, with thumb grip, matt finish.

H. Ditto, downward cutting, with thumb grip, matt finish.

I. Zoellner's small hook, with thumb grip, matt finish.

J. Zoellner's rack to hold instruments above, figs. A to I, with three spare clips for additional similar instruments; arranged to protect the knives, etc. during sterilization and afterwards to make the different instruments easily discernible.

K. Zoellner's suction tube, nickel plated with fine detachable end, 5 sizes 18, 20, 22, 24 and 26 s.w.g. × 19 mm ($\frac{3}{4}$ in) long.

L. Spare detachable ends.

M. Zoellner's raspatory, curved on flat, narrow bladed, on metal handle.

N. Ormerod's aural scissors, extra fine, curved upwards, crocodile action, black finished.

O. Ormerod's aural forceps with extra fine circular cup crocodile action jaws, black finished.

P. Ormerod's aural forceps with extra fine elongated cup crocodile jaws, black finished.

Q. Hartmann's aural forceps with extra fine serrated crocodile action jaws, black finished.

R. Aural forceps, extra fine, double cup oval jaws 1·75 mm × 0·75 mm crocodile action, black finished.

S. Scissors, extra fine, crocodile action jaws, black finished.

T. Zoellner's Skin Graft Plate, 152 × 76 mm (6 × 3 in) with three holes 22, 28, 32 mm ($\frac{7}{8}$, $1\frac{1}{8}$ and $1\frac{1}{4}$ in) diameter.

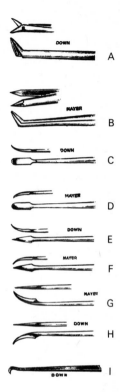

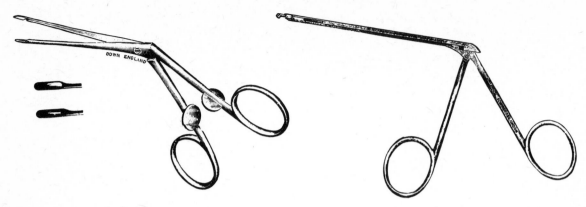

Heath Aural Forceps (Sc. ½)   Wisharts Guillotine Forceps (Sc. ½)   For head of malleus.

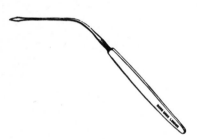

Agnew Myringotome (Sc. ½)

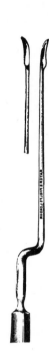

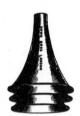

Yearsley Aural Specula (Sc. ½)   Daggets Myringotome (Full size approx.)

99   Jobson Horne Probe (Sc. ⅔)

E.N.T. Nasal Instruments

DOWN BROS. LTD.

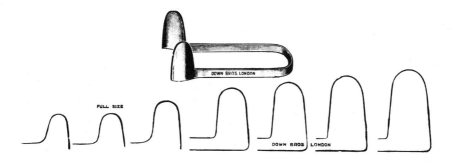

Thudichum Nasal Speculum (Sc. $\frac{1}{2}$)

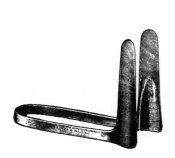

St Clair Thompson Nasal Speculum (Sc. $\frac{1}{2}$)

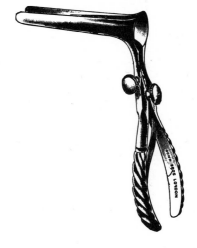

Killian Nasal Speculum,
Available with Screws for
Retaining the blades in
an open position (Sc. $\frac{1}{3}$)

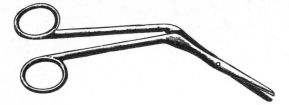

Heymann Angled Nasal Scissors (Sc. $\frac{1}{2}$)

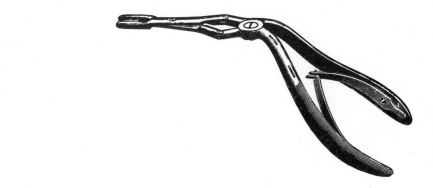

Jansen Middleton Nasal Septum Forceps (Sc. $\frac{1}{2}$)

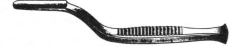

Tilley Nasal Gouge (Sc. $\frac{1}{3}$)

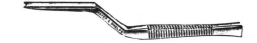

Killian Nasal Gouge (Sc. $\frac{1}{3}$)

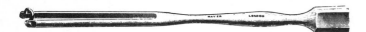

Ballenger Swivel Knife (Sc. $\frac{1}{2}$)

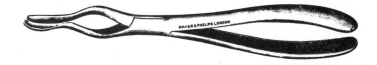

Walsham Nasal Re-Dressing Forceps (Sc. $\frac{1}{3}$)

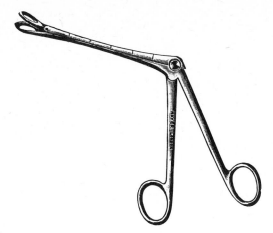

Henckel-Tilleys Punch Forceps (Sc. $\frac{2}{5}$)

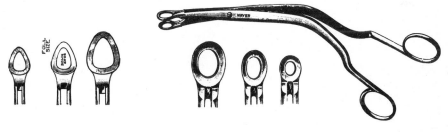

Luc Punch Forceps (Sc. $\frac{1}{3}$)

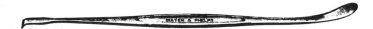

Howarth Nasal Raspatory (Sc. $\frac{2}{5}$)

Hill Nasal Raspatory (Sc. $\frac{1}{2}$)

E.N.T. Tracheal Instruments

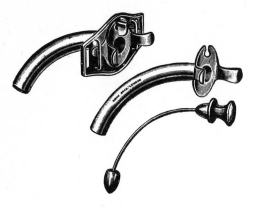

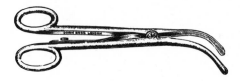

Trousseau Tracheal
Dilating Forceps (Sc. $\frac{2}{3}$)
Sizes available 16–34 Charrière gauge.

Chevalier Jackson Tracheostomy Tubes (Sc. $\frac{2}{3}$)

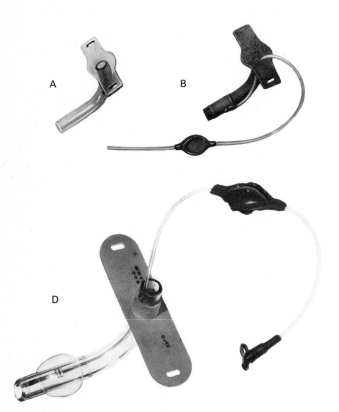

A. Morrant Baker Plastic Tracheostomy Cannula,
with fixed plastic flange slotted for retaining
tape.
B. Morrant Baker Rubber Tracheostomy Cannula,
with fixed rubber flange slotted for retaining
tape and detachable inflatable rubber cuff.
C. James Rubber Tracheostomy Cannula, with
detachable rubber flange slotted for retaining
tape and fixed inflatable rubber cuff.
D. Portex Cuffed Plastic Tracheostomy Tube.

Tracheostomy Cannula or Tubes (Sc. reduced)
Sizes available: A, B and C, 27, 30, 33, 36, 39 and 42 Charrière gauge or 3 to 12 Magill tube scale.

E.N.T. Antrum Instruments

DOWN BROS. LTD.

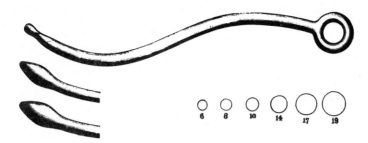

Watson-Williams Set of Bougies (Sc. Full size approx.)

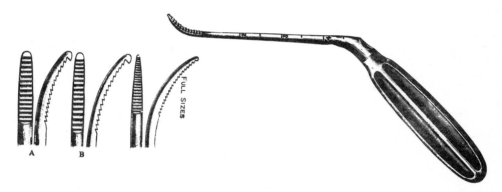

Watson-Williams Frontal Sinus Rasp (Sc. $\frac{1}{2}$)

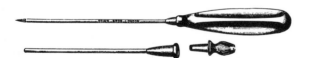

Tilley Lichwitz Antrum Trocar and Cannula (Sc. $\frac{2}{5}$)

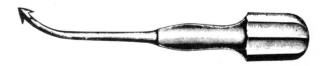

Tilley Antrum Trocar (Sc. $\frac{2}{5}$)

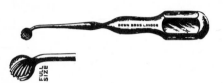

Tilleys Antrum Burrs (Sc. $\frac{1}{3}$)

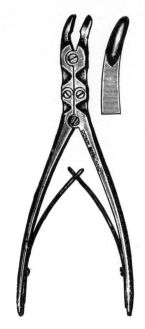

Luer Jansen Gouge or Punch Forceps (Sc. $\frac{1}{2}$)

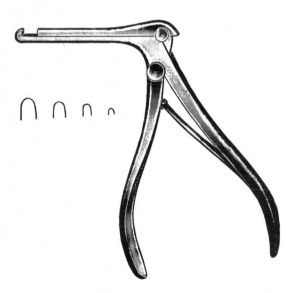

Kerrisons Rongeur, Upward Cutting (Sc. $\frac{1}{2}$)

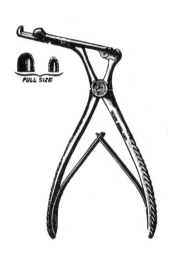

Citelli Gouge or Punch Forceps (Sc. $\frac{1}{3}$)

E.N.T. Tonsil Instruments

DOWN BROS. LTD.

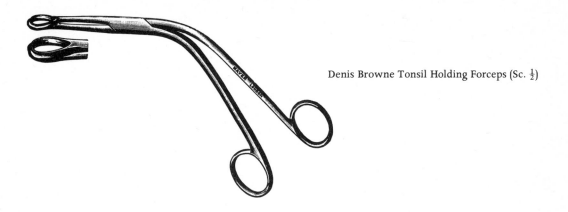

Denis Browne Tonsil Holding Forceps (Sc. $\frac{1}{2}$)

Poppers Haemostatic Tonsil Guillotine (Enculeator) (Sc. $\frac{1}{3}$)

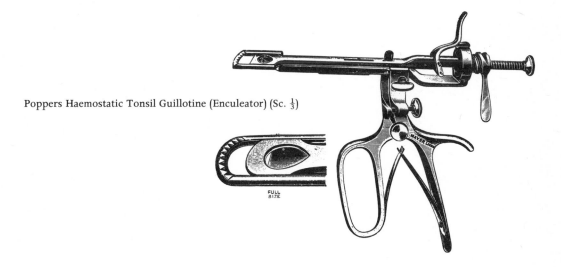

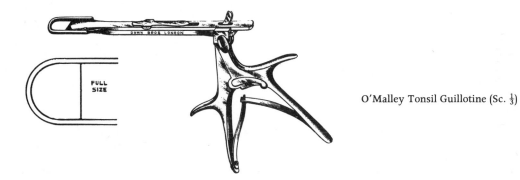

O'Malley Tonsil Guillotine (Sc. $\frac{1}{3}$)

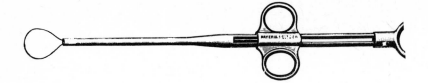

Eves Tonsil Snare (Sc. $\frac{2}{5}$)

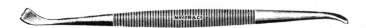

Gwynne Evans Tonsil Dissector (Sc. $\frac{1}{2}$)

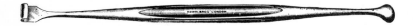

Mollinson Tonsil Dissector and Pillar Retractor (Sc. $\frac{1}{2}$)

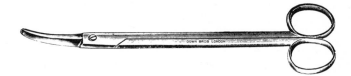

Woods Curved Tonsil Scissors (Sc. $\frac{1}{2}$)

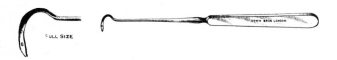

Irwin Moores Tonsil Needle (Sc. $\frac{1}{3}$)

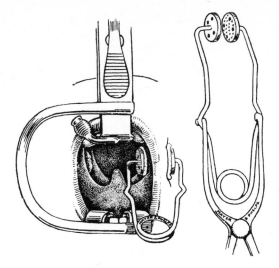

Beneys Tonsil Compressor (Sc. $\frac{2}{3}$)

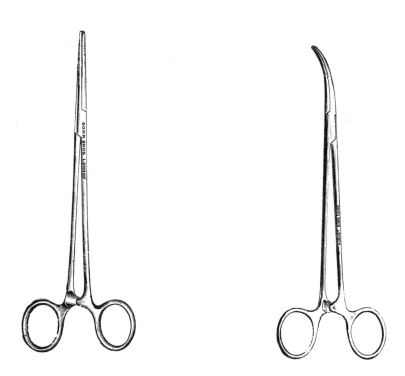

Birkett Tonsil Artery Forceps (straight and curved) (Sc. $\frac{1}{2}$)

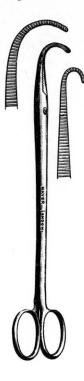

Negus Tonsil Artery Forceps (curved) Sc. $\frac{1}{2}$

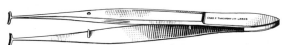

Barraquer Fixation Forceps (Sc. $\frac{3}{4}$)

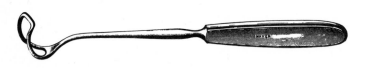

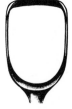

FULL SIZE

Barnhills Adenoid Curette (Sc. $\frac{1}{2}$)

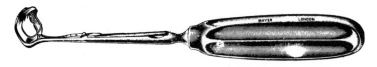

St Clair Thompson Adenoid Curette (Sc. $\frac{1}{3}$)

Gastric and Intestinal Instruments

CHAS. F. THACKRAY LTD.

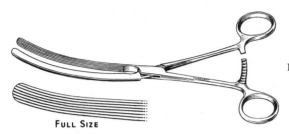

Doyen Intestinal Clamp (Curved Occlusion) (Sc. $\frac{1}{3}$)

FULL SIZE

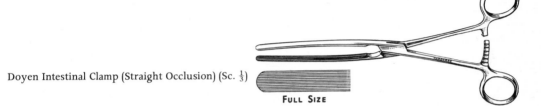

Doyen Intestinal Clamp (Straight Occlusion) (Sc. $\frac{1}{3}$)

FULL SIZE

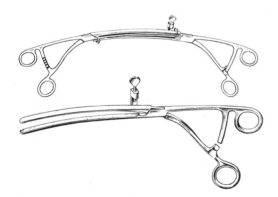

Lane Twin Stomach Clamp (Occlusion) (Sc. $\frac{1}{4}$)

Lloyd Davies Rectal Excision Clamp (Sc. $\frac{1}{4}$)

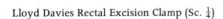

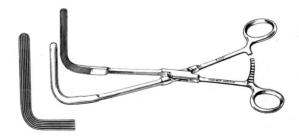

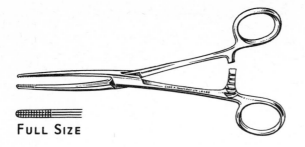

FULL SIZE

Seton Pringles Intestinal Clamp (Sc. $\frac{1}{3}$)

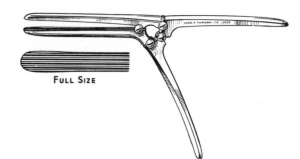

FULL SIZE

Payr Intestinal Clamp (Crushing) (Sc. $\frac{1}{3}$)

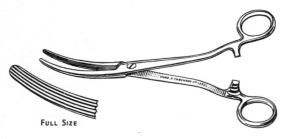

FULL SIZE

Parker-Kerr Intestinal Clamp (Crushing) (Sc. $\frac{1}{4}$)

De Martel Intestinal Clamps (Crushing) (Sc. $\frac{1}{4}$)

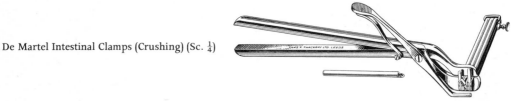

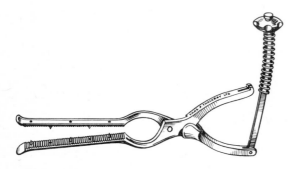

Mikulicz Enterotome (Crushing) Sc. $\frac{2}{3}$

Gall-Bladder and Common Bile Duct Instruments

CHAS. F. THACKRAY LTD.

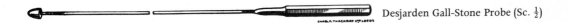

Desjarden Gall-Stone Probe (Sc. $\frac{1}{2}$)

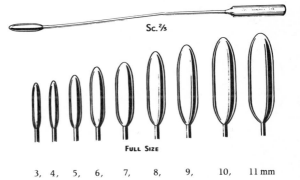

Bakes Common Bile Duct Dilators (Sc. $\frac{2}{3}$)

Sc. $\frac{2}{3}$

FULL SIZE

3, 4, 5, 6, 7, 8, 9, 10, 11 mm

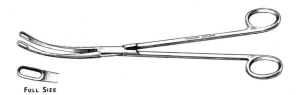

Desjardin Gall-Stone Forceps (Sc. $\frac{1}{3}$)

FULL SIZE

Moynihan Malleable Gall-Stone Probe and Scoop (Sc. $\frac{1}{4}$)

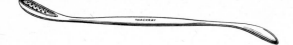

Moynihan Gall-Stone Scoop (Sc. $\frac{2}{5}$)

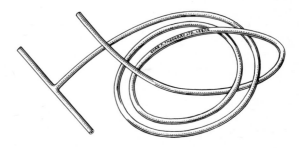

Kehr 'T' Tube (Sc. $\frac{1}{3}$)

Sizes available: 12, 15, 18, 21, 24 and 27 Charrière gauge. Rubber or plastic.

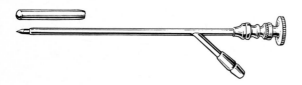

Ochsner Gall-Bladder Trocar (Sc. $\frac{1}{2}$)

Genito-Urinary Instruments, Catheters, etc.

ESCHMANN BROS. & WALSH LTD.

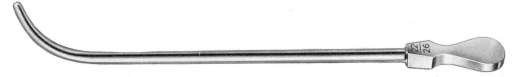

155   Clutton Bougie (Sc. ½)

Sizes available: 00/1, 0/2, ½/3, 1/4, 2/5, 3/6, 4/7, 5/8, 6/9, 7/10, 8/11, 9/12, 10/13, 11/14, 12/15, 13/16, 14/17, 15/18 Charrière gauge. Stainless steel.

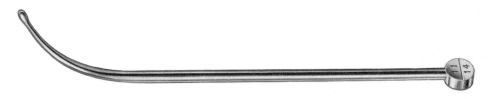

Lister Bougie (Sc. ½)

Sizes available: 6/10, 8/12, 10/14, 12/16, 14/18, 16/20, 18/22, 20/24, 26/30 and 28/32 Charrière gauge. Stainless steel.

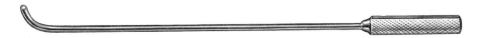

Clutton Bladder Sound (Sc. ½)

Sizes available: 9, 12, 15 and 18 Charrière gauge. Stainless steel.

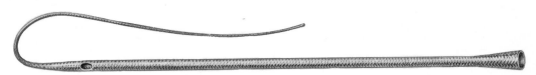

Harrison 'Whip' Catheter (Sc. ⅔)

Sizes available: 5 to 27 Charrière gauge. Rubber.

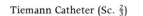

Nélaton Catheter (Sc. $\frac{2}{3}$)

Sizes available: 8 to 30 Charrière gauge. Rubber or plastic.

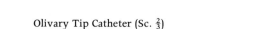

Tiemann Catheter (Sc. $\frac{2}{3}$)

Sizes available: 10 to 26 Charrière gauge. Rubber or plastic.

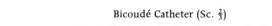

Olivary Tip Catheter (Sc. $\frac{2}{3}$)

Sizes available: 5 to 30 Charrière gauge. Plastic.

Coudé Catheter (Sc. $\frac{2}{3}$)

Sizes available: 5 to 30 Charrière gauge. Plastic.

Bicoudé Catheter (Sc. $\frac{2}{3}$)

Sizes available: 5 to 30 Charrière gauge. Plastic

Harris Catheter (Sc. $\frac{2}{3}$)

Sizes available: 9 to 45 Charrière gauge. Rubber or plastic.

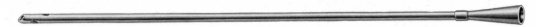

'Whistle Tip' Catheter (Sc. $\frac{2}{3}$)

Sizes available: 9 to 45 Charrière gauge. Rubber or plastic.

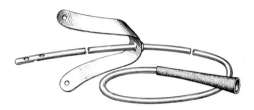

Gibbons Catheter (Sc. $\frac{2}{3}$)

Sizes available: 4 to 24 Charrière gauge. Plastic.

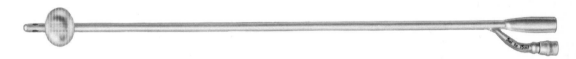

Foley Self-Retaining Catheter (Sc. $\frac{1}{2}$)

Sizes available: 5 to 15 ml balloon, 14 to 26 Charrière gauge. Latex or Plastic.

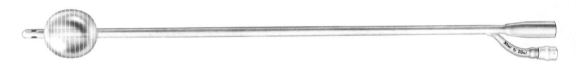

Foley Self-Retaining Catheter, Haemostatic (Sc. $\frac{1}{2}$)

Sizes available: 30 to 50 ml balloon, 14 to 26 Charrière gauge. Latex or Plastic.

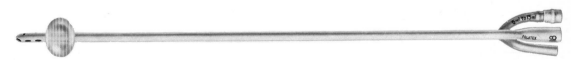

Alcock-Foley Irrigating Catheter (Sc. $\frac{1}{2}$)

Sizes available: 14 to 26 Charrière gauge. Latex or Plastic.

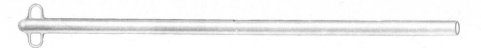

Malecot Self-Retaining Catheter (Sc. ½)

Sizes available: 9 to 48 Charrière gauge. Rubber.

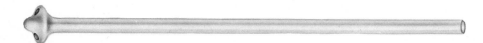

De Pezzer Self-Retaining Catheter (Sc. ½)

Sizes available: 12 to 39 Charrière gauge. Rubber.

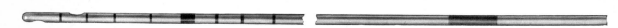

Ureteric Catheter Cylindrical (enlarged)

Marked with black or red bands to distinguish right and left.
Sizes available: 3 to 12 Charrière gauge. Plastic.

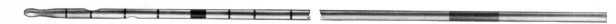

Ureteric Catheter Olivary (enlarged)

Marked with black or red bands to distinguish right and left.
Sizes available: 3 to 12 Charrière gauge. Plastic.

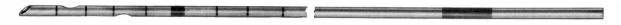

Ureteric Catheter Flute End (enlarged)

Marked with black or red bands to distinguish right and left.
Sizes available: 3 to 12 Charrière gauge. Plastic.

CHAS. F. THACKRAY LTD.

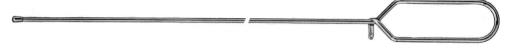

Catheter Introducer (Sc. ⅔)

Genito-Urinary, Prostatectomy and Bladder Instruments

CHAS. F. THACKRAY LTD.

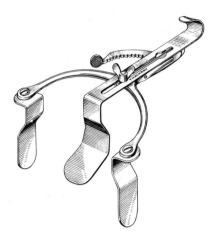

Millen Bladder Retractor (Sc. $\frac{1}{4}$)

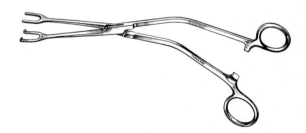

Millen Modified Young Ligature
Holding Forceps (Sc. $\frac{1}{4}$)

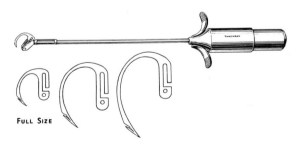

FULL SIZE

Millen Boomerang Needle
Holder and Needles (Sc. $\frac{1}{3}$)

Gynaecological Instruments

ESCHMANN BROS. & WALSH LTD.

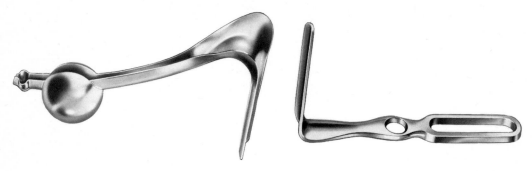

Auvard Vaginal Speculum (Sc. $\frac{1}{4}$)   Landon Vaginal Speculum (Sc. $\frac{1}{3}$)

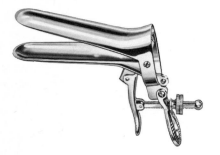

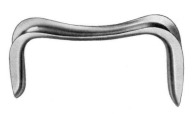

Cuscoe self-retaining vaginal speculum (Sc. $\frac{1}{3}$)   Sims Vaginal Speculum (Sc. $\frac{1}{4}$)

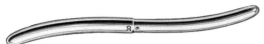

Hawkin Ambler Uterine Dilators (Sc. $\frac{1}{3}$)   Heggar Uterine Dilator Double Ended (Sc. $\frac{1}{3}$)

Sizes available: 3/6 mm. diameter.   Sizes available: 2 to 24 mm.

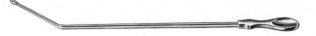

Simpson Uterine Sound (Sc. $\frac{1}{4}$)

Sizes available: 11·5 in. or 28·75 cm. length.

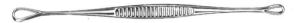

Sims Uterine Curette (Sc. $\frac{1}{4}$)

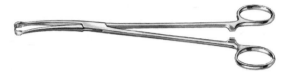

Teale Vulsellum Forceps (Sc. $\frac{1}{3}$)

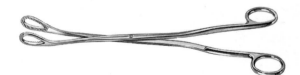

McClintock Ovum Forceps (Sc. $\frac{1}{3}$)

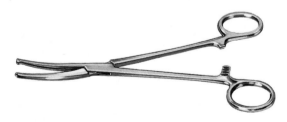

Maingot Hysterectomy Clamps (Sc. $\frac{2}{3}$)

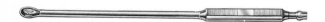

Playfair Probe (Sc. ½)

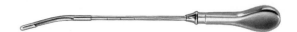

Sharman Endometrial Biopsy Curette (Sc. ⅓)

Rheinstater Flushing Curette (Sc. ⅓)

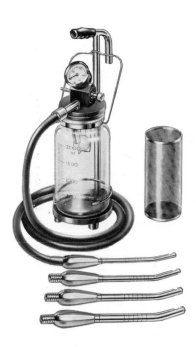

Intra-Uterine Suction Tube and Apparatus (Reduced Size)

Neurosurgical Instruments

DOWN BROS. LTD.

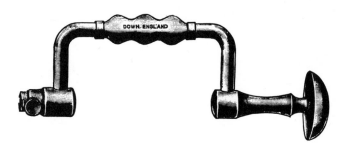

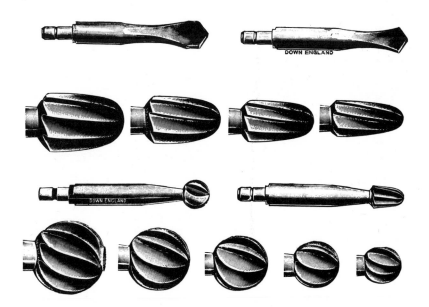

Hudson Brace (Sc. $\frac{1}{2}$) Perforator (Sc. $\frac{1}{3}$)
Spherical and Cylindrical Burrs (Full Size approx.)

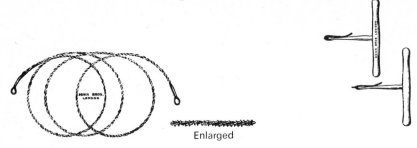

Enlarged

Gigli Wire Saw and Handle (Sc. $\frac{1}{2}$) (Used in pairs)

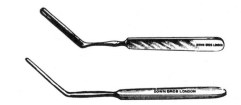

Sergeant-Horsley Dura Mater Separator (Sc. $\frac{1}{3}$)

Cairn-De Martel Wire Saw Guide (Sc. $\frac{1}{3}$)

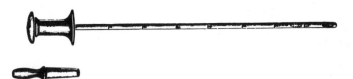

Jefferson Ventricular Cannula and Tubing Connection (Full size approx.)

Dandys Ventricular Drainage Cannulis (Full size approx.)

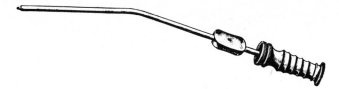

Adson Fraser Brain Suction Tube (Sc. $\frac{1}{2}$)

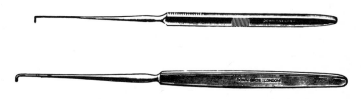

Adson Nerve Hooks (Sc. $\frac{1}{3}$)

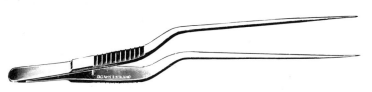

Loves Nerve Root Hook (Sc. $\frac{1}{3}$)

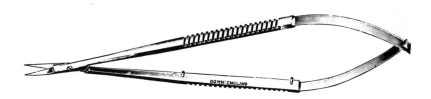

Jacobsons Micro Spring Scissors (Sc. $\frac{2}{3}$)

Bayonet Shaped Fine Dissecting Forceps (Sc. $\frac{2}{3}$)

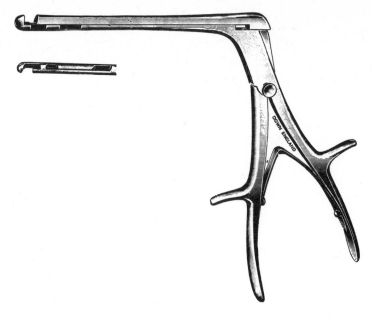

Duggans Rongeur (Sc. $\frac{1}{2}$)

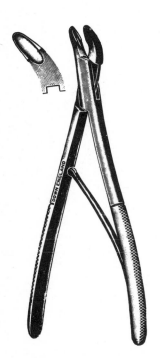

Wilm Gouge Forceps (Sc. $\frac{1}{2}$)

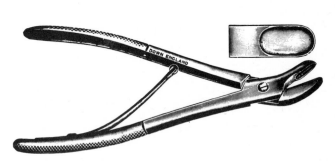

Trotters Rongeur (Sc. $\frac{1}{2}$)

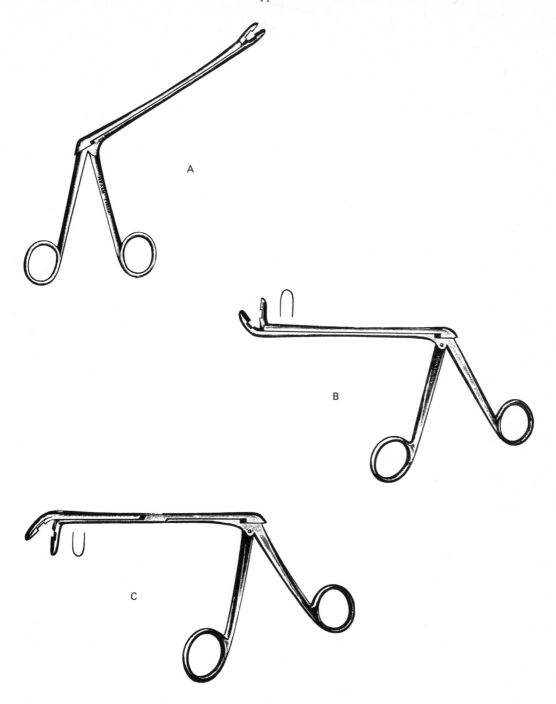

Cushing Rongeur. For Pituitary Body (Sc. $\frac{1}{2}$)

    A. Straight.
    B. Angled forwards.
    C. Angled backwards.

Cushing-McKenzie Silver Haemostasis Clips (Full size approx.)

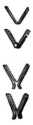

Olivecronia-Norlens Haemostats Clips (Full size approx.)

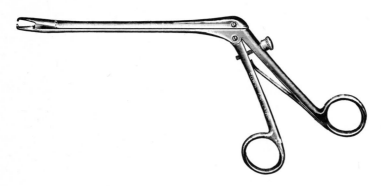

Clip Applying Forceps (Sc. $\frac{1}{2}$)

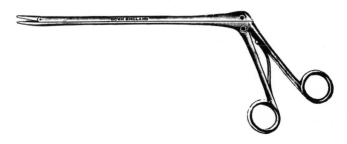

Patterson-Ross Clip Applying Forceps (Sc. $\frac{1}{2}$)

Ophthalmic Instruments

CHAS. F. THACKRAY LTD.

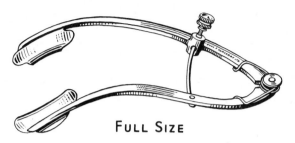

FULL SIZE

Lang Eye Speculum (Full size)

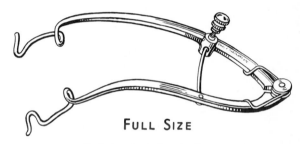

FULL SIZE

Clark Eye Speculum (Full size)

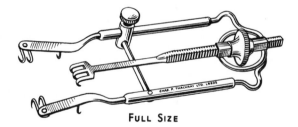

FULL SIZE

Bishop-Harman Lachrymal Retractor (Full size)

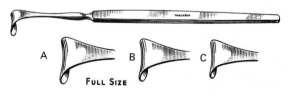

A   B   C

FULL SIZE

Desmarres Retractors (Sc. $\frac{2}{3}$)
(Sizes A, B and C)

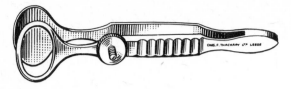

Wilde Entropion Forceps (Sc. $\frac{3}{4}$)

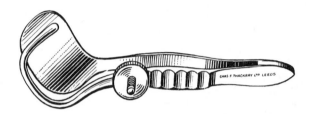

Snellen Entropion Forceps (Sc. $\frac{3}{4}$)

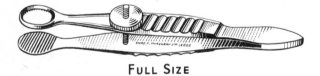

FULL SIZE

Greene Tarsal Cyst Forceps (Sc. $\frac{3}{4}$)

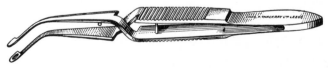

Castroviejo Capsule Forceps (Sc. $\frac{3}{4}$)

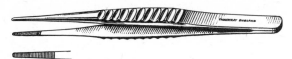

Fixation Forceps (Non-Toothed) (Sc. $\frac{2}{3}$)

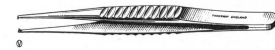

Fixation Forceps (Toothed) (Sc. $\frac{2}{3}$)

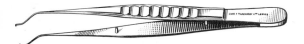

Traquair Iris Forceps (Sc. $\frac{3}{4}$)

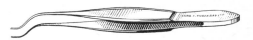

Barraquer Iris Forceps (Sc. $\frac{3}{4}$)

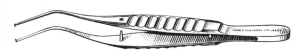

Swann Neck Iris Forceps (Sc. $\frac{3}{4}$)

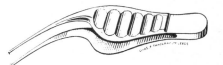

Fischer-Arlt Iris Forceps (Full Size)

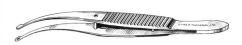

Arruga Capsule Forceps (Sc. $\frac{1}{2}$)

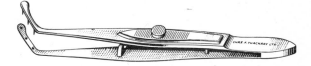

Prince Strabismus Forceps (Sc. $\frac{3}{4}$)

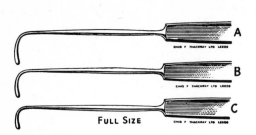

Graefe Strabismus Hooks (Full size)

A. Large;   B. Medium;   C. Small

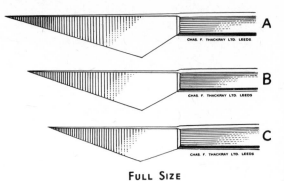

Beer Cataract Knives (Full size)

(Sizes A, B and C)

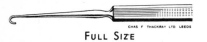

Graefe Cataract Knife (Full size)

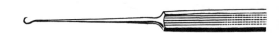

Snellen Vectis (Full size)

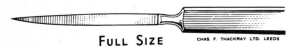

Tyrrel Iris Hook (Full size)

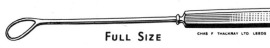

Lens Hook (Full size)

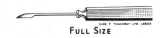

Ziegler Iridotomy Knife (Full size)

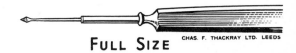

Bowman Cataract Needle (Full size)

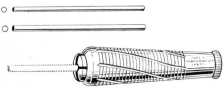

Elliot Sclerectomy Trephine (Full size)

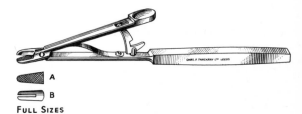

Silcock Needle Holder with Two Shapes of Jaws (Sc. $\frac{1}{2}$)

Orthopaedic Instruments, Bone Holders, etc.

ZIMMER ORTHOPAEDIC LTD.

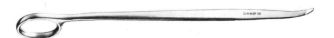

Trethowan (Ring) Bone Lever (Sc. $\frac{1}{3}$)

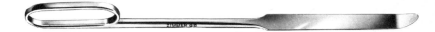

Lane Bone Lever (Sc. $\frac{1}{3}$)

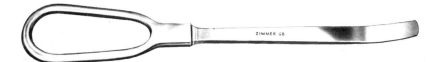

Bristow Bone Lever (Sc. $\frac{2}{3}$)

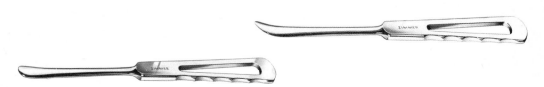

St Thomas' Bone Levers (Sc. $\frac{1}{2}$)

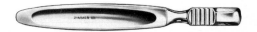

Faraboeuf Rugine (Sc. $\frac{2}{3}$)

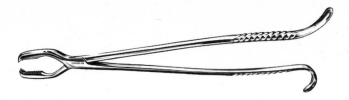

Lane Bone Holding Forceps (Sc. $\frac{1}{4}$)

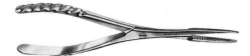

Necrosis Forceps (Straight) (Sc. $\frac{1}{3}$)

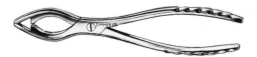

Fergusson Lion Bone Holding Forceps (Sc. $\frac{1}{4}$)

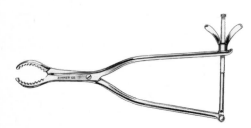

Hey Groves Bone Holding Forceps with Self-Retaining Screw (Sc. $\frac{1}{4}$)

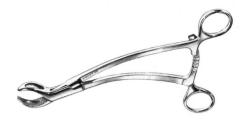

Burns Bone Holding Forceps (Sc. $\frac{1}{4}$)

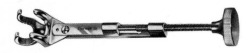

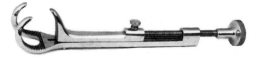

Lowman Self-Retaining Bone Holding Clamps (Sc. $\frac{1}{3}$)

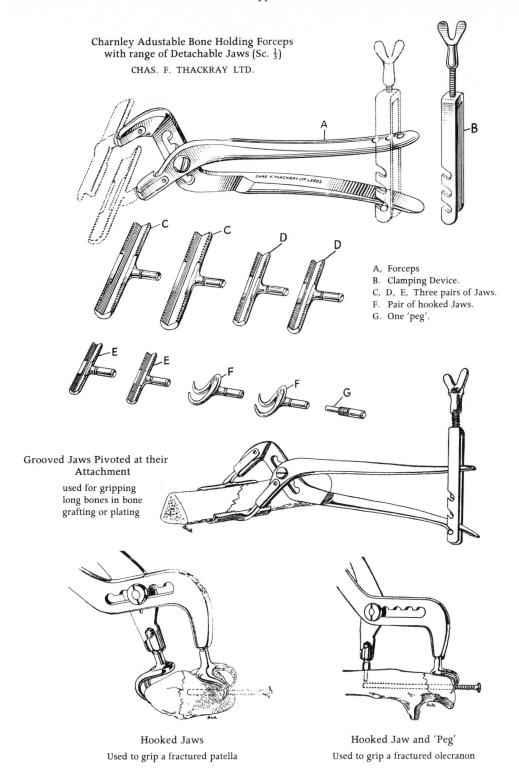

Charnley Adustable Bone Holding Forceps
with range of Detachable Jaws (Sc. $\frac{1}{3}$)

CHAS. F. THACKRAY LTD.

A, Forceps
B. Clamping Device.
C, D, E, Three pairs of Jaws.
F. Pair of hooked Jaws.
G. One 'peg'.

Grooved Jaws Pivoted at their Attachment

used for gripping long bones in bone grafting or plating

Hooked Jaws

Used to grip a fractured patella

Hooked Jaw and 'Peg'

Used to grip a fractured olecranon

Bone Cutting Forceps, etc.

ZIMMER ORTHOPAEDIC LTD.

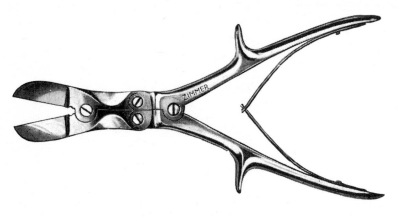

Horsley Bone Cutting Forceps (Sc. $\frac{1}{2}$)

(Compound action)

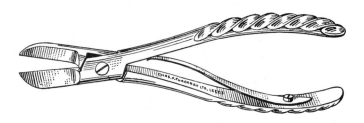

Liston Bone Cutting Forceps (Sc. $\frac{1}{2}$)

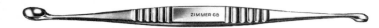

Volkmann Curetting Spoon (Sc. $\frac{1}{2}$)

(Double end. Four sizes A, B, C and D)

CHAS. F. THACKRAY LTD.

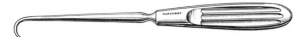

Bone Hook (Sc. $\frac{1}{3}$)

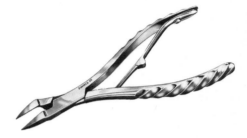

Stamms Bone Cutting Forceps (Sc. $\frac{1}{2}$)

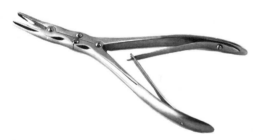

Jansen-Zaufel Bone Rongeur (Compound Action) (Sc. $\frac{1}{2}$)

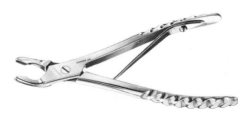

Wilms Gouge Forceps (Sc. $\frac{1}{2}$)

Hand Saws and Mallet

ZIMMER ORTHOPAEDIC LTD.

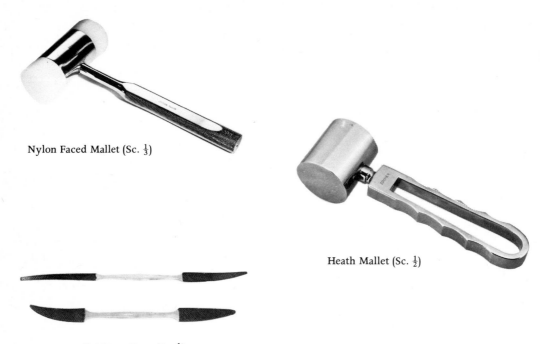

Nylon Faced Mallet (Sc. $\frac{1}{3}$)

Heath Mallet (Sc. $\frac{1}{2}$)

Puttitype Rasp (Sc. $\frac{1}{4}$)

HOWMEDICA (UK) LTD.

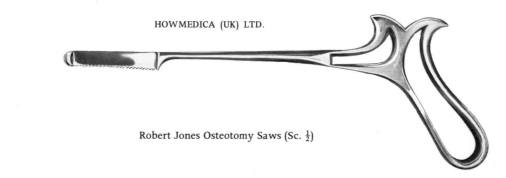

Robert Jones Osteotomy Saws (Sc. $\frac{1}{2}$)

ZIMMER ORTHOPAEDIC LTD.

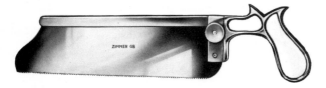

Sergeant Amputation Saw (Sc. $\frac{1}{4}$)

Hand Drills

ZIMMER ORTHOPAEDIC LTD.

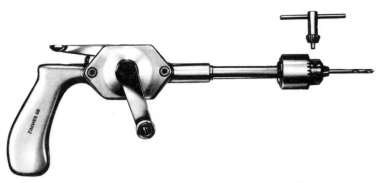

Pistol-Grip Hand Drill with Jacobs Chuck (Sc. $\frac{2}{5}$)

($\frac{1}{4}$ inch capacity)

This drill has a 2-to-1 gear ratio and is cannulated for the entire length to accommodate Steinmann pins, Kirschner wires, long-shank drills and screwdriver bits. Release of the thumb-operated lever at the top of the drill instantly stops the turning of the gears and locks the chuck.

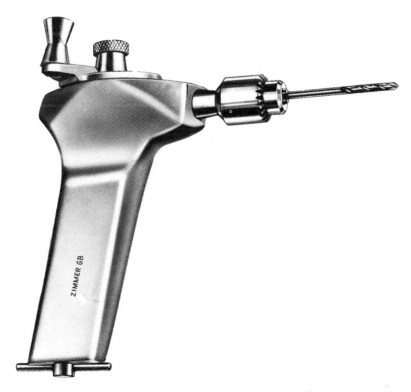

Micro Hand-Drill with Jacobs Chuck (Sc. $\frac{5}{9}$)

(4 mm ($\frac{5}{32}$ in) capacity, 2 to 1 gear ratio)

For use in confined operative fields. Insert shows chuck key fits into base of handle.

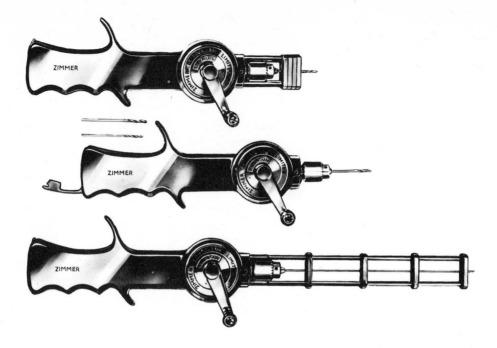

Kirschner Hand Drill with Jacobs Chuck (Sc. $\frac{1}{4}$)

(4 mm ($\frac{5}{32}$ in) capacity, 2 to 1 gear ratio)

A. Twist drill mounted in chuck, showing telescopic extension collapsed.
B. Twist drill mounted in chuck, telescopic extension removed.
C. Kirschner wire mounted in chuck, telescopic extension fully extended to support wire
    NOTE.—Telescopic extension is drilled to take a wire of ·0625 inch maximum diameter.

Air Drill

HOWMEDICA (U.K.) LTD.

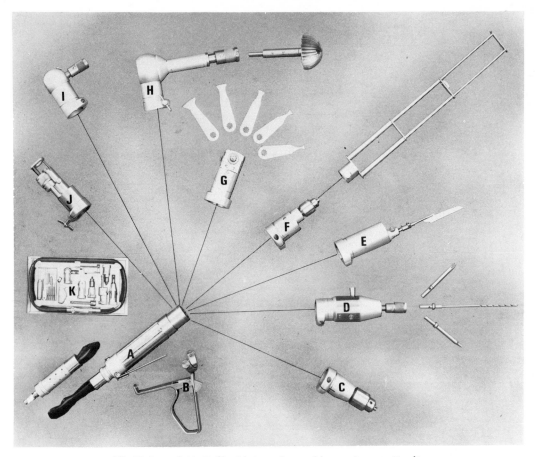

The Universal Air Drill with interchangeable attachments (Sc. $\frac{1}{4}$)

A. Driver/handpiece with attached hose. Consists essentially of an air driven motor with a high torque utilising 180 litres of air per minute at 86 pounds per square inch. The hose assembly provides for the intake and the exhaust of pressurized air which is carried away from the operation area. The appropriate speeds for operating the various attachments are determined automatically by the instrument. In addition, speeds can be varied by the hand throttle control.

B. Pistol grip.

C. Drill attachment with universal Jacobs chuck, driven at a speed of 320 r.p.m., suitable for bone drills or burrs up to 12 mm diameter.

D. Drive attachment for screwdriver bits. Driven at a speed of 260 r.p.m., this attachment will operate with either a right-hand or left-hand drive as has a torque slip mechanism to prevent torque overload.

E. Oscillating saw attachment.

F. Drill attachment with universal Jacobs chuck, driven at a speed of 700 r.p.m. is suitable for bone drills and burrs up to 4mm diameter. Is also suitable for the insertion of Kirschner wires (telescopic wire guide shown).

G. Oscillating saw attachment which operates in an axial pattern.

H. Drill attachment for acetabular reamers, driven at a speed of 80 r.p.m.

I. Drill attachment for flexible intramedullary reamers, driven at a speed of 170 r.p.m.

J. Skull trepan operates at a speed of 400 r.p.m. The trepan shuts off automatically as soon as the skull is perforated. An outer supporting plate prevents further burr penetration.

K. Sterilisation case (size reduced) for universal air drill and attachments.

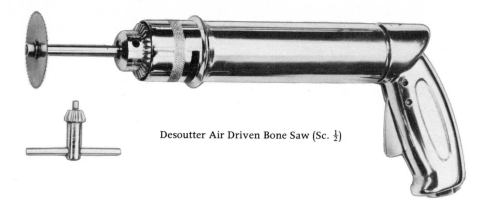

Desoutter Air Driven Bone Saw (Sc. $\frac{1}{2}$)

Screwing and Plating

CHAS. F. THACKRAY LTD.

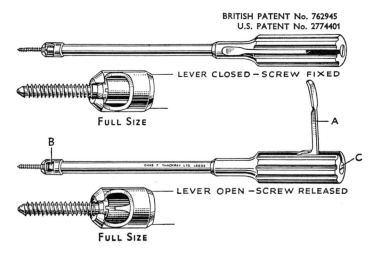

BRITISH PATENT No. 762945
U.S. PATENT No. 2774401

LEVER CLOSED—SCREW FIXED

FULL SIZE

A

B

C

LEVER OPEN—SCREW RELEASED

FULL SIZE

Williams Improved Automatic Screwdriver (Sc. $\frac{1}{3}$)

This instrument facilitates the fixing of screws during bone surgery. It is an adaptation of an existing accepted pattern (Burns) in which the screw fixing device at the base of the handle has been replaced by a quick-action lever recessed in the handle. The lever (A) is closed or opened to fix or release a screw from the shaped sleeve (B) in the end of the tubular shaft. This lever is centrally placed in relation to the screw slot and is suitable for both left- and right-handed operators.

The upper illustration shows the screwdriver ready for use; the spring-loaded driving shaft has been pushed forward to engage the slot of the screw head; the lower illustration shows the lever (A) open and the screw head disengaged.

Standard screws such as Sherman's or Lane's patterns can be used with this instrument (up to 4 mm ($\frac{5}{32}$ in) external diameter of thread with a head diameter of 7·1 mm ($\frac{5}{32}$ in). The shaped sleeve at the distal end accommodates a wide variation in shapes of screw heads.

It is possible to use the instrument to drive a screw fully home after it has been released, and in this case the lever (A) is closed so that the screwdriver protrudes from the sleeve. However, some surgeons use an ordinary Lane's screwdriver to complete this manoeuvre.

A special feature of the instrument is the adjusting screw (C) in the base of the handle. This screw is adjusted to give the lever (A) a firm fixation on the screw head. Once this screw is set correctly it need not be altered unless a screw with a larger or smaller head is required.

The use of this instrument was described in the *Lancet*, June 15, 1957, p. 1225.

ZIMMER ORTHOPAEDIC LTD.

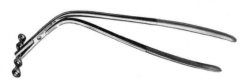

Lane Plate-Holding Forceps (Sc. $\frac{1}{3}$)

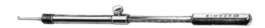

Screw Depth Gauge (Sc. $\frac{1}{5}$)

This is used to determine the length of the screw needed to penetrate the bone. The end of the gauge is inserted in the drilled hole and hooked over the bone surface. By releasing the thumb screw, the sleeve may be advanced snugly against the bone or bone plate. When the screw is tightened, the sleeve will remain in position as the gauge is withdrawn. Calibrations on the stem barrel indicate the length of screw required. Another form of screw depth gauge, the Crawford Adams type, is illustrated in Figure 340, page 428, but in this case a thumb screw is not provided and the length of screw is determined before the gauge is withdrawn from the drill hole.

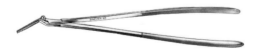

Screw-Holding Forceps (Sc. $\frac{1}{3}$)

Kuntscher Intramedullary Nailing of Femur

ZIMMER ORTHOPAEDIC LTD.

A

B

Kuntscher Intramedullary Femoral Nails (Reduced)

S.Mo. (EN 58J). Stainless steel

A. Single slot
B. Slotted and pointed each end.

These are clover-leaf in section and are supplied either slotted and pointed at one or both end, the latter being essential if the nails are to be inserted by the retrograde method.

Standard sizes available:
12 mm width; lengths of 36 to 52 cm in 2 cm steps.
9, 10 and 11 mm width; lengths of 32 to 52 cm in 2 cm steps.
8 mm width; lengths of 14 to 42 cm in 2 cm steps.
6 mm width; lengths of 14 to 34 cm in 2 cm steps.

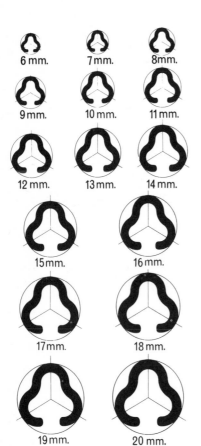

6 mm.   7 mm.   8 mm.
9 mm.   10 mm.   11 mm.
12 mm.   13 mm.   14 mm.
15 mm.   16 mm.
17 mm.   18 mm.
19 mm.   20 mm.

Cross section.

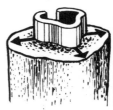

CLOVERLEAF SECTION

Kuntscher Medullary Nails are produced with a cloverleaf profile to achieve axial and longitudinal elasticity.

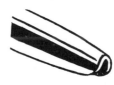

TAPERED ENDS

Specially tapered conical points encourage a free passage through the medullary canal and reduce the possibility of impacting.

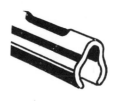

SLOT IN THE ENDS

To provide an adequate slot, for extraction, with minimum weakening of the section, Zimmer Kuntscher Nails are *punched* and not milled.

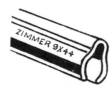

ELECTRIC ETCHING

Diameter and length are marked by an electric etching process, which is chemically clean.

Characteristics.

ZIMMER ORTHOPAEDIC LTD.

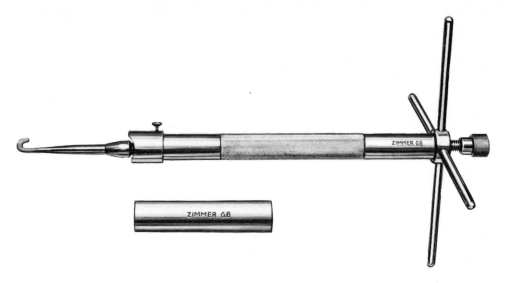

Brigden Extractor for Kuntscher Nails (Sc. $\frac{1}{4}$)

Designed to extract Kuntscher nails although it can be used with an adaptor on Hansen Street nails. Due to the length of the capstan arms, considerable extraction force can be exerted. To accommodate extra-long nails, a special extension tube is available and is illustrated beside the instrument.

The use of this extractor was described by J. H. Penrose, F.R.C.S., in the November 1959, British issue of the *Journal of Bone and Joint Surgery*.

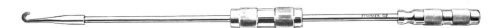

Kuntscher Nail Sliding Hammer Extractor (Sc. $\frac{1}{5}$)

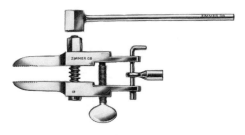

Newman-Kuntscher Nail Extractor (Sc. $\frac{1}{4}$) Used with Sliding Hammer Extractor

Screws and Bolts

Illustrations—ZIMMER ORTHOPAEDIC LTD.

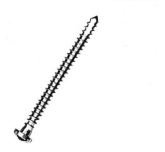
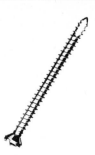
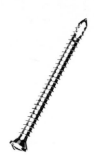

Sherman Bone Screws (Full size approx.)

S.Mo. (EN 58J). Stainless steel, Titanium or Vitallium.

Fine and coarse thread, with self-tapping point and single or cross slotted head.

Supplied in two diameters: 3·6 mm ($\frac{9}{64}$ in) and 4 mm ($\frac{5}{32}$ in).
Lengths available in 10 mm to 51 mm in approx. 3 mm steps, 57 mm, 64 mm, 70 mm, 76 mm, 83 mm, 89 mm, 95 mm and 102 mm.
$\frac{3}{8}$ to 2 in, in $\frac{1}{8}$ in steps, $2\frac{1}{4}$, $2\frac{1}{2}$, $2\frac{3}{4}$, 3, $3\frac{1}{4}$, $3\frac{1}{2}$, $3\frac{3}{4}$ and 4 in.

Technical Data—

$\frac{9}{64}$ in (3·6 mm) diameter screws:

    Head diameter: $\frac{15}{64}$ in (·234 in or 5·9 mm).
    Outside thread diameter: $\frac{9}{64}$ in (·140 in or 3·6 mm).
    Root thread diameter: $\frac{7}{64}$ in (·109 in or 2·8 mm).
    Threads per inch (fine thread): 32
    Threads per inch (coarse thread): 20.
    Recommended drill size. No. 31 (·120 in or 3 mm).

$\frac{5}{32}$ in (4 mm) diameter screws:

    Head diameter: $\frac{9}{32}$ in (·281 in or 7·1 mm).
    Outside thread diameter: $\frac{5}{32}$ in (·156 in or 4 mm).
    Root thread diameter: just under $\frac{1}{8}$ in (·116 in or 2·9 mm).
    Threads per inch (fine thread): 32.
    Threads per inch (coarse thread): 20.
    Recommended drill size: $\frac{9}{64}$ in (·140 in or 3·6 mm).

A   B   C   D

Varieties of Screw Heads (Enlarged Views)

A. Single slot, available in all varieties of screws both S.Mo. (EN 58J). Stainless steel, Titanium and Vitallium.

B. Cross slot, available in Sherman screws S.Mo. (EN 58J). Stainless steel and Titanium.

C. Hexagonal recessed slot.

D. Phillips recessed head, available in Phillips screws Vitallium, which have an identical shaft to $\frac{9}{64}$ in diameter Sherman screws. (These are now available as DuoDrive screws on which a single slot, suitable for an ordinary screwdriver, is superimposed over the cross recess.

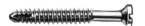   Sc. 5/7

Transfixion Screw

S.Mo. (EN 58J). Stainless steel, Titanium or Vitallium.

Partially coarse thread with self-tapping point and single slotted head.

Supplied in one diameter: 4·4 mm ($\frac{11}{64}$ in).
Lengths available: 45 mm ($1\frac{3}{4}$ in), 51 mm (2 in), 57 mm ($2\frac{1}{4}$ in), and 64 mm ($2\frac{1}{2}$ in), (Vitallium; 45 mm ($1\frac{3}{4}$ in), 51 mm (2 in), 57 mm ($2\frac{1}{4}$ in), 64 mm ($2\frac{1}{2}$ in), 70 mm ($2\frac{3}{4}$ in), and 76 mm (3 in), S.Mo. (EN 58J).

Technical data—

    Head diameter: $\frac{9}{32}$ in (·116 in or 2·9 mm).
    Outside thread diameter: just over $\frac{11}{64}$ in (·177 in or 4·5 mm).
    Root thread diameter: just under $\frac{9}{64}$ in (·135 in or 3·4 mm).
    Threads per inch: 20 (S.Mo.); 18 (Vitallium).
    Recommended drill size: $\frac{9}{64}$ in (·140 in or 3·6 mm).

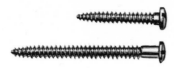

Wood Type Thread Bone Screws

S.Mo. (EN 58J). Stainless steel, Titanium or Vitallium.

Fully and partially coarse threaded with tapered point, single
slotted head.
SLIGHTLY REDUCED

Supplied in two diameters: 2·8 mm ($\frac{7}{64}$ in) Vitallium, and 3·6 mm ($\frac{9}{64}$ in) S.Mo. (EN 58J), stainless steel
Titanium or Vitallium.
Lengths available: 2·8 mm ($\frac{7}{64}$ in) diameter, 10 mm ($\frac{3}{8}$ in), 13 mm ($\frac{1}{2}$ in), 16 mm ($\frac{5}{8}$ in) and 19 mm ($\frac{3}{4}$ in);
3·6 mm ($\frac{9}{64}$ in) diameter, 19 mm ($\frac{3}{4}$ in), 22 mm ($\frac{7}{8}$ in), 25 mm (1 in), 29 mm ($1\frac{1}{8}$ in), 32 mm, $1\frac{1}{4}$ in),
38 mm ($1\frac{1}{2}$ in) and 38 mm ($1\frac{1}{2}$ in) and 45 mm ($1\frac{3}{4}$ in).

Technical Data—

2·8 mm ($\frac{7}{64}$ in) diameter screws:
Head diameter: $\frac{1}{4}$ in (·25 in or 6·4 mm).
Outside thread diameter: $\frac{5}{64}$ in (·109 in or 2·8 mm).
Root thread diameter: $\frac{5}{64}$ in approx. (·078 in or 2 mm).
Threads per inch: 22
Recommended drill size: $\frac{3}{32}$ in (·093 in or 2·4 mm).

3·6 mm ($\frac{9}{64}$ in) diameter screws:
Head diameter: $\frac{15}{64}$ in (·234 in or 5·9 mm).
Outside diameter: $\frac{9}{64}$ in (·140 in or 3·6 mm).
Root thread diameter: just under $\frac{7}{64}$ in (·100 in or 2·5 m
Threads per inch: 20.
Recommended drill size: $\frac{7}{64}$ in (·109 in or 2·8 mm).

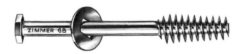

Johannson Lag Screw

S.Mo. (EN 58J). Stainless steel or Vitallium.

Very coarse thread for one-third of shaft approximately
tapered point, single slotted hexagon head.

Sc 5/7

Supplied in one shaft diameter: 4 mm ($\frac{5}{32}$ in).
Lengths available: 41 mm ($1\frac{5}{8}$ in), 57 mm ($2\frac{1}{4}$ in) and 76 mm (3 in).

Technical Data—

Head diameter: $\frac{5}{16}$ in A/f hexagon (·312 in or 8 mm).
Outside thread diameter: $\frac{11}{32}$ in (·343 in or 8·7 mm) tapering to about $\frac{3}{16}$ in (·187 in or 4·8 mm).
Root thread diameter (shaft): $\frac{5}{32}$ in (·156 in or 3·9 mm).
Threads per inch: 10.
Recommended drill size: $\frac{3}{16}$ in (·187 in or 4·8 mm) for about $\frac{1}{8}$ in through the bone cortex followed by
$\frac{5}{32}$ in (·156 in or 4 mm) for total depth of screw being inserted.

Coventry Infant Lag Screw S.Mo. (EN 58J) Stainless steel (Reduced size)

Developed by R. J. Brigden for Mr J. H. Penrose, FRCS, consultant orthopaedic surgeon at Coventry and Warwickshire Hospital, England.

D. HOWSE & CO.

Cannulated Cortex Reamer.

Overall Length 102 mm (4 in).

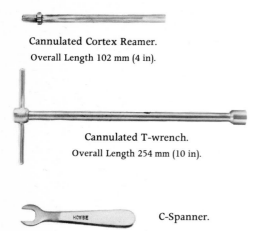

Cannulated T-wrench.

Overall Length 254 mm (10 in).

C-Spanner.

Overall Length 102 mm (4 in). *For holding Lag Screw whilst tightening Nut*

Cannulated Threaded Handle. Overall Length 152 mm (6 in).

Guide Wire. Diameter ·062 in. Length (102 mm (4 in).

Plate Benders. *TUFNOL* handle. Overall Length 216 mm (8½ in) (2 parts).

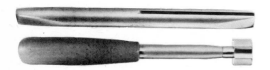

Cannulated Lag Screw with Nut.

Thread Diameter 6·3 mm (·250 in). Core diameter 4 mm (·160 in).
Lengths: 19 mm (¾ in), 22 mm (⅞ in), 25 mm (1 in).

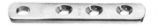

Cannulated Lag Screw with Nut.

Thread Diameter: 6·3 mm (·250 in). Core Diameter 6·3 mm (·16 in).
Shank Diameter: 5·1 mm (·21 in).
Lengths: 29 mm (1⅛ in), 32 mm (1¼ in), 35 mm (1⅜ in), 38 mm
    (1½ in), 41 mm (1⅝ in), 45 mm (1¾ in), 48 mm (1⅞ in), 51 mm
    (2 in), 57 mm (2¼ in), 64 mm (2½ in).

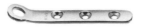

Standard Plate.

used with 2·8 mm ($\frac{7}{64}$ in) screws.
Sizes:
2 hole × 51 mm (2 in) overall;   3 hole × 60 mm (2⅜ in) overall;
                                      4 hole × 76 mm (3 in) overall.

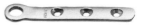

Standard Plate—Straight.

used with 2·8 mm ($\frac{7}{64}$ in) screws.
Sizes:
2 hole × 51 mm (2 in) overall;   3 hole × 60 mm (2⅜ in) overall;
                                      4 hole × 76 mm (3 in) overall.

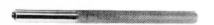

Heavy Duty Plate.

used with 3·6 mm ($\frac{9}{64}$ in) or 4mm ($\frac{5}{32}$ in) screws.
Sizes:
2 hole × 51 mm (2 in) overall;   3 hole × 60 mm (2½ in) overall;
                                      4 hole × 76 mm (3⅛ in) overall.

Heavy Duty Plate—Straight.

used with 3·6 mm ($\frac{9}{64}$ in) or 4 mm ($\frac{5}{32}$ in) screws.
Sizes:
2 hole × 51 mm (2 in) overall;   3 hole × 60 mm (2½ in) overall;
                                      4 hole × 76 mm (3⅛ in) overall.

The use of a rigid blade plate for varus and valgus osteotomies in children has two disadvantages. Firstly the blade component has to be hammered home into the neck which is unnecessarily traumatic in a child, and secondly when performing a varus osteotomy the osteotomy has to be completed first. This subsequently involves driving the blade into the now mobile upper fragment which can prove difficult. Both these difficulties can be overcome by the use of a coarse threaded screw and plate as illustrated. The screw is cannulated and can be introduced over a guide wire if desired. When the screw has been satisfactorily placed in the neck the osteotomy is performed.

During the application of the plate complete control of the angle of the upper fragment can be maintained by temporarily screwing a threaded handle on to the screw in place of the nut. When the plate has been screwed onto the shaft of the femur the handle is removed and the nut applied, giving rigid fixation. No hammering is necessary and the ease of application and subsequent removal is striking.

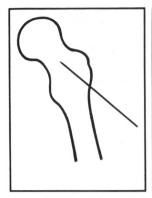

The Guide Wire is inserted in the desired position

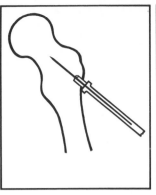

The hole in the cortex is cut with the Cannulated Cortex Reamer over the Guide Wire

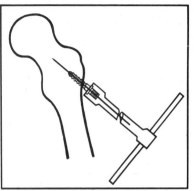

The Lag Screw is inserted over the Guide Wire with the Cannulated T-wrench

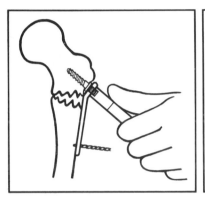

The angle of the upper fragment is controlled by temporarily screwing the Threaded Handle on to the Lag Screw in place of the Nut

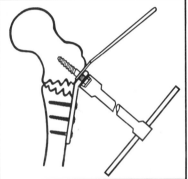

Holding the Lag Screw with the C-spanner the Nut is tightened with the T-wrench

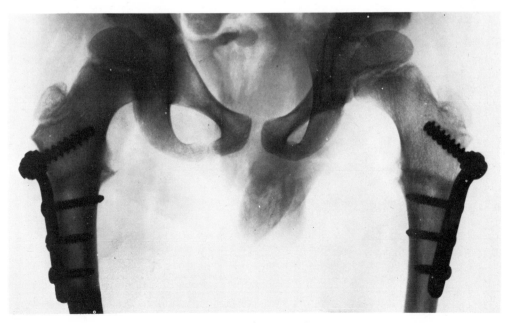

Photograph taken from original X-Ray

Bone Plates

ZIMMER ORTHOPAEDIC LTD.

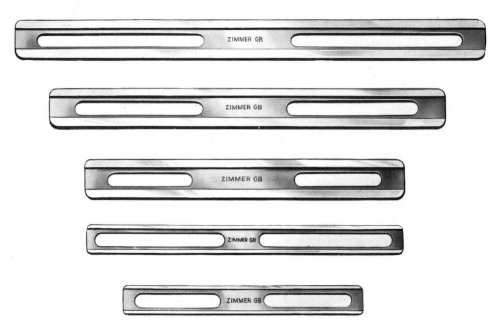

Egger Bone Plates (Sc. $\frac{5}{6}$)   S.Mo. (EN 58J). Stainless steel, Titanium or Vitallium.

Technical data—

Sizes available:

Plates (with slots to accommodate $\frac{9}{64}$ in (3·6 mm) diameter screws):
S.Mo. (EN 58J). Stainless steel, Titanium or Vitallium: Width, $\frac{1}{2}$ in (0·5 in or 12·8 mm); thickness, $\frac{1}{8}$ in (·125 in or 3·2 mm); lengths of 4, 5 and 6 in (wide).

S.Mo. (EN 58J). Stainless steel and Titanium: Width, $\frac{3}{8}$ in (·375 in or 9·5 mm); thickness, $\frac{1}{8}$ in (·125 in or 3·2 mm); lengths of 3 or 4 in (narrow).
Vitallium: Width, $\frac{13}{32}$ in (·406 in or 10·3 mm); thickness, $\frac{1}{8}$ in (·125 in or 3·2 mm); lengths of 3 or 4 in (narrow).

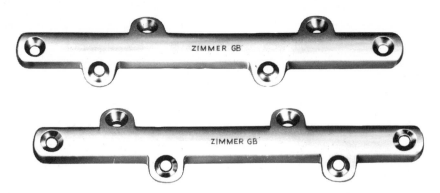

Hicks Lugged Antirotation Bone Plates (Slightly enlarged)

S.Mo. (EN 58J). Stainless Steel or Vitallium.
For fractured shaft of ulna or radius.

Technical data—
Length: 76 mm (3 in). Left and right hand.

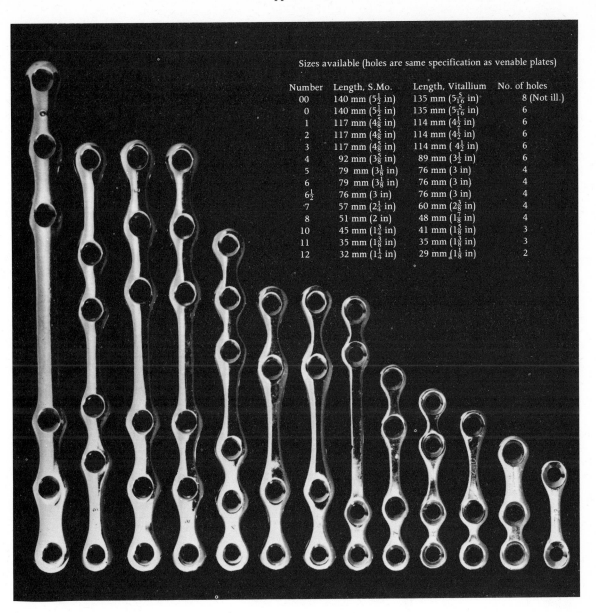

Sizes available (holes are same specification as venable plates)

Number	Length, S.Mo.	Length, Vitallium	No. of holes
00	140 mm ($5\frac{1}{2}$ in)	135 mm ($5\frac{5}{16}$ in)	8 (Not ill.)
0	140 mm ($5\frac{1}{2}$ in)	135 mm ($5\frac{5}{16}$ in)	6
1	117 mm ($4\frac{5}{8}$ in)	114 mm ($4\frac{1}{2}$ in)	6
2	117 mm ($4\frac{5}{8}$ in)	114 mm ($4\frac{1}{2}$ in)	6
3	117 mm ($4\frac{5}{8}$ in)	114 mm ($4\frac{1}{2}$ in)	6
4	92 mm ($3\frac{5}{8}$ in)	89 mm ($3\frac{1}{2}$ in)	6
5	79 mm ($3\frac{1}{8}$ in)	76 mm (3 in)	4
6	79 mm ($3\frac{1}{8}$ in)	76 mm (3 in)	4
$6\frac{1}{2}$	76 mm (3 in)	76 mm (3 in)	4
7	57 mm ($2\frac{1}{4}$ in)	60 mm ($2\frac{3}{8}$ in)	4
8	51 mm (2 in)	48 mm ($1\frac{7}{8}$ in)	4
10	45 mm ($1\frac{3}{4}$ in)	41 mm ($1\frac{5}{8}$ in)	3
11	35 mm ($1\frac{3}{8}$ in)	35 mm ($1\frac{3}{8}$ in)	3
12	32 mm ($1\frac{1}{4}$ in)	29 mm ($1\frac{1}{8}$ in)	2

Sherman Bone Plates

S.Mo. (EN 58J). Stainless steel or Vitallium.

DOWN BROS.

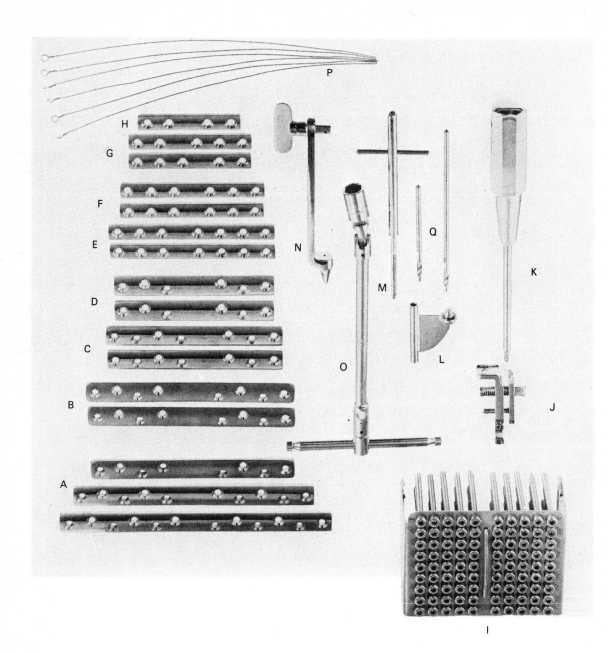

Muller type Compression Bone Plating Set (Reduced size). Titanium

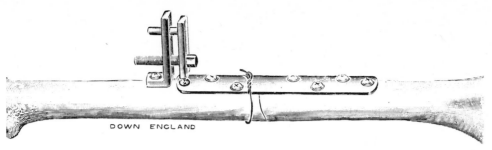

DOWN ENGLAND

Heavy Duty Femur Plates:

A size 8 in × 12 hole × 6 s.w.g. (1 only).
   size 7 in × 10 hole × 6 s.w.g. (1 only).
   size 6 in × 8 hole × 6 s.w.g. (1 only).

Normal duty femur plates:

B size 6 in × 8 hole × 9 s.w.g. (2 only).
C size 5 in × 7 hole × 9 s.w.g. (2 only).
D size $4\frac{1}{2}$ in × 6 hole × 9 s.w.g. (2 only).

Tibial Plate:

E size $4\frac{5}{8}$ in × 7 hole × 10 s.w.g. (2 only
F size 4 in × 6 hole × 10 s.w.g. (2 only
G size $3\frac{3}{8}$ in × 5 hole × 10 s.w.g. (2 only
H size $2\frac{3}{4}$ in × 4 hole × 10 s.w.g. (1 only

Fitzgerald Screws, thread 4·5 mm. diam. (outside):

I 25 mm (1 in), 28 mm ($1\frac{1}{8}$ in), 31 mm ($1\frac{1}{4}$ in), 34 mm ($1\frac{3}{8}$ in), 38 mm ($1\frac{1}{2}$ in), 41 mm ($1\frac{5}{8}$ in), 44 mm ($1\frac{3}{4}$ in), 47 mm ($1\frac{7}{8}$ in), 50 mm (2 in).

Instruments:

J Co-aptation Device
K Fitzgerald Screwdriver with hexagonal end.
L Drill guide for use with $\frac{5}{32}$ in drill.
M Tap for bone screws 4·5 mm. diam. 20 tpi.

N Wire tightener.
O Box spanner with universal joint for use with co-aptation device.
P Six only 11 in lengths Titanium wire 20 gauge.
Q Twist Drills $\frac{5}{32}$ in diam. 3 in and 5 in long.

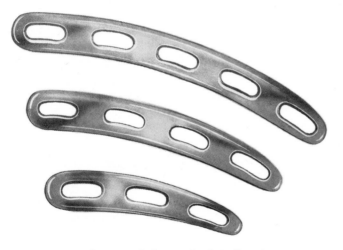

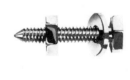

Wilson Spinal Plates and Bolt (Full Size) S.Mo. (EN 58J). Stainless steel or Vitallium.

Technical data—

Sizes available:

Plates with holes or slots (illustrated): Lengths, 64 mm ($2\frac{1}{2}$ in), 76 mm (3 in), 89 mm ($3\frac{1}{2}$ in) and 102 mm (4 in).

Bolts supplied in one diameter: 3·2 mm($\frac{1}{8}$ in). Lengths available: 13 mm ($\frac{1}{2}$ in), 16 mm ($\frac{5}{8}$ in), 19 mm ($\frac{3}{4}$ in), 22 mm ($\frac{7}{8}$ in), 25 mm (1 in), 32 mm ($1\frac{1}{4}$ in), and 38 mm ($1\frac{1}{2}$ in).

Hexagon head diameter: $\frac{5}{16}$ in. A/f hexagon (·312 in or 8 mm).

Outside thread diameter: $\frac{1}{8}$ in (·125 in or 3·2 mm).

Threads per inch: 32.

Recommended drill size: Usually right-angled awl or contra-angle dental drill size $\frac{1}{8}$ in (·125 in or 3·2 mm).

Nuts: Hexagon shape, diameter $\frac{5}{16}$ in. A/f hexagon (·312 in or 8 mm).

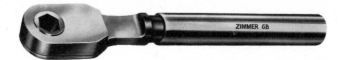

Ratchet Spanner (Full size)
for spinal bolts

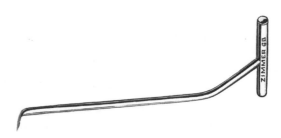

Right-Angled Awl (Sc. $\frac{1}{3}$)
for spinal bolts

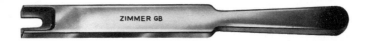

Nut Holders (Sc. $\frac{1}{3}$)
for spinal bolts

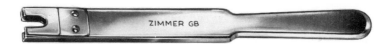

Spinal Plates

ZIMMER ORTHOPAEDIC LTD.

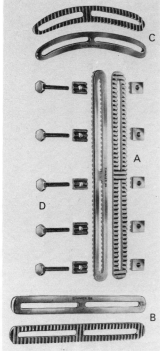

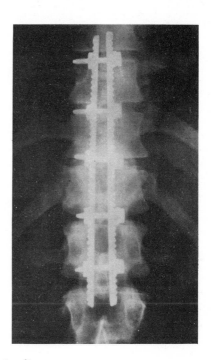

Meurig Williams Spinal Plates (Sc. $\frac{2}{5}$)
Patent No. 780652. S.Mo. (EN 58J). Stainless steel.

A and B, Spinal plates, straight, 5 and 6 in.
C, Spinal plates, curved, for lumbosacral fusion, available in sizes 102 mm (4 in), 127 mm (5 in) and 152 mm (6 in).
D. Spinal bolts with serrated nuts and washers, length, $\frac{3}{4}$ in.

Bolts:
Outside diameter of thread: $\frac{1}{8}$ in. ($\cdot$125 in or 3$\cdot$2 mm).
Threads per inch: 32.
Diameter of hexagon nut: $\frac{5}{16}$ in. A/f hexagon ($\cdot$312 in or 8 mm).
Recommended drill size: Usually right-angled awl or contra-angle dental drill, size $\frac{1}{8}$ in ($\cdot$125 in or 3$\cdot$2 mm).

To hold a dislocation of the spine in the reduced position it is desirable to obtain the maximum fixation which is possible only if all the bolts are anchored through bone. It is therefore essential to select plates of sufficient length to extend along at least five vertebrae, allowing the bolts to pass through two of the spinous processes above and two below the affected vertebra for preference, which then becomes the central point of fixation.

The Meurig Williams plates are said to have a distinct advantage over conventional plates because, being slotted over almost the entire length, it is possible to introduce all the fixation bolts through bone. This is not always possible with conventional plates due to the difficulty of lining up the holes in the plates opposite the spinous processes. Very often two bolts have to be introduced through the interspinous ligaments with consequent risk of the plates cutting out.

This apparatus enables serrated washers and nuts with bolts matching the serrations in the plates to be used in order to ensure that a positive fixation is obtained, thereby overcoming the natural tendency for longitudinal movement in the slotted plates, so that the spine remains stable in the reduced position.

Femoral Neck Nails

HOWMEDICA (UK) LTD.

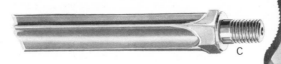

A.   McLaughlin Plate

B.   Locking Collar – Self Locking Nut

C.   McLaughlin Nail

McLaughlin Plate Assembly (For nails with external thread) (Sc. approx full size)

Includes:
Lengths: 38 mm ($1\frac{1}{2}$ in), 57 mm ($2\frac{1}{4}$ in), 82·5 mm ($3\frac{1}{4}$ in), 95 mm ($3\frac{3}{4}$ in), 114 mm ($4\frac{1}{2}$ in), 133 mm ($5\frac{1}{4}$ in), 203 mm (8 in).
Holes: 2, 3, 4, 5, 6, 7, 12.

Lengths: 76 mm (3 in), 82·5 mm ($3\frac{1}{4}$ in), 89 mm ($3\frac{1}{2}$ in), 95 mm ($3\frac{3}{4}$ in), 102 mm (4 in), 108 mm ($4\frac{1}{4}$ in), 114 mm ($4\frac{1}{2}$ in), 121 mm ($4\frac{3}{4}$ in), 127 mm (5 in), 133 mm ($5\frac{1}{4}$ in), 140 mm ($5\frac{1}{2}$ in), 146 mm ($5\frac{3}{4}$ in), 152 mm (6 in).
The Vitallium McLaughlin nail is four-flanged and cannulated to accept a 2·4 mm ($\frac{3}{32}$ in) guide wire.

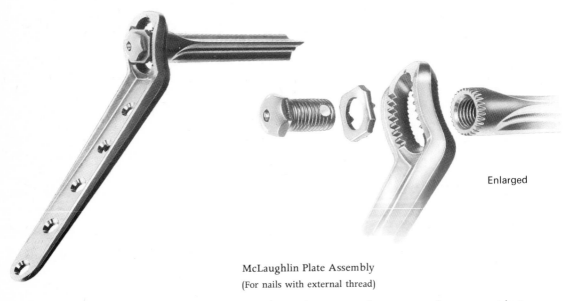

Enlarged

McLaughlin Plate Assembly

(For nails with external thread)

Lengths: 38 mm ($1\frac{1}{2}$ in), 57 mm ($2\frac{1}{4}$ in), 82·5 mm ($3\frac{1}{4}$ in), 95 mm ($3\frac{3}{4}$ in), 114 mm ($4\frac{1}{2}$ in), 133 mm ($5\frac{1}{4}$ in), 203 mm (8 in).
Holes: 2, 3, 4, 5, 6, 7, 12

Thornton Nail, Smith-Petersen type

Smith-Petersen type

Lengths: 76 mm (3 in), 82·5 mm ($3\frac{1}{4}$ in), 89 mm ($3\frac{1}{2}$ in), 95 mm ($3\frac{3}{4}$ in), 102 mm (4 in), 108 mm ($4\frac{1}{4}$ in),
114 ($4\frac{1}{2}$ in), 121 m ($4\frac{3}{4}$ in), 127 mm (5 in), 133 mm ($5\frac{1}{4}$ in), 140 mm ($5\frac{1}{2}$ in), 146 mm ($5\frac{3}{4}$ in), 152 mm (6 in).
The Vitallium Thornton nail is designed with a serrated head and is cannulated to accept a 2·4 mm
($\frac{3}{32}$ in) guide wire.

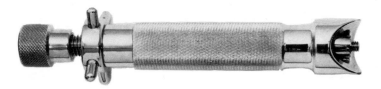

Smith-Petersen Nail, Driver/Extractor (Sc. $\frac{1}{2}$)

(ZIMMER ORTHOPAEDIC LTD.)

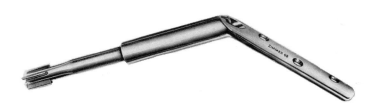

Pugh Hip Nail (Self-Adjusting) Sc. $\frac{2}{3}$)

S.Mo. (EN 58J). Stainless Steel.

Plate Lengths: 25 mm (1 in), 51 mm (2 in), 76 mm (3 in), 102 mm (4 in), 127 mm (5 in) and 152 mm (6 in).
Angle 135°
Machined from 13 mm (·5 in) diameter material, cannulated for 2·4 mm ($\frac{3}{32}$ in) guide wire.

This technique has been devised to give a more desirable and adequate fixation of the nail and plate
combination for fractures of the neck of the femur, inter and subtrochanteric fractures, with additional
advantages over the commonly used nails or nail and plate combinations. The nail is designed to telescope
within the tube, thereby keeping the fracture constantly impacted. To accomplish this, the nail must
have sufficient clearance to slide readily, but at the same time, must have enough resistance to prevent
the nail from falling out of the head should a little absorption occur at the trifin portion at the end of the
nail. The resistance is furnished by means of a friction ring so constructed that the nail will not slide
unless a few pounds of pressure is exerted on the end of the nail. This ensures sliding action without
binding.

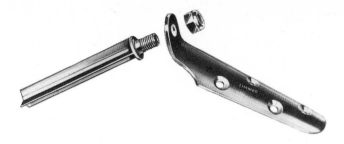

McKee Trifin Nail and Intertrochanteric Plate (Sc. $\frac{2}{3}$)

S.Mo. (EN 58J). Stainless steel, Titanium or Vitallium.

Sizes available:

75 mm to 150 mm lengths in 5 mm steps. Nail: 3 to 6 in lengths in $\frac{1}{4}$ in steps; diameter, 13 mm (·5 in). Plates: Available with a single slot, four slots, four holes or six holes. The nail is cannulated to receive a 2·4 mm ($\frac{3}{32}$ in) guide pin and the male screw thread is 7 mm diameter, 1 mm pitch to take a locking nut.

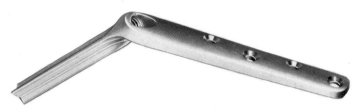

Modified Jewett Nail Plate (Sc. $\frac{2}{3}$)

Vitallium. S.Mo. (EN 58J). Stainless steel, Titanium.

Sizes available:

Plate Length 102 mm (4 in). 4 Holes.
Angles: 120°, 125°, 130°, 135°, 140°, 150°, 160°.
Nail Length 76 mm (3 in), 82·5 mm (3$\frac{1}{4}$ in), 89 mm (3$\frac{1}{2}$ in), 95 mm (3$\frac{3}{4}$ in), 102 mm (4 in), 108 mm (4$\frac{1}{4}$ in), 114 mm (4$\frac{1}{2}$ in), 121 mm (4$\frac{3}{4}$ in), 127 mm (5 in).

Plate Length 127 mm (5 in). 5 Holes.
Angles 130°, 135°, 140°, 150°.
Nail Length 76 mm (3 in), 82·5 mm (3$\frac{1}{4}$ in), 89 mm (3$\frac{1}{2}$ in), 95 mm (3$\frac{3}{4}$ in), 102 mm (4 in), 108 mm (4$\frac{1}{4}$ in), 114 mm (4$\frac{1}{2}$ in), 121 mm (4$\frac{3}{4}$ in), 127 mm (5 in).

Plate Length   Plate Length 152 mm (6 in). 6 Holes.
Angles 130°, 135°, 140°, 150°
Nail Length: 76 mm (3 in), 82·5 mm (3$\frac{1}{4}$ in), 89 mm (3$\frac{1}{2}$ in), 95 mm (3$\frac{3}{4}$ in), 102 mm (4 in), 108mm (4$\frac{1}{4}$ in), 114 mm (4$\frac{1}{2}$ in), 121 mm (4$\frac{3}{4}$ in), 127 mm (5 in).

Plate Length 203 mm (8 in). 7 Holes.
Angle 130°.
Nail Length 76 mm (3 in), 82·5 (3$\frac{1}{4}$ in), 89 mm (3$\frac{1}{2}$ in), 95 mm (3$\frac{3}{4}$ in), 102 mm (4 in).

Plate Length 254 mm (10 in). 9 Holes.
Angle 130°.
Nail Length: 76 mm (3 in), 82·5 mm (3$\frac{1}{4}$ in), 89 mm (3$\frac{1}{2}$ in), 95 mm (3$\frac{3}{4}$ in), 102 mm (4 in).

Diameter of Nail 12·7 mm ($\frac{1}{2}$ in). Thread $\frac{1}{4}$ in-20.
The Jewett nail-plate has a three-flanged nail. It is cannulated to accept a 2·4 mm ($\frac{3}{32}$ in) guide wire.

HOWMEDICA (UK) LTD.

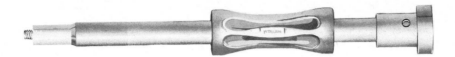

Driver/Extractor (Sc. $\frac{1}{2}$)
For Internal Threaded Hip Nails.

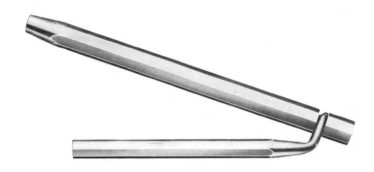

McKee Nail Driver/Extractor (Sc. $\frac{1}{2}$)

Hip Prosthesis for Arthroplasty Operations

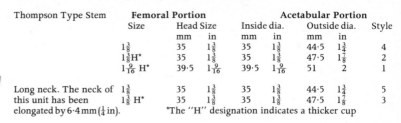

A McKee-Farrar Total Hip Prosthesis (Micro-fitting)

Thompson Type Stem

	Femoral Portion			Acetabular Portion				
Size	Head Size			Inside dia.		Outside dia.		Style
	mm	in		mm	in	mm	in	
$1\frac{3}{8}$	35	$1\frac{3}{8}$		35	$1\frac{3}{8}$	44·5	$1\frac{3}{4}$	4
$1\frac{3}{8}$H*	35	$1\frac{3}{8}$		35	$1\frac{3}{8}$	47·5	$1\frac{7}{8}$	2
$1\frac{9}{16}$ H*	39·5	$1\frac{9}{16}$		39·5	$1\frac{9}{16}$	51	2	1

Long neck. The neck of $1\frac{3}{8}$ 35 $1\frac{3}{8}$ 35 $1\frac{3}{8}$ 44·5 $1\frac{3}{4}$ 5
this unit has been $1\frac{3}{8}$ H*   35 $1\frac{3}{8}$ 35 $1\frac{3}{8}$ 47·5 $1\frac{7}{8}$ 3
elongated by 6·4 mm ($\frac{1}{4}$ in).   *The "H" designation indicates a thicker cup

The McKee-Farrar Total Hip Prosthesis provides the surgeon with a technologically sophisticated appliance designed to replace both sides of the hip joint. It consists of a Vitallium femoral prosthesis and a Vitallium acetabular cup. The cup and stem are designed for fixation by means of quick-acting Surgical Simplex P cement.

micro-fit interchangeable components

The articulating surfaces of the McKee-Farrar components are manufactured by proprietary techniques to close tolerances and an extremely fine surface finish. These new techniques permit interchangeability of components of identical cup and head size . . . thus providing to the surgeon the convenience of selecting the proper femoral stem and neck length *after* the acetabular component is firmly fixed.

B McKee-Farrar Total Hip Prosthesis (Minneapolis stem)

Sizes available:

	Femoral Portion:			Acetabular Portion			
Size	Head Size			Inside dia.		Outside dia.	
	mm	in		mm	in	mm	in
$1\frac{5}{8}$	41·5	$1\frac{5}{8}$		41·5	$1\frac{5}{8}$	51	2

The femoral component consists of a Minneapolis hip prosthesis. It is normally restricted to cases where an osteotomy has been performed and pain has not been relieved. It can also be used where the upper part of the femoral shaft is damaged.

C Austin Moore Self Locking Hip Prosthesis

Vitallium. S.Mo. (EN 58J)
Stainless steel. Titanium.

Head Diameter		Stem Length Vitallium		Stem Length S.Mo. (EN 58J)	
mm	in	mm	in	mm	in
38	$1\frac{1}{2}$	127	5		
41	$1\frac{5}{8}$	127	5	127	5
43	$1\frac{11}{16}$	127	5		
45	$1\frac{3}{4}$	127	5	127	5
46	$1\frac{13}{16}$	140	$5\frac{1}{2}$		
48	$1\frac{7}{8}$	140	$5\frac{1}{2}$		
49	$1\frac{15}{16}$	140	$5\frac{1}{2}$	140	$5\frac{1}{2}$
51	2	152	6		
52	$2\frac{1}{16}$	152	6	140	6
54	$2\frac{1}{8}$	152	6		
57	$2\frac{1}{4}$	152	6	140	6
60	$2\frac{3}{8}$	152	6		
64	$2\frac{1}{2}$	152	6		

Seat width 25 mm (1 in).   Stem thickness 10 mm ($\frac{1}{8}$ in).

D Charnley Total Hip Prosthesis (Chas. F. Thackray)

	Head Diameter		Stem Length		Cup O.D.	
	mm	in	mm	in	mm	in
	22	$\frac{7}{8}$	117	$4\frac{5}{8}$	43	$1\frac{11}{16}$
w/small Cup	22	$\frac{7}{8}$	117	$4\frac{5}{8}$	40	$1\frac{9}{16}$
straight narrow stem	22	$\frac{7}{8}$	121	$4\frac{3}{4}$	43	$1\frac{11}{16}$
straight narrow stem small cup	22	$\frac{7}{8}$	121	$4\frac{3}{4}$	40	$1\frac{9}{16}$

The Charnley Type Total Hip Prosthesis is a low friction replacement prosthesis for arthroplasty of the hip joint. A two-piece appliance, it combines the tissue compatibility of a Vitallium femoral prosthesis with the low friction characteristics of an ultra-high molecular weight polyethylene cup. The femoral head portion is ground to a virtually perfect spherical shape and polished to an optical mirror finish. The cup is double wrapped and sterilized by gamma radiation. A radiopaque Vitallium wire over the cup permits determination of the position of the cup post-operatively.

The Howse Total Hip Prosthesis

D. HOWSE & CO.

Sizes available

No. 607S small   **No. 607E** small, extended neck   **No. 607L** large

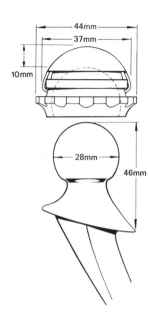 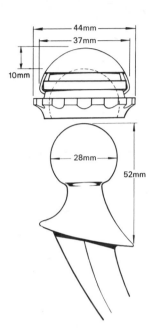 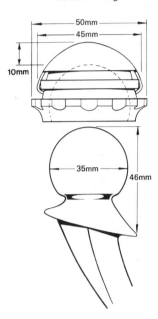

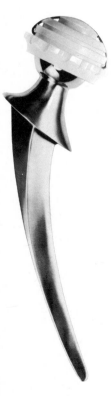

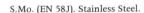

S.Mo. (EN 58J). Stainless Steel.

The Howse Prosthesis is a metal-to-plastic bearing prosthesis. The femoral part is made of stainless steel EN58J, the acetabular cup of high density polyethene (RCH 1000). The combination of these two materials has proved the best for bearing surfaces. The femoral head is subjected to a special optical lapping and polishing process and is truly spherical with a superfinish in terms of micro-inches.

The cup is larger than half a sphere. The depth of its internal surface, spherically shaped, is greater than the radius of the sphere of the femoral head. A slight decrease in the thickness of the external wall of the collar allows the introduction of the head, which is held firmly by the cup after reduction. This characteristic of the prosthesis avoids post-operative dislocation and allows immediate mobilisation of the hip.

The Hose sockets are fitted with a radio-opaque marker.

The size of the internal surface of the cup has been calculated to meet exactly the size of the head at 37°, that is why at room temperature we seem to have too tight a fit between the two parts.

Whatever approach the surgeon decides on, he will find the ease of insertion advantageous, and be able to position the cup well into the acetabulum without removing and weakening the natural structure or having to insert screws or nails, etc.

The prosthesis, received assembled and sterilised by gamma radiation, is ready for immediate use, thus avoiding possible damage during sterilisation. However, should the prosthesis be exposed to infection, the cup can be re-sterilised by boiling, formaldehyde vapour or ethylene oxide gas (it should not be autoclaved) it is inadvisable to re-sterilise by a second exposure to gamma radiation.

The acetabulum should be thickly lined with acrylic resin in the usual way, care being taken to push the resin into the anchoring cavities. The cup is then inserted using the cup inserting instrument (the cup clips onto the adaptor and can be held firmly without fear of dropping off). It is important that the cup and its collar be entirely covered with cement.

The femoral neck is prepared as for the insertion of a Thompson Prosthesis. We would recommend, to avoid any possible damage to the very finely finished head of the prosthesis, that it is not punched in, but pressed into the cortex by pushing onto the flat provided below and behind the actual head of the prosthesis.

Reduction is very simple and easy.

The socket must be cleaned of clots and blood. The inferior limb being placed in horizontal position and internally rotated with an increasing traction and thumb pressure on it, the head is lead in front of the socket.

The limb is put at about 30° of adduction and while releasing traction the head will go into the socket, and as it expels the air a characteristic noise will be heard which guarantees a perfect reduction.

''This prosthesis has been developed with a view to obtaining the continued advantages of both the all-metal types and the metal and plastic types. It has the great advantages of the low friction and low wear characteristics of the metal on plastic prosthesis with the addition of a vacuum effect which positively maintains the head reduced in the acetabulum, this greatly reducing the risks of subsequent dislocation.

It has also taken the greater head size of the all-metal type. The larger head size gives a much lower loading per square centimeter of bearing surface. As a result the rate of wear is greatly diminished. The greater linear velocity at the periphery of a larger head on the hip movement is a relatively unimportant factor compared with the decreased loading per square centimeter.

In order to obtain the best advantage of the large weight bearing surface it is suggested that the largest size of cup should be used that will sit snugly into the acetabulum. It is important, however, that the acetabular portion should sit well within the old acetabulum and the largest cup should not be used if it does not fit inside the acetabulum.''

Mr. A. J. G. Howse, F.R.C.S. Consultant Orthopaedic Surgeon at the Central Middlesex Hospital, London.

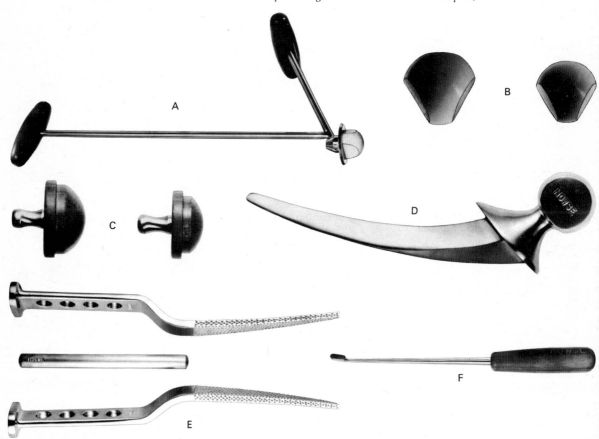

A. Cup holder. Stainless steel. *TUFNOL* handle. Overall length 35 cm.

B. Adaptors. To screw on holder. Nylon (may be sterilised by autoclaving). The cup clips onto the adaptor and can be held firmly without fear of dropping off.

C. Socket size gauges. *TUFNOL*. With detachable heads for screwing onto cup holder if desired.

D. Test femoral stem. Stainless steel.

E. Left and right broaches with Tommy bar. Stainless steel. Overall length 25 cm.

F.   H. Harris Bone curette. Stainless steel. *TUFNOL* handle. Overall length 29 cm.

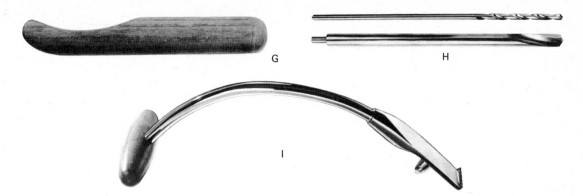

G
H
I

G. Femoral pusher. *TUFNOL*. Overall length
   15 cm.
H. Twist drills. Stainless steel.
   6·6 mm × 250 mm long.
   11 mm × 250 mm long.
I. Braddock retractor. Stainless steel
   handle. Overall length 28 cm. This
   retractor has a serrated claw edge that
   grips the back of the acetabulum. The

protruding pin fits into the intramedullary cavity exposed by the
removal of the femoral head. This
enables the femur to be levered away
from the acetabulum and held under
control by an assistant, allowing the
surgeon unrestricted access to the
acetabulum.

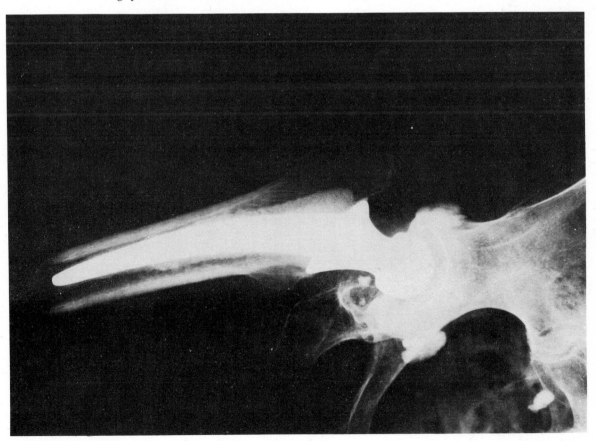

Post-operative X-ray

Staples and Arthrodesis Clamps

ZIMMER ORTHOPAEDIC

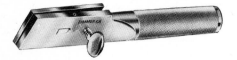

Staple Driver/Inserter (Sc. $\frac{1}{4}$)

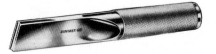

Staple Punch or Set (Sc. $\frac{1}{4}$)

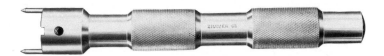

Müller Staple Driver Inserter (Sc. $\frac{2}{3}$)

(Staple fitted in position for insertion.)

S.Mo. (EN 58J) Stainless steel
  2·4 mm ($\frac{3}{32}$ in) diameter
16 mm ($\frac{5}{8}$ in) width × 19 mm ($\frac{3}{4}$ in) length
22 mm ($\frac{7}{8}$ in) width × 19 mm ($\frac{3}{4}$ in) length

1·2 mm ($\frac{1}{16}$ in) diameter
16 mm ($\frac{5}{8}$ in) width × 19 mm ($\frac{3}{4}$ in) length
22 mm ($\frac{7}{8}$ in) width × 19 mm ($\frac{3}{4}$ in) length

Vitallium

16 mm ($\frac{5}{8}$ in) width × 16 mm ($\frac{5}{8}$ in) or 22 mm ($\frac{7}{8}$ in) length
22 mm ($\frac{7}{8}$ in) width × 16 mm ($\frac{5}{8}$ in) or 22 mm ($\frac{7}{8}$ in) length
10 mm ($\frac{3}{8}$ in) width × 16 mm ($\frac{5}{8}$ in), 22 mm ($\frac{7}{8}$ in) or 29 mm ($1\frac{1}{8}$ in) length

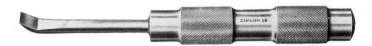

Staple Extractor (Sc. $\frac{2}{3}$)

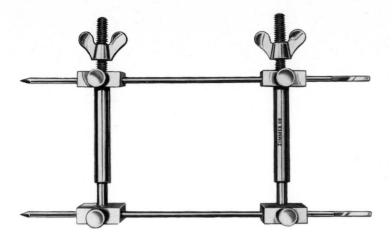

Charnley Compression Clamps (Pair) (Sc. $\frac{1}{2}$)

These clamps are used with two Steinmann pins (S.Mo. (EN 58J) stainless steel), length 204 mm (8 in), diameter, 4 mm ($\frac{5}{32}$ or 4·8 mm $\frac{3}{16}$ in)

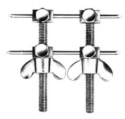

Royal National Orthopaedic Hospital Miniature Clamps

For compression athrodesis of the knee.

Osteotomy Plates

ZIMMER ORTHOPAEDIC LTD.

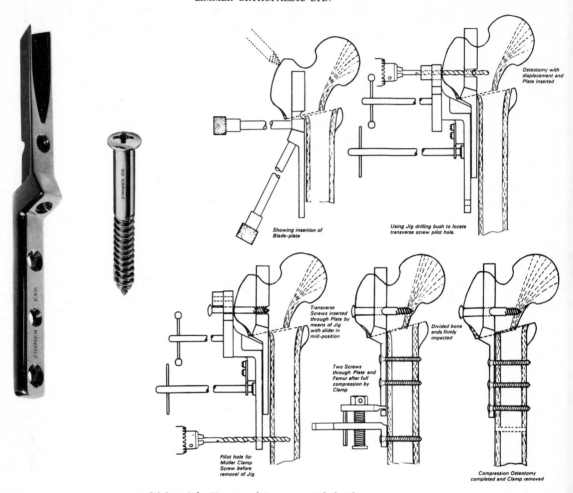

Showing insertion of Blade-plate

Using Jig drilling bush to locate transverse screw pilot hole.

Osteotomy with displacement and Plate inserted

Transverse Screws inserted through Plate by means of Jig with slider in mid-position

Divided bone ends firmly impacted

Two Screws through Plate and Femur after full compression by Clamp

Pilot hole for Müller Clamp Screw before removal of Jig

Compression Osteotomy completed and Clamp removed

Wainwright-Hammond Osteotomy Blade Plates

By means of minor modifications and the addition of a transfixing transverse screw, a well tried and highly successful blade plate for high femoral osteotomy now provides complete rigidity of fixation in compression which is ideal for rapid union. The advantages of the Wainwright-Hammond Osteotomy Blade Plate include maximum stability, the possibility of early post-operative mobilisation and minimal pain combined with absolute safety and the reduction of blood loss from divided bone surfaces.

No. 490AL—Long—Blade length 57 mm ($2\frac{1}{4}$ in).
 Plate length 76 mm (3 in).
No. T.490A—Standard—Blade length 51 mm (2 in).
 Plate length 76 mm (3 in).
No. T.490B—Small—Blade length 45 mm ($1\frac{3}{4}$ in).
 Plate length 76 mm (3 in).
No. T.491—Transverse Screws—Lengths 51 mm (2 in),
 57 mm ($2\frac{1}{4}$ in), 64 mm ($2\frac{1}{2}$ in), 70 mm ($2\frac{3}{4}$ in).

Screw head—Phillips recessed.

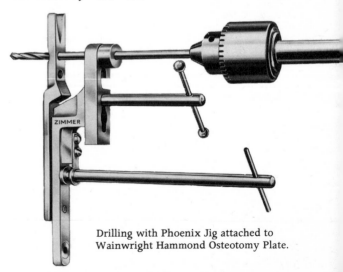

Drilling with Phoenix Jig attached to Wainwright Hammond Osteotomy Plate.

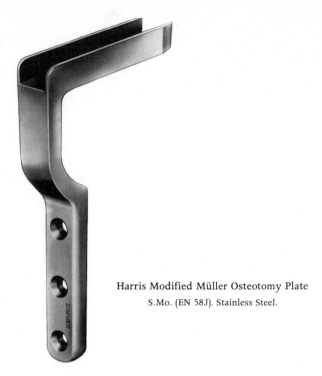

Harris Modified Müller Osteotomy Plate

S.Mo. (EN 58J). Stainless Steel.

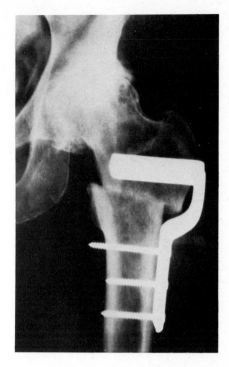

Post-operative radiograph

Sizes available:

41 mm ($1\frac{5}{8}$ in) 45 mm ($1\frac{3}{4}$ in), 48 mm ($1\frac{7}{8}$ in), 51 mm (2 in), 54 mm ($2\frac{1}{8}$ in).

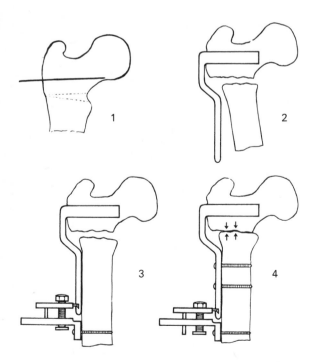

1 Insertion of Guide Wire.
   Note wedge to be removed for
   varus osteotomy.

2 Appliance inserted parallel
   to proximal cut surface of
   the osteotomy and at least
   2·5 cm (1 in) above it.

3 Muller clamp in position.
   Note the gap at the
   osteotomy.

4 Osteotomy compressed.

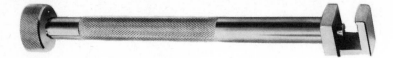

Introducer

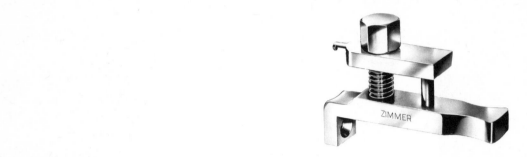

Müller Type Compression Clamp

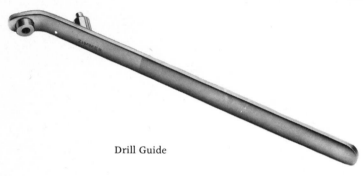

Drill Guide

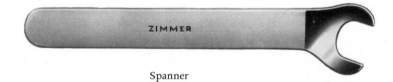

Spanner

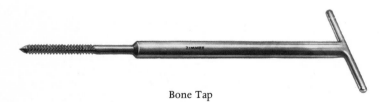

Bone Tap

Plastic Instruments

CHAS. F. THACKRAY LTD.

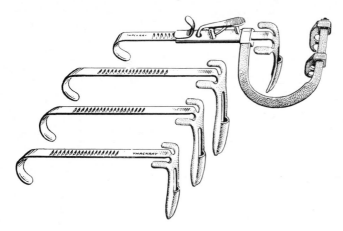

Kilner Dott Insulated Mouth Gag with East Grinstead Blades

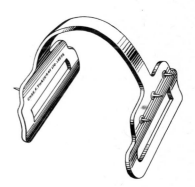

Denis Browne Hare Lip Traction Bow (Full size)

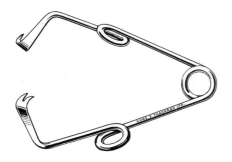

Kilner Spring-Action Retractor (Full size)

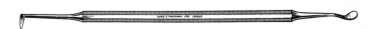

Mitchell Trimmer

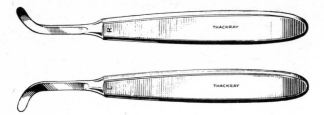

Cleft Palate Raspatories, Right and Left (Curved) (Sc. $\frac{1}{2}$)

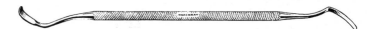

Double End Cleft Palate Elevator (Angled to side and on flat) (Sc. $\frac{1}{2}$)

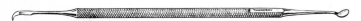

Cleft Palate Sharp Hook and Raspatory (Sc. $\frac{1}{2}$)

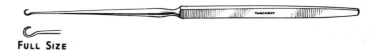

FULL SIZE

Gillies Skin Hook (Sc. $\frac{2}{3}$)

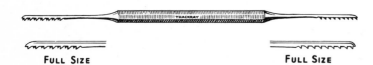

FULL SIZE   FULL SIZE

Robbe Otoplasty Cartilage Rasp (Sc. $\frac{2}{3}$)

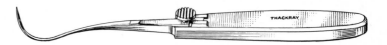

Reverdin Needles (Sc. $\frac{1}{2}$)

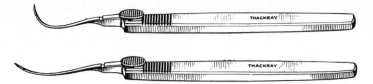

Reverdin Needles (Sc. $\frac{1}{2}$)

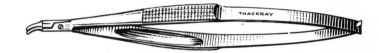

Barraquer Needle Holder (Sc. $\frac{1}{2}$)

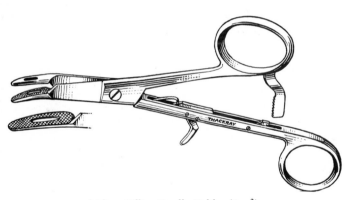

Milton Gillies Needle Holder (Sc. $\frac{2}{3}$)

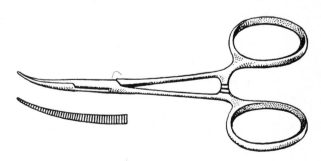

Micron Artery Forceps (Sc. $\frac{1}{2}$)

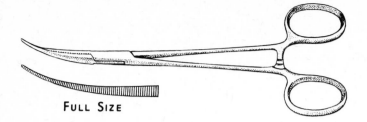

Micron Artery Forceps (Sc. $\frac{1}{2}$)

FULL SIZE

Yasargil Micro Vessel Clips (Full Size)

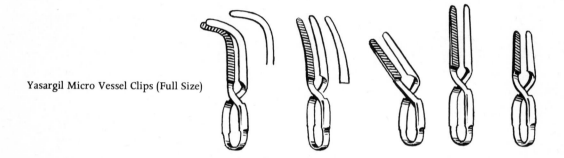

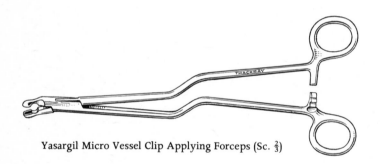

Yasargil Micro Vessel Clip Applying Forceps (Sc. $\frac{2}{3}$)

Hoskin Forceps (Full size)

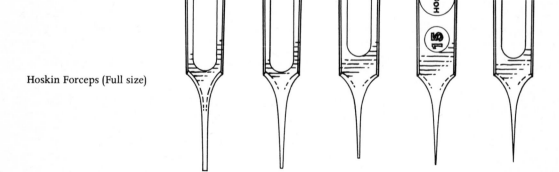

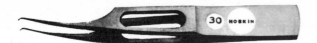

Micro Groove Forceps Curved (Sc. $\frac{2}{3}$)

Micro Groove Forceps Straight (Sc. $\frac{2}{3}$)

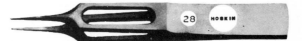

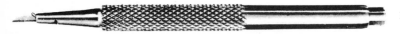

Razor Blade Fragment Holder (Full size)

Micro Scissors Straight (Sc. $\frac{1}{2}$)

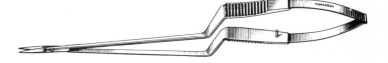

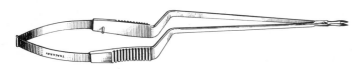

Micro Scissors Curved on Flat (Sc. $\frac{1}{2}$)

Prendville Hand Table (Sc. $\frac{1}{2}$)

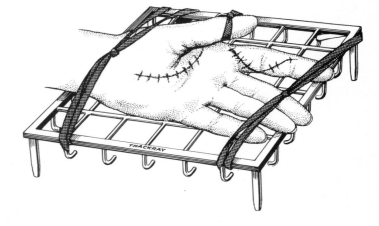

Thoracic Instruments (General)

CHAS F. THACKRAY LTD.

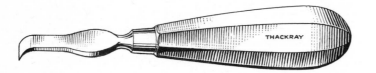

Nelson Rib Raspatory (Sc. $\frac{2}{3}$)

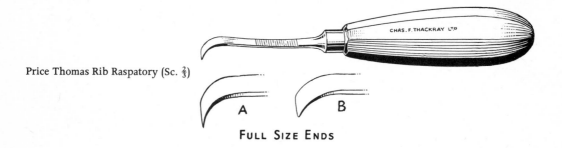

Price Thomas Rib Raspatory (Sc. $\frac{2}{3}$)

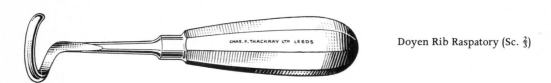

A   B

FULL SIZE ENDS

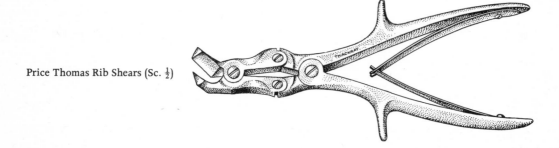

Doyen Rib Raspatory (Sc. $\frac{2}{3}$)

Price Thomas Rib Shears (Sc. $\frac{1}{2}$)

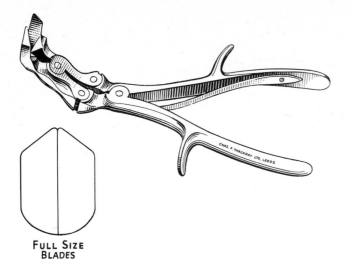

FULL SIZE
BLADES

Tudor Edwards Rib Shears for Anterior Ends (Sc. ⅓)

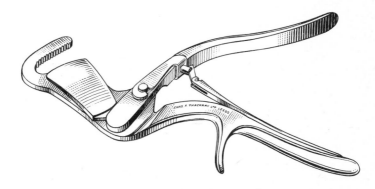

Lebesches Sternum Shears (Sc. ⅓)

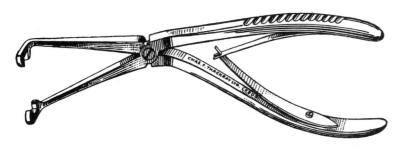

Morriston Davies Rib Approximator (Sc. ⅓)

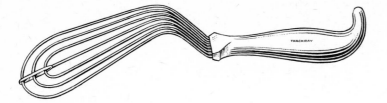

Allison Lung Retractor (Sc. $\frac{1}{3}$)

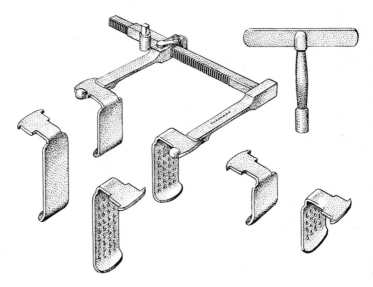

Tudor Edwards Double Rib Spreader With Key (Sc. $\frac{1}{4}$)

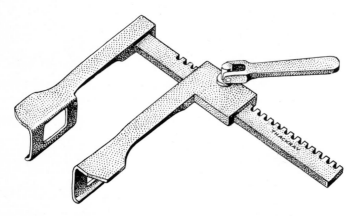

Buckley's Modification of Finochietto's Rib Spreader (Sc. $\frac{1}{3}$)

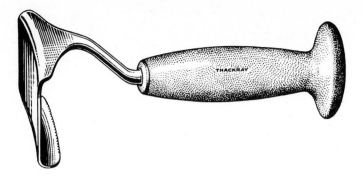

Tudor Edwards Scapula Retractor (Sc. $\frac{1}{2}$)

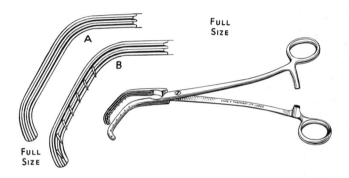

Price Thomas Bronchus Clamp (Sc. $\frac{1}{3}$)

A. Plain jaws.   B. 'Spiked' jaws.

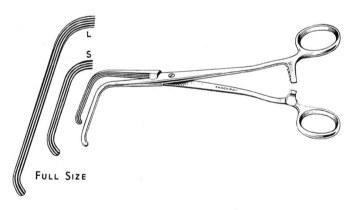

Bickford Bronchus Clamp ($\frac{1}{3}$)

L. Large jaws.   S. Small jaws.

Thoracic Instruments (Cardio-Vascular)

CHAS. F. THACKRAY LTD.

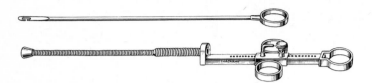

Rumel Flexible Cardio-Vascular Tourniquet (Sc. $\frac{1}{3}$)

DOWN BROS. LTD.

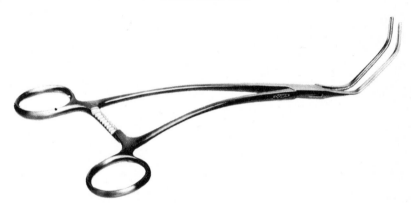

De Bakey Tangential Occlusion Clamp Attraugrip Jaws (Sc. $\frac{1}{2}$)

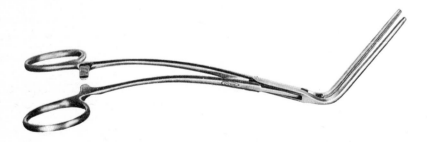

De Bakey Multipurpose Obtuse Angle Occlusion Clamps Atraugrip Jaws (Sc. $\frac{1}{2}$)

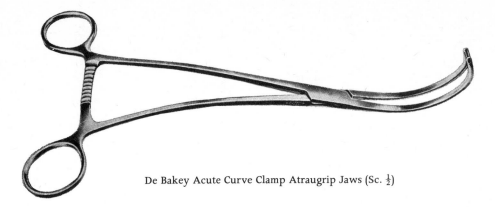

De Bakey Acute Curve Clamp Atraugrip Jaws (Sc. ½)

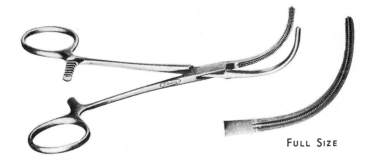

FULL SIZE

De Bakey Peripheral Clamp Atraugrip Jaws (Sc. ½)

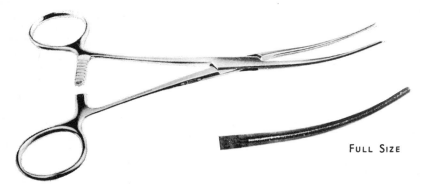

FULL SIZE

De Bakey/Bainbridge Peripheral Clamp Atraugrip Jaws (Sc. ½)

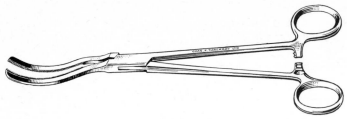

Potts Clamp (Sc. ½)

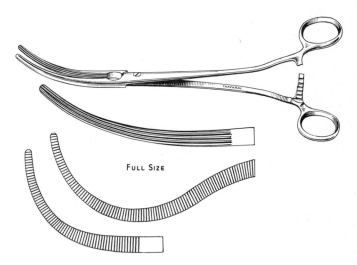

Crafoord Coarctation Clamps, Longitudinally Grooved Jaws, Medium Curved and Long Curved Jaws (Sc. ½)

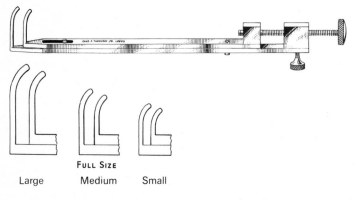

Large   Medium   Small

Blalock Pulmonary Artery Clamp (Sc. ½)

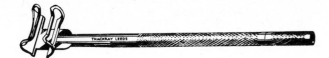

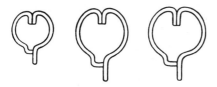

FULL SIZES

Potts Aortic Clamp (Sc. $\frac{1}{2}$)

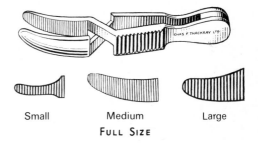

Small   Medium   Large

FULL SIZE

Diffenbach Artery Forceps (Bulldog Clamps)

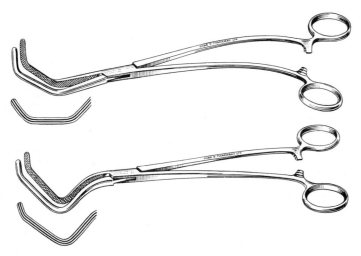

Satinsky Anastomosis Clamp with Cross or Longitudinal Serrations (Sc. $\frac{1}{3}$)

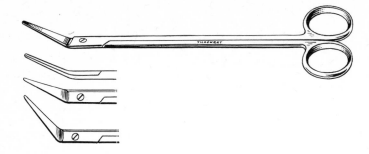

Potts-Smith Scissors (Three types) (Sc. $\frac{1}{2}$)

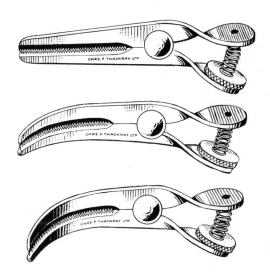

Potts Bulldog Clamps (Three types) (Full size)

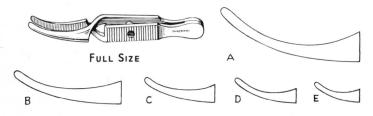

Blalock Bulldog Clamps (Five sizes, A to E)

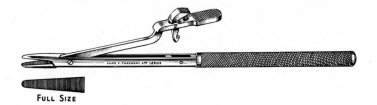

FULL SIZE

Potts-Smith Needle Holder (Sc. $\frac{1}{3}$)

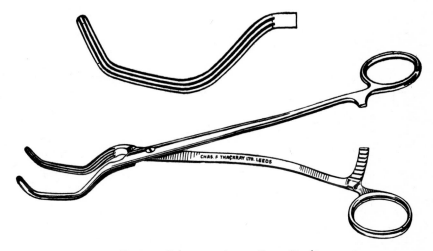

Nystrom Pulmonary Artery Clamp (Sc. $\frac{1}{2}$)

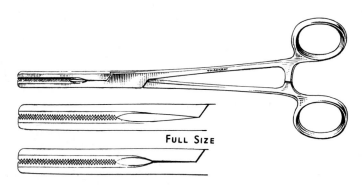

FULL SIZE

Potts Aortic Coarctation Clamp (Sc. $\frac{1}{2}$)

Vascular (Transfusion, etc.)

CHAS. F. THACKRAY LTD.

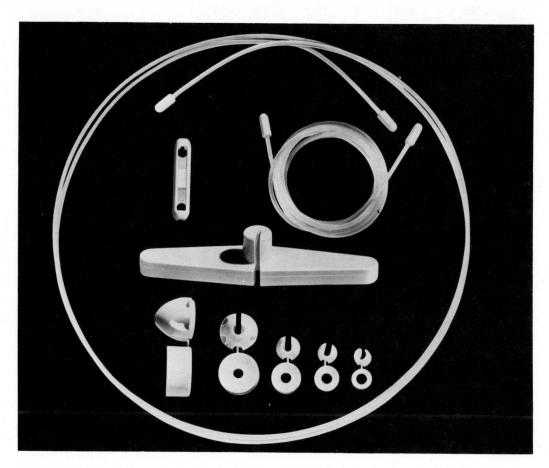

Armour Sterile Disposable Vein Stripper

Made from nylon the instrument consists of two cables 90 cm in length which can be used separately or joined to make one cable 180 cm in length. Five 'stripping' olives are provided each with an integral locking device sizes 15·9 mm, 12·7 mm, 9·5, 8·0 mm and 6·3 mm.

The set is packed ready sterile in double wrapped peelable transparent envelopes.

ESCHMANN BROS. & WALSH LTD.

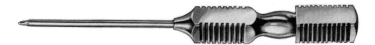

Frankis Evans Intravenous Needle (Full size)

Sizes available in 45 mm ($1\frac{3}{4}$ in) × 16 B.W.G. cannula.

CHAS. F. THACKRAY LTD.

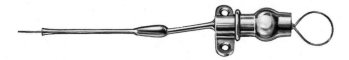

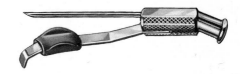

Hamilton Bailey Intravenous Cannula
Size available: Adult, child and infant.

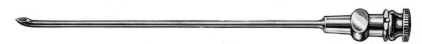

Mitchell Self-Sealing Intravenous Needle (Full Size)
Sizes available: 38 mm ($1\frac{1}{2}$ in) × B.W.G. 18 and 19 B.W.G.

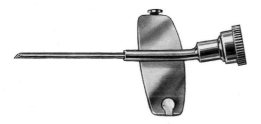

Gordh Intravenous Needle (Full size)
Size available: 27 mm ($1\frac{1}{16}$ in) × 20 B.W.G.

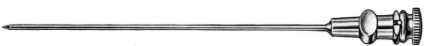

Tuony Spinal Analgesia Needle (Full size)
Size available: 83 mm ($3\frac{1}{4}$ in) × 16 G.

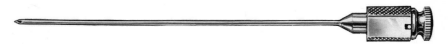

Howard Jones Spinal Analgesia Needle (Full size)
Size available: 85 mm ($3\frac{1}{8}$ in) × 19 G.

Pannett Spinal Analgesia Needle (Full size)
Size available: 76 mm (3 in) × 21 G.

Suction Nozzles

CHAS. F. THACKRAY LTD.

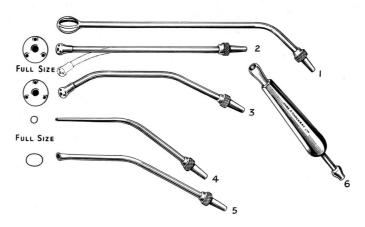

Universal Suction Set (Sc. $\frac{1}{3}$)

1. Abdominal suction tube.
2. Malleable suction tube with perforated tip.
3. Yankauer suction tube.
4. Bent suction tube with round open end.
5. Bent suction tube with oval open end.
6. Universal handle, with socket to take any of the cone-fitting mounts of suction tubes Numbers 1 to 5.

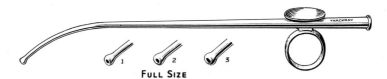

Magill Suction Nozzles (Three sizes of ends) (Sc. $\frac{1}{2}$)

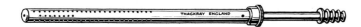

Wheeler or Poole Abdominal Suction Nozzle (Sc. $\frac{1}{2}$)

Index

INDEX

Printed by T. & A. Constable Ltd., Edinburgh, Scotland.